Editor   Dev Maulik

Associate Editor   Ivica Zalud
for Gynecology

**Doppler Ultrasound
in Obstetrics and Gynecology**

Editor   Dev Maulik

Associate Editor   Ivica Zalud
for Gynecology

Doppler Ultrasound in Obstetrics and Gynecology

2nd Revised and Enlarged Edition

With 521 Figures
and 112 Tables

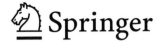 Springer

Editor
DEV MAULIK, MD, Ph.D.
Winthrop University Hospital
Department of Obstetrics and Gynecology,
159 First Street
Mineola, NY 11501
USA

Associate Editor for Gynecology
IVICA ZALUD, MD, Ph.D.
Kapiolani Medical Center for Women and Children
1319 Punahou Street
Honolulu, HI 96826
USA

ISBN-10 3-540-23088-2 Springer-Verlag Berlin Heidelberg New York
ISBN-13 978-3-540-23088-5 Springer-Verlag Berlin Heidelberg New York

ISBN 0-387-94240-8 Springer-Verlag New York Berlin Heidelberg, First edition

Library of Congress Control Number: 2005923619

Springer is a part of Springer Science + Business Media

springeronline.com

© Springer-Verlag Berlin Heidelberg 2005
Printed in Germany

Editor: Dr. Ute Heilmann, Springer-Verlag, Heidelberg
Desk editor: Wilma McHugh, Springer-Verlag, Heidelberg
Production: ProEdit GmbH, Elke Beul-Göhringer, Heidelberg
Cover design: Estudio Calamar, F. Steinen-Broo, Pau/Girona, Spain
Typesetting: K+V Fotosatz GmbH, Beerfelden
Reproduction of the figures: AM-production GmbH, Wiesloch

Printed on acid-free paper
21/3151beu-göh   5 4 3 2 1 0

To the loving memory of my mother

Tara Devi

(1910–1994)

Preface

It is with great pleasure we offer the second edition of "Doppler Ultrasound in Obstetrics and Gynecology" to our readers. We remain deeply appreciative of the success of the first edition with its continuing enthusiastic reception from our readers.

Impressive advances have occurred in diagnostic Doppler sonography since the publication of the first edition of the book. With the ever-increasing emphasis on evidence-based medicine, the clinical applications of fetal Doppler ultrasound have become progressively more refined, although significant uncertainty still continues in many areas, providing opportunities for future investigations. Ultrasound technology and instrumentation have become increasingly more sophisticated and user friendly. Exciting technological innovations and breakthroughs, such as the emergence of real-time three-dimensional sonography, are offering huge potentials for Doppler assessment of the cardiovascular system. These advances have provided a powerful rationale for bringing the book up to date so that it may continue to serve our readers in the future. In this process, we have comprehensively and critically examined the information contained in the first edition, and revised and expanded it as deemed appropriate.

The second edition now boasts 40 chapters, expanded from 34 chapters in the previous edition. This results from the inclusion of eight new chapters and condensation of three gynecology chapters into one. In addition, there have been substantial revisions of the other preexisting chapters. To give the readers an overall sense of the contents, these changes are summarized here. The introductory chapters continue to deal with the basic principles of Doppler sonography, hemodynamics, fetal and maternal cardiovascular physiology, and biosafety and have been extensively revised. We have added two new chapters, one reviewing the venous hemodynamics and the other dealing with three-dimensional color and power Doppler ultrasound. The subsequent chapters have been significantly strengthened by the addition of with six new chapters dealing with the following topics: intrauterine blood flow; postnatal neurological development; clinical application of cerebral Doppler sonography; Doppler ultrasound examinations of the fetal coronary circulation, the umbilical venous flow, and the fetal pulmonary venous circulation; four-dimensional B-mode and color Doppler fetal echocardiography; and three-dimensional Doppler sonography in gynecology. The three previous separate chapters on Doppler ultrasound for benign gynecological disorders, ectopic pregnancy, and infertility have been combined into one single more cohesive and concise chapter. After implementation of these additions and revisions, the book now has 521 illustrations and 112 tables. Moreover, all the illustrations including the color plates are now incorporated in the text, which should significantly improve the ease of perusal for our readers.

In this complex and extensive endeavor, we have been greatly assisted by internationally recognized experts in the field who have generously and enthusiastically participated in this venture despite their enormous responsibilities and hectic schedules. I am truly obliged to my colleagues who were instrumental in making the first edition a success and who have updated their chapters for the second edition to reflect the changes that have developed in their areas of expertise. I am particularly indebted to those authors who, in addition to updating their chapters from the first edition, have kindly contributed new chapters. I take this opportunity to welcome the 23 new authors who have substantially contributed to enriching this edition. As well as those authors who have added new chapters to the book, several of the new authors have rewritten and updated chapters from the first edition. I am truly grateful to Dr. Ivica Zalud for his professional and editorial assistance in reorganizing and updating the chapters on gynecological Doppler ultrasound. I remain forever indebted to all my distinguished colleagues not only for their support in making this second edition a reality but also for their scholarly activities that continue to energize the progress in this field.

Finally, all our efforts will be worthwhile if our readers find this new edition of the book useful and stimulating for their education and clinical practice. It would be especially gratifying if the contents inspire and assist new investigations that make further progress in the development of Doppler sonography with the aim of improving women's health.

Summer 2005   Dev Maulik

Acknowledgements

I would like to express my gratitude to Springer-Verlag GmbH & Co., Heidelberg, for the publication of this book, and in particular Dr. Ute Heilmann, Executive Editor Clinical Medicine at Springer-Verlag, for her enthusiastic support and for facilitating the completion of this second edition and Wilma McHugh, Medical Desk Editor, for her help in production work. I would also like to express my sincere thanks to Wendie Irving, my editorial assistant at Winthrop-University Hospital, for her invaluable assistance and tireless dedication in the preparation of this book.

Finally, most of my activities related to this project occurred in the evenings and the weekends at home. I am deeply appreciative and thankful to my wife Shibani and our children, Devika and Davesh, for their encouragement and support during this long process.

Contents

**38 Three-Dimensional Doppler Ultrasound
in Gynecology**   557
Ivica Zalud, Lawrence D. Platt

**39 Doppler Ultrasonography
for Benign Gynecologic Disorders,
Ectopic Pregnancy, and Infertility**   569
Ivica Zalud

**40 Doppler Ultrasonography
for Gynecologic Malignancies**   599
Ivica Zalud

Authors

Amon Amit, MD
Department of Pathology, Rambam Medical Center,
Haifa 31096, Israel

Philippe Arbeille, MD, PhD
Unité INSERM 316, CHU Trousseau,
37044 Tours, France

Domenico Arduini, MD
Department of Obstetrics and Gynecology,
University di Roma "Tor Vergata", Ospedale Fatebenefratelli,
Isola Tiberina 39, 00186 Rome, Italy

Ray O. Bahado-Singh, MD
Department of Obstetrics and Gynecology,
University of Cincinnati College of Medicine,
231 Albert Sabin Way, Cincinnati, OH 45267, USA

Ahmet Alexander Baschat, MD
Center for Advanced Fetal Care,
Department of Obstetrics,
Gynecology and Reproductive Sciences,
University of Maryland, Baltimore,
22 South Greene Street, Baltimore, MD 21201, USA

Gabriel Carles, MD
Department of Obstetrics and Gynecology,
Hopital de Saint Laurent du Maroni 97320, France

Rabih Chaoui, MD, Prof.
Department of Obstetrics and Gynecology,
Charité Medical School, Humboldt University,
Schumannstrasse 20/21, 10098 Berlin, Germany

Chin-Chien Cheng, MD
Department of Obstetrics and Gynecology,
University of Cincinnati College of Medicine,
231 Albert Sabin Way, Cincinnati, OH 45267, USA

Murielle Chevillot, MD
Départent Obstetrique et Gynecologie,
CHU Bretonneau, 37044 Tours, France

Yoshihide Chiba, MD, PhD
National Cardiovascular Center, 5-7-1 Fujishirodai,
Suita, Osaka 565-8565, Japan

Laura Detti, MD
Department of Obstetrics and Gynecology,
University of Cincinnati College of Medicine,
234 Albert Sabin Way, Cincinnati, OH 45267, USA

Enrico M. Ferrazzi, MD
Professor and Chairman, Department of Obstetrics
and Gynecology, Institute for Clinical Sciences Sacco,
University of Milan, Via G.B. Grassi 74, 20157 Milan, Italy

Reinaldo Figueroa, MD
Department of Obstetrics and Gynecology, Winthrop
University Hospital, 259 First Street, Mineola,
NY 11501, USA

Emanuel P. Gaziano, MD
Abbott Northwestern Hospital, 800 East 28th Street,
Minneapolis, MN 55407, USA

Edwin R. Guzman, MD
Department of Obstetrics and Gynecology, MOB 4th Floor,
St. Peter's University Hospital, 254 Easton Avenue,
New Brunswick, NJ 08903-0591, USA

Ursula F. Harkness, MD, MPH
Department of Obstetrics, Gynecology
and Women's Health
University of Minnesota
420 Delaware Street SE
Minneapolis, Minnesota, 55455, USA

Kai-Sven Heling
Department of Obstetrics and Gynecology,
Charité Medical School, Humboldt University,
Schumannstrasse 20/21, 10098 Berlin, Germany

Philippe Herve, MD
Unité INSERM 316, CHU Trousseau, 37044 Tours, France

James C. Huhta, MD
All Children's Hospital, 880 Sixth Street South, Suite 280,
St. Petersburg, FL 33701, USA

Joseph Itskovitz-Eldor, MD, DSc
Department of Obstetrics and Gynecology,
Rambam Medical Center, Haifa 31096, Israel

Karim D. Kalache, MD
Department of Obstetrics and Gynecology,
Charité Medical School, Humboldt University,
Schumannstrasse 20/21, 10098 Berlin, Germany

Toru Kanzaki, MD
Department of Obstetrics and Gynecology, Faculty
of Medicine, Rambam Medical Center, Technion,
Israel Institute of Technology, Haifa 31096, Israel

Torvid Kiserud, MD, PhD
Institute of Clinical Medicine, Department of Obstetrics
and Gynecology, University of Bergen, 5021 Bergen, Norway

Eftichia Kontopoulos, MD
Department of Obstetrics, Gynecology, and Reproductive
Sciences, UMDNJ-Robert Wood Johnson Medical School,
125 Paterson Street, New Brunswick, NJ 08901, USA

Franka Lenz, MD
Department of Obstetrics and Gynecology,
Charité Medical School, Humboldt University,
Schumannstrasse 20/21, 10098 Berlin, Germany

David Ley, MD
Department of Obstetrics and Gynecology,
Lund University Hospital, 22185 Lund, Sweden

Alain Locatelli, MD
Station INRA-PRMD, Nouzilly, 37380 Monnaie, France

Andrzej Lysikiewicz, MD, PhD
Department of Obstetrics and Gynecology,
Winthrop University Hospital, 259 First Street, Mineola,
NY 11501, USA

Giancarlo Mari, MD
Department of Obstetrics and Gynecology
Hutzel Hospital/Wayne State University
4707 St. Antoine Boulevard
Detroit, Michigan, 48201, USA

Karel Maršál, MD, PhD
Department of Obstetrics and Gynecology,
Lund University Hospital, 221 85 Lund, Sweden

Dev Maulik, MD, PhD
Department of Obstetrics and Gynecology,
Winthrop University Hospital, Mineola, NY 11501, USA

Hein Odendaal, MBChB FCOG(SA), FRCOG, MD
Department of Obstetrics and Gynecology, Faculty
of Health Sciences, University of Stellenbosch,
Stellenbosch, South Africa

William J. Ott, MD, FACOG
Division of Maternal Fetal Medicine, St. John's Mercy
Medical Center, Professor, Clinical Obstetrics,
Gynecology and Women's Health, St. Louis University
Medical School, St. Louis, Missouri, USA

Frank Perrotin, MD
Department of Obstetrics and Gynecology,
CHU Bretonneau, 37044 Tours, France

Lawrence D. Platt, MD, FACOG
Department of Obstetrics and Gynecology, David Geffen
School of Medicine, University of California at Los Angeles,
Center for Fetal Medicine and Women's Ultrasound,
Los Angeles, California 90048, USA

Serena Rigano, MD, PhD
Institute for Clinical Sciences Sacco,
University of Milan, Milan, Italy

Giuseppe Rizzo, MD
Department of Obstetrics and Gynecology,
University di Roma "Tor Vergata", Ospedale Fatebenefratelli,
Isola Tiberina 39, 00186 Rome, Italy

Maria Segata, MD
Department of Obstetrics and Gynecology,
University of Cincinnati College of Medicine,
231 Albert Sabin Way, Cincinnati, OH 45267, USA

Genevieve Sicuranza, MD
Department of Obstetrics and Gynecology,
Winthrop University Hospital, Mineola, NY 11501, USA

Israel Thaler, MD
Department of Obstetrics and Gynecology,
Rambam Medical Center, Haifa 31096, Israel

Gerald Tulzer, MD
Department of Pediatric Cardiology, Children's
Hospital of Linz, Herrenstrasse 20, 4020 Linz, Austria

Jean-Claude Veille, MD
Department of Obstetrics and Gynecology, Albany
Medical Center, MC 74, 43 New Scotland Avenue,
Albany, NY 12208, USA

Sharon R. Weil-Chalker, MD
Department of Pediatrics, Abington Memorial Hospital,
1200 Old York Road, Abington, PA 19001, USA

Zeev Weiner, MD
Department of Obstetrics and Gynecology, Haemek
Medical Center, Afula, Israel

Ivica Zalud, MD, PhD
Fetal Diagnostic Center, Rm 540, Kapiolani Medical
Center for Women and Children, 1319 Punahou Street,
Honolulu, HI 96826, USA

Chapter 1

Doppler Sonography: A Brief History

Dev Maulik

The origins of modern medical technology may be traced to nineteenth-century europe, when the industrial revolution ushered in sweeping changes in every aspect of life. Of all the momentous discoveries and inventions of this period, there was one relatively obscure scientific event that laid the foundation for the subsequent development of Doppler technologies in the twentieth century – the discovery of a natural phenomenon that came to be known as the Doppler effect. Another critical event was the discovery of the piezoelectric phenomenon by Pierre Curie and Jacques Curie, which enabled the development of ultrasonic transducers many decades later. This chapter briefly describes the origin of the Doppler theory during the nineteenth century and traces the development of diagnostic Doppler ultrasound technology during the second half of the twentieth century to the present.

Christian Andreas Doppler and the Doppler Theory

The *Doppler effect* is defined as the observed changes in the frequency of transmitted waves when relative motion exists between the source of the wave and an observer. The frequency increases when the source and the observer move closer and decreases when they move apart. The phenomenon bears the name of its discoverer, Christian Andreas Doppler, an Austrian mathematician and physicist (Fig. 1.1), born to Johann Evangialist and Therese Doppler on November 29, 1803 in Salzburg, Austria. The house in which he was born and raised still stands across the square from the family home of Wolfgang Amadeus Mozart in the Markart Platz. For nearly a century Doppler's Christian name has been consistently misquoted in the literature as Johann Christian. Doppler was baptized on the day of his birth at the Church of St. Andra, which was originally in close proximity of the Doppler home. Eden [1] conducted a thorough search for Doppler's birth and baptismal records and found them still preserved in the Church of St. Andra, which had moved to a new location in Salzburg in 1898. These documents conclusively established that Doppler had been christened Christian Andreas. It

appears, however, that Doppler never used his second name.

Doppler's father, a master stone mason, was a man of wealth and fame. Because of frail health Doppler was sent to school instead of joining the family trade. In 1822 Johann Doppler requested that Simon Stampfer, a professor at the local Lyceum, evaluate his son's aptitude. Stampfer was impressed with young Christian's scholastic abilities in mathematics and science,

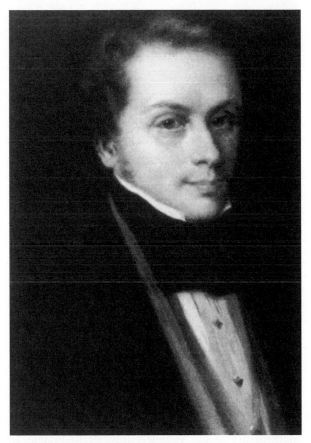

Fig. 1.1. Christian Andreas Doppler. The oil painting was done by an unidentified artist probably at the time of Doppler's marriage in 1836. The original is in the Austrian Academy of Sciences to whom it was donated by Mathilda von Flugl, the great granddaughter of Christian Doppler. (Reprinted from [1], with permission)

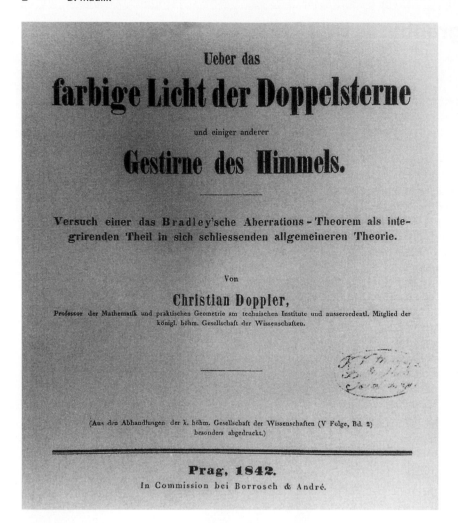

Fig. 1.2. Title page of Christian Doppler's paper titled "On the Coloured Light of the Double Stars and Certain Other Stars of the Heavens." (Reprinted from [1], with permission)

and at his recommendation Doppler was sent to the Polytechnic Institute of Vienna for further education.

Doppler studied mathematics and physics in Vienna for 3 years and then returned to Salzburg where he concluded his education and eventually graduated in 1829. For 4 years he held the position of assistant in higher mathematics at the Vienna Polytechnic Institute. Following this assitantship he experienced difficulty finding an appropriate position, and in 1835 he seriously considered emigrating to the United States. At this point, however, he was offered and accepted the position of Professor of Elementary Mathematics and Commercial Accounting at the State Secondary School in Prague. The following year he was also appointed Supplementary Professor of Higher Mathematics at the Technical Institute in Prague. In 1841 Christian Doppler became a full Professor of Mathematics and Practical Geometry at the latter institution. One year later, on May 25, he presented his landmark paper on the Doppler effect at a meeting of the Natural Sciences Section of the Royal Bohemian Society of Sciences in Prague. Ironically, there were only five people and a transcriber in the audience. The paper was entitled "On the Colored Light of the Double Stars and Certain Other Stars of the Heavens" (Fig. 1.2) and was published in 1843 in the Proceedings of the society [2]. Of 51 papers Doppler published, this one was destined to bring him lasting recognition.

Doppler's work was based on the theory of the aberration of light developed by Edmund Bradley, the eighteenth-century British Astronomer Royal. Doppler established the principle of frequency shift and developed the formula for calculating the velocity from the shift. For elucidating the theoretic background of the principle, Doppler used various analogies and examples primarily based on transmission of light and sound. Although his examples of sound transmission were correct, those involving light transmission were erroneous, as he presumed that all stars emitted only pure white light. He postulated that the color of a star was caused by the relative motions of the star and the earth causing apparent spectral shifts of the emitted white light. The spectrum would shift toward blue if the star approached the earth; conversely, the spectrum would shift to red if the star receded away from the earth. When describing these phenomena Doppler did not take into account preexisting research on light transmission and spectrum. Herschel [3] had already discovered infrared radiation, and Ritter [4] had described ultraviolet radiation; but it appears that Doppler was unaware of these important developments.

Verification of Doppler's Theory

As was to be expected, the paper generated critical responses. The most significant challenge came from a young Dutch scientist working at the University of Utrecht in Holland, Christoph Hendrik Diederik Buys Ballot (Fig. 1.3). In 1844 Buys Ballot proposed to refute the Doppler theory by designing an experiment involving sound transmission as his doctoral research project. Conveniently for him, a new railroad had just been established between Amsterdam and Utrecht, and the Dutch government gave him permission to use this railway system to verify the Doppler effect on sound transmission (Fig. 1.4). The first experiment was designed in February 1845. Two horn players who apparently had perfect pitch were chosen to participate in the experiment. The calibration was accomplished by one musician blowing a note and the other identifying the pitch of the tone. After this calibration was performed, one player was positioned on the train, and the other stood along the track. As the train passed, the stationary musician on the trackside perceived that the note blown by the musician on the train was half a note higher when the train approached him and half a note lower when it moved away. Unfortunately, a raging blizzard forced Buys Ballot to abandon his experiment and to reschedule it in a more temperate season. The results from the first experiment were published within less than a month in a music journal [5].

Buys Ballot conducted the experiment again in early June of the same year [6]. Three teams were stationed along the track. Each team was composed of a horn player, an observer, and a manager. A fourth team was on a flat car behind the locomotive. Buys Ballot positioned himself on the foot plate next to the engineer. This experiment was more sophisticated, but it also encountered environmental complications as the summer heat seriously interfered with the correct tuning of the musical instruments. The musicians originally tried to use one-sixteenth of a single note but failed, and the final experiment was done in eights. The results were remarkable despite all trials and tribulations. The study that set out to re-

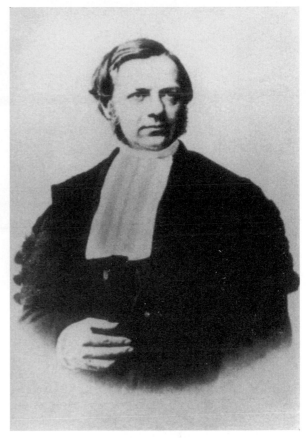

Fig. 1.3. C.H.D. Buys Ballot (1817–1890). (From [40], with permission)

fute the Doppler theory ultimately confirmed it. Buys Ballot proved not only the existence of the Doppler effect in relation to sound transmission but its angle dependency as well. Incredibly, Buys Ballot still refused to accept the validity of the theory for the propagation of light and most of the scientific community of the nineteenth century did not acknowledge the validity of Doppler's theory because of his erroneous interpretation of astronomical phenomena.

As translated by Eden [1], Doppler's response was impressive in its foresight: "I still hold the trust – indeed, stronger than ever before – that in the course of time, this theory will serve astronomers as a welcome help to probe the happenings of the universe, at times when they feel deserted by all other methods" [7]. This statement was prophetic. Since the beginning of the twentieth century, the Doppler principle has been used extensively not only in astronomy but also in the immensely diverse fields of science and technology.

Doppler lived only 10 years after publishing his paper on the frequency shift; however, these few years brought him well-deserved recognition and honor. He

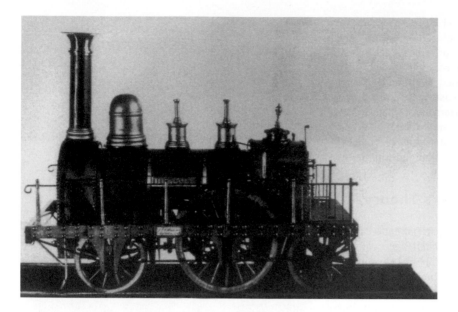

Fig. 1.4. Model of the locomotive (named Hercules) used in the first experiments. (From [40], with permission)

was elected to the membership of the Royal Bohemian Society of Sciences in 1843 and of the highly prestigious Imperial Academy of Sciences in Vienna in 1847. In 1850 he was appointed by Emperor Franz Josef of the Austro-Hungarian Empire to the coveted position of the Chair of Experimental Physics at the University of Vienna. Sadly, however, he was in poor health at this point because of the chronic respiratory disease which was presumed to be "consumption" or pulmonary tuberculosis and which he apparently had contracted in Prague years earlier. With the hope of recuperation he went to the warmer climate of Venice in the winter of 1852, where he died on March 17, 1853 at the age of only 49 in the arms of his wife Mathilde. He was given a grand funeral at the Parish Church of San Giovanni in Bragora and many academic and civil dignitaries were in attendance. A more comprehensive account of Doppler's life is beyond the scope of this review. For those who are interested, I strongly recommend the excellent monograph written by Professor Alec Eden titled *The Search For Christian Doppler* [1].

Technical Utilization of Doppler's Principle

Initial applications of the Doppler principle were mostly for astronomic studies. Over the years the Doppler effect for light and radio waves has yielded information on a cosmic scale, from orbital velocity of planets and stars to galactic rotation and an ever-expanding universe. The principle still serves as a major tool for cosmologic research. With the beginning of the twentieth century, other applications gradually emerged. The first sonar equipment for detecting submarines was developed by Paul Langevin of France, who also pioneered the use of piezoelectric crystals for transmitting and receiving ultrasound waves. This technology was used to detect submarines, initially during World War I and more extensively during World War II. The ensuing decades witnessed widespread application of the principle of the Doppler effect, from road-side radar speed detectors used by the police to the highly sophisticated military defense and weather forecasting Doppler radar systems. Doppler radio signals are used for navigation, surveying, monitoring animal migration, and estimating crop yields. The development of diagnostic Doppler ultrasound technology offers yet another example of the extensive use of the Doppler principle.

Development of Spectral Doppler Ultrasonography

The first medical applications of Doppler sonography were initiated during the late 1950s, and impressive technologic innovations have been continuing ever since. Shigeo Satomura from the Institute of Scientific and Industrial Research of Osaka University in Japan developed the first Doppler ultrasound device for medical diagnostic purposes and reported the recording of various cardiac valvular movements [8]. Based on their experience, Satomura suggested the potential use of Doppler ultrasonography for percutaneous measurement of blood flow. In 1960 he and Kaneko were the first to report construction of an ultrasonic flowmeter [9]. A significant amount of the pioneering work occurred at the University of Washington in

Seattle in the United States. Major driving forces of this group included Robert Rushmer, a physician, and Dean Franklin, an engineer. They initiated the development of a prototype continuous-wave Doppler device in 1959 and reported blood flow assessment using the ultrasound Doppler frequency shift [10]. The Seattle team refined this instrument into a small portable device, and the earliest clinical trials were undertaken during the mid-1960s by Eugene Strandness, who at the time was undergoing training as a vascular surgeon [11].

The first pulsed-wave Doppler equipment was developed by the Seattle research team. Donald Baker, Dennis Watkins, and John Reid began working on this project in 1966 and produced one of the first pulsed Doppler devices [12]. Other pioneers of pulsed Doppler include Wells of the United Kingdom [13] and Peronneau of France [14]. The Seattle team also pioneered the construction of duplex Doppler instrumentation based on a mechanical sector scanning head in which a single transducer crystal performed both imaging and Doppler functions on a time-sharing basis. The duplex Doppler technique allowed the ultrasound operator to determine for the first time the target of Doppler insonation. This development is of critical importance in obstetric and gynecologic applications, as such range discrimination allows reliable Doppler interrogation of a deep-lying circulation, such as that of the fetus and of the maternal pelvic organs. It must be recognized that many others also have made immense pioneering contributions in the development and utilization of diagnostic Doppler sonography, a detailed discussion of which is beyond the scope of this chapter.

The initial attempts involved various invasive and noninvasive modifications of the existing echocardiographic approach, including the use of a sonocontrast agent to obtain information on blood flow patterns during two-dimensional echocardiographic imaging [15] and the development of multichannel duplex Doppler systems [16]. However, the spectral pulsed Doppler ultrasound used in these techniques could produce velocity information only along a single beam line. The development of real-time two-dimensional color Doppler ultrasonography therefore represents a major technologic breakthrough, which became possible because of the introduction of two critical pieces of technology for processing the Doppler ultrasound signal. First was the Doppler sonographic application by Angelsen and Kristofferson [17] of the sophisticated filtering technique of "the moving target indicator" used in radar systems. This filter allows removal of the high-amplitude/low-velocity clutter signals generated by the movement of tissue structures and vessel walls. The second was development of the autocorrelation technique by Namekawa et al. [18]. The autocorrelator is capable of processing mean Doppler phase shift data from the two-dimensional scan area in real time, so two-dimensional Doppler flow mapping is possible (see Chap. 5). In 1983 the Japanese group, which included Omoto, Namekawa, Kasai, and others, reported the use of a prototype device incorporating the new technology for visualizing intracardiac flow [19]. Extensive clinical evaluation of this new approach was carried on in the United States by Nanda and other investigators [20].

Development of Color Doppler Ultrasonography

Spectral Doppler ultrasound interrogates along the single line of ultrasound beam transmission. The hemodynamic information thus generated is limited to unidimensional flow velocity characterization from the target area. This limitation provided the impetus to develop a method for depiction of flow in a two-dimensional plane in real time. Potential clinical utility of such an approach was obvious, particularly for cardiovascular applications to diagnose complex hemodynamic and structural abnormalities associated with acquired and congenital cardiac disease. However, the unidimensional spectral pulsed Doppler method was inadequate to cope with the processing needs of real-time two-dimensional Doppler ultrasonography, which involves analysis of an enormous number of signals derived from multiple sampling sites along multiple scan lines.

Introduction of Doppler Ultrasonography to Obstetrics and Gynecology

The first obstetric application of Doppler ultrasonography consisted in detection of fetal heart movements [21]. Originally developed for fetal heart rate detection, the technique was further developed for noninvasive continuous electronic monitoring of the fetal heart rate. Currently, they constitute the most common uses of Doppler ultrasonography in obstetrics. The systems are based on utilizing relatively simple continuous-wave Doppler ultrasound to determine the fetal heart rate from the fetal cardiac wall or valvular motion. The first application of Doppler velocimetry in obstetrics was reported by FitzGerald and Drumm [22] from Dublin and MacCallum et al. [23] from Seattle. The former are recognized as the first group to publish a peer-reviewed article in this field. These publications were followed by an era if impres-

Table 1.1. Feasibility of Doppler velocimetry of fetal and uteroplacental circulations

Circulation	Year	Author
Umbilical artery	1977	FitzGerald and Drumm [22]
Umbilical vein	1979	Gill and Kossoff [24]
Fetal aorta	1980	Eik-Nes et al. [25]
Uteroplacental	1983	Campbell et al. [26]
Fetal inferior vena cava	1983	Chiba et al. [27]
Fetal cardiac	1984	Maulik et al. [28]
Fetal cerebral	1986	Arbeille et al. [29]
	1986	Wladimiroff et al. [30]
Fetal ductus arteriosus	1987	Huhta et al. [31]
Fetal renal	1989	Vyas et al. [32]
	1989	Veille and Kanaan [33]
Fetal ductus venosus	1991	Kiserud et al. [35]
Fetal coronary artery	1996	Gembruch et al. [36]

sive research productivity during which various investigators [24–36] extended the use of Doppler sonography for assessing the fetal and the maternal circulation (Table 1.1).

In contrast to the prolific publications on the obstetric uses of Doppler sonography, reports on gynecologic applications of the technique did not begin to appear until the mid-1980s. Taylor and colleagues were the first to characterize Doppler waves from the ovarian and uterine arterial circulations utilizing pulsed duplex Doppler instrumentation [37]. This work was followed by reports of transvaginal color Doppler studies [38] and transvaginal duplex pulsed Doppler studies [39] of pelvic vessels. Through the late 1980s and early 1990s, Doppler sonographic research in gynecology steadily expanded.

Conclusion

Discovery of the Doppler effect and its application to medical diagnostics after more than a century is a fascinating example of how our understanding and exploitation of natural phenomena can be translated into tangible advances in medicine. This is also relevant for obstetrics and gynecology as Doppler sonography has enabled us to explore and understand human fetal hemodynamics, which was virtually inaccessible before. As we continue to advance our knowledge, it is important to pause and acknowledge the immense contributions of the pioneers who made it all happen.

References

1. Eden A (1992) The Search for Christian Doppler. Springer, Vienna
2. Doppler C (1843) Uber das farbige Licht der Dopplersterne und einiger anderer Gestirne des Himmels. Abhandl Konigl Bohm Ges Ser 2:465–482
3. Herschel JFW (1800) Experiments on the refrangibility of the invisible rays of the sun. Philos Trans R Soc Lond 90:284–292
4. Ritter JW (1801) Ausfindung nicht lichtbarer Sonnenstrahlen ausserhalb des Farbenspectrums, an der Seite des Violetts. Widerhohlung der Rouppachen Versuche. Wien, Mathemat-Naturw Klasse Sitzungsbericht 79: 365–380
5. Buys Ballot CHD (1845) Bedrog van het gehoororgaan in het bepalen van de hoogte van een waargenomen toon. Caecilia. Algemeen Muzikaal Tijdschrift van Nederlandl Tweede Jaargang No 7:78–81
6. Buys Ballot CHD (1845) Akustische Versuche auf der Niederlandischen Eisenbahn nebst gelegentlichen Bemerkungen zur Theorie des Herrn Prof Doppler. Pogg Ann 66:321–351
7. Doppler C (1846) Bemerkungen zu meiner Theorie des Farbigen Lichtes der Doppelsterne etc, mit vorzuglicher Rucksicht auf die von Herrn Dr Buys Ballot zu Utrecht dagegen erhobenen Bedenken. Pogg Ann 68:1–35
8. Satomura S (1957) Ultrasonic Doppler method for the inspection of cardiac functions. J Acoust Soc Am 29:1181–1183
9. Satomura S, Kaneko Z (1960) Ultrasonic blood rheograph. In: Proceedings of the 3rd International Conference on Medical Elect, London, IEEE, p 254
10. Franklin DL, Schlegel W, Rushmer RF (1961) Blood flow measured by Doppler frequency shift of back scattered ultrasound. Science 134:564–565
11. Strandness DE, Schultz RD, Sumner DS, Rushmer RF (1967) Ultrasonic flow detection – a useful technic in the evaluation of peripheral vascular disease. Am J Surg 113:311–314
12. Baker DW (1970) Pulsed ultrasonic Doppler blood flow sensing. IEEE Trans Sonic Ultrasonics SU-17(3):170–185
13. Wells PNT (1969) A range gated ultrasonic Doppler system. Med Biol Eng 7:641–652
14. Peronneau PA, Leger F (1969) Doppler ultrasonic pulsed blood flowmeter. In: Proceedings of the 8th Conference on Medical and Biological Engineering, pp 10–11
15. Gramiak R, Shah PM, Kramer DH (1969) Ultrasound cardiography: contrast studies in anatomy and function. Radiology 92:939–948
16. Fish PJ (1975) Multichannel direction resolving Doppler angiography (abstract). Presented at the 2nd European Congress of Ultrasonics in Medicine, p 72
17. Angelsen BAJ, Kristofferson K (1979) On ultrasonic MTI mearement of velocity profiled in blood flow. IEEE Trans Biomed Eng BME-26:665–771
18. Namekawa K, Kasai C, Tsukamoto M, Koyano A (1982) Imaging of blood flow using autocorrelation (abstract). Ultrasound Med Biol 8:138–141
19. Omoto R, Yokote Y, Takamoto S et al (1983) Clinical significance of newly developed real time intracardiac

two dimensional blood flow imaging system (2-D-Doppler) (abstract). Jpn Circ J 47:191

20. Omoto R (1989) History of color flow mapping technologies. In: Nanda NC (ed) Textbook of color Doppler echocardiography. Lea & Febiger, Philadelphia, pp 1–5

21. Callaghan DA, Rowland TC, Goldman DE (1964) Ultrasonic Doppler observation of the fetal heart. Obstet Gynecol 23:637–641

22. FitzGerald DE, Drumm JE (1977) Noninvasive measurement of the fetal circulation using ultrasound: a new method. BMJ 2:1450–1451

23. McCallum WD, Olson RF, Daigle RE, Baker DW (1977) Real time analysis of Doppler signals obtained from the fetoplacental circulation. Ultrasound Med 3B:1361–1364

24. Gill RW, Kossoff G (1979) Pulsed Doppler combined with B-mode imaging for blood flow measurement. Contrib Gynecol Obstet 6:139–141

25. Eik-Nes SH, Bruback AO, Ulstein MK (1980) Measurement of human fetal blood flow. BMJ 28:283–287

26. Campbell S, Diaz-Recasens J, Griffin DR et al (1983) New Doppler technique for assessing uteroplacental blood flow. Lancet 1:675–677

27. Chiba Y, Utsu M, Kanzaki T, Hasegawa T (1983) Changes in venous flow and intra-tracheal flow in fetal breathing movements. Ultrasound Med Biol 11:43–49

28. Maulik D, Nanda NC, Saini VD (1984) Fetal Doppler echocardiography: methods and characterization of normal and abnormal hemodynamics. Am J Cardiol 53:572–578

29. Arbeille P, Tranquart F, Body G et al (1986) Evolution de la circulation arterielle ombilicale et cerebrale du foetus au cours de la grossesse. Prog Neonatal 6:30

30. Wladimiroff JW, Tonge HN, Stewart PA (1986) Doppler ultrasound assessment of cerebral blood flow in the human fetus. Br J Obstet Gynaecol 93:471–475

31. Huhta JC, Moise KJ, Fisher DJ, Sharif DS, Wassersturm N, Martin C (1987) Detection and quantitation of constriction of the fetal ductus arteriosus by Doppler echocardiography. Circulation 75:406–412

32. Vyas S, Nicolaides KH, Campbell S (1989) Renal artery flow-velocity waveforms in normal and hypoxemic fetuses. Am J Obstet Gynecol 161:168–172

33. Veille JC, Kanaan C (1989) Duplex Doppler ultrasonographic evaluation of the fetal renal artery in normal and abnormal fetuses. Am J Obstet Gynecol 161:1502–1507

34. Maulik D, Nanda NC, Hsiung MC, Youngblood J (1986) Doppler color flow mapping of the fetal heart. Angiology 37:628–632

35. Kiserud T, Eik-Nes SH, Blaas HG, Hellevik LR (1991) Ultrasonographic velocimetry of the fetal ductus venosus. Lancet 338:1412–1414

36. Gembruch U, Baschat AA (1996) Demonstration of fetal coronary blood flow by color-coded and pulsed wave Doppler sonography: a possible indicator of severe compromise and impending demise in intrauterine growth retardation. Ultrasound Obstet Gynecol 7:10–16

37. Taylor KJW, Burns PN, Wells PNT, Conway DI, Hull MGR (1985) Ultrasound Doppler flow studies of the ovarian and uterine arteries. Br J Obstet Gynaecol 92:240–246

38. Kurjak A, Zalud I, Jurkovic D, Alfrevic Z, Miljan M (1989) Transvaginal color Doppler for the assessment of pelvic circulation. Acta Obstet Gynecol Scand 68:131–135

39. Thaler I, Manor D, Brandes J, Rottem S, Itskowvitz J (1990) Basic principles and clinical applications of the transvaginal Doppler duplex system in reproductive medicine. J In Vitro Fertil Embryol Transfer 7:74–75

40. Jonkman EJ (1980) A historical note: Doppler research in the nineteenth century. Ultrasound Med Biol 6:1–5

Chapter 2

Physical Principles of Doppler Ultrasonography

Dev Maulik

This chapter presents the basic concepts of sound and ultrasound propagation and discusses the physical principles of the Doppler effect and Doppler sonography, which are essential for understanding their diagnostic uses. Although this book focuses primarily on clinical utilization of the diagnostic Doppler technology, developing an understanding of the basic principles is imperative for its proficient use. The following is a brief introduction and is not intended to be a comprehensive treatise on the subject. For a more in-depth discussion, there are several excellent textbooks that comprehensively examine the physics of Doppler ultrasonography [1–4].

Propagation of Sound

Sound is a form of mechanical energy that travels through solid or liquid media as pressure waves (Fig. 2.1). Sound waves are generated when an object vibrates in a medium. For example, percussion causes a drum membrane to vibrate and to generate sound waves in the air. During vibration the forward movement of the sound source causes a pressure rise in the adjacent medium, so the molecules of the medium become crowded. As the source moves backward there is a pressure drop in the medium, so the molecules now move apart. This phenomenon of alternating molecular compression and rarefaction accompanies the waves of sound energy as they propagate along the medium (Fig. 2.2). Although the molecules vibrate, they remain in their original location and are not displaced. Sound travels faster in solids than in liquids and faster in liquids than in gases.

Although usually considered in a unidimensional plane, in reality sound is transmitted in a three-dimensional space. Sound waves from a vibratory source or from a reflector are moving surfaces of high and low pressures. These surfaces are called *waveforms*. The shape of a waveform depends on the shape of the source or the interface. Thus a plane waveform emanates from a flat source and a spherical waveform from a spherical source. With Doppler ultrasonics, the scattered waveform is spherical, as red blood cells (RBCs) behave as spherical sources during the scattering of an incident beam.

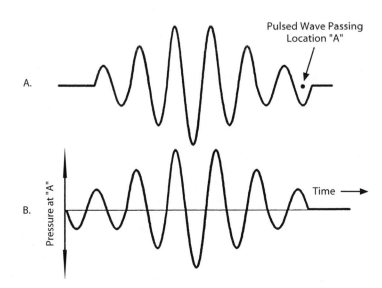

Fig. 2.1 A, B. Propagation of sound. **A** Passage of a sound pulse through point "A" in the medium. **B** Consequent changes in the pressure at that point

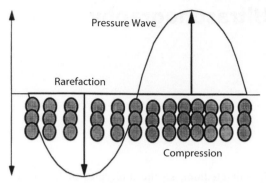

Fig. 2.2. Propagation of sound. Compression and rarefaction of the molecules in a medium associated with the propagation of a pressure wave related to sound or ultrasound transmission. *Horizontal axis* represents the distance; *vertical axis* represents the magnitude of pressure wave deflections around the baseline. Upward deflection represents the positive pressure changes and downward deflection the negative pressure changes

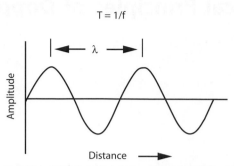

Fig. 2.3. Wavelength of sound. *Horizontal axis* represents the distance and the *vertical axis* the magnitude of pressure wave deflections around the baseline. The peak-to-peak distance (λ) between the consecutive pressure waves is one wavelength

Propagation Speed of Sound

The *propagation speed* of sound in a medium is the rate of change of position of the sound wave in unit time in that medium. It is called *velocity* when the direction of motion is also specified. The speed of ultrasound propagation in a medium is directly related to the bulk modulus of elasticity and density of the medium. A change in transmitting frequency within the range of clinical usage does not alter the speed. Although speed of sound is affected by temperature, no appreciable effects are known in clinical applications. With diagnostic ultrasonography, the propagation speed information is used to compute the depth distance from the echo return time. It is also a component of the Doppler equation that allows determination of speed of the scatterer from the Doppler frequency shift. The average propagation speed of ultrasound in soft tissues is approximately 1,540 meters per second (m/s).

Wavelength, Frequency, Pulse

The *wavelength* of sound is comprised of one cycle of compression and rarefaction. Therefore it is the distance between a pair of consecutive peaks or troughs of adjacent pressure waves (Fig. 2.3). The *frequency* of sound is the number of such cycles occurring in 1 s. One *cycle* is called a hertz (Hz). Wavelength and frequency are inversely related:

$$\lambda = c/f$$

where λ represents the wavelength, c the speed of sound, and f the frequency. As the propagation speed

of sound in tissue is known and is relatively constant, one can determine the frequency from the wavelength and vice versa (Table 2.1). The duration of one cycle, or wavelength, of sound is called its *period* (Fig. 2.4). Period is measured in seconds and microseconds. It is inversely related to the frequency:

$$T = 1/f$$

where T is the period, and f is the frequency of sound.

Pulsed Doppler (both spectral and color flow mapping) and pulse echo imaging systems transmit ultrasound waves in pulses. The number of such pulses transmitted per second is known as the *pulse repetition frequency* (PRF) (Fig. 2.5). The length of one ultrasound pulse is known as the *spatial pulse length* (Fig. 2.6). Pulse length varies according to the mode of ultrasound. With pulsed Doppler ultrasound, the pulse length ranges from 5 to 30 cycles. In contrast, the length is much shorter for pulsed echo imaging system, as they generate two to three cycles per pulse.

Table 2.1. Frequency and corresponding wavelength of commonly used Doppler transducers in obstetrics

Frequency (MHz)	Wavelength (μm)
2.0	770
2.5	616
3.0	513
3.5	440
4.0	385
4.5	342
5.0	308
5.5	280
6.0	257
6.5	236
7.0	220
7.5	205

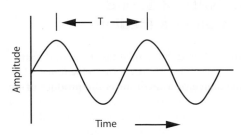

Fig. 2.4. Period of sound. The duration of one wavelength of sound is its period. *Horizontal axis* represents the time and the *vertical axis* the magnitude of pressure wave deflections around the baseline

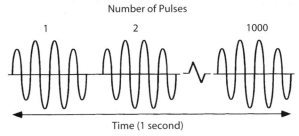

Fig. 2.5. Concept of pulse repetition frequency (PRF). The illustration shows a PRF of 1 KHz (1,000 pulses per second)

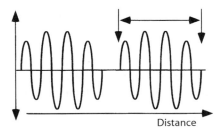

Fig. 2.6. Pulse length, which is the distance in space occupied by one ultrasound pulse. *Horizontal axis* represents the distance and the *vertical axis* the pressure amplitude

For pulsed Doppler applications, the PRF limits the highest velocity that can be measured without creating the artifact known as aliasing. This subject is further discussed in Chap. 3.

Amplitude, Power, Intensity

The maximum variation in pressure generated in a medium by a propagating sound wave is called *pressure amplitude* (Fig. 2.7). Pressure amplitude is directly related to the amount of sound energy emanating from a vibratory source. It is therefore a measure of the strength of sound radiation. The rate of flow of ultrasonic energy through the cross-sectional area of the beam is expressed as its *power*. The *intensity* of a

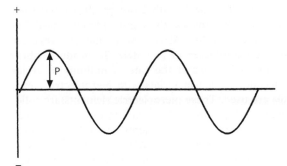

Fig. 2.7. Pressure amplitude of a sound wave. *Horizontal axis* depicts distance or time. *Vertical axis* represents variations in the acoustic pressure. The *plus* and *minus signs* indicate the positive and negative fluctuations of the pressure, respectively. *P*, the amplitude that is the maximum change in the pressure above or below the baseline value represented by the *horizontal line*

sound wave at a location is the rate of flow of energy per unit of cross-sectional area of the beam at that location. It is therefore power divided by beam cross-sectional area. Pressure amplitude is measured using a device called a hydrophone. Intensity (I) is derived from the pressure amplitude (p) as they are directly related:

$$I = p^2/c$$

Intensity is expressed by several descriptor parameters based on its peak and average values.

For continuous-wave Doppler ultrasound, intensity is measured as the spatial peak value (I_{sp}) and the spatial average value (I_{sa}). The former is measured usually at the focal point of the beam, the latter at the cross-sectional location of the beam. For pulsed Doppler ultrasound it is necessary to consider both the spatial and the temporal intensity values. Both peak and average values are measured in various combinations, as follows: spatial peak temporal peak (I_{sptp}), spatial peak temporal average (I_{spta}), spatial average temporal peak (I_{satp}), and spatial average temporal average (I_{sata}). Additional descriptors of pulsed ultrasound intensity include the spatial peak pulse average intensity (I_{sppa}), which is the intensity at the spatial peak averaged over the pulse length. These measures of sound energy of a transmitted Doppler ultrasound beam are important for biosafety considerations and are discussed in Chap. 6.

Ultrasound and Piezoelectric Effect

Audible sound frequency ranges from approximately 10 Hz to 20 KHz. Sound with a frequency of more than 20 KHz is inaudible to the human ear and is known as *ultrasound*. With Doppler ultrasound used for medical diagnostics, the commonly employed frequency range is 2–10 MHz. The frequency range for obstetric transducers in 2–5 MHz. To produce vibrations or oscillations at the rate of millions of cycles per second, special materials with piezoelectric properties are used. These piezoelectric elements are solid, nonconducting substances that demonstrate physical properties whose measurements are different along different axes (anisotropic). When compressed in certain directions, these elements undergo electrical polarization, and a corresponding voltage is generated that is proportional to the pressure. Conversely, when such an element is subjected to an electric field it exhibits mechanical distortion by an amount proportional to the applied field. This phenomenon is known as the *piezoelectric effect* (Fig. 2.8). The piezoelectric effect allows interconversion between sound and electricity and forms the basis for the construction of Doppler and other types of ultrasound transducer. The naturally occurring piezoelectric elements include crystals such as quartz, tourmaline, and rochelle salt. Synthetic ceramic elements employed in the construction of Doppler and other ultrasound transducers are polycrystalline substances consisting of tetravalent metal ions such as zirconium or titanium embedded in a lattice of bigger divalent metal ions such as lead or barium, and oxygen. The most common piezoelectric ceramics include barium titanium trioxide and lead zirconium trioxide. More recently, synthetic single crystals are being developed which include lead zirconate niobate/lead titanate, barium titanate trioxide, and lithium niobate trioxide. These newer single elements demonstrate much greater strain, which is directly related to their performance.

Characteristics of Sound Transmission in a Medium

The resistance offered by a medium to sound transmission is known as its *acoustic impedance*. The acoustic impedance of a medium is the product of its density and the velocity of sound, and it is measured in rayl units. Most soft tissues demonstrate only minor variations in their acoustic impedance [5]. For example, the impedance rayl values for blood, brain, kidney, and muscle are 1.61×10^5, 1.58×10^5, 1.62×10^5, and 1.70×10^5, respectively. In contrast, bones possess a significantly higher acoustic impedance (7.8×10^5). The significance of acoustic impedance lies in the fact that it is the impedance inhomogeneities in tissues that give rise to echoes, which form the basis for ultrasonic imaging and Doppler velocimetry. The boundary between adjacent media with differing acoustic impedance values is called an *acoustic interface*. The characteristics of sound transmission change at the interface. Such changes include reflection and refraction. The amplitude of reflection is directly proportional to the magnitude of impedance difference at the interface. However, even minor differences in acoustic impedance generate echoes. When impedance inhomogeneity exists across an acoustic interface, a variable portion of an ultrasound beam is reflected. At most soft tissue interfaces it involves only a small portion of the ultrasound energy, with the rest being transmitted and reaching the medium beyond the interface (Fig. 2.9). In contrast, thick bone offers a large acoustic mismatch in relation to the surrounding soft tissue medium, so a major portion of the ultrasound energy is reflected. This situation inevitably results in markedly diminished transmission of the beam, and the resultant "acoustic

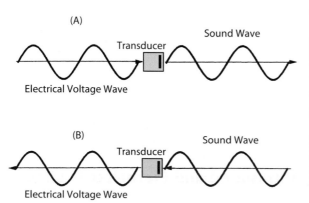

Fig. 2.8 A, B. Piezoelectric effect. **A** Conversion of the electrical energy to sound energy. **B** Conversion of sound to electrical energy

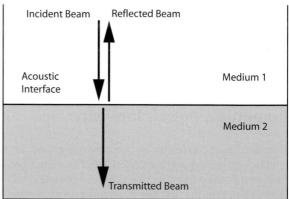

Fig. 2.9. Reflection and transmission of sound at the interface acoustically mismatched in medium 1 and medium 2. In this example the beam strikes the interface perpendicularly

shadow" affects optimal imaging of structures lying posterior to the bone. At most tissue interfaces, an incident beam is echoed in different directions, a process known as *diffuse reflection*. In relation to Doppler ultrasonic reflections, however, an entirely different phenomenon occurs, known as *scattering*. This phenomenon is discussed below.

When an ultrasound beam travels with an oblique angle of incidence across an interface, the beam path deviates and the angle of transmission differs from the angle of incidence (Fig. 2.10). The phenomenon is similar to refraction of light. Refractive deviation in the beam path may compromise image quality. For pulsed Doppler duplex applications, where two-dimensional gray-scale imaging is used for placing the Doppler sample volume in deep vascular locations, refraction may lead to error. However, the propagation speed of sound does not vary appreciably in most soft tissues; therefore only minimal refraction occurs at most tissue interfaces. For example, an ultrasound beam passing through a muscle-blood interface at an incident angle of $30°$ undergoes only a $0°47'$ refractive deviation [2].

Progressive decline in the pressure amplitude and intensity of a propagating ultrasonic wave is known as *attenuation*. Attenuation is caused by many factors, including absorption, scattering, reflection, and wave front divergence. *Absorption* is the phenomenon whereby sound energy is converted to heat and is therefore responsible for thermal bioeffects. Attenuation is also affected by the transmitting frequency of a transducer: the higher the frequency, the greater the attenuation. It limits the use of high-frequency transducers for Doppler interrogation of deep vascu-

lar structures. These considerations influence the choice of a transducer for a specific use. Thus for Doppler examinations of fetal circulation, a 5-MHz transducer may by less efficient for obtaining adequate signals than a 2-MHz transducer.

Doppler Effect

The Doppler effect is the phenomenon of observed changes in the frequency of energy wave transmission when relative motion occurs between the source of wave transmission and the observer. The change in the frequency is known as the Doppler frequency shift, or simply the Doppler shift:

$$f_d = f_t - f_r$$

where f_d is the Doppler shift frequency, f_t is the transmitted frequency, and f_r is the received frequency. When the source and the observer move closer, the wavelength decreases and the frequency increases. Conversely, when the source and the observer move apart, the wavelength increases and the frequency decreases. The Doppler effect is observed irrespective of whether the source or the observer moves (Fig. 2.11). The principle is applicable to all forms of wave propagation. The utility of the Doppler effect originates from the fact that the shift in frequency is proportional to the speed of movement between the source and the receiver and therefore can be used to assess this speed. The Doppler effect is observed irrespective of whether the source or the observer moves.

Doppler Ultrasound

For sound transmission, the Doppler shift sound is of a higher frequency when the source and the receiver move closer and of a lower frequency when they re-

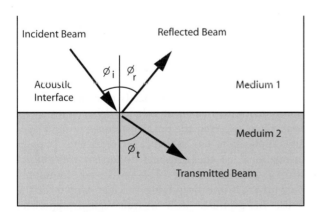

Fig. 2.10. Reflection, refraction, and transmission of sound. The beam, in this example, is encountering the acoustic interface obliquely. A portion of the incident sound is reflected back, and the rest is transmitted. The angle of reflection (Φ_r) equals the angle of incidence (Φ_i). The transmitted sound is refracted. The angle of refraction (Φ_t) depends on the angle of incidence and the propagation speeds of sound in medium 1 and medium 2

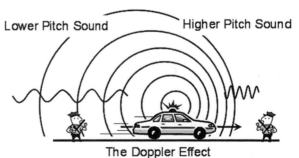

Fig. 2.11. Graphic depiction of the Doppler shift when a source of sound transmission moves away or toward a stationary observer

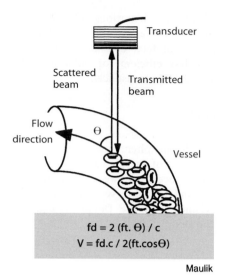

Transducer

Scattered beam

Transmitted beam

Flow direction

θ

Vessel

$$fd = 2 (ft. Θ) / c$$
$$V = fd.c / 2(ft.\cos Θ)$$

Maulik

Fig. 2.12. Doppler effect when an ultrasound beam interrogates circulating blood. *fd* Doppler shift, *ft* transmitted beam, *V* velocity of blood flow, *c* speed sound propagation in tissue, *θ* angle of incidence between the ultrasound beam and the direction of blood flow

cede. The phenomenon of the Doppler effect is also observed when an ultrasound beam encounters blood flow (Fig. 2.12). With blood circulation, millions of red blood cells (RBCs) act as moving scatterers of the incident ultrasound. In this circumstance the erythrocytes act first as moving receivers and then as moving sources [6], forming the basis for the Doppler equation:

$$f_d = 2f_t\, v/c$$

where f_d represents the Doppler frequency shift, f_t the frequency of the incident beam (transducer frequency), v the velocity of the scatterer in a given direction, and c the propagation speed of sound in the medium. Note that the transmitted ultrasound undergoes double Doppler shift before returning to the receiving transducer, the scatterer acting first as a receiver and then as a transmitter. This phenomenon accounts for the factor of 2 in the above equation.

If the direction of the incident beam is at an angle (θ) to the direction of blood flow, the v in the Doppler equation is replaced by the component of the velocity in the direction of the flow (obtained by the cosine of the angle, cos θ):

$$f_d = 2f_t \cdot \cos θ \cdot v/c$$

To determine the velocity of the scatterer, the equation can be rewritten as follows:

$$v = f_d \cdot c/2f_t \cdot \cos θ$$

Thus if the angle of beam incidence and the Doppler shift are known, the velocity of blood flow is also known, assuming that the transducer frequency and the velocity of sound in tissue remain relatively constant (Fig. 2.12). The above equation forms the basis for clinical application of the Doppler principle.

Backscattering

We briefly alluded to a special category of sound reflection called scattering. The process of ultrasonic scattering is analogous to scattering of light by gas molecules and is known as *Rayleigh scattering* [7, 8]. Light so reflected is called Tyndall light and is responsible for the blue sky. Interestingly, it was inquiry into the cause of blue sky at the turn of the century by a group of scientists, including Lord Rayleigh and Tyndall, that led to our understanding of this phenomenon [9]. Rayleigh scattering occurs when energy waves traveling through a medium encounter reflectors whose size is much smaller than the wavelength of the propagating energy; a portion of the energy is then reflected in all directions. The scattered energy wave is spherical in shape irrespective of the shape of the scatterer.

One characteristic of Rayleigh scattering is that the power, or intensity, of the scattered energy (I) is proportional to the fourth power of the frequency (f).

$$I \sim f_4$$

The frequency dependence of scattering power has important consequences for selecting the appropriate transducer frequency for Doppler applications. Increasing the incident ultrasonic frequency immensely amplifies the power of the reflected echoes. Thus raising the transducer frequency from 3 MHz to 4 MHz leads to fivefold augmentation of the scattered echo intensity. Ironically, this increase also limits the ability of the transducer to sample deep-lying circulations, as a higher frequency leads to greater attenuation. Obviously, one must balance these contrary effects when selecting the optimal frequency for a specific application. For example, for most fetal Doppler insonations via the maternal abdomen, transducers with a frequency range of 2–4 MHz are commonly used to reach the deep-lying vascular targets in the fetus. In contrast, with a transvaginal approach, where the transducer lies in close proximity to pelvic structures, such as the uterine or ovarian arteries, the use of a higher frequency (e.g., 5 MHz) increases the Doppler sensitivity without significant attenuation of the beam.

When a propagating ultrasonic wave encounters an acoustic interface, reflection occurs. Scattering takes place when the size of the interface is smaller than the incident sound wavelength. Such an interface is known as a *point target*. In regard to Doppler shift, the scatterer is significantly smaller than the wavelength and is in motion. The Doppler-shifted ultrasound reflecting from such a moving scatter propagates in all directions (Fig. 2.13). Obviously, it also reaches any receiving transducer at the source of transmission. The process of scattered ultrasound returning to the source-receiver is called *backscattering*.

It is well accepted that the primary sources of scattering in blood are the circulating RBCs [10]. These cells are so numerous that the contribution of the other formed elements of blood, such as white blood cells and platelets, to scattering ultrasound is inconsequential. An RBC has a biconcave discoid shape with a mean diameter of 7.2 µm and a mean thickness of 2.2 µm. In comparison, the wavelength of Doppler ultrasound for diagnostic applications varies from 1540 µm to 154 µm, corresponding to 1–10 MHz transducer frequency. As is apparent, the RBCs are several magnitudes smaller than the wavelengths, so they can be regarded as point targets. In reality, however, circulating erythrocytes do not act as discrete scatterers but as volumes of randomly distributed point targets. The number of RBCs in such a scattering volume fluctuates around a mean value and causes fluctuations in the scattering power. Turbulent blood flow increases fluctuations in the RBC concentration and is therefore associated with increases in the scattering power and consequently the power of the Doppler shift signal [10]. In regard to whole blood, it has been experimentally demonstrated that

the scattering power becomes maximum at a hematocrit range of 25%–30% [10]. At higher hematocrit values, the scattering behavior of blood becomes more complex as the RBCs become too crowded and can no longer be treated as randomly distributed scatterers.

In addition to hematocrit, scattering is also affected by the state of red cell aggregation. Spatial variations in the flow field can result in changes in the variance of red cell packing and backscattering cross section which will influence the Doppler power at a given frequency [11]. In this circumstance, the mean Doppler frequency will not necessarily be proportional to the mean flow through the sample volume and may affect volumetric flow quantification and the power mode display of color Doppler. Scattering is also dependent on certain characteristics of the transmitted ultrasound including the frequency and the angle of insonation [12]. The phenomenon is a complex subject and a comprehensive review is beyond the scope of this chapter.

Magnitude of Doppler Shift

Relative velocities of the sound and the scatterers are important determinants of the magnitude of the Doppler frequency shift. In regard to blood flow, the speed of RBCs is significantly less than the speed of sound in a biologic medium. Consequently, the Doppler shift is much smaller than the incident ultrasonic frequency. Assuming a sound propagation speed of 1,540 m/s in soft tissues, the Doppler shift for a given blood flow speed and the transducer frequency can be calculated from the Doppler equation. This exercise is illustrated in Table 2.2, which lists the Doppler frequency shifts for most obstetric transducer frequencies (2–7 MHz) at blood flow speeds of 25, 50, and 75 cm/s. As is evident, the frequency shifts are approximately 1/1,000 their corresponding transducer frequencies. Furthermore, the Doppler shifted sound

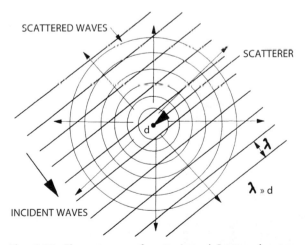

Fig. 2.13. Phenomenon of scattering. *d* Scatter, λ wavelength of the incident beam. The *large arrow* shows the direction of propagation of the incident ultrasound. The *smaller arrows* radiating from *d* indicate the directions of scattering. Note that scattering occurs when the wavelength is much greater than the size of the reflector ($\lambda \gg d$)

Table 2.2. Doppler frequency shifts for various transducer frequencies at three blood flow velocities and an insonation angle of 0°

Transducer frequency (MHz)	Doppler shift at three flow velocities (KHz)		
	at 25 cm/s	at 50 cm/s	at 75 cm/s
2	1.3	0.7	1.9
3	1.9	1.0	2.9
4	2.6	1.3	3.9
5	3.2	1.6	4.9
6	3.9	1.9	5.8
7	4.6	2.3	6.8

Labels in figure: SCATTERED WAVES, SCATTERER, INCIDENT WAVES, $\lambda \gg d$, d

is well within the limits of human hearing as its frequency is in the kilohertz range.

Angle Dependence of Doppler Shift

It is evident from the Doppler equation that the greatest frequency shift occurs when the transmitted ultrasound beam is parallel to the flow axis; and when the beam intersects the vessel, it is the component or the vector of the RBC velocity along the beam path that contributes to the Doppler effect. This vector is determined from the cosine of the beam-vessel angle and is incorporated into the Doppler equation (see above). As the angle increases, the frequency shift proportionately decreases. When the angle exceeds 60°, the fall in the Doppler shifted frequency exceeds 50%. When the angle reaches 90°, the Doppler shift is virtually nonexistent. However, minimal Doppler signals may still be generated because of beam divergence and nonuniform flow in the vessel.

As the angle of insonation decreases, the frequency shift increases; and maximum Doppler shift is obtained, at least in theory, when the angle becomes zero with the ultrasound beam being parallel to the flow axis. In reality, however, as the angle drops below 30°, significant reflection of the incident beam

occurs at the interface between blood and the vessel wall, and the Doppler sensitivity becomes seriously compromised. Thus the lower limit of the angle for desirable Doppler interrogation is 30°. In contrast to general vascular applications, the phenomenon of loss of sensitivity with a low angle is not observed in cardiac Doppler insonations. With fetal and postnatal Doppler echocardiography, optimal Doppler waveforms are obtained when the incident beam is aligned with the vessel axis in pulmonic or aortic outflow tracts. Apparently, complex cardiac anatomy does not reflect the incident beam the same way as do peripheral vessel walls.

As is apparent from the Doppler equation, the estimation of blood flow speed from the Doppler shift requires a reliable measurement of the angle of insonation. Although the Doppler shift is angle-dependent, flow speed calculated from the Doppler shift is not affected, in theory, by the magnitude of the angle. This situation, however, assumes ideal circumstances – such as insonation of a uniform flow in a straight vessel of uniform diameter – which one does not encounter often in reality. Therefore the desirable angle range for flow speed estimation remains, as indicated above, 30°–60°. Measurement of the angle in a duplex Doppler device is usually accomplished with apparent ease. The operator uses the two-dimensional image to

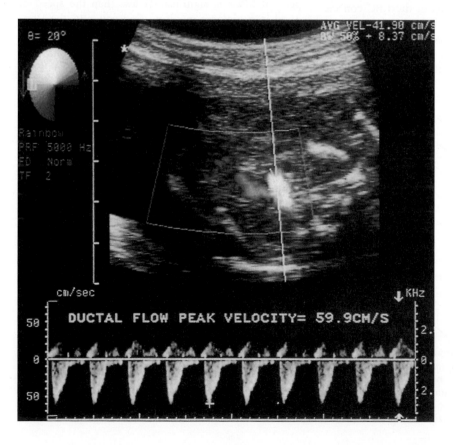

Fig. 2.14. Duplex Doppler interrogation. *Top*: Two-dimensional Doppler flow image of the fetal ductus arteriosus. The *oblique vertical line* is the cursor representing the beam path. The Doppler sample volume (*two short horizontal lines*) is placed at the ductal site, which shows high-speed blood flow. The *small oblique line* at the sample volume is the angle indicator. *Bottom*: Angle-corrected Doppler shifts from the ductus. The *right margin* of the panel shows the frequency scale in kilohertz. The *left margin* of the panel shows the blood flow velocity scale in centimeters per second

align an angle indicator cursor with the vessel axis (the presumed flow axis) and determines the angle it incurs with the beam path indicator cursor (Fig. 2.14). The device computes this angle and produces the velocity information in real time. The procedure is subjective, and the precision of the measurement obviously depends on operator skill.

Determination of the flow velocity may be clinically useful during fetal echocardiographic examination, as abnormal flow velocities in the pulmonary artery, aorta, or ductus arteriosus may assist in identifying structural or functional abnormalities. A reliable measurement of the Doppler angle is also a requirement for measuring volumetric blood flow and inaccuracies in measuring the angle can introduce significant errors in this measurement. Finally, an optimal angle is important for an appropriate interpretation of Doppler waveforms from the arteries that demonstrate continuing forward flow during the end-diastolic phase, as a large angle may artificially reduce the magnitude of the end-diastolic frequency shift. This point is of critical importance when assessing an umbilical arterial circulation in which a reduced or absent end-diastolic frequency shift may indicate fetal jeopardy. The challenge of the angle of insonation in Doppler sonography has prompted significant research on the development of angle-independent ultrasound technology for circulatory investigations; this is further discussed in Chap. 4.

References

1. Wells PT (1977) Biomedical ultrasonics. Academic Press, Orlando, FL
2. McDicken WN (1981) Diagnostic ultrasonics: ultrasonic in tissue. In: Principles and use of instruments (2nd ed). Wiley, New York, pp 54–70
3. Evans DH, McDicken WN, Skidmore R, Woodcock JP (1989) Doppler ultrasound: physics, instrumentation and clinical applications. Wiley, New York
4. Kremkau FW (1990) Doppler ultrasound: principles and instruments. Saunders, Philadelphia
5. Goss SA, Johnston RL, Dunn F (1978) Comprehensive compilation of empirical ultrasonic properties of mammalian tissues. J Acoust Soc Am 64:423–457
6. Atkinson P, Woodcock JP (1982) Doppler ultrasound. Academic Press, London
7. Lord Rayleigh (1871) Scientific papers 8 and 9. Philos Mag 41:107, 274, 447
8. Van de Hulst HC (1982) Light scattering by small particles. Dover, New York
9. Van de Hulst HC (1952) Scattering in the atmospheres of the earth and planets. In: Kuiper GP (ed) The atmospheres of the earth and planets. University of Chicago Press, Chicago
10. Shung KK, Sigelman RA, Reid JM (1976) Scattering of ultrasound by blood. IEEE Trans Biomed Eng BME-23:460–467
11. Bascom PA, Cobbold RS (1996) Origin of the Doppler ultrasound spectrum from blood. IEEE Trans Biomed Eng 43:562–571
12. Fontaine I, Cloutier G (2003) Modeling the frequency dependence (5–120 MHz) of ultrasound backscattering by red cell aggregates in shear flow at a normal hematocrit. J Acoust Soc Am 113:2893–2900

Chapter 3

Spectral Doppler:
Basic Principles and Instrumentation

Dev Maulik

Spectral Doppler ultrasound velocimetry involves systematic analysis of the spectrum of frequencies that constitute the Doppler signal. This chapter presents a general perspective on Doppler signal anlyses and describes the spectral Doppler ultrasound devices commercially available for clinical use. They include continuous-wave (CW) Doppler, pulsed-wave (PW) Doppler, and duplex Doppler devices. Within the realm of obstetric usage, the application needs are diverse and require various choices of equipment. For example, fetal Doppler echocardiography requires advanced duplex ultrasound instrumentation, which combines the capabilities of high-resolution two-dimensional imaging with the PW Doppler mode and an acoustic power output appropriate for fetal application. For umbilical arterial hemodynamic assessment, simpler, substantially less expensive CW Doppler equipment with a spectral analyzer may be sufficient. It is essential therefore that one develop a basic understanding of the implementation of Doppler ultrasound technology.

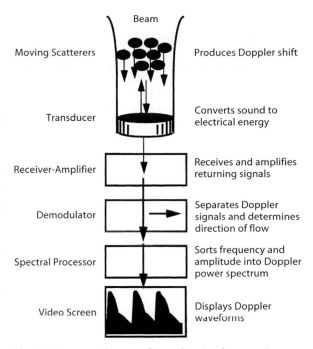

Fig. 3.1. Sequential steps of Doppler signal processing

Doppler Signal Processing

As discussed in Chap. 2, the Doppler frequency shift signal represents the summation of multiple Doppler frequency shifts backscattered by millions of red blood cells (RBCs). The RBCs travel at different speeds, and the number of cells traveling at these speeds varies as well. As the speed of the scatterers determines the magnitude of the frequency shift and the quantity of the amplitude, the Doppler signal is composed of a range of frequencies with varying amplitude content. Moreover, the total received Doppler signal contains low-frequency and high-amplitude signals generated by tissue movements and high-frequency noise generated by the instrumentation. Obviously, systematic processing is necessary before the Doppler shifted frequencies can be used clinically. The Doppler signal is processed in sequential steps (Fig. 3.1), consisting of reception and amplification, demodulation and determination of directionality of flow, and spectral processing.

Reception-Amplification

The returning signals are first received and amplified by a radiofrequency (RF) receiving device. Amplification is necessary, as the Doppler frequency shift generates weak electrical voltage at the receiving transducer.

Demodulation

The total received and amplified echoes contain not only the Doppler-shifted frequencies but also the carrier frequency, which is the frequency of the incident beam. During the next step, the Doppler-shifted frequencies are extracted from the carrier frequency. This process is known as *demodulation*. There are various methods of demodulation [1], among which the coherent phase quadrature procedure is commonly employed. Phase quadrature implies that one signal is one-fourth of a cycle out of phase or delayed compared to the other. With this technique the incoming signals are mixed with the direct and the one-fourth of a cycle (90°) phase-shifted reference electrical signals. With coherent demodulation, the reference signal is supplied by the master oscillator, which is a voltage generator whose primary function is to produce the driving frequency for the source transducer. Demodulation results in generation of a direct and a quadrature output. When the flow is toward the transducer, the direct signal lags the quadrature signal by one-fourth of a cycle. When the flow is away from the transducer, the direct signal leads the quadrature signal by one-fourth of a cycle.

Direction Discrimination

The resulting directional separation of the flow, however, is not complete and requires additional processing. The latter is achieved by frequency domain processing in which the demodulator outputs are mixed with the direct and quadrature (phase shifted by one-fourth of a cycle) outputs of a voltage generator. The resultant single-channel output separates the forward and reverse flow signals. With the pilot frequency of the quadrature oscillator providing the baseline, or zero frequency, the flow toward the transducer is presented as the positive Doppler shift and the flow away as the negative Doppler shift. The next step is comprised of removing the undesirable frequency components from the demodulated Doppler signal by digital filtration.

High-Pass and Low-Pass Filters

The total signal input of a Doppler system is comprised of not only Doppler frequency shift signals from the target vessel but also low-frequency/high-amplitude signals originating from moving adjacent structures such as vessel walls and cardiac valves. It also contains high-frequency noise contributions from within the instrumentation. Obviously the frequencies from the extraneous sources represent error components of the total signal, and their reduction or elimination improves the signal quality. Electronic digital filters are used to accomplish this objective. By and large, two types of filter are used: a high-pass filter and a low-pass filter.

The purpose of a high-pass filtering system is to eliminate the extrinsic low-frequency components of Doppler signals, which arise predominantly from the vessel walls or other adjacent slow-moving structures (Fig. 3.2). For peripheral vascular applications this type of processing often improves the signal quality. Such low-frequency signals may also originate from the slow-moving boundary layer of blood flow adjoining the vascular wall. Moreover, with low-impedance circulations where forward flow continues through the end of the diastolic phase, the important end-dia-

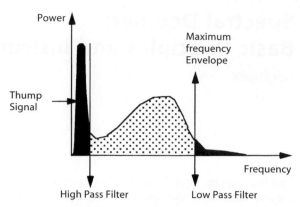

Fig. 3.2. Doppler amplitude-frequency (power) spectrum illustrating the concept of high- and low-pass filtering. *Vertical axis* represents the amplitude or the power of the spectrum. *Horizontal axis* represents the frequency scale. The *left dark area* of the spectrum indicates signals arising from slow-moving tissue structures such as the vessel wall (thump signal). The *right dark area* shows high-frequency noise in the spectrum. The *vertical downward arrows* indicate the frequency cutoff levels of the high- and low-pass filters

stolic velocity information is lost, which may lead to the erroneous inference of compromised or absent end-diastolic velocity. The importance of this situation can be appreciated from the fact that absent or reverse end-diastolic flow is associated with high perinatal mortality and morbidity. Obviously, for most fetal applications the high-pass filter should be either turned off or kept at the lowest setting, preferably at 50 Hz and not exceeding 100 Hz. With most Doppler instruments the high-pass filter is adjustable.

A low-pass filter allows frequencies only below a certain threshold to pass, thereby removing any frequencies higher than that level (Fig. 2). This threshold is set higher than the maximum frequency shifts expected in a circulation. Such low-pass filters, in general, improve the signal-to-noise ratio. However, if the low-pass filter is set at an inappropriately low level, it may eliminate valuable high-frequency information from a high-velocity circulation, which in turn leads to underestimation of the maximum and mean frequency shifts.

Doppler Spectral Analysis

The steps described above generate demodulated and filtered Doppler frequency shift signals displayed as a complex, uninterpretable waveform consisting of variations of amplitude over time (Fig. 3.3). Spectral analysis converts this waveform to an orderly array of constituent frequencies and corresponding amplitudes of the signal. The amplitude approximately represents the

Fig. 3.3. Demodulated Doppler signal prior to spectral processing. The signal was derived from the umbilical arteries

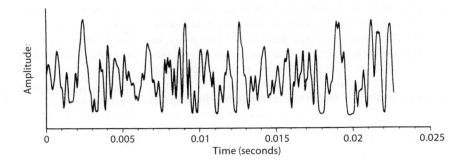

number of scatterers traveling at a given speed and is known as the *power of the spectrum*. A full spectral processing that provides comprehensive information on both the frequency and its average power content is called the *power-spectrum analysis*. As circulation is a pulsatile phenomenon, the speed of flow varies with time, as does the Doppler frequency shift generated by the flow. Spectral processing must therefore estimate temporal changes in the Doppler power spectrum.

Of the various approaches for spectral processing, Fourier analysis and autoregression techniques are commonly used at present. The Fourier-based approaches are usually used for Doppler spectral analysis, whereas autoregression techniques are usually employed for two-dimensional Doppler flow mapping.

Fourier Transform Spectral Analysis

Fourier transform is a powerful mathematic technique for spectral analysis of constantly repeating cyclic phenomena, such as alternating electrical current, sound waves, or electromagnetic waves. Baron Jean Baptiste Joseph Fourier, a French mathematician of the Napoleonic era, first described this approach in 1807. The process breaks down a complex periodic signal or waveform into its constituent frequencies of specific amplitudes and phases (Fig. 3.4). The spectrum of a periodic signal, such as that obtained from Doppler insonation, consists not of discrete values but of a continuous function distributed over the range of the constituent frequencies. For practical implementation, however, samples are drawn so a finite, or discrete, series of frequency points are chosen for analysis. It is called the *discrete* Fourier transform. The *fast* Fourier transform (FFT) is a computer programming sequence for rapid digital implementation of the discrete Fourier transform [2]. FFT processing significantly reduces computational need and is a highly effective tool for power spectral analysis of the Doppler signal [3, 4]. FFT-based Doppler analysis has been used extensively for assessing various circulatory system, including the carotid [5] and umbilical

Fig. 3.4. Principle of Fourier transform analysis. The complex flow waveform (*A*) is transformed into its constituent since waves of different frequencies and phases (*a1, a2, a3, a4, a5*). *Vertical axis* shows the flow magnitude, and *horizontal axis* shows time. The process converts a time domain phenomenon into a frequency domain phenomenon

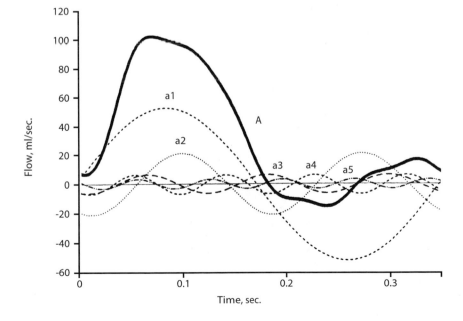

arterial [6] hemodynamics; and it is the current industry standard for Doppler ultrasound devices used for medical diagnostic applications. The number of discrete frequency components usually analyzed varies between 64 and 512. Maulik et al. described a 256-point FFT analysis for umbilical arterial velocimetry yielding a frequency resolution of 31.25 Hz (1.23 cm/s) [7]. For most perinatal applications, a 64-point FFT analysis is adequate. The initial step involves sampling the demodulated signal at given intervals and then digitizing the sampled signals, converting them to numeric values. It is achieved by an analog-to-digital converter. For the next step, the digitized data are processed by the FFT processor, which determines the power spectrum of the sample. Each spectrum is computed over a time window, and a number of consecutive overlapping time windows are averaged to prevent spectral loss. This procedure, regrettably, also compromises the spectral resolution. It should be appreciated that the FFT-derived power spectrum is an approximation of the true spectrum, is relatively noisy, and demonstrates a considerable amount of variance. The latter can be reduced to some extent by various windowing and averaging techniques. Figure 3.5 shows a three-dimensional display of the Doppler power spectrum from the umbilical artery generated by FFT processing.

Limitations of FFT Spectral Analysis

There are basic limitations of the FFT approach for spectral processing of the Doppler signal. They include spectral variance and intrinsic spectral broadening.

Spectral Variance

The Doppler frequency spectrum from an arterial circulation varies with the changing hemodynamics of the cardiac cycle. Therefore the duration of the Doppler signal sample for FFT analysis during which the flow condition, and therefore the power spectrum, can be considered unchanging is limited. For an arterial circulation it is usually 10–20 ms. In the fetus the assumption of the spectral nonvariance may be valid for only 5 ms because the faster fetal heart rate pro-

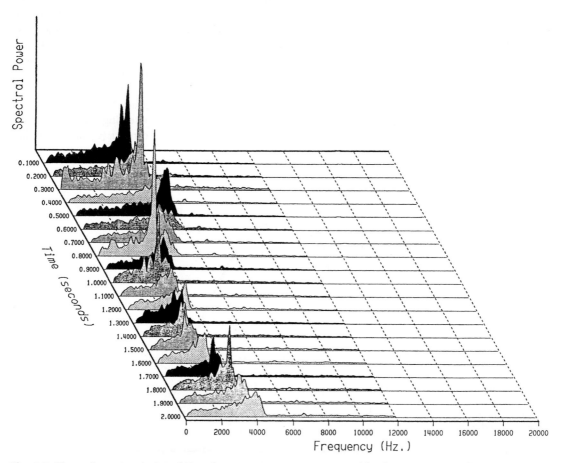

Fig. 3.5. Three-dimensional plot of Doppler power spectrum generated by fast Fourier transform analysis. The spectrum was obtained from the umbilical circulation

duces faster temporal changes in the blood flow speed and in the power spectral density. A shorter temporal length of the sample ensures spectral nonvariance. However, the shorter the duration of the Doppler data segment, the worse is the frequency resolution. A signal segment of 5 ms gives a resolution of only 200 Hz, whereas increasing the duration to 20 ms improves the resolution to 50 Hz. Prolonging the duration, however, introduces uncertainty regarding the constancy of the power spectrum density. Under this circumstance, FFT processing does not function reliably, as it is based implicitly on the assumption of spectral constancy for the duration of the sample.

Intrinsic Spectral Broadening

When a single scatterer moves at a constant speed across an ultrasound beam of limited width, the resultant Doppler spectrum has a range of frequencies instead of a single frequency. Because the phenomenon of broadening the Doppler spectrum is caused by the inherent properties of the measurement system, it is known as *intrinsic spectral broadening* (also *transit time broadening*). Spectral broadening mostly encompasses the following phenomena: (1) transit time broadening caused by the inhomogeneity of the ultrasound field causing amplitude fluctuations of the returning echo; this produces a range of frequencies distributed around the centroid Doppler shift frequency; (2) geometric broadening which results from the changing angles of insonation incurred by the scatterer as it moves across the beam; (3) nonstationery broadening caused by the changes in velocity during the sampling time; and (4) velocity gradient broadening originating from the changes in velocity within the sampling volume [8]. The problem of spectral broadening is compounded by the contribution from multiple moving RBCs traversing the ultrasound beam. The RBCs do not act as discrete scatterers but as volumes of randomly distributed scatterers. The number of RBCs in such a scattering volume in an ultrasonic field varies continually and randomly around a mean value, which causes swings in the scattering power. The consequences are similar to the spectral broadening of the Doppler signal observed with a single moving scatterer.

Spectral broadening is affected by the beam width, pulse length, and angle of insonation. Wider and more homogeneous beams, longer pulses, and smaller angles of insonation narrow the spectral spread. Obviously, the situation is worse with the short-gate pulsed Doppler ultrasound applications, where a scatterer can traverse only a part of the beam of a transmitted short pulse. The consequent transit time broadening effect generates a significant degree of ambiguity regarding the true distribution of velocity

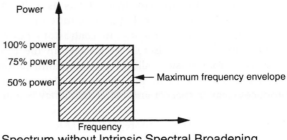

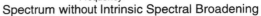

Spectrum without Intrinsic Spectral Broadening

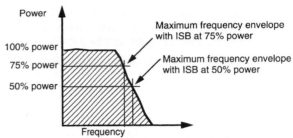

Spectrum with Intrinsic Spectral Broadening

Fig. 3.6. Amplitude-frequency spectrum from a circulation with a parabolic flow velocity profile. *Top*: Ideal spectrum with an even distribution of amplitudes (scattering power) at various frequencies, indicating erythrocytes traveling at various speeds. *Bottom*: Effect of spectral broadening on the maximum frequency defintion of the same spectrum. *ISB* intrinsic spectral broadening

in the sample volume. The main clinical significance of spectral broadening is that it potentially compromises the prercision of the maximum frequency shift envelope (Fig. 3.6). The mean frequency definition, however, is not affected, as the distribution of the frequencies around the mean shift is symmetric.

Analog Fourier Spectral Analysis

Analog fourier spectral analysis allows fast spectral processing of the Doppler signals utilizing analog techniques as opposed to the digital approach of FFT. One such implementation, known as Chirp Z analysis, is also a discrete Fourier transform-based method and requires less computing power and offers a wide dynamic signal processing range.

Autoregression Analysis

Although Fourier-based methods dominate, alternative approaches for Doppler spectral processing are available. These methods are theoretically capable of eliminating many of the inherent disadvantages of the FFT method. Kay and Marple comprehensively described the autoregressive approach for spectral analysis [9]. Such procedures have been widely used for spectral analysis of speech and other periodic phenomena. The autoregression method acts as a digital filter and assumes the signal at a given time to be the sum of the previous samples. In contrast to power quantification of the discrete frequencies in the FFT analysis, autoregression allows power quantification of all the frequencies of the spectrum. Moreover, it produces cleaner spectra and better frequency resolution than those generated by FFT processing.

We have evaluated autoregressive (AR), moving average (MA), and autoregressive moving average (ARMA)-based spectral processing approaches as possible alternatives to the FFT analysis [10]. Compared to the FFT processing, these parametric techniques produce cleaner spectra. The AR model estimates maximum frequency well, and the MA model indicates velocities at which most scatterers (erythrocytes) travel. The ARMA shows the potential of producing superior spectral analysis by combining the advantages of the AR and MA models. These parametric methods depend on appropriate system identification of the data.

Continuous-Wave Doppler Ultrasonography

A continuous-wave (CW) Doppler transducer continuously transmits and receives ultrasonic signals. A CW Doppler system essentially consists of a double element transducer for both emitting and receiving signals, a radiofrequency receiver amplifier for the acquisition and amplification of the electrical voltage signals from the receiving transducer, a voltage generator that provices the driving frequency of the emitting transducer and the reference frequency for the demodulator, a demodulator that extracts the Doppler shifted frequencies from the total echo signals, and a direction detector that completely separates the signals of the forward flow from those of the backward flow. Details of these components of Doppler signal analyses and subsequent spectral processing are described at the outset of this chapter. The transducer assembly encases two piezoelectric elements; one continuously emits ultrasound and the other continuously receives the backscattered echoes (Fig. 3.7). For most transducers, the emitting and receiving elements are either rectangular or half-circle in shape. There may also be a concentric arrangement with a central circular element surrounded by a ring element. The elements are positioned in such a manner that their faces sustain a suitable angle to each other, and consequently there is an overlap between the transmitted ultrasound field generated by the emitting element and the sensitive zone for the receiving element.

A CW Doppler setup does not have range discrimination, and any movement within the sensitive re-

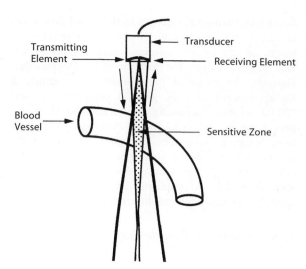

Fig. 3.7. Continuous-wave Doppler transducer

gion causes backscattering and consequently Doppler shift of the incident beam. If the beam interrogates more than one vessel, the Doppler signals from all the vessels merge to form a composite display. The only discrimination that exists is that the signals from a deep location are more attenuated because of the longer transmission path through tissues. A CW system is sensitive also to the movements of nonhemodynamic objects in its path, such as pulsating vascular walls or moving cardiac structures. These sources of Doppler shift produce high-amplitude/low-frequency signals, which may overwhelm a receiver–amplifier of limited dynamic range. This situation leads to loss of important hemodynamic signals. The problem can be resolved by ensuring an extended dynamic range of the receiver and by use of an appropriate high-pass filter, as described above.

Continuous-wave Doppler ultrasound instruments are used extensively in obstetrics for nonvelocimetric applications, such as fetal heart rate detection and external electronic fetal heart rate monitoring. For velocimetric applications, CW devices with a spectral analyzer are used for insonation of the umbilical arteries and often the uterine arteries. Despite the inherent absence of range discrimination, Doppler signals from the umbilical or uterine arteries can be obtained with relative ease. Moreover, the equipment is substantially less expensive than the duplex pulsed Doppler devices and requires less expertise to operate. However, CW Doppler instruments are infrequently used at present for fetal surveillance.

Pulsed-Wave Doppler Ultrasonography

With the PW Doppler setup, a single transducer crystal emits pulses of short bursts of ultrasound energy (Fig. 3.8). Between the pulses the same crystal acts as the receiving transducer. As the velocity of sound in soft tissues is virtually constant, the time interval between transmission and reception of the ultrasound beam determines the distance, or range, of the target area from the transducer. Thus the location of the target area can be selected by varying this time delay. This process is known as *range gating*.

A simplified description of the pulsed Doppler ultrasound system is presented: As mentioned above, the same transducer crystal acts as both the transmitter and the receiver of ultrasound signals. A master oscillator generates a reference signal at the resonant frequency of the transducer. An electronic gate controls the transmission of the signal to the transducer, so a pulse of only a few cycles reaches it. The rate at which the pulses are generated (pulse repetition frequency) is determined by an electronic device called the pulse repetition frequency generator. The generator also controls the delay gate, which in turn controls the range gate and therefore the time interval between the ultrasonic transmission and reception. As described above, a demodulating system extracts the Doppler frequency shifts from the carrier frequency. The Doppler signals thus produced are stored, integrated, and updated with the signals from the next pulse. After appropriate filtering, the signals are now ready for audio output and spectral analysis. A more complete review of the pulsed Doppler system has been presented by Evans and associates [1].

Doppler Sample Volume

The three-dimensional region in the path of the transmitted ultrasound beam from which the frequency shift signals are obtained is called the Doppler *sample volume* (DSV). For the CW Doppler system, the totality of the superimposed region represents the DSV and is therefore of no relevance. For the PW Doppler system, the range-gated zone from which the backscattered echoes are received constitutes the sample volume. The DSV is an important consideration for PW Doppler applications because its location and axial dimension can be controlled by the examiner. The examiner therefore has the ability to interrogate a target area of appropriate location and size and to obtain more precise spatial velocity information. This subject is discussed further below.

The length of the DSV along the ultrasonic beam axis is known as its axial dimension. The lateral measurable limits of the beam, perpendicular to the beam axis, define its transverse dimension, or width. The shape resembles a pear or a teardrop (Fig. 3.9). The axial dimension is determined by the pulse length or duration as sensed by the receiving transducer and is therefore dependent on the duration of the transmitted ultrasonic pulse and the time window during which the receiver gate is open. As the last two factors are amenable to controlled variations, the axial dimension of the DSV can be altered by the operator. Many current duplex systems allow sample length variations, from 1.5 to 25.0 mm.

The transverse dimension of the DSV is determined by the ultrasonic beam width, which approximates the diameter of the transducer face in the near field. In the

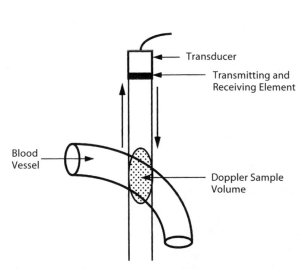

Fig. 3.8. Pulsed-wave Doppler transducer

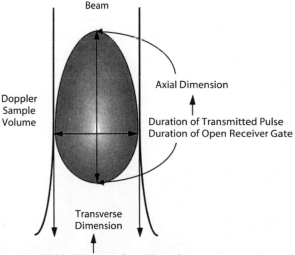

Fig. 3.9. Doppler sample volume and the factors controlling its dimensions

far field the beam progressively diverges. In this circumstance, the angle of beam divergence, which depends on the wavelength and the transducer radius, dictates the transverse dimension of the DSV. Obviously, the width of the DSV is better defined in the near field than in the far field. Consequently, operating in the near field ensures greater certainty of velocity assessment. In contrast to the sample length, the sample width is not amenable to ready manipulation. However, owing to progress in transducer technology, including acoustic focusing, a few instruments allow controlled variations of the beam width in the far field and therefore of the transverse dimension of the DSV.

The dimensions of the sample volume can significantly affect the accuracy of velocity assessment. A sample volume that is large in relation to the dimensions of the target vessel can significantly compromise the range resolution of the measured velocities and lower the signal-to-noise ratio [11]. Conversely, a sample size smaller than the vascular dimension can diminish the sensitivity of the system. Moreover, depending on its relative size and location in the lumen of a large vessel, the assessed velocity profile can be significantly distorted. This subject is further discussed in Chap. 4.

Artifacts of Spectral Doppler Sonography

Limitations of Fourier-based spectral analysis have been described in a previous section of this chapter. There are additional device-dependent false representations of the Doppler information that may compromise interpretive clarity. These artifacts are discussed herein.

Nyquist Limit

A major problem of the PW Doppler system is its inherent limitation in accurately representing Doppler shifts from circulations with high-speed flow. A PW Doppler is essentially a sampling tool for a cyclic phenomenon. The sampling rate is the pulse repetition frequency of the Doppler system; the cyclic phenomenon is the Doppler shift frequencies generated by blood flow. The relation between the pulse repetition frequency and appropriate measurement of the maximum frequency shift is dictated by Shannon's theorem on sampling, which states that for unambiguous measurement of a periodic phenomenon the maximum frequency must not exceed half the sampling rate [12], which amounts to a minimum of two samples per cycle of the highest frequency. This maximum frequency threshold is known as the *Nyquist frequency* or *Nyquist limit*. The relation is expressed in the following equation:

$$f_{max} = f_{pr}/2$$

where f_{max} is the maximum frequency measurable without ambiguity (Nyquist limit), and f_{pr} is the sampling rate or the pulse repetition frequency.

Ambiguity in frequency resolution occurs when the PW Doppler beam interrogates a vessel with such a high blood flow velocity that the maximum frequency content of the Doppler signal exceeds the Nyquist limit. In this circumstance, the frequency cannot be estimated precisely. The frequency component in excess of the limit is subtracted from the Nyquist frequency and is negatively expressed (Fig. 3.10). This phenomenon is known as the *Nyquist effect*. It is also

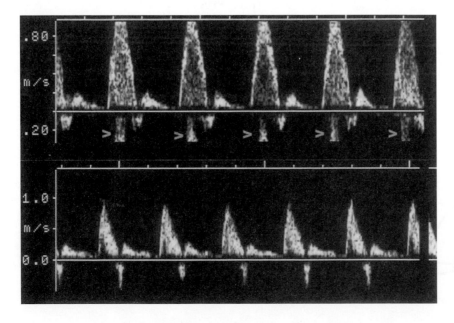

Fig. 3.10. Example of aliasing and its correction. *Top* Aliased waveforms. Note the abrupt termination of the peak portion of the waveforms and the display of these peaks in the *lower part* of the panel below the baseline (*horizontal arowheads*). *Bottom*: Correction of aliasing of the waveforms by increased pulse repetition frequency

known as *aliasing*, as it produces a representation of the frequency shift that is false in terms of magnitude and direction.

Aliasing does not pose a problem with most fetal PW Doppler measurements, particularly those involving the umbilical and cerebral circulations. However, the phenomenon may be observed when a high-velocity flow is encountered in fetal intracardiac and aortic circulations.

Implications of Aliasing

Aliasing distorts the spectral display with an abrupt discontinuity at the Nyquist limit. The aliased part of the signal is displaced into the opposite frequency range of the display (Fig. 3.10). Such distortion also affects the audio output of the Doppler signal. The problem can be corrected in a number of ways.

1. The Nyquist limit can be raised by increasing the pulse repetition frequency, thereby resolving aliasing. However, this measure may introduce range ambiguity, as the Doppler signals from varying depths may be received at the same time.

2. Shifting the baseline resolves the problem by increasing the positive frequency range and decreasing the negative frequency range in the display. It effectively extends the maximum velocity limit, and the spectra are displayed in the same direction without ambiguity.

3. As the operating frequency of the transducer is directly proportional to the magnitude of the Doppler shift, reducing the former may lower the maximum frequency enough for the elimination of aliasing without changing the sampling rate.

4. Increasing the angle of insonation between the Doppler beam and the flow axis reduces the maximum Doppler shift, which may eliminate aliasing.

If these measures are inadequate for resolving aliasing, one may use a CW Doppler setup, which is not limited by the Nyquist frequency and does not produce aliasing, although rane resolution is lost with this approach.

Range-Velocity Resolution

The maximum range, or depth, at which the velocity of blood flow can be measured accurately by a PW Doppler system is limited. As the distance on the target from the transducer increases, more total time is required for a transmitted ultrasound pulse to travel to the target and the backscattered echo to return to the source. The device must wait this period of time before transmitting the next pulse. If more than one pulse propagates in the target at the same time, the PW Doppler system is incapable of determining the

spatial origins of the different returning echoes, resulting in range ambiguity. To avoid this problem, the interpulse interval must be increased with the greater depth of the target vessels. Obviously, the maximum depth at which PW Doppler measurement can be performed without range confusion is limited by the interpulse interval. This relation is shown in the following equation:

$$D_{max} = c \cdot T_p/2$$

where D_{max} indicates the maximum depth of the target vessel, c is the velocity of sound in soft tissue, and T_p is the interpulse interval. As the pulse repetition frequency (f_{pr}) is the reciprocal of the interpulse interval, the equation can be expressed as:

$$D_{max} = c/2f_{pr}$$

The pulse repetition frequency also determines the maximum allowable Doppler frequency shift and therefore the blood flow velocity that can be measured without producing aliasing. It follows therefore that the deeper the PW Doppler sampling location, the lower the maximum measurable velocity.

For the above consideration, it has been assumed that the frequency of the transmitted ultrasound is fixed. However, another variable comes into play when the ultrasound frequency can be changed. The lower the ultrasonic frequency, the lower the attenuation and the greater the maximum depth at which the Doppler measurement can be made. Given a maximum sampling depth, an upper limit is established for the pulse repetition frequency and correspondingly for the Nyquist frequency. It follows therefore that for a given sampling depth and pulse repetition frequency, higher flow velocities can be measured using lower transmitted frequencies. For most obstetric applications, a transducer frequency of 3–4 MHz provides the best Doppler output.

It is interesting to consider the CW Doppler operation as a special case of the pulsed mode, where the pulses are transmitted at an exceedingly high speed, theoretically, at an infinite pulse repetition frequency. Obviously, no range information is available for the received pulses, as it becomes impossible to relate a given reflection to any particular pulse. However, because of the theoretically infinite pulse repetition frequency, the Nyquist limit for the Doppler frequency shift is also infinite. With the DW Doppler system, then, there are no limits on the maximum measurable velocity.

Mirror Imaging

With the artifact of mirror imaging a Doppler device falsely represents unidirectional flow as bidirectional flow. The artifactual flow is depicted as a mirror image of the true flow on the opposite side of the baseline (Fig. 3.11). The problem afflicts both CW and PW Doppler systems and is caused by leakage of the Doppler signal from one directional quadrature channel to the other (quadrature channel cross-talk), so the signals are duplicated. Although there is directional ambiguity, there is no subtraction and relocation of Doppler spectral information as encountered with the Nyquist effect. Quadrature cross-talk can occur with high-velocity flows, excessive gain setting, preponderance of high-amplitude Doppler signals, and paradoxically also with low-velocity flows.

The mirror imaging artifact may be eliminated by decreasing the gain, which reduces the quadrature cross-talk. Increasing the high-pass filter may also improve the problem by removing the high-amplitude/low-frequency signals and decreasing the signal leakage in the quadrature channels. Increasing the angle of insonation may also effectively prevent quadrature leakage while interrogating high-speed circulations. Finally, prior knowledge of the target circulation should prevent erroneous interpretation of the Doppler tracing.

False depiction of a unidirectional flow as bidirectional due to system limitation should be distinguished from the situation where the Doppler beam insonates a true bidirectional flow system and consequently the Doppler waveforms appear on both sides of the baseline. For example, a Doppler beam with a sufficiently long sample volume interrogating the umbilical cord may encounter flows in the adjacent loops of the umbilical arteries in opposite directions relative to the transducer, and the Doppler waveform is correctly depicted on either side of the baseline. Similar nonartifactual mirror imaging may also occur when a focused pulsed Doppler beam intersects the flow axis at a right angle, and the same unidirectional flow is toward the transducer in one part of the beam and away from the transducer in the other part. The Doppler tracing in this situation is correctly bidirectional in relation to the transducer and is depicted as such.

Duplex System

Principles of the Duplex Doppler System

A duplex ultrasound system combines the modality of a real-time two-dimensional pulse-echo imaging of anatomic structures with that of a Doppler ultrasound system. Although the inherent range resolution feature of a PW Doppler system potentially allows collection of Doppler signals from a specific vascular target, this capability is hardly useful unless a method exists for placing the Doppler sample volume at the desired vascular location. A duplex system resolves this problem. The imaging mode offers the

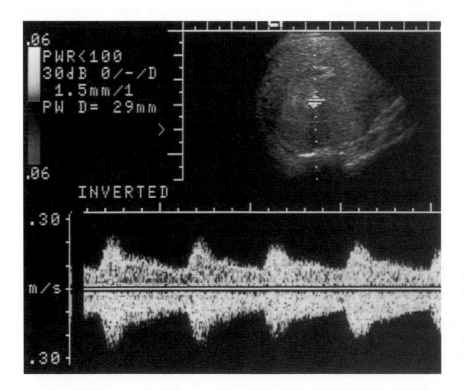

Fig. 3.11. Example of mirror imaging of the doppler waveform obtained from the uterine artery. *Top*: Two-dimensional image shows placement of the Doppler sample volume (*horizontal bars*). *Bottom*: Doppler frequency shift waveforms. The mirror image is seen on the *lower side* of the baseline

anatomic information so the Doppler sample volume can be placed at the target from which the Doppler frequency shift or velocity information can be obtained. It is achieved by employing a technique similar to that used for M-mode echocardiography. An electronically produced cursor line can be directed across any targeted component of the two-dimensional real-time cross-sectional image (Fig. 3.12). The cursor line indicates the Doppler beam path. The location of the Doppler sample volume is indicated on the cursor line by a marker, which can be an arrow, a small variably sized solid rectangle, or other shape. This location can be moved along the cursor line. Moreover, the axial dimension of the sample volume can be varied in most duplex instruments.

Experience with fetal Doppler echodiography illustrates the significant advantages of duplex Doppler for fetal circulatory assessment [13]. A two-dimensional echocardiographic scan allows pulsed Doppler interrogation of complex intracardiac flow channels and outflow tracts. Similarly, it would be impossible to perform reliable Doppler assessment of fetal aortic or middle cerebral circulations without the guidance of two-dimensional imaging. Doppler evaluation of these vascular systems is based entirely on duplex technology, which offers the only choice for interrogating most circulatory targets of the fetus. The only exception is the umbilical artery, which can be readily insonated with CW Doppler without duplex imaging guidance. Most duplex ultrasound instruments include the additional modalities of CW Doppler and M-mode ultrasound; and high-end duplex instruments also include two-dimensional Doppler color flow mapping.

Optimal Configuration of a Duplex System: Imaging Versus Doppler System

One of the major challenges of configuring a duplex ultrasound system lies in reconciling the conflicting needs of optimally performed imaging and the Doppler scanning components. For imaging, spatial resolutions is of basic importance. System features (e.g., short pulses, well-damped transducers, and wide-band receivers) contribute significantly to improving the image resolution. These factors are therefore important considerations for pulsed echo imaging. However, because of the low amplitude of the backscattered Doppler signals, the optimal performance of a Doppler system is mostly dependent on its sensitivity, not on spatial resolution. In contrast to the imaging needs, the sensitivity of a Doppler system is enhanced by longer pulses, which by interrogating larger clusters of RBCs increase the amplitude of returning signals and improve the sensitivity. The sensitivity is increased by reducing the transducer damping and using narrow-band receivers.

It is obvious that the optimal configuration of a transducer system for duplex application is a trade-off between the conflicting needs of imaging and Doppler sonography. For the latter, lower frequencies are preferred as they ensure adequate depth penetration and minimize the changes of producing range-velocity ambiguity. Higher frequencies, on the other

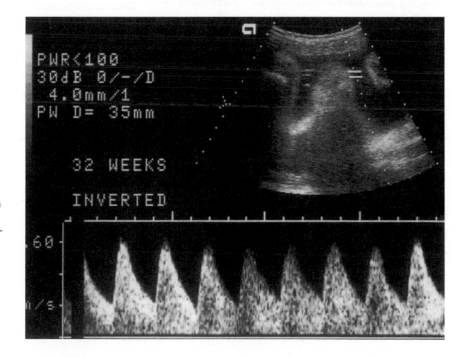

Fig. 3.12. Typical example of a duplex Doppler display. *Top*: Two-dimensional gray-scale image. The spectral Doppler beam path is indicated by the *dotted cursor line*. The Doppler sample volume is indicated by *two white lines*. *Bottom*: Spectral Doppler frequency shift waveforms from the sampled umbilical arterial location

hand, compromise Doppler sensitivity. In contrast, low frequencies reduce spatial resolution, which is of central importance for imaging. These factors are important considerations when choosing appropriate transducers for fetal Doppler applications where deep-lying small vascular structures demand both sufficient spatial resolution and adequate Doppler sensitivity. Obviously, depending on the specific use of a duplex system, varying degrees of compromise are needed between these competing needs.

Duplex Implementation

Efficient integration of imaging and Doppler functions in a duplex transducer assembly offers a significant challenge for engineering innovation. Any comprehensive description of the current state of duplex Doppler transducer technology is beyond the score of this chapter. Therefore only a brief account of the Doppler implementation of the duplex probes is presented in this section. These transducers can be classified into two broad categories according to the mechanism of scanning and focusing: (1) mechanical sector scanners, and (2) electronic array scanners, in which electronic means are employed for scanning and focusing.

Mechanical sector scanners use electric motors to rotate or oscillate the active transducer elements for sweeping the ultrasound beam to scan the tissue plane. Alternatively, a mirror may be used to sweep the beam, while the transducer element remains stationary. For duplex function, most mechanical systems use the same transducer elements for both imaging and Doppler scanning. In a mechanical sector system, the comparatively greater dimension of the transducer crystals and acoustic focusing favor improved image resolution and Doppler sensitivity. The inherent disadvantage of a mechanical system where the same elements are used for both imaging and Doppler scanning is the discontinuity between these two functions. Thus, during the actual Doppler recording, the fetus may move, so that the Doppler sample volume may no longer be at the desired target. Mechanical sector transducers are no longer used in obstetrical duplex Doppler applications, which now invariably involve electronic array transducers.

Electronic Array Scanner

In contrast to the mechnical scanners, electronic array transducers contain multiple piezoelectric elements (128 or more), and the ultrasonic scanning beam is formed by electronically controlled firing of these elements [4–17]. Over the years these transducers have evolved in terms of the complexity of their construction and the sophistication of their opera-

tion. The beam formation, steering, focusing, and aperture control are electronically implemented. Currently, several varieties of electronic array transducers are available. They are classified according to the arrangement of the piezoelectric elements in the transducer assembly and the electronic mechanism of beam formation. The elements may be arranged in the transducer assembly: (1) in a straight line, which constitutes a linear array transducer (Fig. 3.13): (2) in a convex arc, in which case the assembly is labeled as a convex array transducer, (3) in concentric rings, called the annular array (Fig. 3.14); and (4) in a two-dimensional rectangular space for three-dimensional sonography, usually termed a two-dimensional array or matrix array. The last one is discussed further in Chap. 34. According to the electronic mechanism of producing the scanning beam, there are two types of array transducer: (1) the sequenced array, which op-

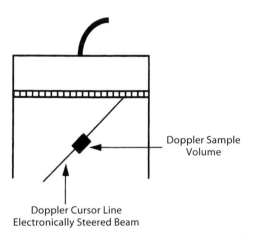

Fig. 3.13. Linear sequenced array transducer. The Doppler cursor line is shown to be electronically steered across the rectangular field of imaging

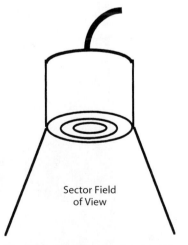

Fig. 3.14. Annular array transducer

erates by sequentially triggering batches of piezoelectric elements for scanning the beam; and (2) the phased array, which electronically triggers all or most of the piezoelectric elements as a group during a given pulse. Time delays (known as *phasing*) are used in consecutive pulses to form the scanning beam. For both of these arrays, the beam is focused by appropriate phasing, or time delay, of the piezoelectric elements. A specific transducer may have mixed features; for example, a linear sequenced array has phasic operation for focusing, or an annular array focuses electronically but scans mechanically. Currently, the following electronic array transducers are most frequently used in obstetric applications.

1. *Convex sequenced array* (Fig. 3.15). The piezoelectric elements are arranged in a convex arc and are fired sequentially in small groups as with the previous two categories. They are also known as curvilinear, curved, or radial array transducers (Fig. 3.15). The field of image is sectorshaped. This design allows a small transducer footprint with a wide field of imaging at depth – a combination of features particularly usuful for obstetric scanning. Furthermore, the wide field of view is achieved without the grating lobe problem of the linear phased array. With the phased convex sequenced array, the focusing is achieved by phasing of the firing sequence. Doppler insonation is performed by a batch of phased elements that can be steered in the sector field of exposure.

2. *Linear phased array*. This configuration is also known as the phased or electronic sector array. As the name implies, the piezoelectric elements are arranged in a straight line, and the beam is formed by the simultaneous phased firing of all the elements. Focusing and steering is accomplished electronically by the phased triggering of the elements. The field of image created by a linear phased array is sector-shape. Although these transducers do not often provide optimal imaging for general obstetric applications, they are useful for fetal cardiac imaging. The Doppler ultrasonic beam is produced by a batch of elements that are phased and can be steered within the scanned image area to interrogate the target vessel.

Integration of the Doppler and Imaging Functions in Array Transducer

We referred earlier in the chapter to the conflicting needs of opitmal transducer frequency for imaging and Doppler sonography. In many current duplex systems the problem has been addressed by providing dual-frequency transducers, a higher operating frequency for imaging, and a lower frequency for Doppler ultrasound. The latter improves the Doppler sensitivity and sets a higher Nyquist limit, whereas the former improves spatial resolution for imaging. For example, the transducer has 3.5 MHz for imaging function and 2.5 MHz for Doppler insonation. Such an arrangement has been possible only since the ad-

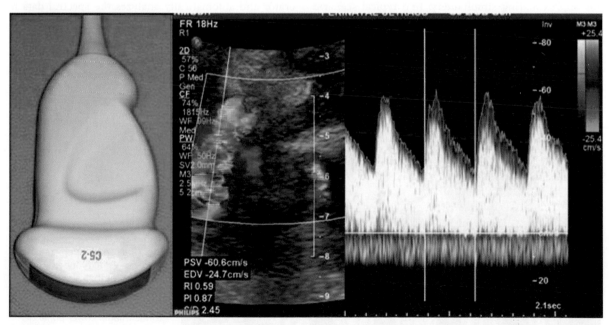

Fig. 3.15. Convex sequenced array transducers. *Left panel*: Example. *Middle panel*: Color flow image of the umbilical circulation demonstrating placement of the Doppler sample volume. The Doppler parameters are noted in *the left* lower corner. *Right panel*: Doppler frequency shift waveforms of the umbilical artery. The *vertical cursors* in this panel define one cardiac cycle

vent of broad bandwidth electronic array transducers and advanced processing capability.

In contrast to mechanical scanners, electronic transducer array scanners are capable of seemingly simultaneous execution of imaging and Doppler functions. The simultaneous operation, which is only apparent and not real, can be achieved by several methods. With one such technique, alternate pulses are shared between the two-dimensional imaging mode and Doppler sonography. This technique is similar to that used when performing simultaneous imaging and M-mode scanning. However, it reduces the Doppler pulse repetition frequency and therefore the Nyquist limit, which results in significant restriction in the maximum velocity that can be measured without aliasing. The two-dimensional imaging, frame rate is also slowed. To address the aliasing problem, a modified time-sharing approach limits the time for imaging in favor of the time for Doppler scanning. However, this method produces slow, sweeping images, which restrict the utility of the imaging guidance and are visually disconcerting for the operator [18].

A more efficient solution, used with the current generation of devices, consists in devoting more scanning time to imaging than to Doppler sonography, so a single but full image frame can be formed. The Doppler data lost during this interval is simulated from the preceding recorded spectrum by an interpolation algorithm, known as the missing signal estimator. Although it still reduces the imaging frame rate, the results are superior to those of other alternatives for approximating simultaneity. In a typical scenario,

the Doppler scan is performed for 10 ms, followed by pulse echo imaging for 20 ms. During the 20-ms interruption, the missing Doppler spectrum is interpolated from the immediate prior recording and is displayed without discontinuity. The system performs this routine with great swiftness many times a second, which allows Doppler shift assessment along with the imaging guidance to continuously verify the source of Doppler signals [19]. Obviously, this level of system performance is possible only in an electronic array with powerful processors and efficient algorithms.

Multiple-Gate and Multiple-Sample Doppler Systems

With a multiple-gate Doppler system, the standard PW Doppler system is enhanced so multiple receiver channels are range-gated sequentially. It allows multiple-point velocity assessment along the beam path. This technique, however, still does not provide comprehensive velocity information encompassing the scanned plane. With a multiple-sample Doppler system, the above approach is extended so multiple lines are sampled at several gate levels in a sequence. The process is complex, requires intensive computing, and its use has been mostly experimental. Relatively recently, a multigated, multisample spectral Doppler system has been reported [20]. The system rapidly acquires multiline, multigated Doppler waveforms from the region of interest as determined by the operator and automatically analyzes the spectral data to

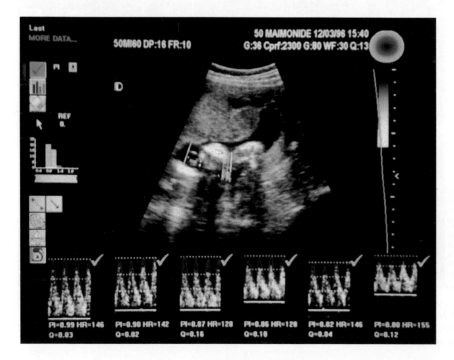

Fig. 3.16. Multigated simultaneous spectral Doppler imaging. *Upper panel* depicts color-coded pulsatility index (*PI*) map from the umbilical cord. Each pixel represents a PI value at the sampled site on the anatomic image. *Lower panel* displays selected spectra from which the color pixels originated. (Courtesy of Dr. S. Haberman)

determine the maximum frequency shift envelopes. Various Doppler indices are determined automatically and displayed either spatially as color-coded superimpositions over the gray-scale two-dimensional anatomical image or as a statistical distribution histogram of the indices in the scanned area (Fig. 3.16). Although the reproducibility of the new modality has been confirmed in relation to the umbilical artery, its utility remains to be confirmed.

Doppler Display

During operation, the Doppler information is displayed on a monitor screen. The details of the display vary according to the type of instrumentation and manufacturer. The CW Doppler instruments obviously have simpler displays (Fig. 3.11) in comparison with duplex Doppler systems (Fig. 3.12). During real-time Doppler interrogation, the spectral display scrolls from the right of the screen to the left with time, as progressively newer spectral information is added to the display. In addition to the spectral waveform, a CW Doppler display also includes the zero line, the frequency (or velocity) scale in the vertical axis, and the time scale in the horizontal axis. The spectral display area also includes the cursor lines for measuring the peak systolic or end-diastolic frequency shifts. Additional information is shown outside the spectral display window but within the screen area. It may include measures of the frequency shift including the peak systolic and end-diastolic components, Doppler indices, and various indicators of the system function.

A duplex Doppler system display is complex because of its extended function, encompassing both imaging and Doppler modes. Moreover, M-mode capability and both CW and PW Doppler modes are integrated into these systems. With more advanced systems, color Doppler flow mapping is also included. Compared with the imaging and M-mode instruments, these devices must convey to the operator a far greater amount of information. To maintain user-friendliness, the devices employ a software menu approach to their system control, which is usually reflected in the control panel display and the monitor display, so the operator is guided through the multiplicity of functions with relative ease. In the Doppler mode the monitor screen should display not only the spectra, the data of examination, and the patient's identity but comprehensive Doppler information as well, including transducer frequency, mode of Doppler, depth and size of the sample volume, angle of insonation, frequency or velocity mode, pulse repetition frequency, and Nyquist limit. It is imperative to indicate the filter and gain settings and to offer some meaningful information on the power output of the transducer. The latter is needed to ensure that the fetus is not exposed to a high level of ultrasonic energy when a lower output is sufficient to yield the desired information. Most current instruments include real-time energy output displays, the thermal index and the mechanical index, which indicate to the operator the potential for producing any biological effects in soft tissue. This is discussed in Chap. 8. Both manufacturers and users must be cognizant of these biosafety considerations. A number of options are available for archival storage of the Doppler information, including video recording and hardcopy prints, thermal printouts, photographic recording, and computer storage. When choosing the appropriate storage modality, many factors should be considered, including the needs of an indivdual practice, cost-benefit issues, archival integrity, and the ease of retrieval.

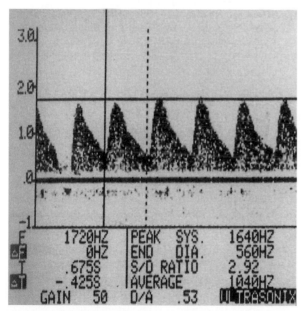

Fig. 3.17. Continuous-wave Doppler sonogram derived from the umbilical arteries. It was obtained with a free-standing Doppler device without duplex imaging guidance. *Vertical axis* represents the magnitude of the Doppler shift in kilohertz and the *horizontal axis* the time. *Bottom*: Peak systolic (*S*), end-diastolic (*D*), and average frequency shift (*A*) values. The indices (*S/D*, *D/A*) are also shown

Summary

The backscattered echo signals from a vascular source consist of the carrier and the Doppler shifted frequencies along with noise generated from various sources. To obtain clinically useful information, it is necessary to generate Doppler waveforms by systematically processing these signals. The steps involve reception and amplification of the returning signals, separation of the Doppler-shifted frequencies and determination of the directionality of flow in relation to the transducer, and spectral processing, which sorts the frequencies of the signal and determines their amplitude content. In addition, appropriate filtering is performed to eliminate the low-frequency/high-amplitude signals from tissue-sources and the high-frequency noise signals from the device. Doppler interrogation is performed by either CW Doppler transducers, which do not have range resolution, or PW transducers, which are capable of sampling a specific vascular location. Each approach has significant advantages and limitations. However, CW Doppler devices are seldom used at present for fetal investigation. Duplex Doppler ultrasonography combines two-dimensional imaging with the Doppler modality that allows image-guided interrogation of vascular targets. This capability is particularly useful for fetal investigation. Of the various types of duplex transducers, the convex sequenced array and the linear phased array are commonly used for obstetrics and gynecology.

References

1. Evans DH, McDicken WN, Skidmore R, Woodcock JP (1989) Doppler ultrasound: physics, instrumentation and clinical applications. Wiley, Chichester
2. Cooley JW, Tukey JW (1985) An algorithm for the machine calculation of complex Fourier series. Math Comp 19:297–301
3. Brigham EO (1974) The Fast Fourier Transform. Prentice Hall, Englewood Cliffs, NJ
4. Macpherson PC, Meldrum SJ, Tunstall-Pedoe DS (1981) Angioscan: a spectrum analyzer for use with ultrasonic Doppler velocimeters. J Med Eng Technol 5:84–89
5. Johnston KW, Brown PM, Kassam M (1982) Problems of carotid Doppler scanning which can be overcome by using frequency analysis. Stroke 13:660–666
6. Maulik D, Saini VD, Nanda NC, Rosenzweig MS (1982) Doppler evaluation of fetal hemodynamics. Ultrasound Med Biol 8:705–710
7. Welch PD (1967) The use of fast Fourier transform for the estimation of power spectra: a method based on time averaging over short, modified periodogram. IEEE Trans Audio Electroacoust AU-15:70–73
8. Hoskins PR (2002) Ultrasound techniques for measurement of blood flow and tissue motion. Biorheology 39:451–459
9. Kay SM, Marple SL (1981) Spectrum analysis – a modern perspective. Proc IEEE 69:1380–1419
10. Kadado T, Maulik D, Chakrabarti S (1994) Comparison of parametric and nonparametric spectral estimation of continuous Doppler ultrasound shift waveforms. IEEE Proc Digit Sig Process WS 6:145–148
11. Gill RW (1985) Measurement of blood flow by ultrasound: accuracy and sources of error. Ultrasound Med Biol 11:625–631
12. Jenkins GM, Watt DG (1969) Spectral analysis. Holden Day, London
13. Maulik D, Nanda NC, Saini VD (1984) Fetal Doppler echocardiography: methods and characterization: methods and characterization of normal and abnormal hemodynamics. Am J Cardioil 53:572–578
14. Bom N, Lancee CT, Honkoop J, Hugenholtz PC (1971) Ultrasonic viewer for cross-sectional analysis of moving cardiac structures. Biomed Eng 6:500–507
15. Eggleton RC, Johnston KW (1974) Real time mechanical scanning system compared with array techniques. IEEE Proc Sonics (Ultrasonics Cat No 74-CH 0896-1; 16)
16. VonRamm RC, Thurston FL (1976) Cardiac imaging using a phased array ultrasound system. Circulation 53:258–262
17. Kremkau FW (1989) Transducers. In: Diagnostic ultrasound. Saunders, Philadelphia, pp 65–104
18. Hatle L, Angelsen B (1985) Blood velocity measurement. In: Doppler ultrasound in cardiology. Lea & Febiger, Philadelphia, pp 32–73
19. Angelsen BAJ, Kristoffersen K (1983) Combination of ultrasound pulse echo amplitude imaging and Doppler blood velocity measurement. In: Proceeding of cardiac Doppler Symposium. Martinus Nijhoff, The Hague. Clearwater, Florida
20. Haberman S, Friedman Z (1998) Multigated simultaneous spectral Doppler imaging: a new ultrasound modality. Obstet Gynecol 92:299–302

Chapter 4

Spectral Doppler Sonography: Waveform Analysis and Hemodynamic Interpretation

Dev Maulik

The spectral Doppler power waveform contains an immense amount of hemodynamic information from the sampled circulation. As we saw in Chap. 3, the spectral information consists of three fundamental variables: frequency, amplitude, and time. Spectral frequency reflects the speed of blood flow. The amplitude approximately represents the number of scatterers traveling at a given speed and is also known as the power of the spectrum. Amplitude depends on the quantity of moving red blood cells (RBCs) in the sample and therefore reflects the volume of blood flow. The time over which the frequency and amplitude vary is the third variable. A comprehensive depiction of the Doppler spectrum is therefore three-dimensional (see Chap. 3). Such a display is complex, however, and not particularly useful for clinical application. Fortunately, there are alternative approaches for effectively characterizing the spectral waveform, including two-dimensional sonograms and various frequency envelope waveforms. These approaches can be utilized to evaluate various aspects of hemodynamics of flow, ranging from the presence and directionality of flow to downstream impedance. This chapter discusses these subjects and other related issues.

Spectral Doppler Sonogram

A typical two-dimensional sonographic display of Doppler frequency shift waveforms from the umbilical circulation is shown in Fig. 4.1. Each spectrum of the Doppler shift is depicted in a vertical line whose vertical dimension represents the magnitude of the

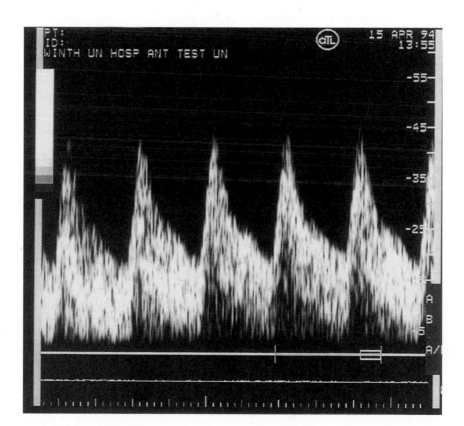

Fig. 4.1. Spectral Doppler waveform from the umbilical arteries. *Vertical axis* represents the magnitude of the Doppler frequency shift. *Horizontal axis* represents time. Brightness of the tracing indicates the amplitude of the Doppler spectrum. Note that the recording is scrolled from right to left as new information is continuously added to the right end of the spectral display

frequency; the image intensity or brightness represents the amplitude. Each successive spectrum is added to the right of the previous spectrum as the display is scrolled from right to left. Thus the horizontal axis indicates the temporal dimension of the Doppler recording. When sampled from an arterial circulation, a Doppler waveform depicts one cardiac cycle. The left limit of the wave corresponds with the onset of systole, the zenith of the wave with peak systole, and the right limit with the end of diastole. In a two-dimensional Doppler sonogram, only the frequency and time are quantitatively depicted, whereas the amplitude, or power of the spectrum, is expressed only qualitatively. The directionality is depicted in terms of whether the flow is toward or away from the transducer. The flow toward the transducer is shown as an upward deflection from the baseline and flow away as a downward deflection; this configuration may be reversed in the display. The hemodynamic interpretation and utilization of the various characteristics of the Doppler wave sonogram are discussed later in this chapter.

Doppler Frequency Shift Envelopes

Although the full power spectral display of the Doppler signal as described above provides a comprehensive account of the dynamics of flow velocity, often more limited and focused spectral information based on the various envelope definitions of the Doppler frequency shift waveform is used (Fig. 4.2). Of the various envelopes, the maximum and mean frequency shift waveforms are most commonly used for clinical applications. These envelopes and an additional one, the first moment, are discussed here.

Maximum Frequency Shift Envelope

The maximum frequency shift envelope may be derived manually by outlining the spectral waveform or electronically by analog or digital techniques. Many devices allow superimposition of the maximum frequency envelope over the spectral display waveform. It should be noted that most Doppler descriptor indices are based on the maximum frequency shift values (see below), although most indices are usually determined without defining the total envelope. This envelope is not significantly affected by uneven insonation so long as the ultrasound beam includes the fastest flow within the lumen. It is also resistant to the flow velocity profile of the circulation, the attenuation variation between blood and soft tissue, the signal-to-noise ratio, and the high-pass filter. The maximum frequency envelope is susceptible to spectral broadening as the definition of maximum frequency in relation to the spectral power becomes im-

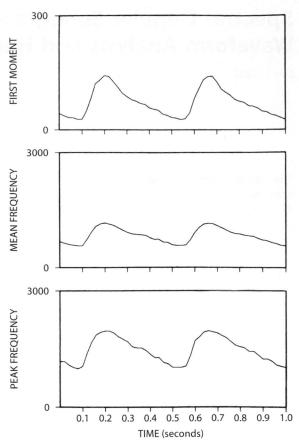

Fig. 4.2. Descriptor envelopes of the Doppler frequency shift waveform. (Reprinted from [2] with permission)

precise, and the maximum frequency values form a gradual slope at the various cutoff levels of peak power (see Fig. 3.6).

Mean Frequency Shift Envelope

Under the ideal circumstances of complete and uniform insonation of the target vessel, the mean frequency provides an indirect estimate of mean flow velocity; corrected for angle of insonation, it yields actual velocity values. The accuracy of the mean frequency depends on the velocity profile and is compromised when a vessel is incompletely insonated. The envelope is affected by the differential attenuation of sound between blood and tissue, which favors transmission of Doppler signals from the center of the vascular lumen; it results in false elevation of the mean frequency. It is also susceptible to high-pass filtering, which increases the mean frequency estimate by eliminating low-frequency signals along with the tissue-derived clutter signals. The mean frequency has the advantage of being unaffected by spectral broadening because of the symmetric nature of the spectral spread.

First Moment Envelope

Of the additional definitions of the Doppler envelope, the first moment of the Doppler power spectrum is of particular interest. The Doppler-shifted frequency is proportional to the speed of the backscattering erythrocytes, and the power of a Doppler spectrum is proportional to the density of erythrocytes moving at a corresponding speed. On this theoretic basis, Saini and associates [1] proposed that being a summation of the power-frequency product the first moment represents the integrated cell count-velocity product within the sample volume and is therefore indicative of instantaneous volumetric flow. Maulik and colleagues [2] investigated the potential of the first moment-derived Doppler waveform from the umbilical artery and observed that the first moment-based pulsatility index was twice that derived by the maximum frequency shift envelope. This phenomenon may be explained by the relative flattening of the velocity profile during early systole and by changes in the arterial diameter.

The utility of first moment remains uncertain. Although this approach contains more hemodynamic information, its practical application is limited by the impracticality of ensuring uniform insonation. Moreover, as pointed out by Evans and coinvestigators [3], the total power of the Doppler spectrum may be affected by many factors other than the vascular cross-sectional dimension.

Hemodynamic Information from Doppler Sonography

The Doppler frequency shift estimates, but does not directly measure, blood velocity. Doppler ultrasound can generate a wide range of hemodynamic information, including the presence of flow, directionality of flow, flow velocity profile, quantity of flow, and the state of down-stream flow impedance.

Flow Detection

Identification of the presence of blood flow is one of the common uses of Doppler ultrasound. Pulsed duplex Doppler insonation, especially with the two-dimensional color flow mapping mode, is capable of identifying flow that has multiple utilities in clinical practice. For example, color Doppler insonation is used to identify loops of umbilical cord in the amniotic cavity, especially when gray-scale imaging is inconclusive (Fig. 4.3). This information is useful for conducting invasive procedures, such as amniocentesis or cordocentesis, and for evaluating the amniotic fluid volume. In the human fetus, detection of anom-

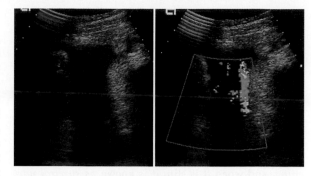

Fig. 4.3. Color Doppler identification of umbilical vessels. *Left*: Gray-scale imaging shows apparently cord-free amniotic fluid space. *Right*: Color Doppler interrogation shows the presence of the umbilical cord in this space

alous flow using pulsed Doppler echocardiography may significantly supplement the two-dimensional echocardiographic technique for diagnosing cardiac abnormalities (see Chap. 33). For example, Doppler ultrasound detection of flow in an echo-deficient area adjacent to the main pulmonary artery of the fetus was noted to assist the diagnosis of congenital aneurysm [4].

A major application of duplex Doppler flow identification is the diagnosis of proximal vein thrombosis. An absent or anomalous flow in a proximal vein suggests complete or partial occlusion. The technique has been used to assess peripheral vascular competence with varying degrees of success. However, caution should be exercised when interpreting failure to detect Doppler shift because in this circumstance the flow may be present but not within the sensitivity of the Doppler device. The maternal and fetal placental circulation offer prime examples of this problem. Although these circulations carry an immense amount of blood flow, Doppler interrogation fails to produce any recognizable Doppler shifts from most of the placental mass. Recent introduction of the power mode of color Doppler ultrasound has significantly improved the capability of recognizing slow- and low-flow states. This subject is further discussed in Chap. 6.

Flow Direction

The demodulation technique allows determination of the directionality of flow; forward and reverse flows are displayed on the opposite sides of the baseline. Flow directionality provides basic hemodynamic information that can be of significant clinical utility. For perinatal applications, flow directionality allows assessment of the status of continuing forward flow during end-diastole in umbilical and uteroplacental circulations. Absence or reversal of this end-diastolic forward flow is of ominous prognostic significance and is further discussed in Chap. 25. Depiction of flow directionality during echocardiographic assessment may assist in recognizing pathology. For example, atrioventricular valvular incompetence may be diagnosed from the demonstration of reverse flow during systole at the tricuspid or mitral orifice.

Flow Velocity Profile

Doppler shift spectral range may reflect the velocity profile of blood flow in the insonated vessel. When the spectral range is wide it is called *spectral broadening*, and when it is slim it is known as *spectral narrowing*.

Spectral narrowing usually indicates a flat or plug flow velocity profile in which most RBCs are moving at a similar speed; it is usually seen in large vessels. For obstetric applications, this flow profile is encountered in fetal ventricular outflows (Fig. 4.4). Spectral narrowing is seen during the early systolic phase (from the outset to peak systole) in a great vessel as the ventricular ejection force at its prime imparts similar speeds of flow to the RBCs; however, such an appearance may be artifactual because of the steepness of the trace [5]. Spectral narrowing is also observed when the sample volume size is smaller than the lumen, and it is placed in the center of the lumen where the flow speed is fastest.

Spectral broadening is seen with a parabolic flow where the RBCs travel at a wide range of speeds and produce a wide range of Doppler-shifted frequencies. In a parabolic velocity profile, the RBCs travel at varying speeds, with the cells at the center of the vessel traveling at the highest velocity and those near the vascular wall at the lowest velocity because of the viscous drag. Such a wide distribution of RBC velocities provides uniform broadening of the Doppler spectral display, which is usually encountered in small vessels, such as the uterine and ovarian arteries. Figure 4.5 shows an example of spectral broadening of the Doppler waveform. In obstetrics, blunted parabolic flow is seen in the umbilical arteries. It is also encountered in a turbulent flow characterized by a wide distribution of RBC speed across the vascular lumen. Finally, as noted with spectral narrowing, partial insonation of an artery may also lead to spectral broadening. If a small sample volume is placed near the wall of a large vessel, spectral broadening occurs as the flow layers toward the vessel wall show wider speed distribution.

Doppler Flow Quantification

Measurement of volumetric blood flow remains a parameter of fundamental hemodynamic importance. There are various noninvasive sonographic methods for quantifying flow. Of these, Doppler ultrasound velocimetry still remains the standard modality. There are also non-Doppler-based ultrasound technologies for measuring volumetric blood flow without some of the limitations of the Doppler technique. These approaches are discussed below.

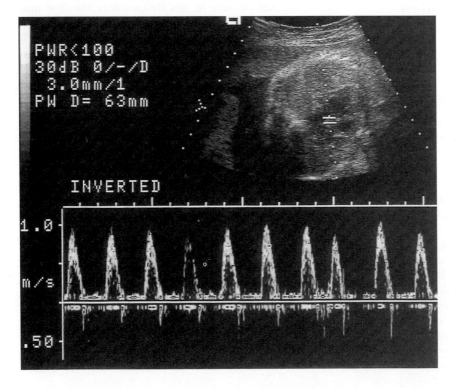

Fig. 4.4. Spectral narrowing. *Top*: Two-dimensional image of the fetal heart with the Doppler sample volume placed at the left ventricular outflow. *Bottom*: Doppler waveforms. Note the spectral narrowing of the waveforms

Fig. 4.5. Spectral broadening.
Top: Flow-guided placement of
the Doppler sample volume in
the uterine artery. Note the
spectral broadening of the
waveform

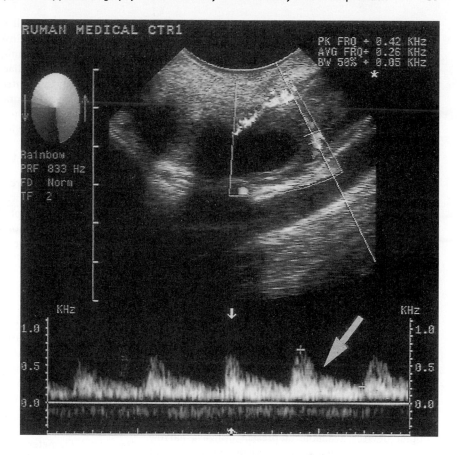

Principle of Doppler Flowmetry

The Doppler flowmetric technique has been used to
measure umbilical venous flow [6], descending aortic
flow [7], and fetal right and left ventricular outputs
[8]. The theoretical basis of Doppler flow quantification is as follows (Fig. 4.6). The volumetric flow in a
given instant (Q) is the product of the spatial mean
velocity across the vascular lumen at that instant
($\bar{v}(t)$) multiplied by the vascular cross-sectional area
at that instant (A(t)):

$$Q(t) = \bar{v}(t)A(t) \tag{1}$$

The mean velocity is estimated from the mean Doppler frequency shift ($\bar{f}_d$) by Doppler velocimetry provided the angle of insonation (θ) is also known:

$$\bar{v}(t) = \bar{f}_d(t)c/2\,f_t \cos\theta \tag{2}$$

where f_t is the transducer frequency and c is the
speed of sound in blood. The equation (1) can now
be rewritten as follows:

$$Q(t) = (\bar{f}_d(t)c/2\,f_t \cos\theta)A(t) \tag{3}$$

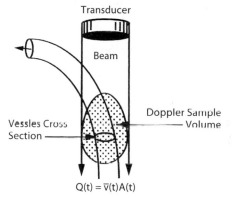

Fig. 4.6. Doppler sonographic volumetric quantification.
Graphic depiction of the principle of even insonation technique. *Q* volumetric flow in a given instant, $\bar{v}(t)$ spatial
mean velocity across the vascular lumen at that instant,
A(*t*) vascular cross-sectional area at that instant

Arterial circulation is pulsatile. Therefore the volumetric flow passing through the arterial tree fluctuates through the cardiac cycle. The temporal average
flow over the cardiac cycle is obtained from the temporal average product of the instantaneous mean velocity (mean frequency shift) and the vascular cross-
sectional area.

Doppler Velocity Measurement

There are several sonographic approaches to Doppler measurement of blood flow velocity. These include the uniform insonation method and the assumed velocity profile method.

Uniform Insonation Method

In this approach, a duplex Doppler ultrasound device is used to insonate uniformly and completely the lumen of the target vessel, and to determine the instantaneous mean frequency shift, the cross-sectional area of the vessel, and the angle of insonation. The Doppler sample volume needs to be large enough to encompass the entire vascular cross-sectional area but not to include the surrounding structures. It is also assumed that the angle of insonation is constant over the entire sample volume.

Error in estimating mean frequency shift can be due to uneven insonation, intrinsic spectral broadening, blood-tissue attenuation difference, high-pass filter, and poor signal-to-noise ratio. Of these, uneven insonation is potentially the most significant contributor. For example, partial insonation of a vessel in the periphery of the lumen will underestimate the mean frequency, whereas similar insonation in the center of the lumen will overestimate it. Most duplex Doppler devices available at present utilize a narrow beam for Doppler insonation and therefore may not be able to uniformly insonate the whole vessel even in the fetus.

Assumed Velocity Profile Method

A modification of the uniform insonation, the assumed velocity profile technique attempts to address the problem related to the mean frequency measurement by estimating the mean velocity from the time-averaged maximum frequency shift value. In this approach, the velocity profile across the flow cross-sectional area is assumed rather than measured, and maximum frequency shift data from a point target are translated into mean frequency shift values. The mean velocity is estimated by multiplying the angle-corrected instantaneous maximum frequency shift with an arbitrary calibration factor and is based on the assumption that the flow velocity profile is either flat or parabolic. In case of a flat profile, the calibration factor has a value of 1 as the mean and maximum velocities are theoretically the same. However, when the profile is parabolic, the mean velocity is half of the maximum velocity and the calibration factor has a value of only 0.5. Although this technique obviates to some extent the problem of mean velocity determination, the underlying assumptions regarding the flow velocity profile often do not exist in reality and the technique still suffers from the other limitations of the uniform insonation method. An example of the use of this technique which describes the measurement of fetal cardiac output is given in Chap. 32. This approach may introduce inaccuracies in quantifying flow. These errors are related to measuring of the mean frequency shifts, the vascular luminal cross-sectional area and the angle of insonation.

Determination of Vascular Luminal Area

The cross-sectional area of the vessel lumen may be measured from the two-dimensional image or from the M-mode tracing of the vessel. The radius, which is half the diameter of the luminal cross section is measured first and the area is estimated according to the equation:

$$A = \pi r^2 \tag{4}$$

where A is the cross-sectional area and r is the radius. This equation assumes that the vascular cross section is circular in shape. This assumption, however, is erroneous as the shape of the vascular lumen is more ellipsoidal than circular, and the shape and the dimensions of the arterial cross section are known to vary during the cardiac cycle. The problem is confounded by the fact that any error in measuring the vessel diameter is significantly amplified in the volumetric flow value. Because of these limitations, measurement of the vascular cross-sectional area is the most significant source of error for Doppler sonographic estimation of volume flow. This is especially relevant for deep-lying smaller fetal vessels. However, the error may be minimized by averaging several measurements of the diameter. Temporal averaging of the diameter during the cardiac cycle is especially important for arterial circulations. Magnification of the digital image of the vessel off line in a computer may also improve the accuracy and has been reported [9]. Simultaneous measurement of the vascular cross section and the mean velocity remains technically challenging. The best sonographic approach for imaging and measuring vascular dimension may not often be optimal for Doppler insonation.

Determination of the Angle of Insonation

Finally, the angle of insonation is an important source of inaccuracy for volumetric flow quantification as the cosine value of the angle ascertains the component of blood flow velocity reflected in the Doppler shift. The higher the angle of insonation, the greater the error of measurement. This is discussed in greater depth in Chap. 2.

Alternative Methods of Doppler Flowmetry

Measured Instantaneous Velocity Profile Method – The Multigated Doppler

In this technique, the individual velocity components across the vascular lumen are measured using multigated pulse-wave Doppler. As in the previous technique, it is also necessary to measure the beam-vessel angle in order to transform the Doppler frequency shift information into velocity data. The summation of these velocity components constitutes the volumetric flow. An advanced implementation of this approach (Cardiosonix, Neoprobe Ltd, Dublin, Ohio, USA) has been reported in which two ultrasound beams set at a fixed known angle are used and numerous small (< 200 mm length) sample volumes at successive depths are collected and analyzed by fast Fourier transform in real time [10] (Fig. 4.7). The angle of insonation and the flow diameter are automatically computed allowing measurement of volumetric flow in real time. This technique is at present limited to assessing superficial vessels such as the carotid arteries and is not available for maternal or fetal applications.

Vector Doppler – Multiple Beam Insonation

Doppler methods as described above measure the component of flow velocity parallel to the vascular axis but not the velocity components from the secondary flows resulting from vessel curvatures, bifurcations, and pulsatility. One of the techniques that attempts to resolve this limitation utilizes multiple transducers to measure multiple velocity vectors in a circulation and is also known as vector Doppler. Systems utilizing a single transmitter and two or more receivers to measure the various velocity vector components have been described [11, 12]. Experiments using a dual-beam vector Doppler system based on a modified linear array show that this system has low dependence on angle and similar reproducibility to that of single-beam systems [13]. These devices are not available yet for clinical use in obstetrics.

Non-Doppler Flowmetry – Time Domain Processing Velocity Measurement

Time domain processing is an emerging field with a tremendous potential for offering a viable alternative to Doppler sonography. The basic implementations of time domain processing for measuring velocity and volume flow are briefly discussed below. Most of these still remain experimental in nature.

Ultrasound B-Flow

As the name implies, this innovative technology is based on B-mode ultrasound and allows imaging of blood flow. It utilizes digital ultrasound which allows encoding of the signals on transmission and decoding of the returning echoes into separate tissue and blood signals. As the echogenicity of blood is substantially lower than that of tissue, the returning signals are processed and equalized to enhance blood flow signals over those from the tissue. Whereas color Doppler duplex ultrasound imaging requires separate activation of the transducer elements for the Doppler

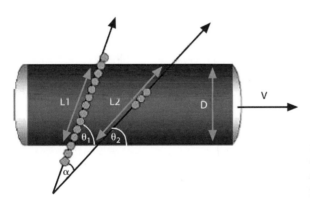

Fig. 4.7. Multigated angle-independent Doppler flow measurement as implemented in a commercial system. Schematic representation of the FlowGuard technology. The ADBF technology uses 2 ultrasound beams (*L1 and L2*) crossing the vessel lumen with a known angle (*θ*) between them and allows the simultaneous acquisition of hundreds of small sample volumes (*small dots*) of less than 200 μm in depth (*D*) along L1 and L2. This in turn authorizes accurate determination of the flow velocity profile, vessel diameter, and isonation angle (*θ*). (With permission from [10])

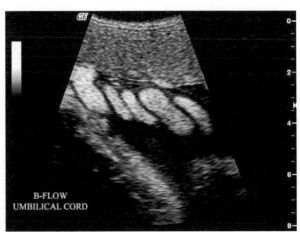

Fig. 4.8. Ultrasound B flow imaging of blood flow in the umbilical vessels. The flow image is simultaneously derived along with B imaging and not superimposed. (With permission from General Electric Health Care System, Milwaukee, WI)

and for the B-mode imaging (see Chap. 6), B-flow approach utilizes the same B-mode scan for both the tissue and the flow imaging. This allows B-flow to achieve high-resolution images at high frame rates without the constraints of Doppler sonography such as aliasing, angle dependence, wall filtering, and the need for complex controls. The safety concerns are also minimized because the acoustic intensity of B-mode ultrasound is lower than that of Doppler. This new modality holds immense potential for clinical application in the perinatal field. An example B-flow image of the umbilical vessels is shown in Fig. 4.8.

Time Domain A-Line Echo Tracking

One of the first commercial implementations of time domain processing, called color velocity imaging (CVI), measured blood flow velocity by determining the distance traveled by a group of RBCs during a known time period (Fig. 4.9) [14–16]. The method is based on cross-correlating the consecutive returning A-line echo signals from an RBC group moving in the beam path. As the interval between the pulses is very short, the cells in the group maintain the same spatial inter-relationship so that their echo signatures remain approximately identical. This allows determination of the distance traveled by the RBC cluster in a given time and therefore the velocity. Volumetric flow is obtained by measuring the spatial average velocity across the vascular lumen and multiplying this value by the cross-sectional area of the functional vascular lumen derived from M-mode tracking of the vessel (Fig. 4.10). The technique was employed also to generate real-time color flow mapping. In vitro and in vivo (animal) validation studies of the technique have confirmed the precision and accuracy of the

technique in measuring velocity and volumetric flow [17]. For velocimetry, both CVI and Doppler methods showed low variance, low intrarater variability (0.03% and 0.09% respectively), high reliability coefficients (97% and 96%, respectively), and a significant correlation ($r = 0.96$; $p < 0.001$). For in vitro flow quantification, CVI and graduated cylinder methods showed low variance, low intrarater variability (0.09% and 0.01% respectively), high reliability coefficients (99.60% and 99.96%, respectively), and a significant correlation ($r = 0.98$, $p < 0.001$). For in vivo flow quantification, CVI and transit time flowmeter showed a significant correlation ($r = 0.96$, $p < 0.001$). Within the limits of the in vitro and in vivo experimental conditions, this study provided the validity of the time domain processing ultrasound technique for measuring peak flow velocity and volumetric flow. In spite of the significant advantages of angle independence and absence of aliasing, the initial promises of this approach have not been realized in clinical use.

Time Domain Speckle Tracking

More recently, time domain processing of blood flow velocity has utilized speckle tracking techniques. Speckle is the manifestation of the variations in the amplitude of the backscattered ultrasound signals from randomly distributed subresolution scatterers. Speckle literally means small spots and gives the mottled appearance to the B-mode ultrasound images resulting from the amplitude fluctuations over time. In Doppler sonography, speckle appears as variations in the Doppler signal amplitude. Speckle degrades the spatial and the contrast resolutions of sonographic images which may be improved by the removal of speckle. However, methods for tracking speckle

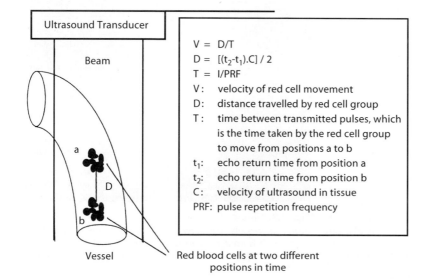

Ultrasound Transducer

Beam

a

D

b

Vessel

Red blood cells at two different positions in time

$V = D/T$
$D = [(t_2 - t_1) \cdot C] / 2$
$T = 1/PRF$
V: velocity of red cell movement
D: distance travelled by red cell group
T: time between transmitted pulses, which is the time taken by the red cell group to move from positions a to b
t_1: echo return time from position a
t_2: echo return time from position b
C: velocity of ultrasound in tissue
PRF: pulse repetition frequency

Fig. 4.9. Principle of time domain processing velocity measurement. (Reprinted from [17] with permission)

Fig. 4.10. Flow quantification by time domain processing. *Top:* Velocity waves. *Bottom:* M-mode imaging of the flow and the outlining of effective flow lumen. Maximum velocity, minimum velocity, and average flow are measured for one cardiac cycle as defined by the cursors *1* and *2*

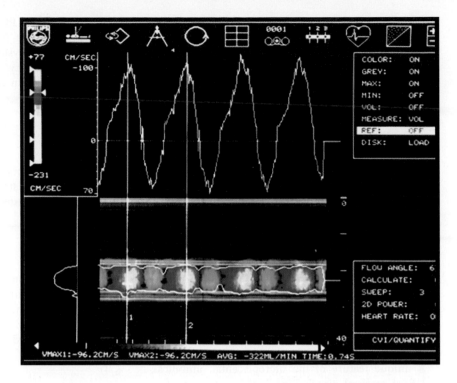

movement are being investigated as a non-Doppler sonographic technique for measuring velocity and therefore blood flow. Speckle patterns remain mostly stable between B-mode image frames and tracking their frame-to-frame displacement allows velocity measurement in a flow (Fig. 4.11) [18]. Theoretically, the technique is capable of measuring both the axial and the lateral flow velocity vectors unencumbered by the angle of insonation, aliasing, or range ambiguities. However, the accuracy of speckle tracking is less for the lateral vectors than for the axial vector aligned with the beam path and several techniques exist for improving the lateral tracking [19]. The speckle tracking principles may also be applied for measuring volumetric flow in the emerging three- or four-dimensional sonography [20]. This approach holds exciting possibilities for real-time flow and perfusion assessment in clinical settings. Speckle tracking technology is not yet commercially available.

Doppler Waveform Analysis and Doppler Indices

Because of the problems related to volumetric flow assessment, there has been a need to seek alternative ways to investigate vascular flow dynamics using the Doppler method. The maximum Doppler frequency shift waveform represents the temporal changes in the peak velocity of RBC movement during the cardiac cycle. It is therefore under the influence of both

Speckle Tracking Velocimetry

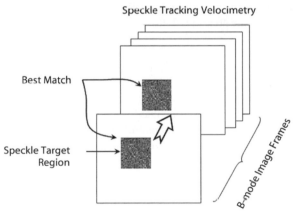

Fig. 4.11. Graphic depiction of speckle tracking velocimetry. The best match of a speckle target region in successive frames determines the distance traveled in unit time. This forms the basis of measuring the velocity and therefore the flow

upstream and downstream circulatory factors [21]. The objective has been to obtain information specifically on distal circulatory hemodynamics. Techniques have been developed for analyzing this waveform in an angle-independent manner. Most of these analytic techniques involve deriving Doppler indices or ratios from the various combinations of the peak systolic, end-diastolic, and temporal mean values of the maximum frequency shift envelope (Fig. 4.12). Because these parameters are obtained from the same cardiac

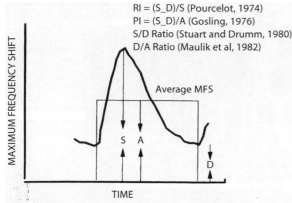

Fig. 4.12. Doppler indices derived from the maximum frequency shift envelope. *S* peak systolic frequency shift, *D* end-diastolic frequency shift, *A* temporal average frequency shift over one cardiac cycle. (Reprinted from [30] with permission)

cycle, the ratios are vitually independent of the angle of insonation.

A unique feature of the uteroplacental, umbilical, and fetal cerebral circulations is the continuing forward flow during diastole so the perfusion of vital organs is uninterrupted throughout the cardiac cycle. This feature develops progressively in the fetoplacental circulation. The essential effects of this phenomenon include not only a progressive increase in the end-diastolic component of the flow velocity but also a concomitant decrease in the pulsatility, which is the difference between the maximum systolic and end-diastolic components (Fig. 4.13). The pulsatility of the flow velocity was originally investigated using Doppler ultrasonography in the peripheral vascular system.

Gosling and King were the first to develop the pulsatility index (PI) as a measure of the systolic-diastolic differential of the velocity pulse [22]. The PI was first derived from Fourier transform data and is

known as the Fourier PI. Subsequently, a simpler version, the peak-to-peak PI (Fig. 4.12), was introduced based on the peak systolic frequency shift (S), the end-diastolic frequency shift (D), and the temporal mean of the maximum frequency shift over one cardiac cycle (A):

$$PI = \frac{S - D}{A} \tag{5}$$

Almost at the same time, Pourcelot reported a similar index, called the resistance index (RI) [23]. It also gave an angle-independent measure of pulsatility:

$$RI = \frac{S - D}{S} \tag{6}$$

where *S* represents the peak systolic and *D* the end-diastolic frequency shift. Stuart and associates [24] described a simpler index for pulsatility in which the numerator is the peak systolic frequency and the denominator is the end-diastolic frequency shift:

$$S/D \tag{7}$$

where *S* represents the peak systolic, and *D* represents the end-diastolic maximum frequency shift. (Originally, it was called the A/B ratio). Because the variations in the end-diastolic frequency shift appear to be the most relevant component of the waveform, Maulik and associates [8] suggested the direct use of this parameter normalized by the mean value of the maximum frequency shift envelope over the cardiac cycle:

$$D/A \tag{8}$$

There has been a proliferation of indices over the years. Most of them refer to the pulsatility of the maximum frequency shift envelope of the Doppler waveform, but some reflect various hemodynamic parameters, such as transit time broadening. For obstetric applications, assessment of the pulsatility and the end-diastolic frequency shift is of clinical importance.

Comprehensive Waveform Analysis

Attempts have also been made to analyze the Doppler waveform in a more comprehensive manner. Maulik and colleagues [2] described a comprehensive feature characterization of a coherently averaged Doppler waveform from the umbilical artery (Fig. 4.14). The measured parameters included the PI and the normalized systolic slope and end-diastolic velocity. In 1983 Campbell and colleagues [25] reported a technique for normalization of the whole waveform, called the frequency index profile. Thompson and as-

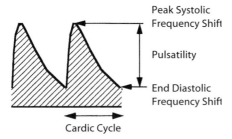

Fig. 4.13. Concept of pulsatility of an arterial velocity waveform. *Vertical axis* represents the velocity magnitude. *Horizontal axis* represents the time

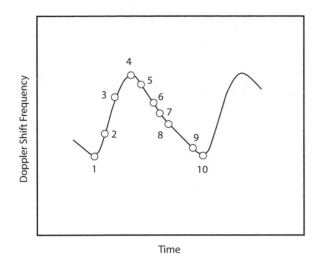

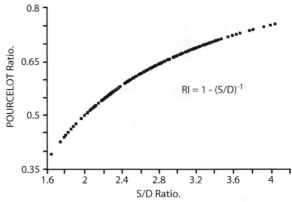

Fig. **4.15.** Correlation between the resistance index (*RI*) and the systolic/diastolic (*S/D*) ratio

Fig. 4.14. Reference points in a typical velocity envelope waveform obtained from the umbilical arteries. *1* trough, *2–3* ascending slope, *4* peak, *5–6* initial descending slope, *8–9* final descending slope, *10* trough. (Reprinted from [2] with permission)

sociates [26] described yet another technique of comprehensive waveform analysis that involved a four-parameter curve-fitting analysis of an averaged waveform. More recently, Maršál reported use of a classification system based on the PI value and end-diastolic flow characteristics [27]. This classification system was superior to other measures of the waveform for predicting fetal distress and operative delivery due to fetal distress. Most of these techniques have not been thoroughly evaluated, and currently there is no evidence that they offer any advantages over the simpler Doppler indices.

Choice of Indices

Of the various indices, the systolic/diastolic (S/D) ratio, RI, and PI have been used most extensively in obstetric practice. Of these, the S/D ratio and RI, being based on the same set of Doppler parameters (peak systolic and end-diastolic frequency shifts), are related to each other as shown in Eq. (8) and Fig. 4.15:

$$RI = 1 - \frac{S}{D} \qquad (9)$$

As the end-diastolic frequency shift declines the S/D ratio rises exponentially; and when the end-diastolic flow disappears the value of the index becomes infinity. Hence the S/D ratio value becomes meaningless beyond a certain point as the fetoplacental flow impedance continues to rise. This behavior of the S/D ratio

is inherent in its formuation and is reflected in its distribution characteristics [28] (Fig. 4.16) and its total variance (Fig. 4.17). Despite these limitations, this index is used extensively in obstetrics, particularly in the United States. The RI values, on the other hand, have defined limits with a minimum value of 0 and a maximum value of 1.0. Unlike the S/D, the RI shows gaussian distribution and is therefore amenable to parametric statistical analyses (Fig. 4.18). The limitation of RI is due to its inability to reflect impedance increases with the reversal of end-diastolic flow. Theoretically, the PI provides more hemodynamic information than the RI and S/D ratio, as it includes data on the whole cardiac cycle in the form of its denominator, which is the time-averaged value of the maximum frequency shift envelope over one cardiac cycle. Furthermore, it expresses hemodynamic alterations associated with absent or reversed end-diastolic flow. In practice, however, computation of the time-averaged value is not as precise as determination of the peak systolic or end-

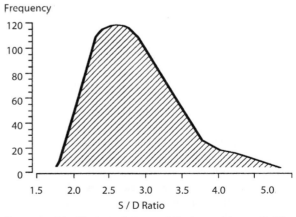

Fig. **4.16.** Distribution of the umbilical arterial systolic/diastolic ratio in the study population. Note its nongaussian distribution. (Based on data from [28])

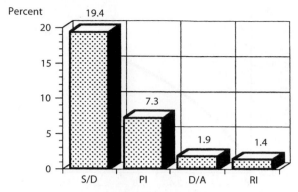

Fig. 4.17. Total variance values (percentage) of the various Doppler indices. *S/D* systolic/diastolic ratio, *PI* pulsatility index, *D/A* diastolic/average ratio, *RI* resistance index. Note that the S/D ratio varies the most and the RI the least under the same hemodynamic conditions

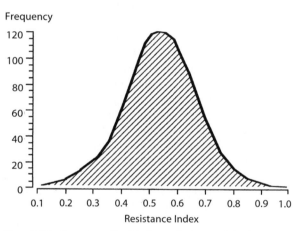

Fig. 4.18. Gaussian distribution of the umbilical arterial resistance index. (Based on data from [29])

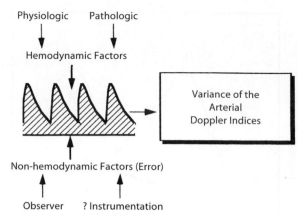

Fig. 4.19. Factors affecting the variance of Doppler indices

diastolic frequency shifts. There has been a paucity of data regarding the relative diagnostic merits of these indices. In a prospective blinded study, Maulik and associates [29] showed that the RI had the best and PI the worst discriminatory performance. This subject is further discussed in Chap. 10.

Sources of Variance of the Doppler Indices

The configuration of an arterial Doppler waveform is modulated by hemodynamic and nonhemodynamic factors [30] (Fig. 4.19). The hemodynamic modulators may be short term or long-term in nature. Examples of short-term factors include any acute changes in the impedance or heart rate; examples of long-term changes in the impedance include those encountered in the umbilical or uterine circulation with the progression of pregnancy. The nonhemodynamic modulators are those related to the examiners and devices,

and they constitute the error component of the variance in the Doppler indices. Intcrobserver and intraobserver variations are the main examples of such errors. The error component of the variance may be systematic or random. The former remains relatively constant from examination to examination. This relative constancy permits it to be considered as predictable when interpreting results. In contrast, random errors are unpredictable and significantly compromise the clinical utility of a test. As an example of the hemodynamic modulation of Doppler waveforms from a circulation, we may briefly consider the sources of variance of the umbilical arterial Doppler indices. Of the various vascular systems of the fetus, the umbilical circulation has been most widely investigated in this regard. The sources of variance that influence the indices through direct or indirect hemodynamic mechanisms include gestational age-related changes in fetoplacental vascular impedance, the site of examination in the cord, fetal breathing, and fetal heart rate. The sources of variance that are not related to any hemodynamic phenomenon and constitute error consist of inter- and intraobserver variations, and interdevice variations. The latter constitute a systematic error. A detailed discussion of the sources of variance of umbilical arterial circulation may be found in Chap. 10.

Hemodynamic Basis of Doppler Waveform Analysis

Studies on the hemodynamic basis of Doppler waveform analysis have, in general, looked for any correlation between the commonly used Doppler indices and independently measured parameters of central and peripheral hemodynamics. The latter included the heart rate, peripheral resistance, and components of arterial input impedance. In addition, the association between placental angiomorphologic changes and the Doppler indices has been investigated by several workers. This section summarizes these findings and presents a brief description of basic hemodynamic concepts relevant for Doppler validation studies.

Experimental Approaches to Hemodynamic Validation of Doppler Indices

Experimental procedures to validate Doppler indices hemodynamically often require not only the direct measurement of relevant hemodynamic parameters, such as pressure and flow, but also controlled alterations of the circulatory state. Such interventions are too invasive to be performed in relation to human pregnancy because of risks to the mother and fetus. This limitation has led to the utilization of physical and animal models. In vitro circulatory simulation exemplifies the physical model and has been used widely to investigate complex hemodynamic phenomena. Nonbiologic materials are used for prototyping circulatory systems for this type of simulation. In an intact organism it may be difficult to perform comprehensive hemodynamic measurements without profoundly altering the physiologic state of the preparation. Indeed, it may be impossible to conduct certain hemodynamic experiments in vivo because of the inherent complexities of modeling. It is also well recognized that the fundamental hydrodynamics principles are equally applicable to explaining circulatory phenomena in a physical simulation and in a biologic system. The principles of in vitro simulation for hemodynamic studies have been comprehensively reviewed by Hwang [31]. More specifically, hemodynamic parameters for designing an in vitro circulatory system for validation the Doppler indices have been reviewed by Maulik and Yarlagadda [32]. Regarding animal models, lamb fetuses and newborns have been used in both acute and chronic preparations. These models have been utilized traditionally to elucidate the circulatory phenomenon in human fetuses.

Arterial Input Impedance: Basic Concepts and Relevance to Doppler Waveform Analysis

The relevant aspects of peripheral circulatory dynamics are briefly reviewed here. Specifically, the basic principle of arterial input impedance and its relevance to Doppler waveform analysis are discussed. Traditionally, opposition to flow has been expressed in terms of peripheral resistance (Z_{pr}), which is the ratio of mean pressure (P_m) to mean flow (Q_m):

$$Z_{pr} = P_m/Q_m \qquad (10)$$

Although peripheral resistance has been the prevalent concept for describing the opposition to flow, it is applicable only to steady, nonpulsatile flow conditions. Flow of blood in the arterial system, however, is a pulsatile phenomenon driven by myocardiac contractions with periodic rise and fall of pressure and flow associated with systole and diastole of the ventricles. The pressure and flow pulses, thus generated, are profoundly affected by the downstream circulatory conditions, specifically the opposition to flow offered by the rest of the arterial tree distal to the measurement point in the peripheral vascular bed. The idea of vascular impedance provides the foundation for understanding this complex phenomenon in a pulsatile circulation. Vascular impedance is analogous to electrical impedance in an alternating current system. Womersley [33] showed that the equations dealing with electrical impedance are applicable to solving the problems of vascular impedance. It should be noted in this context that the idea of vascular resistance is analogous to the principle of electrical resistance in direct-current electrical transmissions.

Closely related to impedance is the phenomenon of wave reflection in a vascular tree. The shape of pressure and flow waves at a specific vascular location results from the interaction of the forward propagating (orthograde) waves with the reflected backward propagating (retrograde) waves [34, 35].

$$P_m = P_o + P_r \qquad (11)$$

$$Q_m = Q_o + Q_r \qquad (12)$$

where P is pressure, Q is flow, m is the measured wave, o is the orthograde wave, and r is the retrograde wave. The presence of reflected pressure and flow waves in the arterial circulation has long been recognized by hemodynamics experts. Comprehensive analysis and understanding of the phenomenon was facilitated by using the analogy of the theory of electrical current transmission. The existence of wave reflections in the circulatory system is evident from the observation that as one obtains samples along the arterial tree from the heart to the periphery the pulsatility of pressure waves progressively increases and that of the flow or flow velocity waves declines. Consequently, pressure and slow waves acquire distinctly differing configurations as they propagate down the arterial tree. The phenomenon has been analyzed mathematically by separating the observed pressure and flow waves into their constituent orthograde and retrograde components [35]. It should be noted that the forward propagating waves of pressure and flow demonstrate the same configuration. When wave reflection occurs, the retrograde flow waves are inverted, but not the retrograde pressure waves. Consequently, the observed pressure waves, which are produced by the summation of orthograde and retrograde waves, show an "additive" effect; in contrast, the observed flow (or flow velocity) waves demonstrate a "subtractive" effect (Fig. 4.20). In the absence of wave reflection, the two waves would have the same shape. Wave reflections arise whenever there is a significant alteration or mismatching of vascular impedance in a circulation. Current evidence suggests that the arterial-arteriolar junctions serve as the main source of wave reflections in an arterial system. Vasodilation decreases impedance and wave reflection. In contrast, vasoconstriction increases impedance and wave reflection. As the Doppler wave represents the flow velocity wave, it is apparent that downstream impedance and wave reflection play a central part in modulating the configuration of this waveform and therefore the descriptor indices. An in-depth discussion of arterial impedance and wave reflection is beyond the scope of this review, although relevant impedance parameters are briefly described below.

The input impedance of an arterial system [32] at a specific vascular site is the ratio of the pulsatile pressure and the pulsatile flow at that location. As the pressure and flow waves are complex in shape, they are first converted by Fourier analysis to their constituent sinusoidal harmonic components. Two parameters are generated: the modulus and the phase (Fig. 4.21). The modulus is the magnitude of the

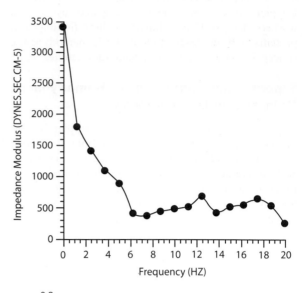

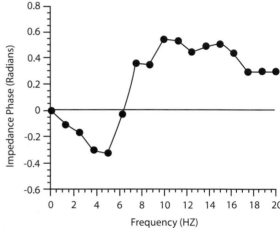

Fig. 4.21. Input impedance modulus (*top*) and phase (*bottom*) as functions of frequency

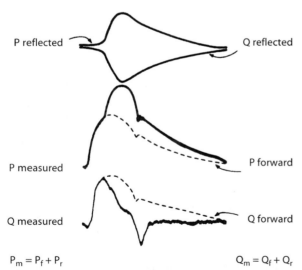

$$P_m = P_f + P_r \qquad Q_m = Q_f + Q_r$$

Fig. 4.20. Influence of pulse-wave reflections on ascending aortic pressure (*P*) and flow (*Q*) waveforms. Incident or forward (*f*) and backward or reflected (*r*) pressure and flow waves are summed to yield measured (*m*) pressure and flow waveforms. The forward pressure and flow waves are identical, as are the reflected waves, except that the reflected flow wave is inverted with an impact on the reflected pressure wave. (From [55] with permission)

pressure/flow harmonic ratios as a function of frequency; the units of measurement for the modulus are dynes·s·cm^{-3} for velocity and dynes·s·cm^{-5} for volumetric flow. The *impedance* phase expresses the phase relation between the pressure and the flow waves as a function of frequency. The phase is measured in negative or positive radians. The descriptors of vascular impedance include the following:

1. *Input impedance* is the opposition to pulsatile flow in an arterial system. Impedance at zero frequency is the peripheral resistance, which represents the steady, nonpulsatile component of vascular impedance.

2. *Characteristic impedance* reflects the properties or characteristics of the arterial system, such as the cross-sectional area, wall thickness, and vasculo-

elasticity. Any discontinuity or change in these properties gives rise to reflections of pressure and flow waves.

3. *Reflection coefficient* expresses the magnitude of the phenomenon of wave reflection in an arterial tree.

These well-established hemodynamic concepts provide the bases for hemodynamic interpretation of fetal Doppler waveforms in various physiologic and pathologic states. As the arterial Doppler wave represents the arterial flow velocity wave, it is apparent that down-stream impedance and wave reflection are among the principal modulators of the waveform and therefore of the descriptor indices. As gestation progresses, umbilical arterial Doppler waveforms demonstrate a continuing increase in the end-diastolic frequency shifts (see Fig. 10.5), which is attributable to a progressive decline in fetoplacental vascular impedance. The latter is necessarily associated with diminished wave reflections, although it has not been feasible to study the phenomenon directly.

Doppler Indices and Peripheral Resistance

Investigations in this field were aimed at establishing a hemodynamic foundation for the Doppler indices in terms of peripheral vascular resistance. In vitro and in vivo models were used. The experimental approach essentially consisted of increasing the circulatory resistance and analyzing the changes in the indices.

Spencer and coinvestigators [36] used an in vitro flow model to validate the Doppler indices in terms of peripheral resistance (mean pressure/mean flow). The flow was reduced in a stepwise fashion using a clamp. The decline in flow led to increases in RI, PI, and S/D ratio. The pressure and pressure waveform remained unchanged. The authors noted that rises in the Doppler indices reflected an increasing peripheral resistance; the RI and PI had a mostly linear increase, whereas the S/D ratio demonstrated an exponential increase. Maulik and colleagues [37] investigated the relation between the various umbilical arterial Doppler indices and umbilical arterial resistance in fetal lambs. The hemodynamic perturbation was induced by mechanical constriction of the umbilical artery, which resulted in declines in flow by 74%–89% and increases in pressure by 8%–23%. The correlation between the Doppler indices and the hemodynamic parameters is shown in Table 4.1, which indicates that with a well-defined obstruction to the downstream flow the indices correlate highly with the downstream hemodynamic parameters, including the peripheral resistance ($p < 0.005$).

Trudinger and associates [38] studied the effects of chronic embolization of the umbilical circulation on

Table 4.1. Correlation coefficients, Doppler indices versus hemodynamic parameters: constriction experiments (from [37] with permission)

Parameter	S/D	PI	RI
Peripheral resistance	0.95	0.89	0.88
Volumetric flow	−0.91	−0.96	−0.97
Pressure	0.81	0.84	0.82

S/D, systolic/diastolic ratio; PI, Pulsatility index; RI, resistance index. All significant at $p < 0.005$.

the umbilical arterial S/D ratio and umbilical circulatory resistance in fetal lambs. Chronic embolization resulted in: (1) increased fetoplacental vascular resistance (0.25–0.35 mmHg·ml^{-1}·min^{-1}); (2) increased umbilical arterial S/D ratios; (3) significant ($p < 0.05$) declines in the umbilical total flow and the umbilical/splanchnic flow ratio (from 3.36 to 1.53). The authors concluded that the umbilical artery flow velocity waveform S/D ratio measures the reflection coefficient at the peripheral vascular bed of the placenta. It should be noted, however, that the reflection coefficient, which has a precise hemodynamic definition (see above), was not measured in these experiments; and no correlations were performed between the hemodynamic parameters and the indices. Nevertheless, the study established a relation between chronic circulatory alteration and the umbilical arterial Doppler waveform. The above findings were corroborated by Morrow and colleagues [39], who observed progressive increases in the umbilical arterial pulsatility consequent to fetoplacental arterial embolization. In this study involving chronically catheterized sheep fetuses, the umbilical arterial S/D ratio correlated significantly ($r = 0.76$, $p = 0.001$) with placental resistance derived from the aortic-inferior vena caval pressure gradient and mean peak velocity.

One of the limitations of these studies was that resistance, rather than impedance, was used to assess the peripheral circulatory state in a pulsatile flow system. Vascular input impedance, however, is the hemodynamic parameter of choice when assessing the opposition to flow in a pulsatile circulation. In contrast, peripheral resistance is applicable only to the nonpulsatile component of a circulation and as such constitutes one of the parameters of arterial impedance.

Doppler Indices and Input Impedance

There have been a few studies investigating the relation between the Doppler indices and vascular impedance using an in vitro model and a neonatal lamb model [40–43].

Maulik and Yarlagadda [40] used an in vitro circulatory simulation system for hydrodynamic validation of the Doppler indices. The in vitro system consisted of a ventricular pump, an "arterial" line, a proximal "arterial" compliance unit, a "fetal placental vascular" branching model, a systemic bypass circuit, and a "venous" line for return of the perfusate into an "atrial" reservoir, which was connected to the pump. The impedance to flow was increased progressively by sequentially occluding the vessels of the branching model. All the indices correlated significantly ($p < 0.01$) with the peripheral resistance and reflection coefficient, indicating that changes in the peripheral resistance and the wave reflections from the downstream circulation are expressed by changes in the Doppler waveform as described by the indices. This study indicated that, within the general confines of a hydrodynamic model characterized by an increasing downstream opposition to a pulsatile flow and by a constant pump function, the descriptor indices of the Doppler waveform are capable of reflecting the state of the downstream flow impedance.

The correlation between vascular impedance and Doppler indices was also investigated in in vivo models. Downing and associates [41] developed a phar-macologic model of hemodynamic alteration using chronic term neonatal lamb preparations (Fig. 4.22). General anesthesia was used for the initial surgical preparation, which allowed in situ placement of a 4-MHz continuous-wave Doppler transducer and a transit time flow transducer on the infrarenal descending aorta. A pressure transducer was introduced retrogradely up to the level of the flow probe by the left femoral artery. Each animal was allowed to recover for 4 days, following which experimental inter-vention was initiated. After baseline recording of the blood pressure, heart rate, aortic flow rate, and Dop-pler waveforms, either vasodilation or vasoconstric-tion was produced with the administration of hydra-lazine or norepinephrine, respectively. The following parameters were measured: peripheral vascular resis-tance, characteristic impedance, reflection coefficient, and PI. The basic hemodynamic changes are shown in Table 4.2. Evidently, vasodilation led to tachycardia, hyperperfusion, and hypotension. Opposite changes were noted with vasoconstriction. Significant in-creases in the PI, peripheral vascular resistance, char-

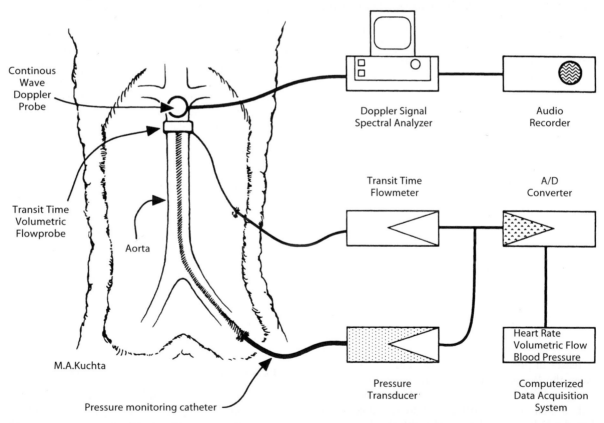

Fig. 4.22. Experimental model. Newborn lambs were in-strumented with indwelling pressure transducers, volu-metric flow probes, and continuous-wave Doppler flow probes around the infrarenal descending aorta. Probe wires were externalized to a flank pouch. During monitoring per-iods, data were collected via the use of a computerized data acquisition system, which permitted conversion of on-line recording of Doppler frequency shift signals, continu-ous aortic blood pressure, and volumetric blood flow. (Re-printed from [43] with permission)

Table 4.2. Alterations of circulatory parameters in response to vasodilation and vasoconstriction (from [41] with permission)

Parameter	Baseline	Hydralazine	Norepinephrine
Heart rate (bpm)	132±15	164±14	82±10*
Mean arterial blood pressure (mmHg)	78±5	55±5*	122±8*
Mean volumetric flow, descending aorta (ml/min)	319±21	405±28*	138±22*

Data are means±SEM. * Significant difference from baseline parameter ($p < 0.005$).

acteristic impedance, and reflection coefficient were seen in response to the administration of norepinephrine, and decreases in PI were noted with the administration of hydralazine. Figure 4.23 depicts the changes in the PI and reflection coefficient and Fig. 4.24 the changes in the input impedance moduli and phase. As is evident, the impedance modulus curve showed distinct changes with vasoconstriction and vasodilation. Further analysis of the data showed a statistically significant correlation between the PI and peripheral resistance. However, changes in the PI did not significantly correlate with the changes in characteristic impedance and reflection coefficient.

The next study investigated this issue [42]. The experimental model was the same as in the previous study. The experimental protocol, however, ensured that the heart rate changes due to vasoactive interventions were pharmacologically suppressed by trimethophan during vasodilation or atropine methylbromide during vasoconstriction. The results are presented in Table 4.3. In response to both vasodilation and vasoconstriction without controlling the reflex heart rate responses, the aortic PI was highly and positively correlated with peripheral resistance ($r = 0.78$, $p < 0.001$) but not with characteristic impe-

dance. However, when the reflex heart rate responses were inhibited, the changes in PI correlated well with peripheral resistance and characteristic impedance ($r = 0.92$, 0.95; $p < 0.001$). It is reasonable to conclude from these findings that the Doppler indices of pulsatility reflect the state of downstream circulation independent of the changes in the heart rate. However, the heart rate does influence the pulsatility and should therefore be taken into consideration. This subject is further discussed below.

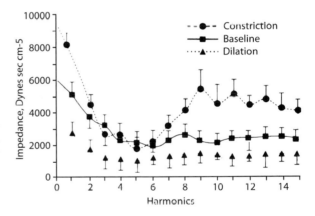

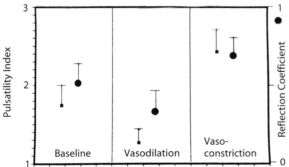

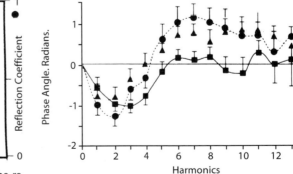

Fig. 4.23. Responses of the pulsatility index (*PI*) and the reflection coefficient (*Rc*) to vasodilation with hydralazine and vasoconstriction with norepinephrine. PI and Rc increased significantly from baseline in response to hydralazine, but Rc was not significantly affected. (From [56] with permission)

Fig. 4.24. Impedance moduli and phase angle during baseline, vasodilation, and vasoconstriction with hydralazine and norepinephrine, respectively. Each curve represents the mean±SEM impedance moduli for all study animals. (From [56] with permission)

Table 4.3. Hemodynamic parameters and Doppler indices in drug-induced vasodilation and vasoconstriction with and without heart rate changes (from [43], with permission)

Parameters	Control	Hydralazine	Hydralazine, trimethophan	Phenylephrine	Phenylephrine, atropine MB
HR	128±10	186±12	130±8	65±7	126±8
PI	1.91±13	1.50±21	1.71±13	2.54±19	2.28±0.21
Z_{pr}	39,960±8,728	12,350±1,210	10,460±961	65,380±8,130	60,840±7,590
Z_o	4010±340	1683±350	1333±410	8960±760	7683±630

HR, heart rate (bpm); PI, pulsatility index; Z_{pr} peripheral resistance; Z_o, characteristic impedance.

Doppler Indices and Central Circulation

Central circulation potentially influences the Doppler waveform and should be an important consideration when interpreting the changes in Doppler indices. The clinical significance of fetal heart rate effect on the indices has been somewhat controversial. Although earlier studies found no significant effect of the heart rate on the Doppler indices [44], several subsequent reports refuted these findings [45, 46]. There is no evidence at present to indicate that correcting the indices for fetal heart rate improves their diagnostic efficacy when the baseline heart rate remains within the normal range. The mechanism of the heart rate effect on the Doppler indices has been well studied in animal and in vitro models. It is well recognized in clinical practice that when the heart rate drops the diastolic phase of the cardiac cycle is prolonged, which results in a decrease in the end-diastolic frequency shift (Fig. 4.25). This condition obviously increases the pulsatility of the waveform,

which is reflected in the descriptor indices, such as the PI or the S/D ratio.

This phenomenon was clearly demonstrated in fetal ovine models in which fetal bradycardia was experimentally induced by either acute uteroplacental flow occlusion [47] or maternal hypoxia [48]. The Doppler indices measured were the RI, S/D ratio, and PI. The duration of the cardiac cycle and its systolic and diastolic times were approximated from the Doppler waveform. In the uteroplacental flow insufficiency model, transient occlusion of the maternal common uterine artery produced statistically significant ($p<0.005$) increases in the Doppler indices and cardiac cycle time. The increases in the Doppler indices disappeared ($p>0.05$) when the latter were corrected for changes in the cardiac cycle time (Fig. 4.26). As expected, the diastolic time was noted to be the principal contributor to the changes in heart rate (Fig. 4.27). The effect of heart rate was also investigated in a chronic ovine model in which changes in the umbilical arterial Doppler waveform

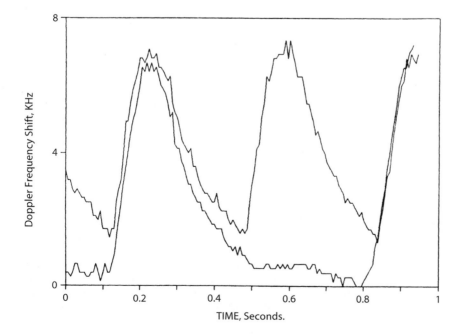

Fig. 4.25. Comparison of the umbilical arterial Doppler waveforms with normal heart rate (125 bpm) and bradycardia (77 bpm). *Vertical axis* represents the magnitude of Doppler frequency shift. *Horizontal axis* represents the time

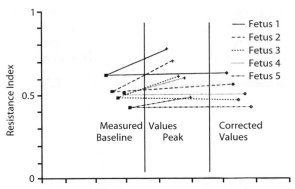

Fig. 4.26. Effect of variations in the cardiac cycle time correction on the resistance index (*RI*). The three divisions in this figure correspond to baseline, measured peak, and corrected values, respectively. Please note that the differences between the baseline and the measured peak values (all significant at $p < 0.005$) disappeared when corrected for fetal heart rate (none significant at $p < 0.005$). (From [47] with permission)

in response to acute maternal hypoxemia were assessed. During the periods of maternal hypoxemia, the fetal heart rate decreased (to < 80 bpm) and umbilical arterial Doppler indices increased ($p < 0.001$). Furthermore, the Doppler indices were highly but negatively correlated with alterations in the fetal heart rate ($p < 0.001$). Analysis of the Doppler waveform phase intervals revealed nearly constant systolic intervals, whereas diastolic intervals varied inversely with the heart rate alterations. Moreover, the umbilical arterial Doppler indices, when corrected for the fetal heart rate changes, were relatively unchanged from

baseline measurements. Both studies confirmed that the fetal cardiac cycle, and therefore the fetal heart rate, plays an important role in shaping the umbilical arterial Doppler waveform. Furthermore, this effect is mediated predominantly via changes in the diastolic phase of the cardiac cycle. There is also evidence that the fetal heart rate may affect the ability of the Doppler waveform analysis to reflect completely the changes in downstream impedance [49]. It should be noted that there is a paucity of information on the central circulatory factors, other than heart rate, that influence the Doppler waveform.

Legarth and Thorup [49, 50] utilized an in vitro model of circulation in which they studied the influence of central and peripheral circulations on the Doppler waveform. The in vitro model allowed independent control over pulse rate, volumetric flow, stroke volume, pressure, and peripheral resistance. The authors observed that the velocity indices changed with the pulse rate, although flow and peripheral resistance were constant. They also noted that the rising slope of the Doppler waveform did not correlate with cardiac contractility as measured by the changes in pressure (the first maximum derivative of the intraventricular pressure: dP/dt).

This finding is intriguing and deserves further investigation. Regarding the effect of resistance on the rising slope, the two parameters did not correlate when the flow was kept constant, but when the pressure was kept constant the rising slope increased significantly with resistance.

These studies emphasize the relative importance of the central circulatory changes to alterations in the Doppler waveform.

Fig. 4.27. Correlation between systolic and diastolic components of the Doppler waveform and the fetal heart rate (*FHR*), which is the reciprocal of the cardiac cycle time. Note that the slope of the diastolic time versus FHR is approximately 9 times greater than the slope of the systolic time versus FHR. (Based on data from [47])

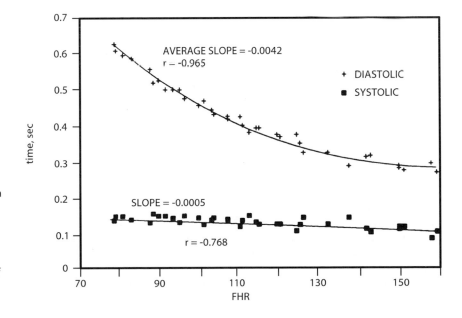

Placental Vascular Changes and Abnormal Doppler Waveforms

The dependence of arterial Doppler waveform on downstream circulatory impedance is also reflected in the pathology of the distal vascular bed. Various investigators reported fetoplacental morphological changes in relation to umbilical arterial velocimetry and pregnancy complications including fetal growth compromise. Giles and coinvestigators [51] correlated fetoplacental histopathological changes with umbilical arterial S/D ratio in women with normal and complicated pregnancies. A statistically significant decrease ($p < 0.01$) in the modal small arterial count (arteries in the tertiary stem villi measuring less than 90 μm in diameter) was observed in abnormal pregnancies with an abnormal Doppler index. The authors suggested fetoplacental vaso-obliterative pathologic processes as the underlying cause of an abnormal Doppler waveform. Subsequently, Krebs and coinvestigators [52] demonstrated that in preterm intrauterine growth restriction pregnancies with umbilical arterial absent end-diastolic flow velocity, the capillary loops were sparse in number and significantly longer, and had significantly less branching and coiling than in the control cases. These findings are more reflective of villous maldevelopment rather than a vaso-obliterative process. This was further corroborated by Todros and associates [53] who demonstrated that, compared with those with positive end-diastolic flow in the umbilical artery, the placentas from growth-restricted fetuses with absent or reverse end-diastolic flow showed a normal pattern of stem artery development, accompanied by significantly decreased capillary angiogenesis and terminal villous development. The authors speculated that these findings suggested fetoplacental adaptive response in the presence of uteroplacental ischemia.

A similar observation has been reported in relation to angiomorphological pathology of the uteroplacental vascular bed and the uteroplacental Doppler waveform. Voigt and Baker [54] performed placental bed biopsies in pregnancies complicated by preeclampsia or otherwise presumed fetal growth restriction delivered by cesarean section. Similar biopsies were also performed in a control group of healthy pregnancies delivered by cesarean section for labor dysfunction or malpresentation. The uteroplacental PI predicted abnormal uteroplacental angiomorphology with significant accuracy.

Based on these observations, the following vascular and hemodynamic mechanism may be suggested for abnormal umbilical arterial Doppler waveforms in pregnancies complicated with fetal growth restriction and highly abnormal umbilical arterial Doppler indices. Abnormal uteroplacental angiogenesis and consequent ischemia leads to fetoplacental villous malde-

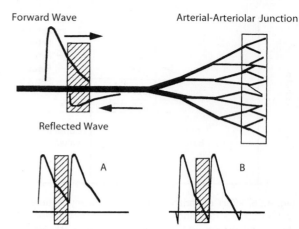

Fig. 4.28. Effect of wave reflection on umbilical arterial Doppler waveforms. Note that as the pulse wave propagation velocity in the fetus is slower than in the adults, retrograde waves affect forward propagating waves during late diastole (*cross-hatched box*). (*A*) Normal waveforms with minimal wave reflection because of low impedance in the fetoplacental arterial circulation. (*B*) Effect of significant wave reflection when fetoplacental impedance becomes high, resulting in the absence or reversal of end-diastolic frequency shift

velopment and deficient angiogenesis and vascularity. These changes result in an increase in the arterial impedance, which is necessarily associated with enhanced pressure and flow velocity wave reflections. The reflected flow velocity waves propagating backward will change the shape of arterial flow velocity waves. A graphic depiction of this concept in relation to umbilical arterial Doppler waveforms is presented in Fig. 4.28.

Summary

Doppler velocimetry offers a wide range of hemodynamic information. Although the technique permits volumetric flow quantification, there are critical concerns regarding the precision of this approach. Assessment of the downstream hemodynamic state is of importance for perinatal application. It is achieved by Doppler waveform analysis, which generates indices describing the pulsatility of the wave. These analytic techniques are based on accepted hemodynamic principles and are supported by experimental evidence on hemodynamic validation of the Doppler indices. As summarized above, the Doppler indices can reflect impedance to flow downstream from the measurement point, although the effect of fetal heart rate changes on the diastolic phase of the cardiac cycle may confound this ability of the indices. In addition, there is angiomorphologic evidence that links abnormal Doppler indices to both the fetoplacental and the uteroplacental vascular pathology.

References

1. Saini VD, Maulik D, Nanda NC, Rosenzweig MS (1983) Computerized evaluation of blood flow measurement indices using Doppler ultrasound. Ultrasound Med Biol 9:657–660

2. Maulik D, Saini VD, Nanda NC, Rosenzweig MS (1982) Doppler evaluation of fetal hemodynamics. Ultrasound Med Biol 8:705–710

3. Evans DH, McDicken WN, Skidmore R, Woodcock JP (1989) Doppler signal processors: theoretical considerations. In: Doppler ultrasound: physics, instrumentation and clinical applications. Wiley, Chichester, p 144

4. Maulik D, Nanda NC, Moodley S, Saini VD, Thiede HA (1985) Application of Doppler echocardiography in the assessment of fetal cardiac disease. Am J Obstet Gynecol 151:951–957

5. Kremkau F (1990) Doppler ultrasound: principles and instrumentation. Saunders, Philadelphia

6. Gill RW (1979) Pulsed Doppler with B-mode imaging for quantitative blood flow measurements. Ultrasound Med Biol 5:223–235

7. Eik Nes SH, Brubakk AO, Ulstein MK (1980) Measurement of human fetal blood flow. BMJ 280:283–284

8. Maulik D, Nanda NC, Saini VD (1984) Fetal Doppler echocardiography: methods and characterization of normal and abnormal hemodynamics. Am J Cardiol 53:572–578

9. Boito S, Struijk PC, Ursem NT, Stijnen T, Wladimiroff JW (2002) Umbilical venous volume flow in the normal developing and growth restricted human fetus. Ultrasound Obstet Gynecol 19:344–349

10. Soustiel JF, Levy E, Zaaroor M, Bibi R, Lukaschuk S, Manor D (2002) A new angle-independent Doppler ultrasonic device for assessment of blood flow volume in the extracranial internal carotid artery. J Ultrasound Med 21:1405–1412

11. Overbeck JR, Beach KW, Strandness DE Jr (1992) Vector Doppler: accurate measurement of blood velocity in two dimensions. Ultrasound Med Biol 18:19–31

12. Dunmire B, Beach KW, Labs K, Plett M, Strandness DE Jr (2000) Cross-beam vector Doppler ultrasound for angle-independent velocity measurements. Ultrasound Med Biol 26:1213–1235

13. Steel R, Ramnarine KV, Criton A, Davidson F, Allan PL, Humphries N, Routh HF, Fish PJ, Hoskins PR (2004) Angle-dependence and reproducibility of dual-beam vector doppler ultrasound in the common carotid arteries of normal volunteers. Ultrasound Med Biol 30:271–276

14. Dotti D, Gatti E, Svelto V, Ugge A, Vidali P (1976) Blood flow measurement by ultrasound correlation techniques. Energia Nucleare 23:571–575

15. Embree PM, O'Brien Jr WD (1985) The accurate ultrasonic measurement of the volume flow of blood by time domain correlation. IEEE Ultrason Symp 963–966.

16. Bonnefus O, Pesque P (1986) Time domain formulation of pulse Doppler ultrasound and blood velocity estimation by cross correlation. Ultrasonic Imaging 8:73–85

17. Maulik D, Kadado T, Downing G, Phillips C (1995) In vitro and in vivo validation of time domain velocity and Flow Measurement Technique. J Ultrasound Med 14:939–948

18. Bohs LN, Friemel BH, McDermott BA, Trahey GE (1993) A real time system for quantifying and displaying two-dimensional velocities using ultrasound. Ultrasound Med Biol 19:751–761

19. Chen X, Zohdy MJ, Emelianov SY, O'Donnell M (2004) Lateral speckle tracking using synthetic lateral phase. IEEE Trans Ultrason Ferroelectr Freq Control 51:540–550

20. Bohs LN, Geiman BJ, Anderson ME, Gebhart SC, Trahey GE (2000) Speckle tracking for multi-dimensional flow estimation. Ultrasonics 38:369–375

21. McDonald D (1974) Blood flow in arteries. Williams & Wilkins, Baltimore

22. Gosling RG, King DH (1975) Ultrasound angiology. In: Macus AW, Adamson J (eds) Arteries and Veins. Churchill-Livingstone, Edinburgh, pp 61–98

23. Pourcelot L (1974) Applications clinique de l'examen Doppler transcutance. In: Pourcelot L (ed) Velocimetric ultrasonore Doppler. INSERM, Paris, p 213

24. Stuart B, Drumm J, FitzGerald DE, Diugnan NM (1980) Fetal blood velocity waveforms in normal pregnancy. Br J Obstet Gynaecol 87:780–785

25. Campbell S, Diaz-Recasens J, Griffin DR et al (1983) New Doppler technique for assessing uteroplacental blood flow. Lancet 1:675–677

26. Thompson RS, Trudinger BJ, Cook CM (1985) Doppler ultrasound waveforms in the fetal umbilical artery: quantitative analysis technique. Ultrasound Med Biol 11:707–718

27. Maršál K (1987) Ultrasound assessment of fetal circulation as a diagnostic test: a review. In: Lipshitz J, Maloney J, Nimrod C, Carson G (eds) Perinatal development of the heart and lung. Perinatology Press, Ithaca, NY, pp 127–142

28. Maulik D, Yarlagadda P, Youngblood JP, Ciston P (1990) The diagnostic efficacy of umbilical arterial systolic/diastolic ratio as a screening tool: a prospective blinded study. Am J Obstet Gynecol 162:1518–1523

29. Maulik D, Yarlagadda P, Youngblood JP, Ciston P (1991) Comparative efficacy of umbilical arterial Doppler indices for predicting adverse perinatal outcome. Am J Obstet Gynecol 164:1434–1439

30. Maulik D, Yarlagadda P, Youngblood JP, Willoughby L (1989) Components of variability of umbilical arterial Doppler velocimetry: a prospective analysis. Am J Obstet Gynecol 160:1406–1409

31. Hwang NHC, Norman A (1977) An engineering survey of problems in cardiovascular flow dynamics and measurements. University Park Press, Baltimore

32. Maulik D, Yarlagadda P (1987) In vitro validation of Doppler waveform indices. In: Maulik D, McNellis D (eds). Doppler Ultrasound Measurement of Maternal-Fetal Hemodynamics. Perinatology Press, Ithaca, NY, p 257

33. Womersley JR (1957) The Mathematical Analysis of the Arterial Circulation in a State of Oscillatory Motion. Technical Report WADC-TR56-614. Wright Air Development Center, Maryland

34. Westerhof N, Sipkema P, Van den Bos GC, Elzinga G (1972) Forward and backward waves in the arterial system. Cardiovasc Res 6:648–656

35. Murgo JP, Westerhof N, Giolma JP, Altobelli SA (1981) Manipulation of ascending aortic pressure and flow ave

reflections with Valsalva maneuver: relationship to input impedance. Circulation 63:122–132

36. Spencer JAD, Giussani DA, Moore PJ, Hanson MA (1991) In viro validation of Doppler indices using blood and water. J Ultrasound Med 10:305–308

37. Maulik D, Yarlagadda P, Nathaniels PW, Figueroa JP (1989) Hemodynamic validation of Doppler assessment of fetoplacental circulation in a sheep model system. J Ultrasound Med 8:177–181

38. Trudinger BJ, Stevens D, Connelly A et al (1987) Umbilical artery velocity waveform and placental resistance: the effects of embolization of the umbilical circulation. Am J Obstet Gynecol 157:1443–1448

39. Morrow RJ, Adamson SL, Bull SB, Knox Ritchie JW (1989) Effect of placental embolization on the umbilical arterial velocity waveform in fetal sheep. Am J Obstet Gynecol 161:1055–1060

40. Maulik D, Yarlagadda P (1990) Hemodynamic validation of the Doppler indices: an in vitro study (abstract). Presented at the International Perinatal Doppler Society: 3rd Congress, Malibu, CA

41. Downing GJ, Yarlagadda AP, Maulik D (1991) Comparison of the pulsatility index and input impedance parameters in a model of altered hemodynamics, J Ultrasound Med 10:317–321

42. Downing GJ, Maulik D (1991) Correlation of the pulsatility index (PI) with input impedance parameters during altered hemodynamics (abstract). J Matern Fetal Invest 1:114

43. Downing GJ, Maulik D, Phillips C, Kadado T (1993) In vivo correlation of Doppler waveform analysis with arterial input impedance parameters. Ultrasound Med Biol 19:549–559

44. Thompson RS, Trudinger BJ, Cook CM (1985) Doppler ultrasound waveforms in the fetal umbilical artery: quantitative analysis technique. Ultrasound Med Biol 11:707–718

45. Mires G, Dempster J, Patel NM et al (1987) The effect of fetal heart rate on umbilical artery flow velocity waveform. Br J Obstet Gynaecol 94:665–669

46. Yarlagadda P, Willoughby L, Maulik D (1989) Effect of fetal heart rate on umbilical artery Doppler indices. J Ultrasound Med 8:215–218

47. Maulik D, Downing GJ, Yarlagadda P (1990) Umbilical arterial Doppler indices in acute uteroplacental flow occlusion. Echocardiography 7:619

48. Downing GJ, Yarlagadda P, Maulik D (1991) Effects of acute hypoxemia on umbilical arterial Doppler indices in a fetal ovine model. Early Hum Dev 25:1–10

49. Legarth J, Thorup E (1989) Characteristics of Doppler blood velocity waveforms in a cardiovascular in vitro model. II. The influence of peripheral resistance, perfusion pressures and blood flow. Scan J Clin Lab Invest 49:459–464

50. Legarth J, Thorup E (1989) Characteristics of Doppler blood velocity waveforms in a cardiovascular in vitro model. I. The model and the influence of pulse rate. Scand J Clin Lab Invest 49:451–457

51. Giles WB, Trudinger JB, Baird PJ (1985) Fetal umbilical artery flow velocity waveforms and placental resistance: pathologic correlation. Br J Obstet Gynaecol 92:31–38

52. Krebs C, Macara LM, Leiser R, Bowman AW, Greer IA, Kingdom JC (1996) Intrauterine growth restriction with absent end-diastolic flow velocity in the umbilical artery is associated with maldevelopment of the placental terminal villous tree. Am J Obstet Gynecol 175:1534–1542

53. Todros T, Sciarrone A, Piccoli E, Guiot C, Kaufmann P, Kingdom J (1999) Umbilical Doppler waveforms and placental villous angiogenesis in pregnancies complicated by fetal growth restriction. Obstet Gynecol 93:499–503

54. Voigt HJ, Becker V (1992) Uteroplacental insufficiency – comparison of uteroplacectal blood flow velocimetry and histomorphology of placental bed. J Matern Fetal Invest 2:251

55. Nichols WW, O'Rourke MF, Avolio AP et al (1987) Age-related changes in left ventricular/arterial coupling. In: Yin FCP (ed) Ventricular/vascular coupling. Springer, Berlin Heidelberg New York, pp 79–114

56. Downing GS, Maulik D (1991) Comparison of the pulsatility index (PI) with input impedance parameters in a model of altered hemodynamics. J Ultrasound Med 10:317–321

Chapter 5

Venous Hemodynamics

Torvid Kiserud

In recent years evaluation of the venous system has become a compulsory part of the haemodynamic assessment of the fetus, but the underlying mechanisms of our Doppler recordings are still incompletely understood. The present chapter is not intended to solve all that, but rather to address important hemodynamic issues from a clinical point of view to help clinicians use and interpret venous Doppler recordings. For the interested reader more extensive discussions of blood flow dynamics are available in the literature [1–5].

Velocity Profile in Veins

Parabolic Blood Velocity Profile and Flow Calculation

In a straight section of the umbilical vein with a steady velocity, the distribution of the velocity across the cross-sectional area of the vessel is assumed to be parabolic with the highest velocity (V_{max}) in the center of the cross section (Fig. 5.1). The ratio of the average velocity across the vessel (V_{mean}) and the V_{max} characterizes the velocity profile. For parabolic flow, the ratio V_{mean}/V_{max} is 0.5.

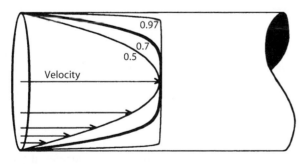

Fig. 5.1. The velocity profile represents the velocity distribution across the vessel and is characterized by the V_{mean}/V_{max} ratio. The steady blood flow in the umbilical vein has a parabolic velocity profile (i.e. ratio 0.5). The accelerated blood at the ductus venosus inlet has a partially blunted velocity profile corresponding to a ratio of 0.7, while at the cardiac outlets the profile is even more blunted (e.g. ratio 0.97). (From [17])

For calculating volume flow we need the averaged velocity across the vessel area. We can derive that by tracing the weighted mean velocity ($V_{w.mean}$) of the Doppler recording. Ideally, with a strictly parabolic flow, the relation would be $V_{w.mean} = V_{mean} = 0.5\ V_{max}$. This is particularly useful since the intensity-weighted mean velocity ($V_{w.mean}$) derived from the Doppler shift is easily influenced by low-velocity signals from the vessel wall or neighboring vessels, or from loss of low-velocity recordings due to filters, or loss of the weakest signals when travelling through the tissues. Secondly, the $V_{w.mean}$ represents the average of the velocities recorded in the sample volume (Doppler gate), which is not identical to the vessel cross-section. The sample volume may cover the vessel incompletely or asymmetrically. The low velocities at the periphery of the vessel are more likely to be underrepresented than the high axial velocities of the center. In short, we have two ways of calculating blood flow:

$$\pi(D/2)^2 V_{w.mean}$$

and

$$\pi(D/2)^2\ 0.5\ V_{max}$$

the latter being the more robust, provided the velocity actually is parabolic.

That may not always be the case. For example, the velocity profile is found to be more blunted the first few centimetres after the umbilical vein has left the placenta [6]. During acceleration or retardation the velocity profile changes, and variation in geometry, branching and curvature alter the velocity profile (Fig. 5.2). These changes are further determined by the viscosity of the blood and dimension of the vessel expressed in the Reynold's number [1]. These facts favor the use of $V_{w.mean}$, which is not dependent on a known profile factor; thus, it has not been determined which method is the best, and the literature has examples of both methods [7–14].

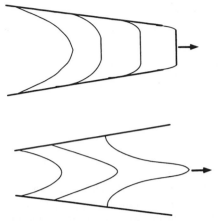

Fig. 5.2. The impact of geometry on the velocity profile. The profile changes from a parabolic shape to a more blunted (flat) shape at converging vessel lumen (*upper panel*). A funnel-shaped geometry with increasing diameter is associated with reduced velocities at the periphery and a more or less maintained axial velocity resulting in a pointed velocity profile (*lower panel*). (From [2])

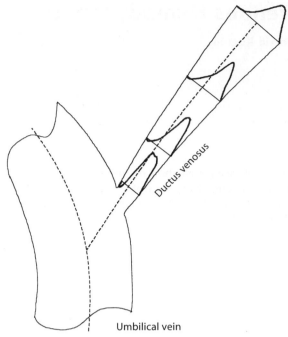

Fig. 5.3. Two-dimensional velocity profile in the ductus venosus predicted by computer modelling (**a**). Note the skewed profile and the small negative velocity component estimated by using the present geometrical details. (From [16])

Factors Modifying the Velocity Profile

The acceleration of blood, as seen in the isthmus of the ductus venosus, also represents a transition of the velocity profile from the parabolic ($V_{mean}/V_{max} = 0.5$) to a more blunted profile (Fig. 5.1). There is now theoretical and experimental proof that the blood velocity profile at the ductus venosus inlet is partially blunted with $V_{mean}/V_{max} = 0.7$ [15–17], which has been used when calculating volume flow in the ductus venosus [12, 13]. This value of the ratio is applicable with the high ductus venosus velocities seen during the second half of pregnancy. It is less certain that it applies to the low velocities of early pregnancy.

Curvature, bifurcation or other changes in blood flow direction cause changes in the velocity profile. The blood starts spiralling along the wall of the curvature and the velocity profile is commonly dislodged towards the periphery of the vessel cross section. Depending on the geometrical details, dimensions and viscosity (i.e. Reynold's number), and the magnitude of the velocity, the velocity profile may show a proportion of negative (reversed) velocity (Fig. 5.3).

It is also worth noting that the velocity and its profile starts to change before the blood has reached the narrow section of a constriction, and gradually returns to parabolic or more pointed velocity profile on the other side of the constriction, again depending on geometrical details (Fig. 5.4). An example would be the physiological constriction of the umbilical vein at the abdominal inlet. The abrupt expansion of the umbilical vein diameter after the constriction at the abdominal wall makes the blood slow down and re-gain parabolic flow within a short distance. In some cases this expansion is extensive and permits vortex formation (whirls) and may be misinterpreted as an aneurysm instead of a "post-stenotic dilatation". In contrast, the tapering geometry of the ductus venosus central to the isthmic inlet maintains the high axial velocity for a longer distance (Fig. 5.4).

During pulsation the velocity profile is continuously changing. That is of particular interest in early pregnancy when the Doppler recording of the ductus venosus is used to identify risk groups of chromosomal aberration. During atrial contraction the velocity may retard to reach the zero line or beyond. Commonly, there may be both positive and negative velocities at the same time (Fig. 5.5, left). Apart from interference of signals from neighboring vessels (umbilical vein or liver), both the negative and positive recordings could be genuine ductus venosus signals representing a transitional change of the velocity profile containing both negative and positive velocities at the same time (Fig. 5.5, right). The degree of such changes depends on the velocity, vessel diameter, viscosity and pulse frequency, and can be predicted by using the Womersley equation [1]; thus, the results of the studies in early pregnancy using the zero or reversed velocity in the ductus venosus recorded during atrial contraction depend on how the velocity is

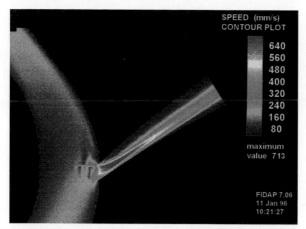

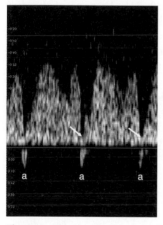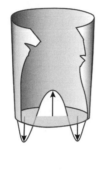

Fig. 5.4. Estimated spatial velocity distribution at the umbilical vein–ductus venosus junction based on a computer model. The velocity increases before the blood has reached the narrow entrance of the ductus venosus. The high axial velocity is maintained for a longer distance compared with the peripheral velocities that are reduced with the growing cross section along the vessel (see also Figs. 5.2, 5.3). (From [32])

Fig. 5.5. Blood velocity recorded at the isthmus of the ductus venosus at 12 weeks of gestation (*left*). During atrial contraction the velocity shows a deflection below the zero line (*a*), but at the same time retaining some antegrade velocity (*arrow*). The reason could be that the velocity profile across the vessel cross section at this moment is transformed and contains both antegrade and retrograde velocities (*right*)

traced and what is actually defined as the minimum velocity during atrial contraction.

Pulsation in Veins

Venous pulsation observed during ultrasound Doppler recording is commonly used for diagnostic purposes. It is a regularly repeated velocity increment or inflection; however, it is worthwhile to keep in mind

that the velocity pulsation of the Doppler recording incompletely describes the pulse wave, excluding such information as variation in volume or cross section, pressure, pulse velocity and direction.

Cardiac Function and Waveform

The waveform of the venous pulse is determined by the function of the heart. Usually there is a systolic peak (during ventricular systole), a diastolic peak (during passive filling of the ventricles) and a diastolic nadir (reflecting the atrial contraction; Fig. 5.6). The more energy put into the pulse, the further out in the system it will reach. That is particularly obvious during atrial contraction. The Frank-Starling mechanism causes an augmented contraction in a distended atrium during fetal bradycardia, and the wave propagating along the veins reflects that. A particularly strong atrial wave is seen in cases of arrhythmia when atria and ventricles happen to beat simultaneously. An augmented atrial wave is also seen in cases with increased afterload and adrenergic drive during hypoxemia [18–23]. Although the atrial contraction wave is the most commonly used sign for cardiac function, there is additional information hidden in the waveform [24, 25].

The smooth systolic peak of the wave of a precordial vein also reflects a normal compliance of the heart. External constricting processes (e.g. high-pressure pleural effusion; Fig. 5.6), particularly a stiffer and less compliant myocardium (e.g. hypoxia, acidosis, cardiomyopathy), gives a quick rise in pressure during systolic filling of the atrium, and a corresponding steep downstroke of velocity resulting in the more pointed systolic peak velocity (Fig. 5.6) [26, 27]. A quick rise in atrial pressure is sometimes caused by a significant tricuspid regurgitation leading to a similar but less acute downstroke during systole.

Reduced compliance of the myocardium is not only reflected in the acute downstroke of the systolic peak but also in the dissociation of the systolic and diastolic peak (Fig. 5.6). The dissociation between the systolic and diastolic peak seems to be a late and ominous sign of myocardial compromise [27, 28].

Transmission Lines

The pulse generated in the heart is not transmitted equally well in all tissues. It travels better along transmission lines, and arteries and veins connected to the heart constitute such transmission lines.

A discontinuation of the transmission line affects the pulse propagation and deprives the venous waveform of its usual details [27, 29]. If the pulmonary vein is not connected to the left atrium but to the portal system, the pulse recorded in the vein no longer reflects

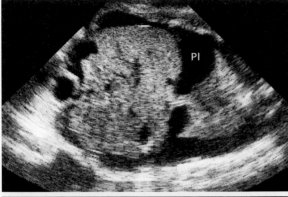

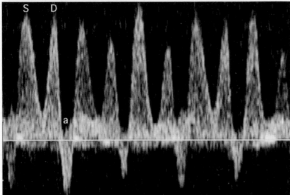

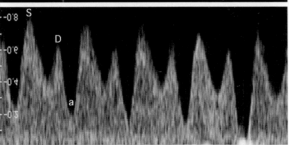

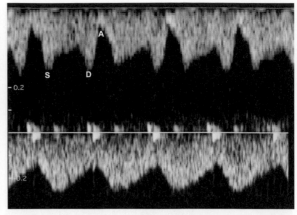

Fig. 5.7. The pressure variation of the left atrium is reflected in the velocity recording of the pulmonary veins (*upper panel*). With the loss of connection the pressure variation is not transmitted into the vein and the velocity pattern reflects instead the general pressure variation in the chest (typical for anomalous pulmonary venous drainage; *lower panel*). *A* atrial contraction wave, *D* diastolic peak, *S* systolic peak. (From [27])

Fig. 5.6. Effect of cardiac compliance on the venous waveform in the ductus venosus. Although a stiff myocardium due to acidosis or hypoxia is the most common cause, in this case it was the fetal pleural effusion (*Pl*) at 30 weeks of gestation (*upper panel*) that had a constrictive effect on the heart. The reduced compliance was reflected in the rapid downstroke of the peak velocity during ventricular systole (*S*) causing the dissociation between S and the diastolic peak (*D; middle panel*). Doppler recording 2 min after the pleural effusion has been drained off (*lower panel*) showed an instantaneous improvement in myocardial compliance (less pointed S and reduced dissociation between S and D), and the end-diastolic pressure was less, signified by the less pronounced atrial contraction wave (*a*)

details of the cardiac events, but rather the general pressure variation of the fetal chest (Fig. 5.7). The Doppler recording thus supports the diagnosis.

Another important transmission line is formed by the inferior vena cava (IVC), ductus venosus and um-

bilical vein (Fig. 5.8a) [30, 31]. Agenesis of the ductus venosus has been shown to interrupt the transmission of the cardiac wave to the umbilical vein [29]. The wave propagating along this line reflects the changes in both the left and the right atrium since the IVC is connected to the left atrium through the foramen ovale in addition to the connection to the right atrium. Conversely, the pulmonary veins reflect predominantly the left atrium, and to some extent the right atrium, depending on the size of the foramen ovale [27].

Wave Reflections

The pulse wave travelling along the transmission line is modified according to the local physical conditions [6, 15, 16, 27, 30, 32–35]. Pulsation at the ductus venosus outlet is more pronounced than at the inlet [36]. The stiffness of the vessel wall is different at the ductus venosus outlet, ductus venosus inlet and intra-abdominal umbilical vein, and so are cross-section and compliance [37]. The single most important mechanism for changing the propagating pulse in the veins is reflections. In much the same fashion as light is reflected or transmitted when the beam encounters a medium with a different density, the pulse wave in the veins is reflected and transmitted when it hits a change in impedance (Fig. 5.8b) [30, 31, 38]. Vascular junctions often represent a significant change in cross section (and thus impedance). The junction between the ductus venosus inlet and the umbilical vein is of great diagnostic interest and has been particularly well examined. During the second half of pregnancy

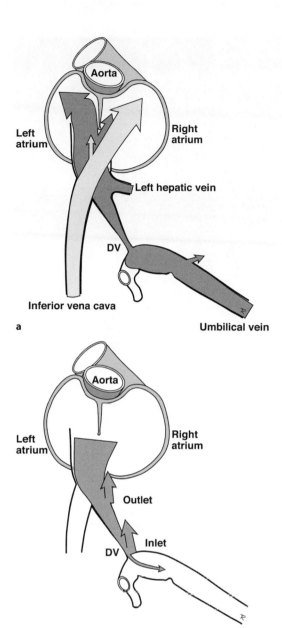

Fig. 5.8. The same veins that direct blood towards the heart (**a**) act as transmission lines for pulse waves generated in the heart. The most studied transmission line is formed by the proximal portion of the inferior vena cava, ductus venosus (*DV*) and the umbilical vein (**b**). The wave is partially reflected at the junctions according to the difference in impedance above and below the junction. Due to the large difference in impedance between the ductus venosus inlet and the intra-abdominal umbilical vein, most of the wave is reflected at this junction. The small wave energy transmitted into the umbilical vein is usually not enough to cause visible velocity pulsation at this site. (From [31], [55])

pulsation is regularly observed at the ductus venosus inlet, but on the other side of the junction, millimeters away, there is no pulsation in the umbilical vein. The reason is reflections [34]. The Reflex coefficient (R_c) determines the degree of reflection and depends on the impedance of the two sections of veins (e.g. Z_{DV}, ductus venosus, and Z_{UV}, umbilical vein):

$$R_c = \frac{\text{Reflected wave}}{\text{Incident wave}} = \frac{Z_{UV} - Z_{DV}}{Z_{UV} + Z_{DV}}$$

In this case, Z_{UV} represents the terminal (distal) impedance in fluid dynamic terms, whereas Z_{DV} represents the characteristic impedance. From a practical point a view, the single most important determinant for impedance is the cross section of the vessel (A):

$$Z = \rho c / A$$

(ρ = density, and c = wave velocity). In the case of the ductus venosus–umbilical vein junction, there is an extraordinary difference in cross section, and thus impedance; the ratio of the diameter of the umbilical vein and the ductus venosus being 4 (95% CI 2; 6) [30]. Correspondingly, most of the wave will be reflected and little energy transmitted further down. The small proportion of the energy transmitted to the umbilical vein is not sufficient to cause visible pulsation. In extreme conditions, such as during hypoxia, the ductus venosus distends [39, 40], and the difference in vessel area between the two sections is reduced, and less wave is reflected and more transmitted (Fig. 5.9a); thus, a larger proportion of the wave arrives in the umbilical vein and may induce pulsation, particularly if the a-wave was augmented in the first place.

In 3% of all recordings there is no pulsation in the ductus venosus, which is a normal phenomenon [41]. The pattern is in many cases caused by the position of the fetus bending forward and thus squeezing the IVC and ductus venosus outlet (Figs. 5.9b, 5.10) [30]. The extensively reduced cross section causes a total reflection of wave at the level of the IVC–ductus venosus junction and hardly any pulse is transmitted further down until the squeeze has been released. A similar effect can probably be obtained by the spontaneous variation in cross section sometimes seen in the proximal portion of the IVC.

Compliance and Reservoir Function of the Umbilical Vein

Another determinant affecting pulsation is the reservoir effect [34]. Whether a pulse that arrives in the umbilical vein induces velocity pulsation depends on the local compliance. The umbilical vein is a sizeable

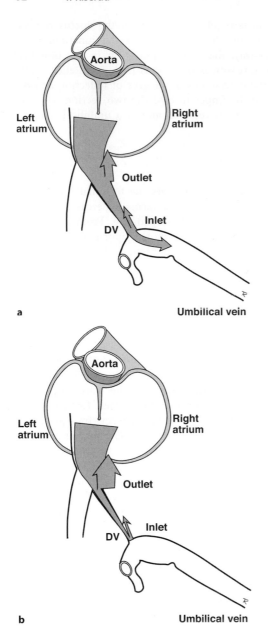

a

b

Fig. 5.9. A distension of the ductus venosus (*DV*) inlet and increased tone in the umbilical vein with reduced diameter reduce the difference of impedance between the two sections. Correspondingly, less reflection and more transmission increase the likelihood that velocity pulsations are observed in the umbilical vein (**a**). When the DV is squeezed right up to the outlet, a larger proportion of the wave is reflected at the level of outlet (**b**) leaving little wave energy to be transmitted further down the transmission line. No pulsation may then be observed at the DV inlet. (From [31])

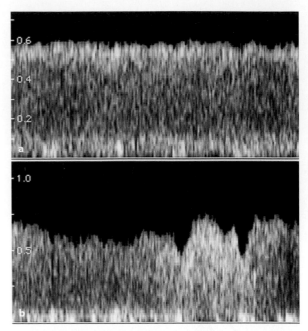

Fig. 5.10. Doppler recording of the ductus venosus blood velocity without pulsation (**a**) due to the fetal position bending forward and squeezing the ductus venosus outlet. The wave has been completely reflected at the junction with the inferior vena cava (see Fig. 9b). Seconds later, a change in fetal position restores the dimension of the vessel and the pulsatile flow pattern (**b**). (From [31])

vessel and acts as a reservoir. The larger and more compliant the reservoir is, the higher wave energy is required to induce a visible pulsation of the blood velocity (Fig. 5.11). Accordingly, pulsation should be a rare event in late pregnancy, whereas the small vascular dimensions in early pregnancy predispose for pulsation. Pulsation in the umbilical vein is a normal phenomenon particularly before 13 weeks of gestation [56]. It follows that an increased tone of the vessel wall (e.g. adrenergic drive, venous congestion) and reduced diameter (e.g. hypovolaemia in fetal hemorrhage) may be accompanied by pulsation in the umbilical vein.

The effect of compliance is particularly well illustrated by the physiological stricture of the umbilical vein at the entrance through the abdominal wall. Once the period of physiological umbilical herniation has been completed at 12 weeks of gestation, there is an increasing tightening of the umbilical ring causing a constricting impact on the vein in quite a few fetuses during the following weeks and months [42–44]. The stricture causes a high velocity, which, interestingly, often pulsates (Fig. 5.12) [45]. Although the pulsation may be a velocity inflection caused by the a-wave, probably a more common waveform would be a smooth increment of velocity caused by the neighboring umbilical arteries. The same phenomenon can be traced in the umbilical cord with increased turgor, angulation or extreme twisting [46]. Another example is the pulsation commonly traced in the left branch

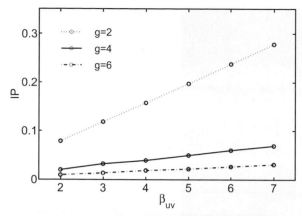

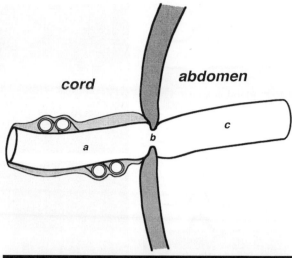

Fig. 5.11. Mathematical model showing how umbilical venous pulsation changes with wall stiffness (β_{UV}), a determinant for compliance. Index of pulsation for the pressure wave (IP=pulse amplitude divided by time-averaged pressure) increases with stiffness. The model also demonstrates the effect of increased diameter ratio between the umbilical vein and ductus venosus ($D_{UV}/D_{DV}=g$) on pressure transmission to the umbilical vein. Increased ratio is associated with less pulsation in the umbilical vein due to increased degree of reflections at the junction. (From [34])

of the fetal portal vein [47, 48]. Compared with the umbilical vein, the left portal branch has a smaller diameter (i.e. compliance), which increases the likelihood for visible pulsation [49].

Direction of Pulse and Blood Velocity

A short velocity deflection of the umbilical venous flow is commonly recognized as the atrial contraction wave; however, pulsations may appear differently and have various causes. Recent research has addressed this part of physiology. One important determinant is the direction of the pulse wave compared with the direction of the blood flow. The concept of wave intensity was introduced to explain the wave in arteries [50], but the concept is equally valid for veins [27, 28, 38]. When the pressure wave travels in the opposite direction of the blood velocity (Fig. 5.13), the pressure wave causes a deflection in the velocity (e.g. atrial contraction wave in the hepatic veins, ductus venosus and umbilical vein); however, if the pressure wave and blood velocity travel in the same direction, the pressure wave will impose a velocity increase (e.g. umbilical artery waveform), an effect also seen in the venous system (e.g. left portal vein; Fig. 5.13).

A particularly instructive example is found at the junction between the ductus venosus and the umbilical vein/portal system (Fig. 5.14) [49]. The pressure wave travels down the ductus venosus in the opposite direction of the blood flow (atrial contraction wave is negative). When the pressure wave enters the umbili-

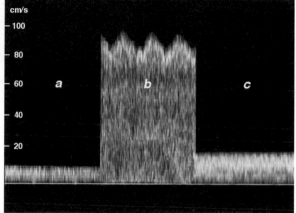

Fig. 5.12. *Upper panel:* The physiological constriction of the umbilical vein at the abdominal inlet (*b*) represents a reduction in compliance compared with the section in the cord (*a*) or intra-abdominal portion (*c*; from [43]). *Lower panel:* High velocity is recorded at the constriction (*b*) compared with outside (*a*) or inside (*c*) the abdominal wall. The pulsation from the neighboring umbilical artery induces velocity pulsation in the vein at the constriction area but not in the neighboring sections where the compliance is higher (*a* and *c*). (From [45])

cal vein it propagates in two directions: down the umbilical vein, or up the left portal vein. In the former case the velocity wave is negative, in the latter it is positive (Figs. 5.13, 5.15). In the compromised fetal circulation the left portal vein also acts as a watershed area between the left and right part of the liver [49]; thus, blood in this section may pendulate or reverse. Depending on the direction of flow in this section, the waveform will turn the same way or be inverted when compared with the umbilical vein pulse.

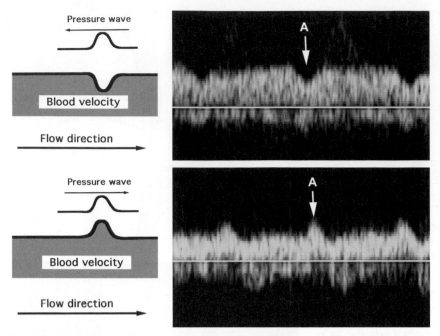

Fig. 5.13. *Upper panel:* When the pressure pulse and velocity travel in *opposite* directions, the resulting velocity change during the pulse will be a deflection. A common example is the atrial contraction wave recorded in the umbilical vein (*A*). *Lower panel:* When the pressure pulse and velocity travel in the *same* direction, the resulting velocity change during the pulse will be an increase. Accordingly, the atrial contraction wave recorded in the left portal vein is recognized as a peak (*A*). For further explanation see Fig. 5.14 and 5.15. (From [28], [49])

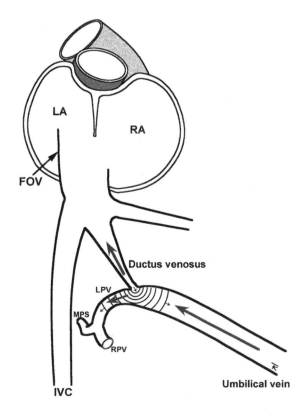

Source of Pulse

Whenever a pulse is generated it will be transmitted into the neighboring structures modified by the local physical conditions. Although the pulse wave commonly carries the "fingerprint" of its source (e.g. cardiac cycle) [20, 21, 51], at some distance such characteristics may have disappeared making the identification of the source less certain. Pulsation in the umbilical vein is of clinical interest if it signifies an augmented atrial contraction that has reached that far out [23, 46, 52–54]; however, the velocity pulse could have been transmitted locally from the umbilical artery, or could have been caused by rapid fetal respiratory movements or any other rhythmic fetal activity.

Fig. 5.14. The pressure pulse emitted from the heart travels along the veins as transmission lines. When the pulse reaches the junction between the ductus venosus inlet and the umbilical vein, the pulse wave continues in two directions: it continues along the umbilical vein *against* the flow direction, or follows the left portal branch (*LPV*) into the liver *with* the flow direction. *FOV* foramen ovale valve, *IVC* inferior vena cava, *LA* left atrium, *MPS* main portal stem, *RA* right atrium, *RPV* right portal branch. (From [49])

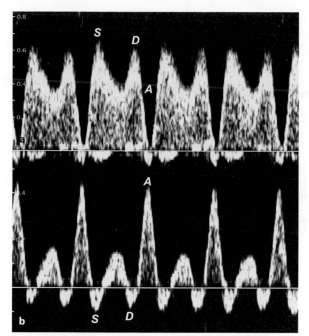

Fig. 5.15. Doppler recording in the ductus venosus (**a**) and the left portal branch (**b**) in a fetus of 25 weeks gestation with placental compromise. For anatomical references see also Fig. 5.14. The ductus venosus recording shows an augmented atrial contraction wave (*A*) reaching the zero line (pulse wave and blood flow have opposite directions). The same wave recorded in the left portal branch is a peak (*A* in **b**) since pulse wave now has the same direction as the blood flow; thus, the entire waveform during the cardiac cycle is found to be reciprocal (mirror image) at the two sites. *D* diastolic peak, *S* systolic peak. (From [49])

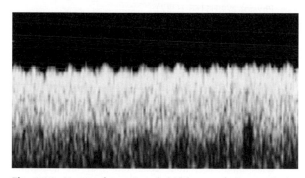

Fig. 5.16. Vortex formation (whirls) recorded as velocity variation, which mimics pulsation, in the umbilical vein. Such whirls tend to occur in large bore vessels with steady velocity, particularly if there is a diameter variation, curvature or bifurcation. The velocity usually does not fit with the heart rate. (From [29])

The vibration of the heart is also transmitted into the liver tissue and beyond and may have impact on the venous flow. Vortices, like whirls in a river, may occur in large veins and cause velocity variation recorded in the Doppler shift (Fig. 5.16). In some cases, infor-

mation on pulse-wave direction, time of the pulse and details of its form does permit the discrimination between sources.

It follows from what is presented in this section that pulsatile venous flow, both in precordial veins and in peripheral veins, such as the umbilical vein and intracranial veins, is determined by cardiac function *and* the local physical properties of the vasculature. All determinants vary with gestational age. Unless these facts are taken into account, we shall not be able to use the diagnostic techniques of venous Doppler recordings to their full potential, but face a commonly occurring risk of misinterpretation.

References

1. Nichols WW, O'Rourke MF (1998) McDonald's blood flow in arteries. Theoretical, experimental and clinical principles. Arnold, London, p 564
2. Burns PN (1995) Hemodynamics. In: Taylor KJW, Burns PN, Wells PNT (eds) Clinical applications of Doppler ultrasound. Raven Press, New York, pp 35–44
3. Fung YC (1984) Biodynamics. Springer, Berlin Heidelberg New York
4. Fung YC (1984) Biomechanics. Springer, Berlin Heidelberg New York
5. Fung YC (1993) Biomechanics. Springer, Berlin Heidelberg New York
6. Pennati G, Bellotti M, Gasperi C de, Rognoni G (2004) Spatial velocity profile changes along the cord in normal human fetuses: can these affect Doppler measurements of venous umbilical blood flow? Ultrasound Obstet Gynecol 23:131–137
7. Gill RW (1979) Pulsed Doppler with B-mode imaging for quantitative blood flow measurement. Ultrasound Med Biol 5:223–235
8. Eik-Nes SH, Maršál K, Brubakk AO, Ulstein M (1980) Ultrasonic measurements of human fetal blood flow in aorta and umbilical vein: Influence of fetal breathing movements. In: Kurjak A (ed) Recent advances in ultrasound diagnosis. Proceedings of the International Symposium on Recent Advances in Ultrasound Diagnosis, vol 2. Excerpta Medica, Amsterdam, pp 233–240
9. Jouppila P, Kirkinen P, Puukka R (1986) Correlation between umbilical vein blood flow and umbilical blood viscosity in normal and complicated pregnancies. Arch Gynecol 237:191–197
10. Kiserud T, Eik-Nes SH, Blaas H-G, Hellevik LR, Simensen B (1994) Ductus venosus blood velocity and the umbilical circulation in the seriously growth retarded fetus. Ultrasound Obstet Gynecol 4:109–114
11. Tchirikov M, Rybakowski C, Hünecke B, Schröder HJ (1998) Blood flow through the ductus venosus in singleton and multifetal pregnancies and in fetuses with intrauterine growth retardation. Am J Obstet Gynecol 178:943–949
12. Kiserud T, Rasmussen S, Skulstad SM (2000) Blood flow and degree of shunting through the ductus venosus in the human fetus. Am J Obstet Gynecol 182:147–153
13. Bellotti M, Pennati G, Gasperi C de, Battaglia FC, Ferrazzi E (2000) Role of ductus venosus in distribution

of umbilical flow in human fetuses during second half of pregnancy. Am J Physiol 279:H1256–1263

14. Barbera A, Galan HL, Ferrazzi E, Rigano S, Józwik M, Pardi G (1999) Relationship of umbilical vein blood flow to growth parameters in the human fetus. Am J Obstet Gynecol 181:174–179

15. Pennati G, Redaelli A, Bellotti M, Ferrazzi E (1996) Computational analysis of the ductus venosus fluid dynamics based on Doppler measurements. Ultrasound Med Biol 22:1017–1029

16. Pennati G, Bellotti M, Ferrazzi E, Bozzo M, Pardi G, Fumero R (1998) Blood flow through the ductus venosus in human fetuses: calculation using Doppler velocimetry and computational findings. Ultrasound Med Biol 24:477–487

17. Kiserud T, Hellevik LR, Hanson MA (1998) The blood velocity profile in the ductus venosus inlet expressed by the mean/maximum velocity ratio. Ultrasound Med Biol 24:1301–1306

18. Reuss ML, Rudolph AM, Dae MW (1983) Phasic blood flow patterns in the superior and inferior venae cavae and umbilical vein of fetal sheep. Am J Obstet Gynecol 145:70–76

19. Hasaart TH, de Haan J (1986) Phasic blood flow patterns in the common umbilical vein of fetal sheep during umbilical cord occlusion and the influence of autonomic nervous system blockade. J Perinat Med 14:19–26

20. Reed KL, Appleton CP, Anderson CF, Shenker L, Sahn DJ (1990) Doppler studies of vena cava flows in human fetuses; insights into normal and abnormal cardiac physiology. Circulation 81:498–505

21. Kanzaki T, Chiba Y (1990) Evaluation of the preload condition of the fetus by inferior vena caval blood flow pattern. Fetal Diagn Ther 5:168–174

22. Kiserud T, Jauniaux E, West D, Ozturk O, Hanson MA (2001) Circulatory responses to acute maternal hyperoxaemia and hypoxaemia assessed non-invasively by ultrasound in fetal sheep at 0.3–0.5 gestation. Br J Obstet Gynaecol 108:359–364

23. Gudmundsson S, Gunnarsson G, Hökegård K-H, Ingmarsson J, Kjellmer I (1999) Venous Doppler velocimetry in relationship to central venous pressure and heart rate during hypoxia in ovine fetus. J Perinat Med 27:81–90

24. Huhta JC (1997) Deciphering the hieroglyphics of venous Doppler velocities. Ultrasound Obstet Gynecol 9:300–301

25. Kiserud T (1997) In a different vein: the ductus venosus could yield much valuable information. Ultrasound Obstet Gynecol 9:369–372

26. Kiserud T (2001) The ductus venosus. Semin Perinatol 25:11–20

27. Kiserud T (2003) The fetal venous circulation. Fetal Maternal Med Rev 14:57–97

28. Kiserud T (2003) Venous flow in IUGR and cardiac decompensation. In: Yagel S, Gembruch U, Silverman N (eds) Fetal cardiology. Dunitz, London, pp 541–551

29. Kiserud T, Crowe C, Hanson M (1998) Ductus venosus agenesis prevents transmission of central venous pulsations to the umbilical vein in the fetal sheep. Ultrasound Obstet Gynecol 11:190–194

30. Kiserud T (1999) Hemodynamics of the ductus venosus. Eur J Obstet Gynecol Reprod Biol 84:139–147

31. Kiserud T (2000) Fetal venous circulation: an update on hemodynamics. J Perinat Med 28:90–96

32. Pennati G, Bellotti M, Ferrazzi E, Rigano S, Garberi A (1997) Hemodynamic changes across the human ductus venosus: a comparison between clinical findings and mathematical calculations. Ultrasound Obstet Gynecol 9:383–391

33. Hellevik LR, Kiserud T, Irgens F, Ytrehus T, Eik-Nes SH (1998) Simulation of pressure drop and energy dissipation for blood flow in a human fetal bifurcation. ASME J Biomech Eng 120:455–462

34. Hellevik LR, Stergiopulos N, Kiserud T, Rabben SI, Eik-Nes SH, Irgens F (2000) A mathematical model of umbilical venous pulsation. J Biomech 33:1123–1130

35. Hellevik LR (1999) Wave propagation and pressure drop in precordial veins. Department of Applied Mechanics, Thermodynamics and Fluid Dynamics. Norwegian University of Science and Technology, Trondheim

36. Acharya G, Kiserud T (1999) Ductus venosus blood velocity and diameter pulsations are more prominent at the outlet than at the inlet. Eur J Obstet Gynecol Reprod Biol 84:149–154

37. Hellevik LR, Kiserud T, Irgens F, Stergiopulos N, Hanson M (1998) Mechanical properties of the fetal ductus venosus and umbilical vein. Heart Vessels 13:175–180

38. Hellevik LR, Segers P, Stergiopulos N et al. (1999) Mechanism of pulmonary venous pressure and flow waves. Heart Vessels 14:67–71

39. Bellotti M, Pennati G, Pardi G, Fumero R (1998) Dilatation of the ductus venosus in human fetuses: ultrasonographic evidence and mathematical modeling. Am J Physiol 275 (Heart Circ Physiol 44):H1759–H1767

40. Kiserud T, Ozaki T, Nishina H, Rodeck C, Hanson MA (2000) Effect of NO, phenylephrine and hypoxemia on the ductus venosus diameter in the fetal sheep. Am J Physiol 279:H1166–H1171

41. Kiserud T, Eik-Nes SH, Hellevik LR, Blaas H-G (1992) Ductus venosus: a longitudinal doppler velocimetric study of the human fetus. J Matern Fetal Invest 2:5–11

42. Kilavuz Ö, Vetter K (1998) The umbilcal ring: the first rapid in the fetoplacental venous system. J Perinat Med 26:120–122

43. Skulstad SM, Rasmussen S, Iversen O-E, Kiserud T (2001) The development of high venous velocity at the fetal umbilical ring during gestational weeks 11–19. Br J Obstet Gynaecol 108:248–253

44. Skulstad SM, Kiserud T, Rasmussen S (2002) Degree of fetal umbilical venous constriction at the abdominal wall in a low risk population at 20–40 weeks of gestation. Prenat Diagn 22:1022–1027

45. Skulstad SM, Kiserud T, Rasmussen S (2004) The effect of vascular constriction on umbilical venous pulsation. Ultrasound Obstet Gynecol 23:126–130

46. Nakai Y, Imanaka M, Nishio J, Ogita S (1997) Umbilical venous pulsation associated with hypercoiled cord in growth-retarded fetuses. Gynecol Obstet Invest 43:6–7

47. Mari G, Uerpairojkit B, Copel JA (1995) Abdominal venous system in the normal fetus. Obstet Gynecol 86:729–733

48. van Splunder IP, Huisman TWA, Stijnen T, Wladimiroff JW (1994) Presence of pulsations and reproducibility of

waveform recording in the umbilical and left portal vein in normal pregnancies. Ultrasound Obstet Gynecol 4:49–53

49. Kiserud T, Kilavuz Ö, Hellevik LR (2003) Venous pulsation in the left portal branch: the effect of pulse and flow direction. Ultrasound Obstet Gynecol 21:359–364

50. Parker KH, Jones CJH (1990) Forward and backward running waves in the arteries: analysis using the method of characteristics. ASME J Biomech Eng 112:322–326

51. Schröder HJ, Tchirikov M, Rybakowski C (2002) Pressure pulses and flow velocity in central veins of anesthetized sheep fetus. Am J Physiol Heart Circ Physiol 284:H1205–H1211

52. Lingman G, Laurin J, Maršál K, Persson P-H (1986) Circulatory changes in fetuses with imminent asphyxia. Biol Neonate 49:66–73

53. Gudmundsson S, Huhta JC, Wood DC, Tulzer G, Cohen AW, Weiner S (1991) Venous Doppler ultrasonography in the fetus with nonimmune hydrops. Am J Obstet Gynecol 164:33–37

54. Nakai Y, Miyazaki Y, Matsuoka Y, Matsumoto M, Imanaka M, Ogita S (1992) Pulsatile umbilical venous flow and its clinical significance. Br J Obstet Gynaecol 99:977–980

55. Kiserud T, Rasmussen S (2001) Ultrasound assessment of the fetal foramen ovale. Ultrasound Obstet Gynecol 17:119–124

56. Rizzo G, Arduini D, Romanini C (1992) Umbilical vein pulsation: a physiological finding in early gestation. Am J Obstet Gynecol 167:675–677

Chapter 6

Sonographic Color Flow Mapping: Basic Principles

Dev Maulik

Color flow mapping consists of real-time depiction of two-dimensional flow patterns superimposed on cross-sectional pulse echo images of anatomic structures [1–3]. The flow patterns are color-coded to present a variety of hemodynamic information. Doppler color flow mapping is based on the estimation of mean Doppler-shifted frequency and does not provide information on peak frequency shift or actual flow. Furthermore, the hemodynamic information provided is qualitative rather than quantitative. Nevertheless, color flow mapping has proved useful for elucidating structural and functional abnormalities of the circulatory system. The technique was first introduced in cardiology practice and has revolutionized noninvasive diagnosis of cardiac pathology. The use of this method has since been extended to other medical disciplines. In obstetrics and gynecology, color flow mapping has been used to investigate fetal and maternal hemodynamics during pregnancy and pelvic vessels in non-pregnant women. Color flow has been found to be useful for elucidating complex cardiac malformations of the fetus, directing spectral Doppler interrogation of fetal cerebral, renal, and other circulations, diagnosing ectopic pregnancy, and assessing pelvic tumor vascularity. It should be recognized, however, that the information generated by Doppler color flow mapping is significantly influenced by the instrumental setting and characteristics. The reliability of the method thus depends on the appropriate use of the device by the operator, who should have a clear understanding of the basic principles of Doppler color flow mapping and its implementation.

In this chapter we describe the basic principles, instrumentation, and limitations of Doppler color flow mapping and present practical guidelines for its use. We also discuss an alternative sonographic color flow mapping technique based on the time domain processing analysis.

Principles of Doppler Color Flow Mapping

Multigated Doppler Interrogation

Doppler color flow mapping is based on multigated sampling of multiple scan lines using bursts of short pulses of ultrasound (Fig. 6.1). Many range-gated samples are obtained for each emitted pulse of ultrasound along a single scan line by opening the receiving gate sequentially to the echo signals arriving from various depths along the scan line. The time needed for the return journey of the echo is used to determine the spatial origin of the returning echoes. Assuming a sound propagation speed of 1,540 m/s in tissue, the echo return time for an emitted sound pulse in 13 ms/cm of tissue depth. Thus a signal from a depth of 5 cm takes 65 ms from the moment of transmission to its return to the transducer. If the second sample is to be obtained from a depth of 10 cm, the range gate is opened at 65 ms after reception of the first sample (130 ms after transmission of the pulse). In reality, many samples are collected, and the consecutive sampling of the signals along the

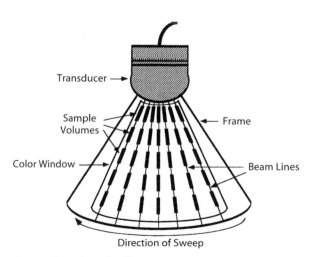

Fig. 6.1. Doppler color flow mapping. Multigated sampling of multiple scan lines sweeping across the field of color Doppler interrogation

scan line is timed according to the depth of the sampling location.

Each returning echo is referenced to its range gate, which identifies it with the spatial location of its origin, and is electronically stored using delay circuitry. After all the echoes from the first pulse are received, a second pulse in phase with the first pulse is sent along the same scan line. Appropriate timing of the pulse repetition is a critical consideration for pulsed Doppler, as transmission of a pulse before the return of the echoes from the previous pulse causes range ambiguity (see Chap. 3). With two-dimensional Doppler color flow mapping, range ambiguity is not permissible. The backscattered echo signals of the second pulse are collected from range locations identical to those of the first pulse and are referenced to their respective range gates. To determine the mean Doppler shift, each echo signal from each pulse sampled from a given range gate is compared with that from the previous pulse sampled from the same gate. Because an enormous amount of samples are collected, the comprehensive spectral processing techniques (see Chap. 3) cannot be implemented in Doppler color flow mapping. Instead, the autocorrelation technique is utilized to obtain the mean Doppler phase shift (see below).

Each scan line is repeatedly sampled using multiple pulses. The latter ranges from 3 to 32, although usually 8–10 pulses are used. The signals from the identical range gates are collected and compared to obtain mean Doppler shifts, which are averaged for each gate. The number of pulses per scan line is called the *ensemble length* (Fig. 6.2). There are several reasons for this repeated sampling of a single scan line. The most important is the fact that blood flow is a continuously changing phenomenon, and the duration of each pulse in Doppler color flow mapping is too short (<2 ms) to provide an acceptable mean

value. As the number of pulses per scan line is increased, the quality of flow information improves in terms of reliability and completeness. Another distinct advantage of increasing the samples is the enhancement of Doppler sensitivity to detect low-velocity circulations. This ability may be useful for gynecologic applications, specifically for detecting ovarian, uterine, or tumor blood flow, where it is more important to detect flow than to be concerned with the temporal resolution. Moreover, as the samples are repeated and averaged against a constant background of noise, the signal-to-noise ratio improves. Multiple sampling also contributes to stabilization of the highpass filter.

Once sampling of a scan line is completed, the next scan line is interrogated in the same manner as described above. The color flow map is completed by multiple scan lines sweeping across the imaging field (Fig. 6.1).

Color Doppler Signal Analysis

Multigated sampling of multiple scan lines of the color flow imaging field generates an enormous amount of data. Color flow mapping requires real-time processing and display of these data. The demands of processing such a vast flow of information cannot be met by the currently available comprehensive spectral analytic techniques, such as fast Fourier transform (see Chap. 3). For example, during the time the Fourier spectral analyzer processes signals from one sample volume, thousands of samples must be processed for color flow mapping. Obviously, color flow mapping requires an alternative approach for Doppler signal analyses [4, 5], which is usually achieved by the autocorrelation technique (Fig. 6.3), which generates mean Doppler shift information, rather than the comprehensive power spectral data generated by full spectral processing. It is important to note that the autocorrelation method does not estimate the peak frequency shift.

The mean Doppler shift is based on phase differences between the echoes generated from consecutive sound pulses transmitted in the same direction and sampled from the same location. *Phase* is defined in physics as a specific degree of progression of a cyclic phenomenon. When two waves are in step, they are in phase. The movement of the scatterer during the elapsed time between the two consecutive pulses causes the resulting echoes to be out of step or phase. The autocorrelator measures this phase difference by multiplying the successive signals. The mean Doppler shift is related to the phase difference, as shown in the following equation:

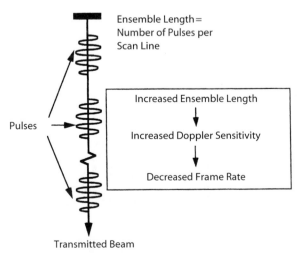

Fig. 6.2. Concept of ensemble length

$$\varphi = 360° \times MF_d/PRF$$

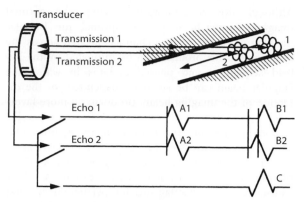

Fig. 6.3. Principle of two-dimensional Doppler signal analysis. During the first ultrasound transmission, the stationary tissue objects and the moving erythrocytes generated echoes (*A1* and *B1*, respectively). During the second transmission echoes are produced again (*A2* and *B2*, respectively). Note that the echoes from the stationary objects remain the same (*A1* and *A2*), whereas those originating from the moving objects (*B1* and *B2*) differ. Correlating the first echo with the next echo cancels the signals from the stationary targets and identifies the signals from the moving scatterers (*C*). This process is repeated with the successive echoes from moving targets to estimate the mean Doppler frequency shift in real time

where φ is the phase angle, MF_d is the mean Doppler frequency shift, and PRF is the pulse repetition frequency. The autocorrelation is achieved by electronically delaying an echo signal, which is then processed with the subsequent echo signal (see above).

Table 6.1. Ultrasound modalities in current diagnostic devices

Two-dimensional real-time gray scale imaging
M-mode
Spectral Doppler
Doppler color flow mapping
Color flow M-mode
Doppler color flow amplitude (power or energy) mode

Instrumentation

The instrumentation for two-dimensional Doppler color mapping consists of multiplex systems that combine multiple ultrasound modalities, providing a comprehensive array of sophisticated diagnostic tools (Table 6.1). It is not surprising that the technology employed in these devices is highly complex, especially in the Doppler color mode. In addition, commercially available devices not only demonstrate a fair degree of diversity in the engineering implementation of the Doppler technology they also differ in the organization and the choice of system controls they offer to the operator. Although a comprehensive discussion is beyond the scope of this chapter, we present here the basic principles of Doppler color flow instrumentation.

Color Flow Processor

The basic components of a color flow signal processing system consist of the following (Fig. 6.4):

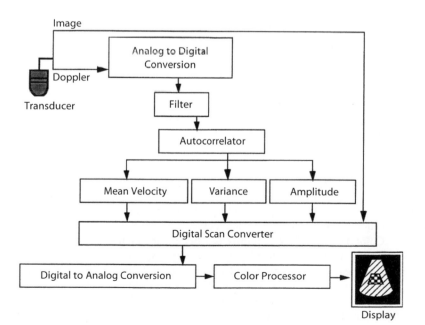

Fig. 6.4. Doppler color flow signal processing system

1. Transducer for transmitting the ultrasound beam and receiving the echoes for both imaging and Doppler analysis.

2. Receiver, which receives and amplifies the incoming signals from the transducer for further processing for gray-scale tissue imaging and for Doppler color flow mapping.

3. Echo information for tissue imaging is processed and converted to digital format. It is stored in the digital scan converter for subsequent integration with color flow mapping.

4. Backscattered echoes for Doppler processing are first converted from analog (electrical voltage variations) data to numeric or digital data.

5. Digitized signals are then subjected to filtering to remove noise generated by stationary and slow-moving tissue structures. The filter is known as the moving target indicator.

6. Filtered data are then analyzed by the autocorrelator to determine the Doppler phase shift. The autocorrelator output consists of three types of information: Doppler mean frequency shift, variance, and Doppler amplitude (power or energy). These data are fed to the digital scan converter, where they are integrated with the tissue image information.

7. Doppler-related data are color-coded by the color processor and the combined gray-scale tissue image, and the Doppler color map is sent to the video display via digital-to-analog conversion.

The above description is only a general outline. The implementation of color Doppler sonography involves highly complex technology and proprietary engineering innovations – information not accessible in the public domain.

Transducers for Doppler Color Flow Mapping

The various types of duplex transducer are discussed in Chap. 3. Among them electronic array systems are used in most devices for color flow mapping. Mechanical transducers do not offer as optimal a platform for Doppler color flow implementation as does simultaneous tissue imaging and Doppler interrogation; and other advanced features, such as beam steering cannot be performed with these transducers. With these devices one must freeze the tissue image before using the Doppler mode. These limitations preclude their use for obstetric Doppler sonography.

Color Doppler flow mapping has been implemented using linear sequenced array, convex sequenced array, linear phased array, and annular phased array transducers. In a linear sequenced array transducer, the scan lines are perpendicular along the length of the transducer face, producing a rectangular field.

Although this configuration provides the optimal imaging approach, it is not optimal for Doppler imaging of vessels or flow channels located across the beam path. This problem can be mitigated by the hybrid sequenced and phased systems in which the Doppler beam can be steered independent of the direction of the imaging beam, producing a more favorable angle of insonation. As all scan lines are parallel to one another, they incur the same angle with a given flow axis. Beam steering reduces the effective aperture and increases the beam thickness; it may compromise the sensitivity and lateral resolution. These transducers are advantageous for peripheral vascular imaging, but they are not particularly useful for obstetric or gynecologic applications.

A modification of the linear sequence design, the convex sequenced array offers distinct advantages over the previous design for obstetric scanning because of its smaller footprint. It also offers a wider field of imaging at depth, and the wider field of view is achieved without the grating lobe problem of the linear phased array. The angle of Doppler insonation is better achieved in the convex than in the linear array despite some of the disadvantages of the former, as previously discussed.

The linear phased array offers a sector-shaped field of image and is useful for cardiologic applications. These transducers, however, are not optimal for fetal imaging applications. They do not provide the wide angle of view at depth and may produce side lobe problems, resulting in spurious flow depiction. Annular array transducers are seldom used for color flow obstetric applications.

Color Mapping

Color flow mapping is based on color-encoding each pixel representing the averaged mean Doppler shift. The color is used to represent the direction, magnitude, and flow characteristics of the sampled circulation. These parameters are qualitative rather than quantitative. The color scheme is based on color classification, which is derived from the fundamental properties of light perception composed of hue, luminance, and saturation.

Color Classification

Hue is the property of light by which the color of an object is classified as the primary colors of red, blue, green, or yellow in reference to the light spectrum. The basic classification is based on the presence or absence of hue. Those colors with hue are termed chromatic colors and include red, orange, yellow, green, blue, and so on. Those without hue are called achromatic colors and include black, gray, and white. The chromatic colors are further classified into groups according to their hue. All hues of red are grouped together, all blues are together, and so on, resulting in a continuous circle of overlapping hues. The human eye is incapable of differentiating between two superimposed primary hues, which led to the discovery that it was possible to produce any given color using a combination of three primary colors. The selection of the three primary hues is arbitrary. Red, blue, and green colors are used in color video displays, including color flow mapping, whereas artists use red, blue, and yellow pigments as their three primary colors.

The next characteristic of light for color classification is *luminance*, which is the brightness: Some of the chromatic colors of a single hue are darker or lighter than others, analogous to the degrees of gray of the achromatic colors. This classification is known as luminance or brightness.

The third property for color grouping is *saturation*, which indicates the combination of a hue of particular brilliance with an achromatic color of the same brightness. The consequent light stimulus depends on the relative amount of the chromatic and achromatic components in which the latter has 0 saturation and the former has a saturation value between 0 and 1.0.

Color Perception

Color is the perception generated by the stimulus of light falling on the retina of the human eye. The eye can distinguish a wide range of gradations of hue and saturation. In contrast, the ability to differentiate various grades of luminance is relatively limited. Therefore refined appreciation of color maps is achieved better with hue and saturation than with luminance. Hues with higher luminance are better perceived by older observers.

In regard to the impact of color blindness on a diagnostician's ability to assess color flow mapping, it should be recognized that about 8.0% of men and fewer than 0.5% of women suffer from varying degrees of deficiency of color perception. Total absence of color vision is rare. Anomalopia is partial color blindness, in which both red and green are poorly recognized. Most color-blind persons find it easier to recognize saturation characteristics of a color flow map because saturation involves mixing of achromatic colors with chromatic hues.

Color Encoding of Doppler Flow Signals

Hemodynamic attributes of the interrogated blood flow are expressed by color encoding of the mean Doppler shift signals. These attributes are the direction of flow in relation to the transducer, the magnitude of velocity, variance of the measured mean parameter (mean Doppler shift), and the amount of scattering power (the amplitude or energy or power of the Doppler shift).

Color Mapping of Direction of Flow

The directionality of flow in relation to the transducer is depicted in the primary colors of red and blue. With most Doppler color flow systems, the default mode depicts the flow toward the transducer as red and the flow away as blue.

Color Mapping of Velocity and the Color Bar

The magnitude of the flow velocity is qualitatively expressed by assigning levels of luminance to the primary hue. The highest velocity flow is depicted by the most luminance and the lowest velocity by the least luminance or black. The highest measurable velocity toward the transducer is shown in the most brilliant red, and the highest measurable velocity away from the transducer in the most brilliant blue. The highest limit of the velocity unambiguously measurable by a Doppler color flow mapping system, based on the pulse Doppler interrogation, is the *Nyquist limit*. As noted before (see Chap. 3), this limit depends on pulse repetition frequency and the depth of Doppler interrogation. The lowest measurable velocity in a color flow mapping device depends on a multiplicity of factors and varies from device to device.

The calibration of the velocity magnitude as a function of luminance gradation is displayed graphically on the video screen as a color bar or circle (Fig. 6.5). It is customary to display the magnitude of the Doppler shift on the vertical axis and the variance (see below) on the horizontal axis. The Doppler shift may be displayed as either frequency or velocity. The velocity information is merely an approximation, as the Doppler angle of insonation is not measurable in color flow mapping. For color flow mapping, it is usually assumed that this angle is zero. The scales are not quantitative, and a particular level of luminance does not reflect a specific single value of Doppler shift but, rather, a range of values. In addition, the color bars of the devices do not have any uniformity of scale for depicting the magnitude of Doppler shift, as the corresponding levels of brightness are assigned arbitrarily and on a nonlinear scale. The baseline, which indicates zero frequency shift, divides the color bar into positive and negative frequency shifts. The baseline is indicated as a black band on the color bar,

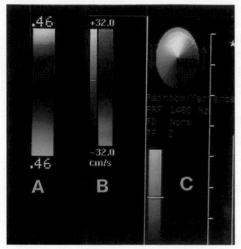

Fig. 6.5. Examples of color indicators from three ultrasound devices (*A, B, C*). The *first two panels* show the color velocity information in the form of a color bar. The flow toward the transducer is encoded in *red*, and flow away from the transducer is encoded in *blue*. The baseline is the *black band* between the two colors. Its vertical dimension varies with the magnitude of the wall filter. The magnitude of velocity is indicated by the brightness of colors, which progressively increases toward the upper and lower ends of the color bar. The magnitude of the velocity is indicated either as Doppler frequency shift (kilohertz) or as velocity (centimeters per second). The *third panel* (*C*) represents the Doppler information as a *color circle*, with the color flow directionality indicated by *arrows*. The color coding in this example is the same as that in the previous examples. The variance information is indicated by the additional mixing of color in the horizontal axis. Examples B and C also include indicators for gray-scale imaging priority

and its location can be adjusted to vary the proportion of positive or negative shifts. The vertical measure of the baseline is variable and reflects the magnitude of the wall filter.

Despite its qualitative nature, the velocity information provided by color flow mapping is of significant clinical utility. Identification of different vessels traversing in close proximity may be facilitated by the luminance and hue of the color display, with the former indicating velocity magnitude and the latter providing directional information. For example, with fetal echocardiography ascending aortic and pulmonary trunk systems can be distinguished and their "crossover" spatial relationship confidently established with the assistance of color flow mapping (see Chap. 32). This information helps to exclude various outflow tract malformations, such as the transposition of great vessels or the common outflow tract. Although this diagnostic information may be obtained through two-dimensional gray-scale imaging alone, addition of color flow mapping significantly augments the diagnostic efficacy. Similarly, the technique eases iden-

tification of the ductus arteriosus, noting the directionality of flow in conjunction with brightness of color because of a high ductal flow velocity. Often the ductal flow velocity exceeds the Nyquist limit so aliasing can be observed, which also assists the process of identification.

Color Mapping of Variance

Variance is statistically defined as a measure of dispersion of the values around the mean. As discussed above, color flow mapping is based on the estimation of mean Doppler shift calculated by autocorrelation from the phase difference between consecutive echo signals. Variance in color flow mapping is the spread of the mean Doppler shift value and is determined statistically by the autocorrelator. Variance information is displayed only when the value exceeds a certain threshold and is achieved by changing the hue. With most devices this change consists in adding green to the primary color. If the flow is toward the transducer, mixing of green with red results in yellow. If the flow is away, addition of green to blue results in cyan color. In either situation, the brightness of the mixed color is determined by the luminance of the primary hue.

The presence of variance above the threshold value may indicate spectral broadening caused by flow turbulence. However, the variance display may also be activated in a nonturbulent flow by variations in the flow velocity. In addition, if the flow velocity exceeds the Nyquist threshold, consequent aliasing may produce mosaic patterns in the color display that may be misinterpreted as turbulent flow.

Formation of a Color Frame

A color frame is a single complete cross-sectional display of a two-dimensional color flow map superimposed on a gray-scale image of the tissue structures produced by one complete sweep of the ultrasound beam. Obviously, there are two primary components of such a frame: the color flow map and the gray-scale image.

Two-Dimensional Color Frame Formation

The color flow map is generated by the multigated interrogation of multiple scan lines sweeping across the target field as discussed above. A two-dimensional B-scan tissue image is formed by pulse echo interrogation of the same scan lines. There are various procedures for achieving this image:

1. Imaging and flow information are sampled from each scan line synchronously and collated in the digi-

tal scan converter. When both imaging and flow mapping fields are completely scanned, the completed frame is displayed with the flow image superimposed on the tissue image.

2. Imaging and flow data are synchronously sampled for each line similar to the previous approach but are displayed sequentially as each line is interrogated rather than when a complete frame is formed.

3. Scanning for tissue imaging is performed first followed by scanning for flow. Flow information is then superimposed on the tissue image.

The composite image frames generated by the above methods are remarkably similar, although there are differences related to the superimposition technique that may compromise the ease of visual perception or interpretation of the hemodynamic information. For example, separate frame formations for the tissue and color flow images may produce a hemodynamically incoherent appearance. Similarly, line-by-line sequential image formation may lead to mixing of consecutive individual frame components, which is seen during frame-by-frame review of the images stored in the memory.

It should be noted that whereas only one pulse per scan line is sufficient for tissue imaging, 3–32 pulses are needed for color Doppler imaging – which is therefore a more time-consuming process. One way to minimize the demand on time is to restrict Doppler flow sampling to an area smaller than the total available field. This color window is superimposed on the gray-scale tissue image, and its size can be manipulated by the operator. A small color window improves Doppler sensitivity and temporal resolution. Therefore it is advisable to restrict the size of this window to the area of interest for Doppler interrogation.

Persistence

Interpolation algorithms may be used to produce temporal averaging of color Doppler information. The process of averaging is known as *persistence*, as it allows more prolonged display or lingering of the color image. It produces a smoother color Doppler image at the cost of losing some detail. Most devices allow selection of different degrees of averaging or persistence. As the color Doppler image remains displayed longer with a higher persistence setting, areas of circulation with a lower flow velocity become more visible in the color map. The application of persistence control may therefore be useful when color mapping such slow-flow conditions as are encountered in the ovarian, placental, and fetal splanchnic circulations. Similarly, as the blood flow velocity declines near the vessel wall because of viscous drag, persistence may produce a more complete outline of a vascular image.

Frame Rate

Frame rate is the number of image frames produced per second. For Doppler color flow mapping, the rate varies from 10 to 60 frames per second. As discussed above, Doppler color flow interrogation places great demand on time. The frame rate (FR) is directly affected by the pulse repetition frequency (PRF); it is inversely influenced by the scan line density (SLD) in the color field and the number of pulses per scan line or the ensemble length (EL):

$$FR = PRF/(SLD \cdot EL)$$

Therefore the frame rate of color imaging can be changed by manipulating these factors, which, however, alters other imaging parameters due to their interdependence. For example, a higher frame rate can be achieved by increasing the PRF, which also limits the depth of interrogation. Similarly, a reduction in the line density not only increases the frame rate, it compromises the spatial resolution; a decline in the number of samples per line also reduces the Doppler sensitivity. These trade-offs should be taken into consideration when ensuring optimal color imaging for a given situation. Thus a low frame rate improves image quality by producing better sensitivity and spatial resolution. Slow flows are better detected with a low frame rate. The latter also allows more effective high-pass filtering, which results in more effective elimination of motion artifacts, such as ghosting. A low frame rate decreases temporal resolution, however, so asynchronous events may be displayed in the same frame. As expected, the problem becomes worse with a high heart rate, as observed in the fetus. A high frame rate improves the temporal resolution, provided the line density and number of pulses per scan line remain adequate to maintain an acceptable spatial resolution and Doppler sensitivity, respectively.

M-Mode Color Frame Formation

In Doppler color M-mode, multigated Doppler sampling is performed on a single scan line sampled 1,000 times per second. The unidimensional tissue and color flow images are scrolled (usually from right to left on the video screen) and therefore are displayed as a function of time (Fig. 6.6). In the time-motion format, the vertical axis represents tissue depth, and the horizontal axis represents time. As with gray-scale M-mode insonation, the spatial location of the beam path is ascertained using two-dimensional color flow imaging. Because of the high sampling rate from a single line, color M-mode insonation provide high Doppler sensitivity and temporal resolution, and it allows reliable timing of the flow

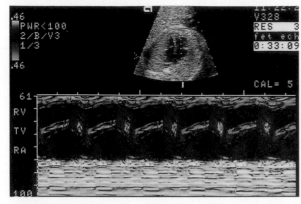

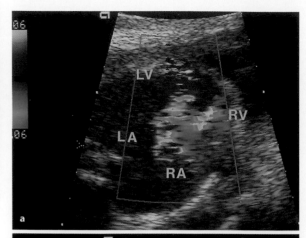

Fig. 6.6. Color M-mode sonogram. *Top*: Two-dimensional color Doppler echocardiogram of the fetal heart (four-chamber view). M-mode cursor is indicated by the *dotted line*. *Bottom*: Color M-mode tracing of flow from the right atrium (*RA*) to the right ventricle (*RV*) across the tricuspid orifice. The movement of the tricuspid valve (*TV*) is visible in the *middle* of the panel. As the flow is toward the transducer, it is coded *red*. Note the aliasing at the tricuspid orifice level (*blue* and *yellow*)

with the events of the cardiac cycle. For this reason, color M-mode sonography is a useful tool for fetal echocardiographic examination.

Operational Considerations

Transducer Frequency

The operating frequency of the transducer is an important contributor to the functional efficacy of the system. A high carrier frequency results in better spatial resolution of the image but reduces the depth of penetration. The Doppler mode is more vulnerable to depth limitation than gray-scale tissue imaging. For most obstetric applications, a frequency of 2–4 MHz provides adequate penetration and resolution and is usually preferred. For transvaginal applications, a higher frequency (5–12 MHz) is used, as penetration is not a problem. Currently, piezoelectric elements capable of resonating at more than one frequency are available, so a single transducer can operate at multiple frequencies. This capability offers a unique advantage for color flow mapping, as a low frequency may be used for the combined tissue imaging and color Doppler mode, and one may then default to a high frequency for tissue imaging to ensure a higher gray-scale resolution.

Pulse Repetition Frequency

Doppler color flow mapping is based on pulsed Doppler insonation. The magnitude of the frequency shift in color flow Doppler sonography therefore depends on the PRF of the transmitted ultrasound. The PRF is

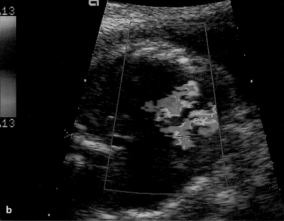

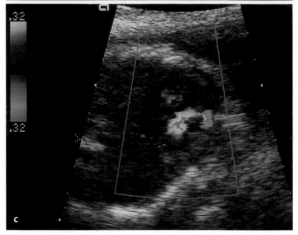

Fig. 6.7 a–c. Effect of pulse repetition frequency (PRF) on the color flow map. The images show atrioventricular flow on the oblique apical four-chamber view of the heart. **a** Low PRF setting resulting in severe aliasing with mosaic patterns and spatial overrepresentation of flow. **b** Effect of a modest increase in the PRF is partially improved image quality. Overrepresentation of flow and mosaic appearance are still present. **c** More appropriate color flow depiction with another substantial increase in the PRF. Note the presence of aliasing across the tricuspid orifice. *RA* right atrium, *RV* right ventricle, *LA* left atrium, *LV* left ventricle

adjustable and should be optimized for specific applications. As the PRF is changed, the range of Doppler shifts for a given PRF is shown in the color bar. The displayed range is a qualitative approximation and cannot be used as quantitative information. The PRF setting should be manipulated to accommodate a changing velocity pattern (Fig. 6.7). A low PRF in the presence of a high-velocity flow results in aliasing of the displayed frequencies. A high PRF, on the other hand, reduces the sensitivity so a low-velocity flow may not be identified. The location of the baseline can be changed to depict optimally the entire range of frequencies encountered in a target vessel in the appropriate direction. As indicated in the previous section, the PRF is related to the frame rate and affects the depth of imaging. These factors should be taken into consideration for increasing the efficiency of color flow imaging.

Doppler Color Flow Gain

The gain control deals with signal amplification. Most color flow devices offer separate gain controls for pulse echo imaging, spectral Doppler, and Doppler color mapping functions. The greater the gain, the more sensitive the Doppler procedure. Appropriate color gain adjustment is essential for generating reliable hemodynamic information. A higher gain setting improves the sensitivity of color Doppler sonography for identifying low-velocity flow states. However, increased gain also amplifies the noise component of the signal (Fig. 6.8), which causes display of misleading information, including the appearance of random color speckles in the color window, overflow of color outside vascular areas, and semblance of mosaic patterns. The latter falsely suggests the presence of turbulence when the flow is nonturbulent. The optimal gain setting should therefore be tailored to the specific examination. As a practical guideline, the gain should be initially increased until random color speckles start to appear; the gain is then reduced until the speckles disappear. Further manipulation should take into account other attributes of the color image and the characteristics of the flow.

High-Pass Filter (Wall Filter)

A high-pass filter eliminates high-amplitude/low-frequency Doppler shift signals generated by movement of the vascular wall, cardiac structures, or surrounding tissues (Fig. 6.8). Such signals, because of their high-power content, obfuscate Doppler signals generated by blood flow. This filter is called *high pass* because it allows high frequencies to pass through for further processing. As discussed in Chap. 4, high-pass filters are an essential part of signal processing in spectral Doppler ultrasonography. They are also an integral part of Doppler color flow mapping. The technique, however, is relatively more complex in this application, as an immense amount of Doppler data must be processed in real time. A filter that simply eliminates low-frequency signals also removes low-velocity blood flow signals with consequent loss of important hemodynamic information. For obstetric and gynecologic applications, low-speed flow is encountered in ovarian and tumor vessels, placental circulation, and fetal splanchnic vessels. The technique used for Doppler color flow application has its origins in radar engineering and is also known as a moving target indicator. The filters can be implemented at various levels of high-pass threshold. The thresholds are defined in terms of either frequency values or predesignated levels optimized for specific applications. The threshold may change automatically as the PRF is increased. With many devices a minimum level of filtering operates at all times.

For proper use of the high-pass filter, the circumstances of its application must be taken into account. Thus investigation of such low-flow systems as are encountered in the ovaries involves little or no filtering. Moreover, unlike the Doppler interrogation of the cardiac circulation, which may be associated with significant high-amplitude/low-velocity signals because of the movement of cardiac structures and surrounding tissues, such clutter signals are not a significant problem during interrogation of the pelvic vessels. The need for the use of high-pass filters in this situation is less compelling. In contrast, careful use of graded high-pass filters may be necessary during fetal echocardiography, as significant tissue movement is often encountered because of a fast fetal heart rate. For optimal use of the filter, one must also take into account other system parameters, especially the frame rate. A high frame rate decreases the processing time and Doppler sensitivity. Therefore a high-pass filter setting should not be used along with a high frame rate, as this combination leads to loss of low-velocity flow signals. As a rule of thumb, a low-level filter should be used for imaging ovarian, pelvic tumor, fetal splanchnic, intrauterine, and placental vessels; a medium level is useful for imaging umbilical or fetal venous flow; and a high level is recommended for fetal intracardiac flow or pelvic vessels such as the internal iliac or uterine arteries.

Although the exact algorithm of filtering is proprietary and varies according to the vendor, the current generation of high-pass filters use multivariate techniques capable of discriminating between low-velocity blood flow and wall motion. Introduction of such filtering techniques has led to the recent resurgence of interest in Doppler amplitude mode (also known as power Doppler or energy Doppler) for col-

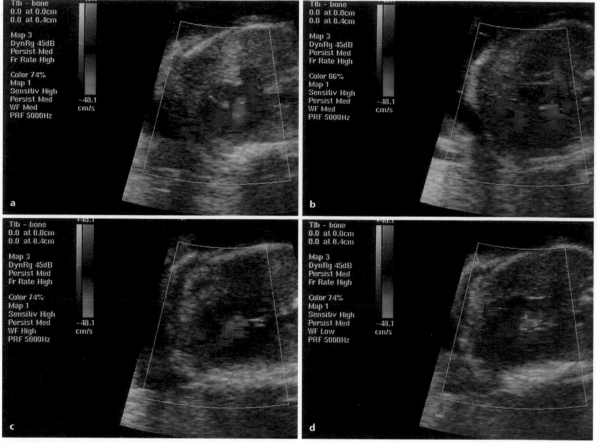

Fig. 6.8a–d. Doppler color gain and wall filter. The examples illustrate the effect of variations in color gain and wall filter on color flow imaging of the fetal heart. The gain, wall filter, and other settings of the image are displayed at the *left upper margin*. **a** Echogram at 74% color gain and medium level of wall filter. **b** Image at 86% color gain and at the same level of wall filter and other settings. Note the overflow of color and the appearance of color speckles. **c, d** Effects of high and low filters, respectively, with the color gain and other attributes maintained at the same level as the image in **a**

or flow mapping, which may be helpful for identifying slow-flow circulations (see below).

Limitations of Doppler Color Flow Mapping

Despite the impressive technologic innovations of Doppler color flow ultrasonography that have revolutionized noninvasive cardiovascular diagnosis, there are important limitations of the method that should be considered. These limitations are inherent in the physical principles and the engineering implementation of the method. They are also responsible for various artifacts that one may encounter during use of this technique. An understanding of these limitations and artifacts is essential for the appropriate use and interpretation of Doppler color flow mapping. The following section discusses these factors, which include aliasing, range ambiguity, temporal ambiguity, problems related to the angle of insonation, tissue ghost signals, and mirror imaging.

Aliasing

As color flow mapping is based on pulsed Doppler insonation, its ability to measure the maximum frequency shift without ambiguity is limited by the PRF rate of the system. The threshold level of Doppler shift beyond which the measurement becomes ambiguous is called the Nyquist limit, and the phenomenon of Doppler shift ambiguity beyond the Nyquist limit is called the Nyquist effect, or *aliasing*. This phenomenon is known as aliasing because it falsely depicts the frequency shift in terms of both magnitude and direction. Aliasing in spectral pulsed Doppler sonography is discussed in detail in Chap. 3.

Aliasing in a color flow system is shown in a spatial two-dimensional plane in which the aliased flow is depicted in reversed color surrounded by the non-aliased flow (Fig. 6.9). This pattern mimics the color flow appearance of separate streams in differing directions. The two patterns, howerver, are clearly distinguishable. In an aliased flow, the higher velocity generates a higher Doppler shifted frequency, which is depicted with greater brightness: the higher the frequency shift, the brighter the color. The brightest level in the color calibration bar (the uppermost for the flow toward the transducer and lowermost for the flow away from the transducer) represents the Nyquist limit. As the velocity, and therefore the frequency shift, exceeds this limit, the color wraps around the calibration bar and appears at the other end as the most luminous color of the opposite direction (Fig. 6.10). For example, flow toward the transducer with an increasing velocity is depicted with an increasingly bright red color changing to yellow (Fig. 6.9). As the Nyquist limit is reached, the color flow shows brightest yellow in the color bar; and as the limit is exceeded, flow is shown in the brightest blue. Thus in an aliased flow, the bright or pale color of one direction is juxtaposed against the bright color of the opposite direction. In contrast, with genuine flow separation the distinct flow streams are depicted in the directionally appropriate colors separated by a dark margin (Fig. 6.11). Note that the hue that demarcates an aliased flow depends on the choice of the color mapping scheme.

When demonstrating aliasing, an apparent contradiction may be seen between the spectral Doppler and the Doppler color flow interrogations. Doppler color flow mapping may show a nonaliased flow pat-

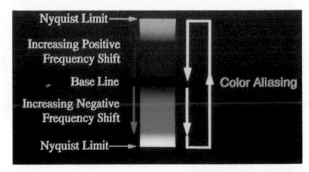

Fig. 6.10. Color Doppler Nyquist effect. The image shows Doppler color flow mapping of the left ventricular outflow. Note the change of color from *red* to *yellow* and then from *bright blue* to *dark blue*. With the declining velocity, blue changes first to yellow and then to red. *LVOT* left ventricular outflow tract

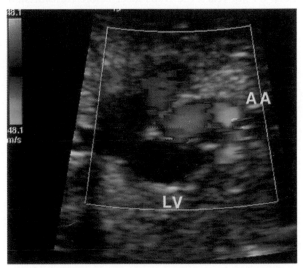

Fig. 6.11. Doppler color flow depiction of change in the direction of flow. The image shows Doppler color mapping of flow through the ascending aorta (*AA*) and the arch of the aorta. In the ascending aorta the flow is toward the transducer and is therefore depicted as *red* according to the color bar setting. As the direction of flow changes, the color becomes *blue* with a dark line separating the two hues. *LV* left ventricle

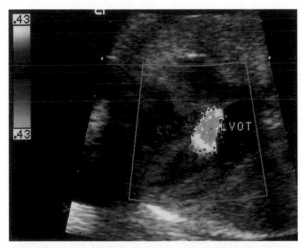

Fig. 6.9. Color Doppler Nyquist effect. The image shows Doppler color flow mapping of the left ventricular outflow. Note the change of color from *red* to *yellow* and then from *bright blue* to *dark blue*. With the declining velocity, blue changes first to yellow and then to red. *LVOT* left ventricular outflow tract

tern when aliasing is observed with the spectral Doppler waveform. This phenomenon is explained by the fact that the mean frequency is less than the peak frequency, and Doppler color flow depiction is based on the use of mean frequency, so the Nyquist limit is not reached as readily as with the peak frequency depiction by the spectral Doppler method.

Color Doppler aliasing can be eliminated by elevating the Nyquist limit, which can be achieved by either increasing the PRF or decreasing the transducer frequency. However, an increasing PRF may eventually result in such shortening of the interpulse interval as to cause range ambiguity of the returning echoes – unless the depth of interrogation is reduced so all the echoes from one pulse are received at the transducer before the next pulse is transmitted. As Doppler color flow mapping technology critically depends on identifying the spatial origin of an echo, color Doppler devices are preset to prevent range ambiguity by automatically reducing the color imaging depth.

Range Ambiguity

The occurrence of range ambiguity in regard to pulsed spectral Doppler sonography is discussed in Chap. 3. Range ambiguity arises when the interpulse interval is short in relation to the depth of the field of insonation, so echoes from deeper sampling locations do not reach the transducer before transmission of the next pulse. These Doppler signals are then treated as the early returning echoes of the second pulse being reflected from a superficial location and are displayed as such. Consequently, spurious color flow is shown in areas devoid of any vascularity. In practise, however, most Doppler color flow devices prevent this problem by automatically reducing the depth when the PRF is increased to the threshold of range ambiguity.

Temporal Ambiguity

Temporal ambiguity occurs when Doppler color flow mapping fails to depict hemodynamic events with temporal accuracy. Specifically, such a situation arises when the frame rate for color flow is too slow relative to the circulatory dynamics. As discussed earlier, the basic unit of color flow depiction is a single frame that, when completed, shows the average mean frequency shifts color-coded and superimposed on the gray-scale tissue image. The flow dynamics are therefore summarized for the duration of one frame. As we noted above, the frame rate is inversely proportional to the number of scan lines and the number of samples per scan line. The slower the frame rate, the better the color image quality in terms of both spatial resolution and Doppler sensitivity. Herein lies the paradox, as a slower rate means longer duration of a frame. As the frame duration increases, there is progressive loss of the ability to recognize discrete hemodynamic events.

This decline in the temporal relevance of the flow map is accentuated by hyperdynamic circulatory states with the rapidly changing hemodynamic phenomena. One may encounter such a situation in the fetal circulation, which is driven by a fast heart rate, normally 120–160 bpm. A faster rate means a shorter cardiac cycle. The shorter the cardiac cycle, the lower

Table 6.2. Relation between frame rate, completed frames per cardiac cycle, and fetal heart rate

Frames per second	Duration of a frame (ms)	Complete frames per cardiac cycle	
		FHR 120 bpm	FHR 160 bpm
10	100	5	3
15	66	7	5
30	33	15	11

FHR, fetal heart rate.

the number of complete frames available for depicting each cardiac cycle (Table 6.2) and the greater the risk of temporal ambiguity. This artifact may be apparent in the simultaneous depiction of temporally sequential circulatory phenomena. For example, with fetal echocardiography one may see in the same frame atrioventricular flow across the mitral orifice and left ventricular outflow into the aortic root. The former is related to ventricular diastole and the latter to ventricular systole. One may also experience temporal ambiguity in color flow devices that form gray-scale and color flow images separately in a frame that may depict discordance between the gray-scale depiction and the color flow mapping of the cardiac events.

Angle of Insonation

Angle dependence of the Doppler shifted frequencies, discussed in Chap. 2 in relation to spectral Doppler sonography, is a critical factor in color flow mapping. With sector scanning, multiple scan lines spread out from the transducer in a fan-like manner. When the sector scanner is used to interrogate a circulatory system in which the direction of flow is across these scan lines in a color window, the angle of insonation between the flow axis and the ultrasound beam changes (Fig. 6.12). The angle is smallest when the flow stream enters in the sector field and progressively rises to 90° as the flow approaches the center of the field. Concurrently, the Doppler-shifted frequencies progressively decline and may become undetectable at the center of the color field (Fig. 6.13).

A sector scanner may also create apparently contradictory directional information in a vessel traversing the color field. As the flow approaches the midline of the field, the flow is depicted in color encoding for flow toward the transducer, which usually is red; as the flow moves away, it is encoded blue. Thus the same vessel shows bidirectional flow (Fig. 6.13). This paradox highlights the basic concept of representation of flow directionality by any Doppler system. The latter does not depict the actual flow direction, merely the vector of flow toward the transducer.

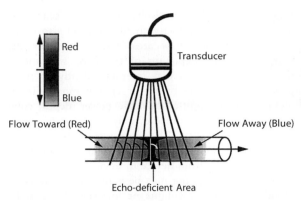

Fig. 6.12. Progressive increase in the angle of insonation and change in color coding of flow as a vessel traverses a sector field

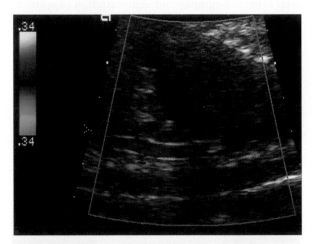

Fig. 6.13. Color Doppler sonogram of the fetal thoraco-abdominal aorta demonstrating the effect of varying angles of insonation in a sector field. Although the flow in reality is unidirectional, the color coding of flow changes as the vessel traverses across the sector field giving a false impression of bidirectional flow. Note also the absence of color flow at the center of the color field as the beam intersects the vessel at a right angle

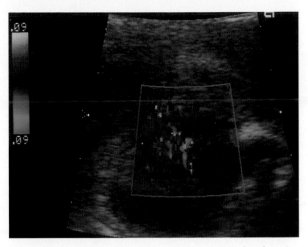

Fig. 6.14. Example of tissue motion-generated color signals unrelated to flow (*horizontal arrow*). The echogram depicts a fetal thoracic cross section at the level of the heart

Wall Motion Ghost Signals

Spurious color flow signals may be generated by movements of the cardiac structures or vascular walls. These signals may be easily distinguished from the blood flow-related color map, as they are of lower frequency, are usually displayed outside the intracardiac or intravascular space, and may be asynchronous with the cardiac or vascular hemodynamic events (Fig. 6.14). These signals are seen more frequently with hyperdynamic circulations with high-speed wall movements. They may also be noted with deep cardiovascular structures whose motion generates Doppler signals; these signals reverberate at various structures and become more visible as the real blood flow signals are attenuated because of the depth. With obstetric applications, this artifact is of relevance mostly in relation to fetal echocardiography. Ghost signals may be reduced by elevating the high-pass filtering threshold, by increasing the PRF (which raises the minimum detectable velocity), or by the reject function (which cuts off low frequencies).

Mirroring

Mirror images of color flow are produced by reflection of the Doppler signal at a vessel wall or other structures so it takes longer to return to the transducer. The system recognizes and depicts the signal as originating from a deeper location than its real source.

Color Mapping of Doppler Amplitude (Doppler Power or Doppler Energy)

The Doppler signal amplitude implies the intensity of the signal and is also referred to as Doppler power or energy. As discussed in Chaps. 3 and 4, Doppler flow signals have three dimensions: (1) frequency, which is proportional to the speed of red blood cell (RBC) movement; (2) amplitude, or intensity, of the signal, which is proportional to the number of RBCs scattering the transmitted ultrasound beam; and (3) time, during which the above two parameters change. Whereas the frequency information and its temporal changes form the basis for clinical application of the Doppler technique, the amplitude data remain largely unutilized. However, amplitude reflects the scattering power and therefore may prove useful in clinical applications. During Doppler color flow processing, the autocorrelator measures the amplitude from the

Table 6.3. Advantages and disadvantages of the Doppler power or energy mode

Advantages
  Increased sensitivity for detecting low-velocity circulatory systems as encountered in splanchnic, placental, or tumor vessels

  Virtual independence of the angle of insonation

  May allow better delineation of flow in vascular channels

  Absence of Nyquist effect

Disadvantages
  Does not provide information on the directionality of flow

  Depth-dependent, so the greater the depth of the vessel, the less available amplitude flow information

phase analysis of the returning echoes. Although it was theoretically possible to produce two-dimensional Doppler color flow mapping based on the intensity of the Doppler signal, it is only recently that the systems have seriously attempted to resolve the technical challenge of producing an amplitude-based map that would be independent of Doppler-shifted frequency. The advantages and disadvantages of the amplitude mode are summarized in Table 6.3 and are discussed further below.

With spectral Doppler analysis the amplitude information is generated by the spectral analysis, which provides complete information on the Doppler power spectrum. It is depicted in the so-called Z axis as brightness of the waveforms. With color flow processing, which is based on phase-difference analysis, the amplitude of the Doppler signal is estimated by the autocorrelator. The output is color-coded and is displayed along with the gray-scale tissue images. The Doppler energy or power display, however, does not indicate directionality of flow in relation to the transducer. In contrast to the frequency mode, which as is apparent from the Doppler equation is angle-dependent, the amplitude mode is virtually unaffected by the angle of insonation.

The amplitude output is affected by the wall (high-pass) filter as it removes high-amplitude/low-frequency Doppler signals generated by tissue movements. If the filter setting were identical to the frequency-based color flow mapping, the amplitude map would offer no more flow information than the former. Current filter algorithms, particularly those utilizing the multivariate approach, have substantially minimized this problem. An appropriate filter setting is essential for optimal color Doppler amplitude imaging (Fig. 6.15). A low threshold of wall filter is needed for identifying low-flow states. Doppler power, or energy, imaging is also affected by the gain

(Fig. 6.15). A high gain results in increased sensitivity for detecting slow-velocity circulations but also in the extension of color flow areas beyond the vascular margin and the depiction of tissue or wall movements. Other factors that interdependently or independently affect the power or energy mode display include the transmitted acoustic power, depth, color sensitivity, preponderance of gray scale (write priority), and persistence. The implementation of these controls and the resultant changes in the amplitude color maps vary from device to device.

Amplitude mapping may be helpful for identifying blood flows of low volume or low velocity. Doppler mean frequency shift based on color mapping may not be sensitive enough to detect such a flow system. Examples of such potential uses in obstetrics include fetal echocardiography and demonstration of splanchnic flow in fetal lungs and placenta. In gynecologic practice, amplitude may optimize our ability to detect flow in pelvic organs such as the ovaries (Fig. 6.16), especially in postmenopausal women. The extent of its clinical utility is still being explored, particularly in assessing tumor vascularity. Three-dimensional reconstruction of the vascular channels has been accomplished utilizing the Doppler amplitude mode. This feature may have potentially promising clinical application. Applications of power Doppler sonography are discussed in Chaps. 7, 39, and 40.

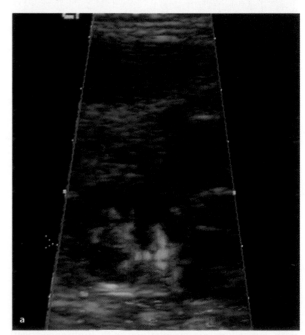

Fig. 6.15a–e. The effects of wall filter and gain on color Doppler amplitude imaging of fetal renal flow. **a** A reasonable amplitude image of renal flow. **b, c** The effect of low- and high-wall filter setting, respectively. **d, e** The effects of low and high gain, respectively

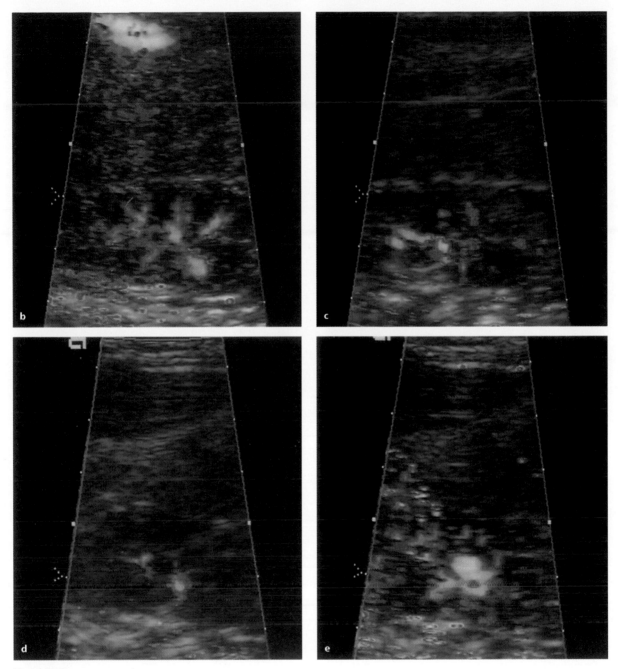

Fig. 6.15 b–e.

Summary

The introduction of Doppler color flow mapping has ushered in an exciting era for diagnostic sonographic imaging. As discussed in the relevant chapters of this book, application of this technique to obstetric and gynecologic imaging has proved highly useful. A prerequisite for optimal utilization of this technique is an in-depth knowledge of its principles and limitations. Furthermore, it is important to appreciate that the appearance of color flow images is influenced by the operational setting of the equipment, which must be taken into account for reliable interpretation. Finally, there are even newer modalities of flow imaging that present exciting possibilities for the future of noninvasive hemodynamic investigation in clinical practice.

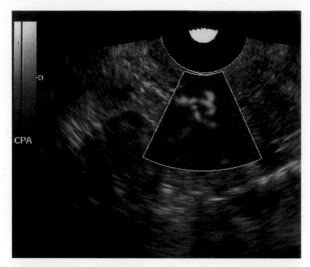

Fig. 6.16. Color Doppler amplitude image of the uterine vessels obtained by transvaginal scanning

References

1. Omoto R, Kasai C (1987) Physics and instrumentation of Doppler color flow mapping. Echocardiography 4:467–483
2. Lee R (1989) Physical principles of flow mapping in cardiology. In: Nanda NC (ed) Textbook of color Doppler echocardiography. Lea & Febiger, Philadelphia, p 18
3. Kremkau FK (1991) Principles of color flow imaging. J Vasc Tech 15:104–109
4. Namekawa K, Kasai C, Tsukamoto M, Koyano A (1983) Real time bloodflow imaging system utilizing autocorrelation techniques. In: Lerski R, Morley P (eds) Ultrasound "82". Pergamon, London, pp 203–208
5. Angelsen BAJ, Kristoffersen K (1979) On ultrasonic MTI measurement of velocity profiles in blood flow. IEEE Trans Biomed Eng 26:665–671

Three-dimensional Color and Power Doppler Ultrasonography of the Fetal Cardiovascular System

Rabih Chaoui, Karim D. Kalache

Introduction

The recent development of fast processors has enabled ultra-rapid calculation and rendering of 3D images and the advent of real-time 3D (also called 4D) ultrasonography. Moreover, using newer systems, fetal structures can now be visualized in different modes including the surface-, the maximum-, the minimum-, and the "X-ray" mode. The fetal vascular anatomy can be examined by using color Doppler and power Doppler ultrasound, power Doppler being superior to color Doppler in visualizing small vessels with low flow; however, the spatial course of the vessels in the human body is best evaluated using 3D ultrasonography. By combining power Doppler and 3D techniques it is possible to study the fetal and placental vessels in relation to surrounding anatomic structures.

Potential fields of application in obstetrics have been reported in the past several years either as single case reports [1–5] or small series [6, 7]. This chapter reviews the technical background and potential fields of application in obstetrical ultrasound.

Technical Background

Equipment

The few commercially available 3D systems have an integrated 3D power Doppler ultrasonography (3D PDU) feature as well, but there are also external workstations adaptable to the different ultrasound systems, offering offline postprocessing analysis and evaluation. Most of our expertise we report in this chapter was acquired by using the Voluson 730 Expert system (General Electrics-Kretztechnik, Zipf, Austria) with an integrated on-line evaluation of volume rendering. Broadband curvilinear transducers with frequencies ranging between 4–8 MHz for the abdominal probe and 5–9 MHz for the vaginal probe were used.

Advantages of Power Doppler for 3D Rendering

Both color and power Doppler ultrasonography are applied in vessel visualization, and practically both can be used for 3D visualization. Power Doppler has, however, various advantages over conventional color Doppler [8, 9] that make it optimal for the 3D mode:

1. Sensitivity in flow detection: amplitude of Doppler signals instead of their frequency shift is analyzed in power Doppler and this was shown to be three to five times more sensitive than conventional color Doppler in visualizing small vessels and low flows [8].
2. Improved noise differentiation: in power Doppler, noise signals are encoded in a uniform color; hence, it is possible to turn the gain all the way up, which fills the entire image with noise, and the vascular signal will still be distinguishable.
3. Better edge definition: power Doppler has a better edge definition in displaying flow. This is because color samples which extend partially beyond the edges are shown in a different color due to the lower signal amplitude.
4. Detection of flow orthogonal to beam: power Doppler is able to detect flow at right angles to the beam. The amplitudes of the positive and negative components of the flow tend to add up, resulting in a powerful signal.

Principle of Data Acquisition, Image Rendering, and Display

The two main aspects which have to be considered when using a 3D imaging system are given below.

Volume Data Acquisition, Image Rendering, and Display

1. During volume data acquisition the information is stored within a volume of interest. The acquired volume is a sequence of a pre-defined number of 2D slices (Fig. 7.1). The system assesses the spatial information of the structures in relation to each other in the different 2D images and allows a 3D

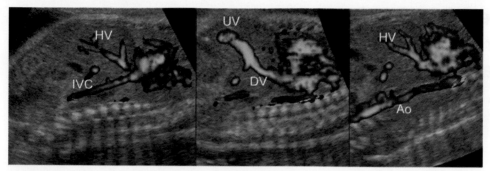

Fig. 7.1. Several longitudinal views are necessary to visualize the different vessels in the upper abdomen such as the hepatic veins (*HV*), inferior vena cava (*IVC*), umbilical vein (*UV*) with ductus venosus (*DV*), and the descending aorta (*Ao*). Compare with Fig. 7.2

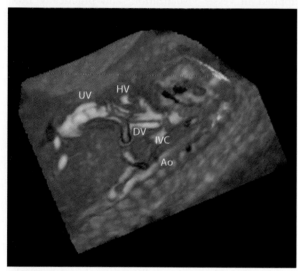

Fig. 7.2. Longitudinal view of thorax and upper abdomen. Three-dimensional power Doppler rendering allows visualization of all vessels described in Fig. 7.1 and their relationship to one another

rendering (Fig. 7.2). Detailed gray-scale information is often not essential and lowers the quality of the rendered 3D power Doppler image; therefore, sufficient knowledge about how vessels are best visualized using power Doppler is a prerequisite to obtaining a good-quality 3D power Doppler image. Even if the method is very sensitive and allows the imaging of small vessels, the optimization of pulse repetition frequency (PRF), filter, insonation angle, and persistence are of major importance. The PRF and filter have to be set as high as necessary in order to visualize only the vessels of interest, since superimposed vessels may lead to confusion and complicates orientation within the 3D volume. Neighboring vessels or noise signals interfering with the region of interest can be erased during off-line reconstruction; however, good quality of the original volume is essential for an optimal rendering.

2. Image rendering is the process of creating a 3D representation of the parameters of interest. Generally, the principle used is the "planar geometric projection" of the 3D image, i.e. a 2D image representing the 3D data as seen in the figures of this chapter. The virtual impression of the third dimension is generally given by the on-line rotation of the image on the screen and by different shadowing of anterior and posterior structures. Different color maps can be used as well as various post-processing features

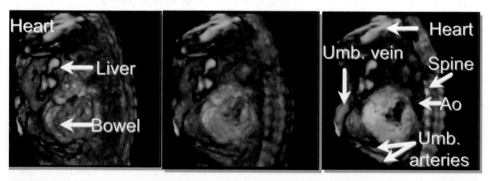

Fig. 7.3. Combined solid and 3D PDU mode with increasing transparency from left to right in a fetus with ascites

such as changing the brightness, threshold, or transparency of color. The examiner can further-more decide whether only vessels of interest are to be visualized or if it is important to have the information of the surrounding structures as well (so-called glass-body rendering). The system allows the examiner to switch progressively between surface and transparent mode, which gives the impression that the vascular tree shines through the surrounding structures (Fig. 7.3).

Limitations of 3D Power Doppler in Prenatal Ultrasound

Similar to other 3D modes, fetal movements are a major cause of artifacts. Other limitations specific to the method are related to the regions of interest and neighboring vessel. In most cases the examiner is choosing a compromise between the vessels of interest with their ramifications and the overlapping from neighboring vessels. Most limitations are still at the level of the heart, where overlapping of color from adjacent structures can limit the understanding of the image. Pulsations of the heart during data acquisition are still difficult to overcome, but the use of a quick sweep by reducing image quality and increasing persistence can reduce these artifacts [3].

Clinical Application

Conventional color Doppler and power Doppler ultrasound are both useful in the assessment of fetal abnormalities involving the cardiovascular system [12]. Application of color Doppler is not only of benefit in the assessment of fetal cardiac anomalies [13, 14], but also for completing diagnosis in many extracardiac conditions [12]. The 3D PDU technique allows spatial analysis of fetal vessels in relationship to their surrounding anatomic structures. In a recent study [6] we examined the application of 3D PDU in prenatal

diagnosis, by comparing 45 normal fetuses and 87 abnormal pregnancies with vascular abnormalities. In the study we used a prototype system (HDI-3000, Philips-ATL, Bothell, Wash.) and satisfactory image information was obtained in only 64% (56 of 87) of the abnormal cases. The following eight anatomical regions were, however, found to be of interest:
1. Placenta
2. Umbilical cord
3. Abdomen
4. Kidneys
5. Lung
6. Brain
7. Fetal tumors
8. Heart and great vessels

The following section summarizes possible applications of 3D color and power Doppler ultrasonography in these different regions.

Umbilical Cord and Placenta

Placental vessels are best visualized in relation to the umbilical cord insertion. The intraplacental vascular tree can be visualized with this method [15]. The umbilical cord can be rendered from its placental (Figs. 7.4, 7.5) to its abdominal insertion including the free loop (Figs. 7.6, 7.7) [6]. From our experience it is the easiest structure to assess using 3D PDU throughout pregnancy. Conditions in which 3D power Doppler might be of some benefit are listed in Table 7.1.

Intraabdominal Vessels

Examination of the intraabdominal structures using 3D Power Doppler is best achieved when examining the abdomen in a longitudinal plane. This approach allows the visualization of the intraabdominal portion of the umbilical arteries (Figs. 7.8, 7.9) and vein with the ductus venosus (Figs. 7.2, 7.3), the portal system, the hepatic veins, the splenic vessels, the inferior vena

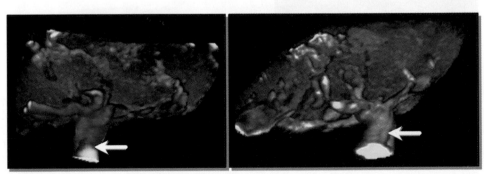

Fig. 7.4. Three-dimensional PDU images of cord insertion in anterior wall placenta. The umbilical cord (*arrow*) is shown entering the placenta with the surface vessels diverging from the site of insertion

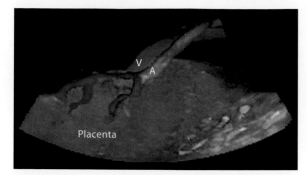

Fig. 7.5. Placenta with central insertion of the umbilical cord as demonstrated with 3D color Doppler ultrasonography. There is a single umbilical artery (*A*). Umbilical vein (*V*)

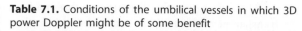

Table 7.1. Conditions of the umbilical vessels in which 3D power Doppler might be of some benefit

Placenta previa
Vasa previa
Insertio velamentosa
Connecting vessels in twin pregnancies (TTTS)
Vessel architecture in intrauterine growth restriction
Single umbilical artery
Nuchal cord
Torsion of umbilical vessels
True and false knot

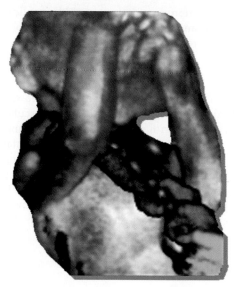

Fig. 7.6. Three-dimensional PDU of a nuchal cord in a 23-week-old fetus

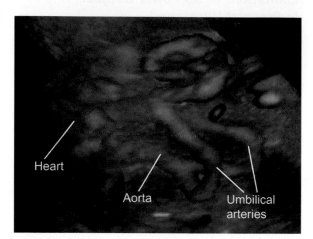

Fig. 7.8. Three-dimensional PDU view of the lower abdomen and pelvis of a normal 23-gestational-week fetus demonstrating both umbilical arteries converging toward the anterior abdominal wall

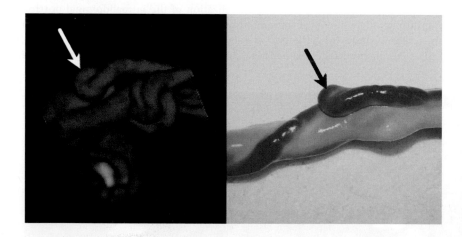

Fig. 7.7. False knot in the free loop of the umbilical cord in prenatal 3D PDU and postnatal finding

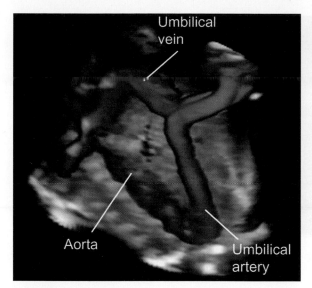

Fig. 7.9. In the same view as Fig. 7.8, 3D PDU demonstrates in this case an agenesis of the left umbilical artery. Only one (dilated right) artery can be seen in its course to the umbilical ring

Table 7.2. Conditions for potential 3D power Doppler application in the abdominal region

Abnormal cord insertion on the abdomen (omphalocele, gastroschisis), abnormal shape of the umbilical vein size (varix or ectasia)
Ductus venosus agenesis with persistent right umbilical vein
Agenesis of the portal vein
Abdominal vessels in malformations, congenital diaphragmatic hernia, severe ascites, etc.
Abnormal course of vessels in isomerism, i.e., interruption of inferior vena cava with azygous continuity
Single umbilical artery and abnormalities in lower abdomen

cava, and the abdominal aorta. Using this technique it is also possible to display the normal course of umbilical arteries around the urinary bladder (Fig. 7.8). Since Doppler studies of the ductus venosus in growth-restricted fetuses is becoming an important field in prenatal medicine, abnormalities of the intrahepatic venous system are frequently detected (Fig. 7.10) [16]. This anatomical region is, however, complex, and it has been shown that 3D Power Doppler can help in the differentiation between anomalies (Table 7.2).

Renal Vessels

The renal vascular tree is best visualized in a coronal plane (Fig. 7.11). Depending on velocity scale setting, vessels can be seen from the main artery with some ramifications to the peripheral cortical vessels including arteries and veins. The visualization of renal vessels is known to increase the accuracy of diagnosis of kidney malformations in the fetus. The examiner should be, however, aware of pitfalls such as the visualization of the ventrally situated abdominal arteries (inferior mesenteric artery and vessels from celiac trunk) that can be misinterpreted as renal arteries. Conditions in which 3D PDU could be of diagnostic value are listed in Table 7.3.

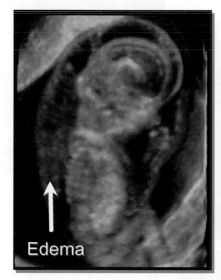

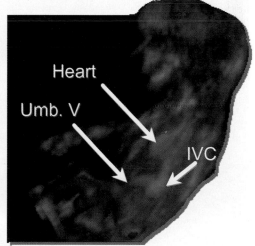

Fig. 7.10. Abnormal course of the intraabdominal umbilical vein and ductus venosus in a fetus with early hydrops at 13 weeks

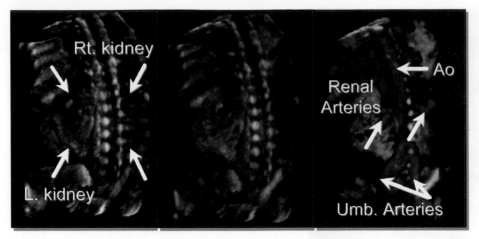

Fig. 7.11. A dorsal view to the fetus in 3D showing the spine and both kidneys. The progressive visualization of power Doppler demonstrates the descending aorta (*Ao*) and the bifurcation of both renal arteries. Ductus venosus is connected directly to the IVC

Table 7.3. Renal anomalies amenable to 3D power Doppler application

Agenesis of one or both kidneys
Horseshoe kidney
Pelvic kidney
Abnormal vessel course in dysplastic renal anomalies

Intracranial Vessels

As with color Doppler two main vascular regions can be examined in 3D mode depending on the insonation plane. A transversal insonation allows easy reconstruction of the circle of Willis (Fig. 7.12), whereas a sagittal approach enables the visualization of the pericallosal artery with its ramifications (Fig. 7.13) [17]. By selecting a lower velocity scale it is possible to obtain impressive images of the cerebral veins and the sagittal sinus. Conditions with possible benefit of 3D power Doppler, such as vein of Galen aneurysm (Fig. 7.14) and others, are listed in Table 7.4.

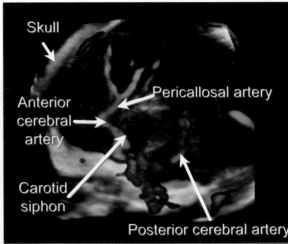

Fig. 7.13. Sagittal approach insonation of the brain enables the demonstration of the pericallosal artery arising from the anterior cerebral artery

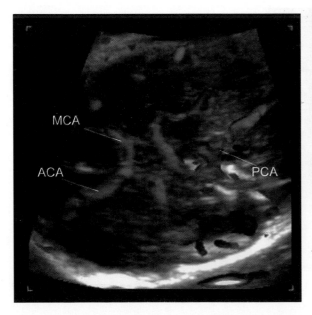

Fig. 7.12. Circle of Willis as demonstrated with 3D PDU, with the anterior (*ACA*), middle (*MCA*), and posterior (*PCA*) cerebral arteries

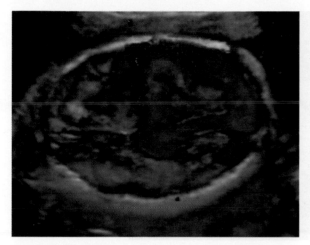

Fig. 7.14. Three-dimensional PDU of a vein of Galen aneurysm at 22 weeks gestation with the dilated vessel between the hemispheres and in the posterior fossa

Table 7.4. Conditions for potential 3D power Doppler application in the intracranial region

Abnormal anterior cerebral artery in agenesis of the corpus callosum
Aneurysm of the vein of Galen
Severe cerebral malformations (holoprosencephaly, hydrocephaly, encephalocele, etc.)

Lung Vessels

Proximal and peripheral lung arteries and veins can be seen from their origin to the peripheral pulmonary segments. Especially the right lung can be as-

Table 7.5. Conditions for potential 3D power Doppler application in the pulmonary region

Cystic lung malformations
Congenital diaphragmatic hernia
Bronchopulmonary sequestration
Vessel anatomy or ramification in lung hypoplasia

sessed even by a less experienced examiner. Potential fields of interest include the analysis of the 3D vessel architecture in cystic lung malformations, congenital diaphragmatic hernia, and in bronchopulmonary sequestration. In the latter condition 3D power Doppler facilitates the visualization of the abnormal systemic vessel that feeds the sequester. Application fields are listed in Table 7.5.

Fetal Tumors or Aberrant Vessels

Aberrant vessels can be visualized in the presence of several malformations such as choriangioma, lymphangioma sacrococcygeal teratoma (Fig. 7.15), and acardiac twin. The visualization of the vascular pattern of fetal tumors is not only interesting because of

Table 7.6. Conditions for potential 3D power Doppler application in tumors and aberrant vessels

Choriangioma
Teratoma
Acrania (TRAP)
Hemangioma
Renal tumors
Cardiac rhabdomyoma

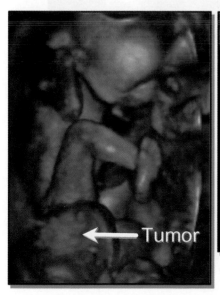
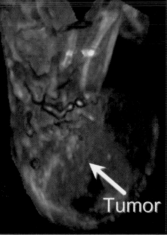

Fig. 7.15. Three-dimensional surface and 3D PDU images of a sacrococcygeal teratoma at 22 weeks gestation. The tumor is not highly vascularized

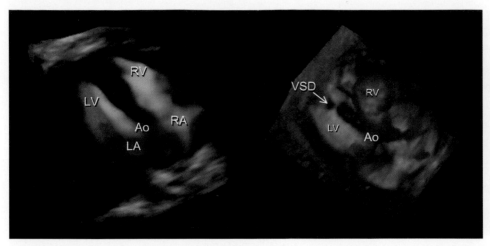

Fig. 7.16. Three-dimensional PDU of a normal four-chamber view (*left*) with right and left atria (*RA, LA*), right and left ventricles (*RV, LV*), and the aortic root. In comparison with the right side, there is a muscular ventricular septal defect (*VSD*) connecting both ventricles

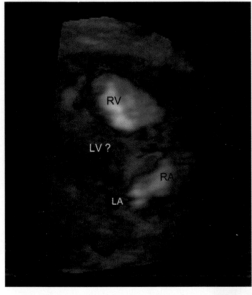

Fig. 7.17. Three-dimensional PDU of a four-chamber view in a fetus with a hypoplastic left heart syndrome. Blood flow enters from the right atrium (*RA*) into the right ventricle (*RV*), but no flow is seen within the left ventricle (*LV*). *LA* left atrium

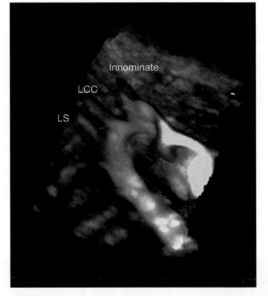

Fig. 7.18. Aortic arch with the origin of the cephalic vessels: the innominate (brachiocephalic) artery; the left common carotid artery (*LCC*); and the left subclavian artery (*LS*)

their risk of cardiac failure due to the presence of arteriovenous fistulae, but also to assess compression or shifting of neighboring organs. Table 7.6 gives a summary of these fields of interest.

Heart and Great Vessels

The 3D rendering of the heart and the great vessels is still a challenge to fetal ultrasound. Reliable volumes are still difficult to obtain under routine scan conditions. According to our experience we think that 3D PDU can be helpful in fetal cardiology in the near future and might facilitate the assessment of spatial arrangement of the heart chambers including their size and shape (Figs. 7.16, 7.17) as we demonstrate in some of the figures in this chapter. Another possible application field is an easier assessment of the course of the great vessels (Fig. 7.18). Crossing of vessels vs parallel course (Fig. 7.19), abnormal course as seen in double aortic arch, right arch with a sling, or simply tortuous hypoplastic aorta or pulmonary artery

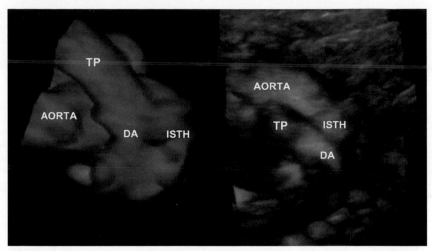

Fig. 7.19. Great vessels of a normal fetus (*left*) and a fetus with transposition of the great arteries (*right*). In the left image the crossing of the vessels is recognized with the course of the aorta under the pulmonary trunk (*TP*) and the connection of the ductus arteriosus (*DA*) at the level of the isthmus (*ISTH*). In transposition both vessels are parallel and the aorta is on the right side of the pulmonary trunk

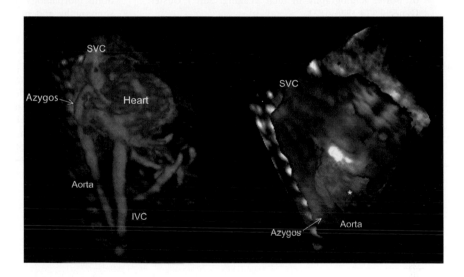

Fig. 7.20. A normal fetus (*left*) compared with a fetus with left isomerism (polysplenia; *right*): On the left the inferior vena cava is seen entering the heart and on the right side of the aorta the tiny azygos vein is recognized connecting with the superior vena cava. In left isomerism there is an interruption of the inferior vena cava (*star*), which is absent on 3D PDU. Venous blood from the inferior part of the body returns via the azygos vein, which is dilated and seen side by side near the aorta

Table 7.7. Conditions for potential 3D power and color Doppler application in fetal echocardiography

Anomalies of the four chambers
Abnormal atrioventricular connection
Malformations of the great arteries in conotruncal malformations such as transposition
Severe tricuspid regurgitation
Aberrant course of vessels such as right aortic arch and double aortic arch

in different anomalies may represent future application fields [18, 19]. Venous anomalies could be of further interest in the future (Fig. 7.20). Table 7.7 summarizes some of these fields of interest.

References

1. Heling KS, Chaoui R, Bollmann R (2000) Prenatal diagnosis of an aneurysm of the vein of Galen with three-dimensional color power angiography. Ultrasound Obstet Gynecol 15:333–336

2. Chaoui R, Zodan-Marin T, Wisser J (2002) Marked splenomegaly in fetal cytomegalovirus infection: detection supported by three-dimensional power Doppler ultrasound. Ultrasound Obstet Gynecol 20:299–302

3. Chaoui R, Kalache KD (2001) Three-dimensional power Doppler ultrasound of the fetal great vessels. Ultrasound Obstet Gynecol 17:455–456

4. Lee W, Kirk JS, Comstock CH, Romero R (2000) Vasa previa: prenatal detection by three-dimensional ultrasonography. Ultrasound Obstet Gynecol 16:384–387

5. Lee TH, Shih JC, Peng SS, Lee CN, Shyu MK, Hsieh FJ (2000) Prenatal depiction of angioarchitecture of an aneurysm of the vein of Galen with three-dimensional color power angiography. Ultrasound Obstet Gynecol 15:337–340

6. Chaoui R, Kalache KD, Hartung J (2001) Application of three-dimensional power Doppler ultrasound in prenatal diagnosis. Ultrasound Obstet Gynecol 17:22–29

7. Lee W, Kalache KD, Chaiworapongsa T, Londono J, Treadwell MC, Johnson A, Romero R (2003) Three-dimensional power Doppler ultrasonography during pregnancy. J Ultrasound Med 22:91–97

8. Fortunato SJ (1996) The use of power Doppler and color power angiography in fetal imaging. Am J Obstet Gynecol 174:1828–1831

9. Rubin JM, Bude RO, Carson PL, Bree RL, Adler RS (1994) Power Doppler US: a potentially useful alternative to mean frequency-based color Doppler US. Radiology 190:853–856

10. Chaoui R, Kalache KD (1998) Three-dimensional color power imaging: principles and first experience in prenatal diagnosis. In: Merz E (ed) 3D ultrasonography in obstetrics and gynecology. Lippincott, Williams and Wilkins, Philadelphia, pp 135–142

11. Ritchie CJ, Edwards WS, Mack LA, Cyr DR, Kim Y (1996) Three-dimensional ultrasonic angiography using power-mode Doppler. Ultrasound Med Biol 22:277–286

12. Chaoui R (2000) Color Doppler sonography in the diagnosis of fetal abnormalitites. In: Nicolaides KH, Rizzo G, Hecher K (eds) Placental and fetal Doppler. Parthenon, London, pp 187–203

13. Chaoui R (2000) Color Doppler Sonography in the assessment of the fetal heart. In: Nicolaides KH, Rizzo G, Hecher K (eds) Placental and fetal Doppler. Parthenon, London, pp 171–186.

14. Chaoui R, McEwing R (2003) Three cross-sectional planes for fetal color Doppler echocardiography. Ultrasound Obstet Gynecol 21:81–93

15. Pretorius DH, Nelson TR, Baergen RN, Pai E, Cantrell C (1998) Imaging of placental vasculature using three-dimensional ultrasound and color power Doppler: a preliminary study. Ultrasound Obstet Gynecol 12:45–49

16. Kalache K, Romero R, Goncalves LF, Chaiworapongsa T, Epinoza J, Schoen ML, Treadwell MC, Lee W (2003) Three-dimensional color power imaging of the fetal hepatic circulation. Am J Obstet Gynecol 189:1401–1406

17. Pooh RK, Pooh KH (2002) The assessment of fetal brain morphology and circulation by transvaginal 3D sonography and power Doppler. J Perinat Med 30:48–56

18. Chaoui R, Kalache KD, Heling KS, Schneider M (2003) 3D-power Doppler echocardiography: usefulness in spatial visualization of fetal cardiac vessels. Ultrasound Obstet Gynecol 22 (Suppl) 45 (Abstract)

19. Chaoui R, Schneider MB, Kalache KD (2003) Right aortic arch with vascular ring and aberrant left subclavian artery: prenatal diagnosis assisted by three-dimensional power Doppler ultrasound. Ultrasound Obstet Gynecol 22:661–663

Chapter 8

Biological Safety of Diagnostic Sonography

Dev Maulik

Introduction

Diagnostic insonation is generally considered to be safe during pregnancy as cumulative experience and epidemiological investigations have failed to demonstrate any causally related adverse effects in the exposed population since its introduction over 40 years ago. Over the decades prenatal utilization of diagnostic ultrasonography has continued to expand [1]. According to the National Vital Statistics, approximately 2.7 million mothers comprising 68% of those who had live births were exposed to diagnostic ultrasound in 2002 in the United States [2]. This represents a 42% increase since 1989 when about 50% of the mothers with live births underwent sonographic scanning. Such a magnitude of exposure requires continuing concern regarding its safety as it has long been recognized that ultrasound exposure can affect biological systems under certain circumstances.

The conventional wisdom has held until recently that the intensity and other acoustic features of diagnostic insonation are insufficient to trigger the known physical mechanisms for bioeffects. This contention has been challenged by theoretical considerations and experimental findings which suggest that such exposure may potentially exert bioeffects, especially tissue heating which may possibly lead to deleterious consequences. In 1997, further concerns were raised when regulatory changes in the United States allowed the Food and Drug Administration (FDA) to give market approval for obstetrical diagnostic ultrasound devices with significantly increased overall upper limits of acoustic energy output (spatial peak temporal average intensity of 720 mW/cm^2) provided that these devices incorporated an acoustic power output display (see below). Even this limit can be surpassed under certain operational conditions, especially during Doppler color flow imaging [3, 4]. Moreover, unlike the United States, most countries do not regulate acoustic output of diagnostic ultrasound instruments which therefore can be equipped with unrestrained acoustic power. This relaxed regulatory policy significantly shifts the responsibility for the safe use of diagnostic ultrasound to sonographers and sonologists who are obliged to respond to this challenge by careful practice and through continuing education. The scientific community remains divided on the issue of continuing the current upper limits of acoustic power output imposed by the FDA as exemplified by the recent educational debate organized by the American Institute of Ultrasound in Medicine (AIUM) where arguments in favor of removing the limits were counterbalanced by continuing concerns and uncertainties regarding safety [5].

Any absolute assurance on the safety of embryonic and fetal exposure to diagnostic ultrasound remains unattainable because of the continuing possibility that a rare or as yet unknown risk may be present from prenatal exposure. However, if biosafety implies the absence of any recognizable adverse effects, then diagnostic ultrasound can surely be considered safe. Furthermore, the theoretical question of hazards from any potential bioeffects must be considered against the benefits that this diagnostic modality offers for optimizing patient care and the risks related to refraining from indicated use.

Extensively updated to address these complex issues, this chapter presents a concise review of the safe use of Doppler sonography in pregnancy and includes the following: the acoustic output of diagnostic ultrasound devices and its regulation; the known physical mechanisms of interaction between ultrasound and biological systems; the bioeffects observed under experimental circumstances; and the current epidemiological evidence regarding its safety. The chapter also recommends guidelines for the safe use of Doppler ultrasound drawing liberally from the current reports and guidelines developed by the various societies and agencies including the following: the National Council on Radiation Protection and Measurements (NCRP) [6], the American Institute of Ultrasound in Medicine (AIUM) [7], the International Perinatal Doppler Society (IPDS) [8], the European Federation of Societies for Ultrasound in Medicine and Biology (EFSUMB) [9], and the World Federation of Societies for Ultrasound in Medicine and Biology (WFSUMB) [10].

Acoustic Output of Diagnostic Ultrasound Devices and Its Regulation

A central issue in the safe use of diagnostic ultrasound is the power output of the instruments. By enacting the Medical Devices Amendment to the US Food, Drug and Cosmetic Act on May 28, 1976, the United States Congress empowered the FDA to control the output limits to the devices through the mandatory premarketing approval process. The approval was based on the manufacturers' ability to demonstrate substantial equivalence of each new device in safety and efficacy to diagnostic ultrasound devices on the market prior to the enactment date. The principle of substantial equivalence in safety was based on the assumption that the pre-enactment devices were safe and was supported by the available scientific data which provided no evidence of independently confirmed adverse significant biological effects in mammalian tissue exposed in vivo to I_{SPTA} below 100 mW/cm^2 [11]. In 1985, the FDA introduced the application specific output standards of substantial equivalence covering four areas of use: cardiac, peripheral vascular, fetal imaging and other, and ophthalmic. In the early 1990s, based on an NCRP technical report called the Output Display Standard (ODS) [12], the AIUM and the National Electrical Manufacturers Association (NEMA) led an initiative to increase the intensity in exchange for on-screen labeling which resulted in a modification of the existing regulation by the FDA. The track 3 option allows devices to increase the overall maximum output limit to 720 mW/cm^2 provided they incorporate the ODS [13]. Equipments used in ophthalmology were exempted. The track 3 devices can have a substantial increase in the power output and it is the responsibility of the sonographer to use the display to limit the intensity of fetal exposure. Given the potential for adverse effects, the need for user education and training in this area can not be overstressed. This provides a compelling rationale for this chapter.

The ODS consists of two risk indicators, a thermal index (TI) for thermal bioeffects, and a mechanical index (MI) for nonthermal bioeffects [12]. The TI was further refined in 1998 adding three tissue-specific TI models [14]. These are further described below:

■ The TI is the ratio of total acoustic power to the acoustic power that would be required to raise temperature by 1°C for a specific tissue model. As a ratio it is dimensionless and provides an estimate of maximum temperature rise rather than the actual increase. Thus a TI of 2 indicates a higher temperature elevation than a TI of 1, but does not imply an actual rise of 2°C in the insonated tissue. There are three tissue-specific thermal indices:
  - TIS = Thermal index for soft tissue is concerned with temperature rise within homogeneous soft tissue.
  - TIB = Thermal index bone is related to temperature elevation in bone at or near the focus of the beam.
  - TIC = Thermal index cranial bone indicates temperature increase of bone at or near the surface, such as during a cranial examination.
■ The MI is also a dimensionless quantity and is derived from the peak rarefactional pressure at the point of the maximal intensity divided by the square root of the center frequency of the pulse bandwidth. It is an indicator of potential nonthermal bioeffects, especially those that are cavitation-related. According to the FDA, the MI may range up to 1.9 except for ophthalmic usage. The higher the value of MI, the higher the risk of a mechanical effect.

The relevance and practical utilization of the indices for safe use of diagnostic sonography are further discussed later.

Mechanisms of Bioeffects

Any review of bioeffects of ultrasound must include considerations of the known mechanisms by which propagating ultrasound reacts with biological systems. The following effects are currently recognized:
1. Thermal effects which are mediated by insonation-induced tissue heating
2. Nonthermal or mechanical effects which include those not related to heat generation.

The thermal and the mechanical effects of diagnostic acoustic exposure and their relevance for the safety of Doppler ultrasound usage are further discussed below.

Thermal Effects

As a beam of ultrasound propagates through a tissue medium, a portion of its energy is absorbed and converted to heat because the frictional forces in the medium oppose the ultrasound-related molecular oscillations. The rate of temperature elevation in the insonated tissue is determined by the balance between the rates of heat production and of heat dissipation. The rate of heat generation depends on the characteristics of the transmitted ultrasound and the tissue medium [15].

Acoustic Characteristics

Generation of heat in the insonated tissue depends essentially on the power and intensity of the ultrasound. Several acoustic features are involved in this process including the following:

a. Acoustic power: The most relevant power parameter for thermal bioeffect is the spatial-peak temporal-average intensity (I_{SPTA}) which, as discussed in Chap. 2, is the highest time-averaged acoustic intensity at any point in the field. The output intensity varies with the application-specific default settings such as fetal, cardiac, or peripheral vascular investigations. The operator can supersede such regulations in choosing the mode. Most devices provide a control for altering the power output. Caution must be exercised in increasing the power indiscriminately as most obstetrical ultrasound examinations can be performed efficiently with the acoustic power set well below the regulatory limits. These issues will be discussed again.

b. Focus: The I_{SPTA} increases with focusing, which concentrates the power in a small area, causing higher intensities and increasing the potential for heating. Most diagnostic instruments employ a focused beam in order to enhance lateral resolution and directionality.

c. Scanning vs stationary beam: The I_{SPTA} intensity is affected by whether the ultrasound device utilizes a scanning or a stationary beam. In the scanning ultrasound modes, which include B-mode and color flow Doppler imaging, the moving beam temporally distributes the acoustic energy over a wide volume of tissue in the scanned area and thus minimizes the risk of tissue heating. In the stationary ultrasound modes, which include spectral Doppler and M-mode, the acoustic power is concentrated linearly along the static ultrasound beam axis, depositing acoustic energy in a significantly smaller volume of tissue for the duration of exposure. In this scenario, the highest elevation of temperature is encountered along the beam axis between the surface and proximal to the focal point, and its location is near the surface if the focal length is long and adjacent to the focal point if the focal length is short.

d. Pulse repetition frequency (PRF): The higher the PRF, the greater the temporal average intensity. The PRF is under the user control, but can change automatically interactively with other controls such as the focal range. Increasing the focal range may automatically elevate the PRF. In spectral pulsed Doppler and color Doppler modes, the PRF is increased to eliminate aliasing which can result in increased I_{SPTA}.

e. Pulse length (also known as the pulse duration or burst length): This directly affects I_{SPTA}. This is relevant for using the pulsed Doppler mode, as a larger Doppler sample volume will increase pulse duration which will increase the intensity. The pulse length is also greater in color flow Doppler than in B-mode imaging.

f. Dwell time: This refers to the duration of ultrasound exposure. The longer the dwell time, the greater the thermal effect. During most fetal examinations the operator moves the transducer around, thereby reducing the duration of exposure in a given location. In using unscanned modes such as spectral Doppler interrogation of the middle cerebral artery, one needs to reduce the scan time deliberately because of the greater risk of thermal effect in this specific instance.

g. Write zoom: In this function, where the image is magnified by rescanning a smaller area of interest in the image plane with more scan lines, the insonated tissue is exposed to a higher concentration of acoustic intensity. Moreover, using the write zoom box at a greater depth will lead to an even higher intensity as this requires a larger aperture involving more transducer elements emitting more power. This is especially applicable to the color flow Doppler color box function where a narrower and deeper color box will increase the intensity and the risk of temperature elevation. This risk is enhanced when color flow Doppler is used along with spectral pulsed Doppler in the duplex mode.

h. Transducer frequency: Higher frequency ultrasound is more avidly absorbed by tissues, increasing the risk of heating. As higher frequency limits the depth of penetration, heating is restricted to the superficial tissues close to the transducer. Moreover, suboptimal depth resolution in this case may prompt the user to increase the power output, which may contribute to tissue heating.

i. The nonlinearity of ultrasound propagation: In ultrasound pulses, especially the high amplitude waves, the compression in the wave propagates faster than the rarefaction, resulting in distortion in the waveform so that the peak of the wave follows the trough very closely. With the compression following the rarefaction very quickly, shock and harmonic components of higher frequencies are generated. This phenomenon is impeded in tissue with higher attenuation such as bone and is facilitated in tissue with lower attenuation such as amniotic fluid or even neural tissue. The higher frequency may lead to significant absorption of energy and conversion to heat. Although such thermal effects have not been demonstrated in the fetus, the potential exists, especially when ultrasound of higher amplitudes propagating through a fluid media develops shock waves with high-frequency harmonics before entering soft-tissue media.

Tissue Characteristics for Thermal Effect

Ultrasound-induced tissue heating is determined by the balance between heat generation and heat loss (Fig. 8.1). The ultrasound-induced temperature increase in biological tissue depends on the inherent acoustic properties of the tissue that determine heat generation. These include its acoustic impedance and the attenuation and absorption of the sound in the tissue which leads to conversion of sound energy to thermal energy. The degree of ultrasound-induced temperature is directly related to the absorption coefficient of the tissue [16, 17]. The actual temperature elevation is also dependent on the factors that control dissipation of heat in the tissue and include tissue perfusion and thermal conduction and diffusion. The impact of tissue heating depends on the mechanisms that control cellular response to heating, the specific types of tissue, and the anatomic configuration, such as proximity to bone. These are discussed below.

Cellular Response to Heating, Acoustic Power, and Temporal Threshold

The cellular and tissue response to hyperthermia has been extensively investigated in relation to cancer therapy. Cells and tissues differ in their response to heat. Nonlethal temperature elevation induces cells to mobilize defensive mechanisms constituting what is known as the heat-shock response. The response essentially involves induction of genes that encode a spectrum of protective proteins known as heat-shock proteins (HSP) [18]. The dominant group in eukaryotic cells is the HSP70 family although other HSP families are also involved. Nonlethal temperature elevations above the normal induce synthesis of the HSPs which then act as molecular chaperones and prevent protein denaturation or aggregation. These protective mechanisms, however, become rapidly ineffective if the tissue temperature exceeds 43 °C. Beyond this threshold the duration and the magnitude of temperature elevation determine the thermal injury, with each degree of temperature elevation reducing the temporal threshold for thermal effect by a factor of 2 [19]. As discussed by Duck [20], these considerations, especially the exponentially decreasing temporal threshold for producing thermal injury with the increasing acoustic power, assist in defining the safe upper limits of power. For example, if insonation with an acoustic power equivalent to a TI of 6.0 raises tissue temperature to 43 °C, and thermal injury occurs after 30 min of such exposure, doubling that acoustic power will markedly reduce the time threshold to only 30 s. This theoretical scenario is based on the available experimental evidence and theoretical analyses. The practical implications are further considered below. As many currently marketed devices are capable of producing a TI of 6.0 [21], great caution should be exercised in using such instruments.

Experimental Evidence of Thermal Effects

Because of the importance of thermal injury in any consideration of ultrasound biosafety and the potential of temperature elevation from the current generation of ultrasound diagnostic devices especially with spectral pulsed Doppler applications, thermal effects have been extensively investigated. Animal studies have demonstrated that embryonic and fetal tissues are more prone to thermal injury during organogenesis with rapidly replicating and differentiating cells [22]. Furthermore, germ cells in the fetal gonads, especially the testes, continue to be vulnerable to temperature elevation; this may compromise future fertility. Hyperthermia is a proven teratogen and thermal teratogenesis is threshold dependent [23]. The spectrum of thermal teratogenic effects include abortion, neural tube defects, decreased brain growth, anophthalmia, cataracts, cleft lip and cleft palate, and heart, skeletal, spinal, vertebral, and dental defects [17].

However, extrapolating experimental findings to clinical situations remains challenging. It is difficult to justify that experimental conditions such as whole-body heating are applicable to the circumstances of clinical diagnostic ultrasound. Nevertheless, these data help to define boundary conditions of safe use. For exposures lasting up to 50 h, no significant biological effects have been observed when temperature

Acoustic Characteristics
Acoustic Power
Frequency
Source Dimensions
Pulse Repetition Frequency
Pulse Duration
Exposure Duration
Transducer Self Heating

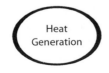

Tissue Characteristics
Acoustic Impedance
Absorption
Perfusion
Heat Conductivity
Heat diffusivity
Speed of Sound
Anatomic Structure

Fig. 8.1. Factors contributing to the thermal effect of ultrasound in a tissue medium

elevation does not exceed 1.5 °C above the normal core temperature. Most evidence shows that developmental injury requires a temperature rise of at least 1.5 °C. Above this threshold, teratogenic effects are determined by the magnitude of the temperature rise and its duration. For temperature increases of 4 °C and 6 °C above normal, the respective limits for the duration are 16 min and 1 min. The lowest temperature value for consistent teratogenesis in mammals has been reported to be 41.5 °C [24].

Acoustic Heating of Fetal Bones

Mineralized bone has the highest coefficient, 10 dB/cm·MHz, and therefore the highest likelihood of thermal effect. Mineralization and ossification of fetal bones begins in the 12th week of pregnancy and progresses with advancing gestation. Drewniak and associates [25] studied the effect of progressive ossification with advancing gestation on ultrasound-induced heat generation in human fetal femur ex utero. By 15 weeks of pregnancy, the rate of temperature rise in the bone was 30 times greater than that in the soft tissue.

Acoustic Heating of Fetal Brain

The average absorption coefficient for neural tissue is 0.2 dB/cm·MHz. Despite its low absorption coefficient, the fetal central nervous system being enclosed in the skull and the spinal canal vertebrae is vulnerable to bone-related heating. Similar risks may also exist for other structures lying close to bone, such as the pituitary gland or the hypothalamus. However, there is conflicting evidence on the actual risk of brain heating from insonation.

Bosward et al. [26] noted in fresh and formalin-fixed fetal guinea-pig brains a mean temperature elevation of 5.2 °C following a 2-min insonation with I_{SPTA} of 2.9 W/cm^2 with a stationary beam in a tank containing water at 38 °C. The greatest temperature rise in brain tissue occurred close to the bone and correlated with both gestational age and progression in bone development. Barnett [27] has recently reviewed the experimental evidence regarding brain temperature elevation and concluded that insonation-induced intracranial heating increases with gestational age concomitant with progressive fetal bone development. Pulsed spectral Doppler ultrasound can produce a biologically significant temperature rise in the fetal brain with approximately 75% of the maximum heating occurring within 30 s. Brain blood flow does not significantly impact heating induced by exposure to a narrow focused ultrasound beam. An insonation-induced temperature rise of 4 °C sustained for 5 min leads to irreversible injury to the fetal

brain, whereas a temperature increase of up to 1.5 °C for 120 s does not elicit measurable electrophysiological responses in the fetal brain.

In contrast to the above findings, others have failed to note any significant temperature elevation in animal models. Stone and associates [28] conducted investigations on the heating effects of pulsed Doppler ultrasound on fetal brain tissue in dead and live animals. Whereas tissue heating was observed at the skull bone-to-brain interface in the dead lamb brain, minimal or no temperature elevation was observed in live lambs. Tarantal and colleagues [24] investigated in vivo temperature elevations in gravid primates (macaques) measured intracranially or at the muscle-bone interface consequent to imaging and pulsed Doppler ultrasonic exposure. This study is one of the very few reports on pulsed Doppler exposure. Utilizing a commercial ultrasound instrument and with varying duration of insonation involving the imaging and the pulsed Doppler mode, the highest temperature elevation observed was 0.6 °C. Both the reports suggest that the presence of tissue perfusion in a living animal may play a protective role by dissipating the heat.

A rare report involving direct thermocouple recording of intracranial temperature in a neurosurgical patient during color transcranial Doppler ultrasound for 30 min failed to demonstrate any temperature elevation either in the brain parenchyma or at the bone/soft tissue interface [29]. A 2.5-MHz transducer was used with the Doppler mode power settings at SPTA of 2,132 mW/cm^2 and a maximum power of 149.3 mW. The ipsilateral tympanic temperature rose by 0.06 °C, indicating an overall increase in brain temperature.

Clinical Significance of the Ultrasound Thermal Effects

Although ultrasound exposure carries the potential for tissue heating, there is no clinical evidence of thermal injury to the human fetus from diagnostic insonation. However, as theoretical risks exist, one must exercise caution especially in using spectral pulsed Doppler ultrasound. The ability of the human body to tolerate limited temperature elevations without any harm is well known. In healthy humans, variations in the body temperature occur under different physiological circumstances such as during physical exercise. However, febrile illnesses may increase the risk enough for extra caution. The fetus is dependent on the mother for heat dissipation mostly through the placental circulation and to some extent across the fetal skin and amniotic fluid to maternal tissues and circulation [30]. The fetus is warmer than the mother [31]. Fetal skin temperature has been shown on average 0.23 °C above the temperature of the uterine wall [32] and fetal core temperature is 0.75 °C above its skin temperature [33].

Miller and Ziskin [23] suggested that the probability of any measurable bioeffects from diagnostic insonation is minimal or nonexistent if the maximum temperature rise remains 2 °C or less in an afebrile subject. Temperature elevations not exceeding 39 °C are most unlikely to induce any fetal abnormalities. However, at higher temperatures, the duration of ultrasound exposure becomes a significant factor. Indeed, as shown in Fig. 8.2, these authors have defined a boundary line based on the temperature rise and exposure duration; below this line, risks of thermal bioeffects are virtually nonexistent. The authors recommended that an ultrasound examination need not be restricted if the combination of temperature elevation and exposure duration remains below this boundary line.

In obstetrical ultrasonography, fetal developmental issues require additional considerations. Fetal vulnerability in the worst case scenario demands prudent practice while not depriving the patient of the benefits of diagnostic ultrasonography. This issue has been discussed extensively by the various international societies who have issued official statements on thermal effects and the safe use of diagnostic insonation.

The WFSUMB endorsed the following recommendations regarding Doppler in 1997:

"It has been demonstrated in experiments with unperfused tissue that some Doppler diagnostic equipment has the potential to produce biologically significant temperature rises, specifically at bone/soft tissue interfaces. The effects of elevated temperatures may be minimised by keeping the time for which the beam passes through any one point in tissue as short as possible. Where output power can be controlled, the lowest available power level consistent with obtaining the desired diagnostic information should be used. Although the data on humans are sparse, it is clear from animal studies that exposures resulting in temperatures less than 38.5 °C can be used without reservation on thermal grounds. This includes obstetric applications" [10].

The 1997 AIUM position on temperature elevation and exposure duration is as follows [7]:

■ "For exposure duration up to 50 hours, there have been no significant biological effects observed due to temperature increases less than or equal to 2 °C above normal.

■ For temperature increases greater than 2 °C above normal, there have been no significant biological effects observed due to temperature increases less than or equal to $6-(\log_{10} t/0.6)$, where t is the exposure duration ranging from 1 to 250 min. For example, for temperature increases of 4 °C and 6 °C, the corresponding limits for the exposure duration t are 16 min and 1 min respectively.

■ In general, adult tissues are more tolerant of temperature increases than fetal and neonatal tissues.

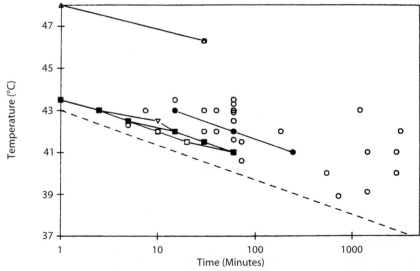

Fig. 8.2. Thermal bioeffects. A plot of thermally produced biological effects that have been reported in the literature in which the temperature elevation and exposure durations are provided. Each data point represents either the lowest temperature reported for any duration or the shortest duration for any temperature reported for a given effect. The *solid lines* link multiple data points relating to the same bioeffect. The *dashed line* represents a lower boundary (t43 = 1) for observed, thermally induced biological effects. (With permission from [23])

Therefore, higher temperatures and/or longer exposure durations would be required for thermal damage."

The position of the International Perinatal Doppler Society, which draws extensively from the existing evidence as well as the deliberations of the other learned societies, published in 2001, is reflected in the following statement:

"In general, Doppler applications (excluding fetal monitoring) present the highest risk of inducing biological effects that are thermally mediated. This follows from the use of longer pulses and higher pulse repetition rates than those used in B-mode gray scale scanned imaging modes. The current FDA regulatory limit for diagnostic ultrasound devices used in the USA for obstetric ultrasound applications is 720 mW/cm^2 intensity (I_{SPTA}) at the tissue of interest, i.e. attenuated according to the beam path length in tissue. For this intensity, the maximum temperature increase in the conceptus may exceed 2 °C. Data from animal experiments have shown that some Doppler equipment can produce a biologically significant temperature rise (>4 °C), especially at bone/soft tissue interfaces such as in fetal examinations in the 2nd and 3rd trimester. Scientific data on effects of whole body hyperthermia show that adverse effects on embryo and fetal development can result from exposure to temperature increases of 2 °C or more above normal body temperature. The risk of adverse effects resulting from a given level of heating increases with duration of exposure" [8].

Mechanical Effects

These bioeffects of ultrasound exposure encompass nonthermal mechanisms, primarily those related to acoustic cavitational phenomena involving expansion and collapse of gas bubbles in tissues. Nonthermal effects also include nonthermal and noncavitational phenomena such as acoustic radiation pressure, force, and torque and acoustic streaming; these will not be discussed in this chapter as their significance in producing biological effects remains unclear.

Cavitation

Cavitation is the formation and growth of bubbles in a liquid. Under certain circumstances the bubbles undergo inertial collapse. Acoustic cavitation relates to cavitational phenomena caused by propagating sound waves on preexisting gaseous nuclei or microbubbles in the exposed medium [34–37]. Two types of cavitational phenomena are recognized: inertial cavitation and stable cavitation.

In inertial cavitation, the rarefaction and compression cycle of propagating ultrasound waves induce expansion and contraction of gaseous micronuclei of appropriate resonant size [38]. At lower ultrasound intensities, as used in diagnostic ultrasound devices, the size of the bubble is bigger during the expansion than during the contraction. This results in gradually increasing dimensions of the bubble until it starts to resonate when it readily absorbs acoustic energy and rapidly expands. A critical threshold is reached when the bubble can no longer absorb energy sufficient enough to maintain its expansion. During the compression, the surrounding fluid rushes into the bubble at a very high speed and the momentum of the fluid jet causes rapid collapse of the bubble. In the final phase of collapse, the energy content of the cavity will be liberated in an extremely minute space, generating intense heat and pressure. The temperatures of a collapsing bubble may exceed 5,000 °C with pressures of hundreds to thousands of atmospheres. The heat and the pressure rapidly dissipate as the phenomenon is very localized, microscopic in size, and less than a microsecond in duration. This phenomenon of nonlinear oscillation and eventual collapse of a resonating bubble in an acoustic field is known as inertial cavitation (Fig. 8.3). In the past, the phenomenon has also been known as transient or collapse cavitation.

If the acoustic pressure amplitude remains less than the initial radius of the bubble, the oscillations are relatively stable. This is known as stable cavitation. Such an oscillating bubble absorbs energy from the incident ultrasonic beam and converts this into heat and spherical waves. These waves then re-radiate from the bubble. The oscillatory motion of a cavity often shows asymmetry because of the distortions produced by an adjacent solid boundary or by surface waves at the bubble-liquid interface. In the adjacent

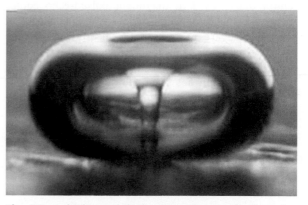

Fig. 8.3. A high-speed flash photomicrograph of an imploding cavity. The asymmetry of implosion is caused by the solid surface near the bubble (depicted by the *straight line*). (With permission from [123])

liquid, the oscillatory motion generates a steady eddying flow, often of high velocity; this phenomenon is known as microstreaming. Intracellular microstreaming can also occur from a vibrating cell membrane close to an asymmetrically oscillating cavity. That stable cavitation can induce bioeffects under experimental conditions has been demonstrated by various investigators [39, 40]. However this type of cavitation has not been shown to be of any significance in bioeffects considerations.

Cavitational phenomenon in a medium related to ultrasound exposure is controlled by many factors including acoustic characteristics of field, ambient factors, and cavitational potential of the medium. These are elaborated below.

Acoustic Characteristics for Cavitation

The critical acoustic factors responsible for producing inertial collapse of a resonating bubble are the maximum rarefaction and compressional pressures. The greater the rarefactional or negative pressure, the more the bubble expands preceding collapse. The greater the compressional or positive pressure, the more intense is the inertial pressure of the collapse. Both factors determine the intensity of the bubble collapse and the consequent severe local disruption. However, positive or negative pressure spikes of very short duration ($< 0.01 \,\mu s$) are not of significance. With pulsed ultrasound, the pulse length, duty cycle and frequency affect cavitation. Shorter pulses and lower pulse repetition frequency increase the cavitational intensity threshold. Indeed, it has been suggested that cavitation may probably be prevented if the pulse duration is sufficiently reduced [41], which has led to the general assumption that with medical diagnostic pulsed echo ultrasound, the pulse duration is too short to produce any cavitational activity. However, it has been demonstrated that microsecond-length pulses used in diagnostic pulsed-echo equipment may cause inertial cavitation if gas nuclei of suitable size are present in the medium and if the acoustic parameters of the ultrasound are appropriate. Moreover, the intensity threshold for producing inertial cavitation has been shown to be 1–10 W/cm^2 for microsecond-length pulses [42]. Temporal maximum intensity far exceeding this level can occur in diagnostic ultrasound imaging. The risk is potentially greater with some pulsed Doppler systems because of the higher pulse repetition frequency and intensity.

Ambient Pressure and Temperature

Ambient pressure and cavitational activity are inversely related, so an increase in the former increases the threshold intensities for cavitation. Conversely, higher temperature facilitates cavitation by decreasing the solubility of gas in the medium which will lead to microbubbles that serve as nuclei for cavitation to occur.

Tissue Characteristics for Cavitation

Prerequisites for cavitational activity are the quantity and size of the gas nuclei present in the medium. As mentioned earlier, even microsecond-length pulses have the potential to induce inertial cavitation, depending on the presence of micronuclei of sufficient size. Unfortunately, gaseous micronuclei are not easily detected. Although it has been disputed in the past, there is ample evidence that strongly suggests the presence of such nuclei in mammalian tissues. Such evidence includes studies on decompression syndrome in humans, experiments with lithotripter in dogs [43], and the observation in mice that application of hydrostatic pressure increased the threshold for sonar-related tissue damage [44]. The presence of such nuclei and insonation-related cavitation has been demonstrated in mammals by Lee and Frizzell [45] who observed hydrostatic pressure and temperature-dependent neonatal mouse hind limb paralysis due to ultrasound exposure. Aerated lung tissue with its blood – gas interface is particularly susceptible to the presence of gas nuclei. This is further discussed below.

Biological Effects of Inertial Cavitation

A collapsing cavity can result in cell lysis, dissociation of water vapor, and generation of free radicals. The mechanism by which inertial cavitation causes cell destruction involves generation of intense local heat and pressure and the generation of shear forces by the bubble implosion [14, 46]. Furthermore, it has recently been suggested that such implosions may occur within the cell; such an event may not lyse the cells but may give rise to free radicals. Continuous-wave high-intensity ultrasound has been shown to produce free radicals in aqueous biological medium by inertial cavitation [47]. The free radicals may affect macromolecules. Thymine base alteration, chromosomal agglomeration, and mutation have been observed in insonated but intact cells. Irreversible deterioration of the enzyme A-chymotrypsin has been reported following production of radicals from insonation-induced cavitation [48]. Similarly, other toxic products such as hydrogen peroxide may induce adverse effects in a biological system. It should be emphasized that these phenomena have been noted mostly during in vitro experiments and never in relation to any human exposure.

Animal experiments have demonstrated lung, kidney, and other organ injuries due to nonthermal effects of ultrasound exposure. Especially relevant is the demonstration of pulmonary capillary hemorrhage and cardiac arrhythmia in nonmammalian and mammalian species from exposure to ultrasound. *Drosophila* larvae are highly susceptible to injury from exposure to high peak intensity (50–100 W/cm^2) pulsed ultrasound only shortly before hatching when they have air in the respiratory system, suggesting a cavitational effect [49]. The mouse lung exposed to pulsed ultrasound demonstrates threshold-dependent hemorrhagic lesions [50]. More relevantly, a primate study corroborates these findings [51]. Appropriately controlled studies were performed in monkeys using a clinical diagnostic ultrasound instrument with combined imaging, and color and pulsed Doppler modes creating maximum power output conditions with peak rarefactional pressure of 3.7 MPa at 4 MHz representing an MI of approximately 1.8. The exposure resulted in multiple well-demarcated circular hemorrhagic focal lesions (0.1–1.0 cm) in the study groups but not in the control groups. Recently, acoustic cavitation as the mechanism for insonation-induced lung hemorrhage has been questioned. It has been suggested relatively recently that lung hemorrhage in the absence of the contrast agents may not be related to acoustic cavitation [52]. It has also been demonstrated recently in a rat model that lung hemorrhage correlates better with in situ (at the lung surface) pulse intensity integral than with in situ peak rarefactional pressure, suggesting a mechanism other than cavitation [53]. Insonation-induced reductions in aortic pressure and ventricular arrhythmia have been reported in the frog and murine hearts [54, 55]. It appears that the former effect may be related to radiation force. No lesions were noted in the cardiac tissues. Comprehensive reviews of these studies are available elsewhere [6, 56].

In a rare study involving humans, ultrasonically induced lung hemorrhage was investigated in 50 patients following routine intraoperative transesophageal echocardiography [57]. The left lung was observed directly by the surgeon. The ultrasound characteristics were: maximum derated intensity in the sound field of 186 W/cm^2, maximum derated rarefactional acoustic pressure of 2.4 MPa, maximum mechanical index of 1.3, and lowest frequency of 3.5 MHz. These criteria are greater than the threshold found for gross lung surface hemorrhage seen in laboratory animals. No lung surface hemorrhage was observed on gross examination. The authors concluded that clinical transesophageal echocardiography, even above the threshold levels for lung hemorrhage in experimental animals, did not cause surface lung hemorrhage apparent on gross observation.

Most of the above and similar evidence is more relevant for neonatal and adult than fetal diagnostic ultrasound. No gas bodies have been shown to exist in the fetus. Although lung tissue, because of its blood–air interface, may be particularly susceptible to cavitational effects, this clearly is not applicable to fetal lung tissue. There are no reported studies demonstrating any cavitational effects in the fetus.

The use of contrast agents, however, presents a different scenario. Contrast agents are encapsulated gas microbubbles that are used to enhance the ultrasound backscattering in echocardiography and vascular imaging. When exposed to ultrasound, the contrast agent gas bodies are activated, destabilize, and form cavitation nuclei, and thus provide the potential for inertial cavitation. Such activation has been implicated in causing hemolysis in whole blood [58], membrane damage in cells in monolayer culture [59], increased cardiac microvascular permeability, petechial hemorrhage, and premature ventricular contractions in rats [60]. There is an ever-increasing body of evidence on the bioeffects of contrast agents and a comprehensive review is beyond the scope of this chapter.

Clinical Significance of Acoustic Cavitation

Although the question of inertial or stable cavitation occurring from diagnostic insonation is entirely speculative, a theoretical possibility exists, as the presence of gaseous nuclei in mammalian tissues has been demonstrated and some diagnostic ultrasound instruments may generate temporal maximum intensities in excess of the cavitational threshold. Even if cavitational phenomena occur, the consequent loss of a few cells, in all probability, may not be significant for most clinical situations. However, even this scant theoretical risk of cavitation should be considered in order to restrict the maximum intensity output of diagnostic imaging especially for the Doppler mode. Consistent with the principles of prudent practice, one should be guided by the MI, which is the best indicator of cavitational potential currently available. An MI value of 1 or lower, considered to be safe for adult and pediatric applications, should also suffice for fetal applications where the risks of cavitation remain very remote. However, the safety concerns are substantially different with regard to the use of contrast agents in obstetrics and their use is clearly contraindicated in obstetrical imaging.

The IPDS recommendation for the prenatal use of Doppler use is as follows: "To avoid cavitation-related biological effects it is important to reduce the peak amplitude, or to use a lower value for MI on equipment that has an ODS. The presence of contrast agents should be taken into account when considering the risk/benefit ratio of an ultrasound examination" [8].

Experimentally Induced Developmental Bioeffects

Although Mackintosh and Davey [61] reported low-intensity ultrasound-induced chromosomal aberrations in human leukocyte culture, subsequent investigators, including Mackintosh and coworkers, did not succeed in reproducing these results, even when the intensities were raised to cavitational threshold [62–64]. Increased sister chromatid exchange in human lymphocytes was reported to occur from experimental ultrasound exposure [65]. The significance of this finding can be appreciated from the fact that such an increase in sister chromatid exchange is regarded as an indicator of chromosomal damage. However, numerous subsequent reports failed to corroborate this. In an in vitro model utilizing fresh human placentas, Ehlinger et al. [66] observed increased sister chromatid exchange in fetal lymphocytes using a clinical diagnostic linear array unit. However, a subsequent investigation [67] and a subsequent review by Miller [68] failed to verify this. It can be reasonably concluded from the available evidence that clinical diagnostic ultrasound exerts no appreciable damaging effects on chromosomes.

Consequences of prenatal insonation on embryonic and fetal development were extensively investigated in animals. Most of the reports demonstrated conflicting outcomes, and thus contributed little to elucidating the risks of prenatal ultrasound exposure. In their excellent review on this subject, Carstensen and Gates [69] observed that more than half the reported investigations failed to demonstrate any developmental bioeffects. Moreover, multigeneration studies have failed to demonstrate any consistent adverse effects in the offsprings of animals exposed to ultrasound in utero [70, 71]. The adverse effects, when noted, included fetal growth restriction [72, 73], increased perinatal loss [74–76], fetal malformations [77, 78], and behavioral teratogenesis, including delayed maturation of grasp reflex. In contrast, there are studies that failed to show fetal growth compromise [79–81], increased malformation [82], increased perinatal mortality [83], and behavioral alterations in the neonate [84].

Epidemiological Evidence of Developmental Bioeffects

It is well known that embryos and fetuses of all mammalian species are highly sensitive to environmental insults. This makes them more vulnerable than adults to the risks of ultrasound-induced bioeffects. Although a number of investigations have been carried out in humans on the developmental effects of ultrasound, the dearth of well-controlled studies dedicated to safety is remarkable. This is understandable because of formidable logistics and financial challenges of such investigations. Furthermore, acoustic specifications of the diagnostic equipment should

Table 8.1. Summary of epidemiological evidence of biological effects of diagnostic ultrasound

Outcome	Study type	Ultrasound	Results	References
General development and neonatal outcome	Observational and randomized trial	Ultrasound and B-mode	No effects	87–94
Fetal movements	Observational	CW Doppler FHR monitor	One study noted increased movements. Other studies did not confirm	95–98
Fetal and infant growth	Observational and randomized trial	Doppler and B-mode imaging	One study showed increased low birth weight. Follow up showed no difference at 1 year. All other studies showed no adverse effect on fetal and infant growth	94, 99–107
Pediatric malignancies	Observational	B-mode imaging	No increased risk in any of the studies	109–113
Neurodevelopment, learning, speech	Observational and randomized trial	B-mode imaging	One study showed higher incidence of delayed speech. Rest of the studies did not confirm this	94, 114–117
Neurodevelopment, sinistrality	Randomized trials and cohort	B-mode imaging	Not increased in general. Increased left handedness in boys by subgroup analysis	118–120

remain comparable during the study period in order to ensure uniformity of exposure conditions, which is unlikely with the rapid evolution of ultrasound technology. Despite these challenges, a substantial body of evidence exists which has been extensively reviewed [85, 86]. A review of human bioeffects is presented below according to selected outcome categories and further summarized in Table 8.1.

General Outcome

It is noteworthy that almost all human epidemiological studies fail to show any demonstrable adverse outcome in the fetus, the neonate, and the infant [87–94]. In 1972, Ziskin [90] reported a survey of clinical applications of diagnostic insonation involving over 121,000 examinations and noted no recognizable adverse effects. The data indicate that the probability of occurrence of a known adverse effect is less than 1 in 400,000 examinations. In the largest study reported [92], the Health Protection Branch of the Canadian Environmental Health Directorate conducted a nation-wide survey of diagnostic ultrasound usage during 1977. This report, which involved 340,000 patients and 1.2 million exposures, failed to identify any adverse effect clearly attributable to insonation. Hellman et al. investigated the risk of insonation-related developmental anomalies in 3,297 exposed mothers, of whom only 1,114 patients were included in the analysis [88]. Mothers were exposed to pulsed or continuous-wave ultrasound between 10 and 40 weeks of pregnancy. The investigators reported no greater frequency of congenital abnormalities in the insonated group than in the general population.

Fetal Movement

Following a report by David and associates that continuous-wave Doppler ultrasound exposure as used in electronic fetal heart rate monitoring increased the mean fetal activity by 90% as measured by fetal movement count [95], several studies failed to confirm such an association [96–98]. Murrills and coinvestigators performed a randomized double-blind controlled trial involving 100 mothers in the study group and 50 in the control group and found no evidence supporting such an effect. The authors attributed the initial reported observation to mechanisms unrelated to continuous-wave Doppler ultrasound exposure.

Birth Weight

The relationship between prenatal diagnostic ultrasound exposure and fetal growth has been investigated primarily or secondarily by several investigators [94, 99–107]. Moore and associates [101] conducted a retrospective cohort study that compared the birth weights of 1,598 exposed and 944 unexposed single live births. Confounding variables associated with both exposure status and birth weight outcome were included in multivariate analysis. Although the frequency of ultrasound scanning and the first exposure during the third trimester were associated with a reduction in birth weight, the most consistent effect on the birth weight appeared to be the indication for an ultrasound examination. The relationship of ultrasound exposure and reduced birth weight appeared to be due to shared common risk factors, which lead to both exposure and a reduction in birth weight. Waldenstrom and associates performed a randomized trial in 4,997 pregnant women of whom 2,482 received routine ultrasound screening at 15 weeks of pregnancy and the 2,515 received the usual prenatal care [102]. In the study group, the frequency of birth weight less than 2,500 g was significantly reduced (59 vs 95, $p = 0.005$) and the mean birth weight was significantly higher (42 g, $p = 0.008$). The authors speculated that the effect may be attributable to reduced smoking in screened women in response to watching their fetus on the scan. Ewigman and coinvestigators performed a randomized clinical trial of prenatal ultrasound involving more than 15,000 pregnancies and did not observe any effect of ultrasound exposure on the birth weight [104]. Newnham and associates investigated the beneficial effects of frequent prenatal ultrasound, both imaging and Doppler, in a randomized trial involving 2,834 women (study group 1,415, control group 1,419) with singleton pregnancies. Sonographic investigations were carried out at 18, 24, 28, 34 and 38 weeks [103]. The only outcome difference noted between the two groups was significantly higher intrauterine growth restriction in the ultrasound group (birth weight 10th centile: relative risk 1.35, 95% confidence interval 1.09–1.67, $p = 0.006$; and birth weight 3rd centile: relative risk 1.65, 95% confidence intervals 1.09–2.49, $p = 0.020$). The primary objective of the study was not to test the effect of ultrasound on fetal growth. Subsequent follow-up of these infants demonstrated no growth differences between the groups at 1 year of age [107]. The issue was studied by Grisso and associates [106] utilizing a case-control approach involving more than 13,000 pregnancies. This retrospective investigation specifically examined the association between prenatal ultrasound exposure and the risk of low birth weight. No adverse effects of ultrasound were noted. The most recent Cochrane Review reported a meta-analysis of nine published trials of ultrasound. Six trials provided information on the incidence of low birth weight (< 2,500 g ms) and the systematic review of the data did not demonstrate any significant effect of prenatal ultrasound on the frequency of low birth weight (Peto odds ratio 0.96, 95% confidence interval 0.82–1.12) [108].

Pediatric Malignancy

The risks of childhood malignancies following prenatal diagnostic ultrasound exposure have been studied by several investigators. The malignant conditions investigated included lymphatic leukemia, myeloid leukemia, and solid tumors. The earlier studies found no association between in utero ultrasound exposure and childhood leukemia or solid tumors [109–112]. More recently, a prospective population-based case-control study from Sweden investigated the relationship between fetal exposure to ultrasound and development of childhood leukemia [113]. The study failed to demonstrate any significant association between single or repeated prenatal insonation and lymphatic or myeloid leukemia developing in infancy and childhood. The respective odds ratios were 0.85 (95% confidence interval 0.62–1.17) and 1.0 (95% confidence interval 0.42–2.40). Corrections for potential confounding variables, such as maternal age, high birth weight, and twin pregnancies, did not influence the results.

Neurodevelopment – General

Investigations in this field have so far yielded assuring results [99, 114–117]. Stark and coinvestigators followed up 425 infants exposed to diagnostic insonation in utero and a control group of 381 unexposed infants for various outcome parameters including neurological outcomes at 7 and 12 years of age [99]. The tests included conductive and nerve measurements of hearing, visual acuity and color vision, cognitive function, behavior, and a complete and detailed neurologic assessment. No significant differences were noted between the study and the control groups. Salvesen and associates [114] examined any association between routine ultrasonography in utero and subsequent brain development in 8- and 9-year-old children of 2,161 women who took part in two randomized, controlled trials of routine ultrasonography during pregnancy. No clear differences were found between the groups with regard to deficits in attention, motor control, and perception or neurological development during the first year of life. The results are very assuring as no association with impaired neurological development was found. The same group [116] also investigated any possible association between routine ultrasonography in utero and reading and writing skills among 8- or 9-year-old children in primary school. The population base was the same as the previous report [114]. Of 2,428 singletons eligible for follow-up, the school performance of 2,011 children (83%) was assessed by their teachers, who were unaware of ultrasound exposure status. A subgroup of 603 children were also tested for dyslexia. There were no statistically significant differences between children screened with ultrasound and controls in the teacher-reported school performance (scores for reading, spelling, arithmetic, or overall performance). Results showed no differences between screened children and controls in reading, reading comprehension, spelling, arithmetic, overall performance, and dyslexia. Kieler et al. [117] investigated the association between ultrasound exposure in early fetal life and impaired neurologic development in childhood in 3,265 children age 8–9 years whose mothers participated in a randomized controlled trial of ultrasound screening during pregnancy in Sweden during 1985–1987. No significant difference in impaired neurologic development between ultrasound-exposed and -unexposed children was found in this study. A Cochrane systematic review of ultrasound in early pregnancy reanalyzed the results of the Scandinavian trials and showed no long-term adverse outcome related to school performance, neurobehavioural function, vision, or hearing as a consequence of prenatal exposure to ultrasound [108].

Neurodevelopment – Sinistrality

Salvesen and colleagues observed a significant increase in non-right handedness among the children in the study group than among those in the control group (odds ratio 1.32; 95% confidence interval 1.02–1.71) [118]. Kieler and associates also studied a possible association between ultrasound screening in early pregnancy and altered cerebral dominance measured by the prevalence of non-right handedness among children, particularly boys [119]. A significant association was found between ultrasound exposure and non-right handedness among boys (odds ratio 1.33; 95% confidence interval 1.02–1.74). The association was, however, confined to analyses comparing exposed and nonexposed boys and no associations were found when the comparisons were performed according to the randomized groups. This study was unable to exclude a possible association between non-right handedness among boys and sonographic exposure in early fetal life. In a subsequent cohort study, the same group of investigators found a significant association between ultrasound exposure and non-right handedness among boys (odds ratio 1.32; 95% confidence interval 1.16–1.51) when ultrasound was offered more widely (1976–78), whereas no such association was found during the initial phase of routine screening with ultrasound (1973–75) (odds ratio 1.03; 95% confidence interval 0.91–1.17) [120]. The effect was estimated as an extra three left-handers among 100 male births.

The most recent Cochrane Review of the trials observed that although fewer of the ultrasound exposed children were right-handed, this was not confirmed by analysis of long-term follow-up data [108]. However, the possibility of such an effect may exist if exposure of male children to early ultrasound is considered separately regardless of the actual group of assignment in the study. The reviewers concluded that this finding may have been "a chance observation that emanated from the large number of outcome measures assessed, or from the method of ascertainment; alternatively, if it was a real consequence of ultrasound exposure, then it could imply that the effect of diagnostic ultrasound on the developing brain may alter developmental pathways. No firm conclusion can be reached from available data, and there is a need to study these children formally rather than to rely on a limited number of questionnaire responses obtained from the parents".

Clinical Significance

The evidence as discussed above is overwhelmingly reassuring. The position of the AIUM is as follows [121]: "Based on the epidemiologic evidence to date and on current knowledge of interactive mechanisms, there is insufficient justification to warrant a conclusion that there is a causal relationship between diagnostic ultrasound and adverse effects." However, there is a limitation to the current epidemiological evidence of safety, which has been summarized in the International Perinatal Doppler Society Guidelines [8]. The current epidemiological data are based on the use of diagnostic ultrasound devices from the pre-amendment period. However, as discussed at the outset of this chapter, an amendment in the regulatory policy in the USA has enabled the use of substantially increased acoustic outputs, including applications in obstetrics. There are no data from the substantial acoustic exposures delivered by modern ultrasound equipment or from exposures in the early first trimester. This should prompt prudent use of diagnostic ultrasound, especially in the pulsed Doppler mode in a pregnant patient. This is further elaborated in the next section.

Guidelines for Clinical Application

It is assuring that even after years of use, there has not been a single known instance of any identifiable perinatal injury from diagnostic ultrasound usage. This must be recognized as an impressive record of safety. The benefits of diagnostic ultrasound, on the other hand, are remarkable. The technique has extended the scope and precision of diagnostic medi-

cine, and thus has promoted better patient care. This assessment holds true for a wide spectrum of clinical disciplines ranging from cardiology to obstetrics and gynecology.

In spite of this excellent record, the need for continuing vigilance for biosafety is well recognized. That insonation can produce bioeffects is well known, although much of this information is not very relevant for assessing the risks of diagnostic exposure. The epidemiological evidence is very assuring. However, there has been no comprehensive well-controlled, large-scale human study investigating the possibility of subtle, long-term, or cumulative adverse effects of Doppler ultrasound. A matter of recent concern is the increased acoustic power output of the diagnostic ultrasound devices following the changes in FDA regulations [122]. This has renewed the need for caution for pulsed Doppler ultrasound exposure at high intensity and for prolonged periods near fetal bone such as the fetal cranium as would be required for cerebral arterial Doppler interrogation. Similar caution should be exercised for transvaginal Doppler scanning in early pregnancy because close proximity of the transducer to the target tissue and, therefore, reduced attenuation will increase the acoustic energy delivered to the tissue. These risk potentials, although theoretical, should guide us to use diagnostic ultrasound with prudence and clinical judgment. Diagnostic Doppler ultrasound should be used in pregnancy when a medical benefit is expected. Furthermore, as suggested in this chapter, the acoustic exposure conditions should be kept within the limits for obtaining adequate diagnostic information and be guided by the display indicators (MI and TI). Practical guidelines and recommendations have been forwarded by various organizations in this regard. A compilation of the IPDS recommendations are summarized here to serve as guidelines for use of Doppler sonography in obstetrical practice [8]:

1. Care should be taken to ensure that all examinations are performed with the minimum level of acoustic output and dwell time necessary to obtain the required diagnostic information, i.e., use the ALARA (As Low As Reasonably Achievable) principle.
2. Where equipment provides a form of output display, users are encouraged to utilize this feature to help apply the ALARA principle.
3. Users of equipment with an output display should be aware that it is capable of producing far greater intensities in obstetric examinations than equipment that has no output display (i.e., approved through FDA-regulated application-specific limits).
4. Users should take notice of exposure information provided by the manufacturer and minimize exposures to tissue structures containing bone and/or gas.

65. Liebeskind D, Bases R, Mendez R et al (1979) Sister chromatid exchanges in human lymphocytes after exposure to diagnostic ultrasound. Science 205:1273–1275

66. Ehlinger CA, Katayama PK, Roester MR et al (1979) Diagnostic ultrasound increases sister chromatid exchange, preliminary report. Wisc Med J 80:21–25

67. Brulfert A, Ciaravino V, Miller MW et al (1981) Diagnostic insonation of extra-utero human placenta: No effect of lymphocytic sister chromatid exchange. Hum Genet 66:289–291

68. Miller MW (1985) Does ultrasound induce sister chromatid exchanges? Ultrasound Med Biol 11:561–570

69. Carstensen EL, Gates AH (1984) The effects of pulsed ultrasound on the fetus. J Ultrasound Med 3:145–147

70. Manor SM, Serr DM, Tamari I et al (1972) The safety of ultrasound in fetal monitoring. Am J Obstet Gynecol 113:653–661

71. Lyon MF, Simpson GM (1974) An investigation into the possible genetic hazards of ultrasound. Br J Radiol 47:712–722

72. Pizszarello DJ, Vivino A, Maden B et al (1978) Effect of pulsed low-power ultrasound on growing tissues. Expl Cell Biol 46:179–191

73. Stolzenberg S, Torbit CA, Edmonds PD et al (1980) Effects of ultrasound on the mouse exposed at different stages of gestation: Acute studies. Radiat Environ Biophys 17:245–270

74. Cevito KA (1976) Early postpartum mortality following ultrasound radiation. Ultrasound Med 2:535

75. Fry FJ, Erdmann WA, Johnson LK et al (1978) Ultrasound toxicity study. Ultrasound Med Biol 3:351–366

76. Sikov MR, Hildebrand BP (1979) Effects of prenatal exposure to ultrasound. In: Persaud TVN (ed) Advances in the study of birth defects, vol 2. MIT Press, Lancaster, p 267

77. Shimizu T, Shoji R (1973) An experimental Safety Study of Mice Exposed to Low-Intensity Ultrasound. Excerpta Medica International Series No. 227. Excerpta Medica, Amsterdam, p 28

78. Shoji R, Murakami U (1974) Further studies on the effect of ultrasound on mouse and rat embryos. Teratology 10:97–101

79. Murai N, Hoshi K, Kang C et al (1975) Effects of diagnostic ultrasound irradiation during foetal stage on emotional and cognitive behavior in rats. Tohoku J Exp Med 117:225–235

80. Kimmel C, Stratmeyer ME, Galloway WD et al (1983) An evaluation of the teratogenic potential of ultrasound exposure in pregnant ICR mice. Teratology 27:245–251

81. McClain RM, Hoar RM, Saltzman MB (1972) Teratology study of rats exposed to ultrasound. J Obstet Gynecol 14:39–42

82. Warwick R, Pond JB, Woodward B et al (1970) Hazards of diagnostic ultrasonography – a study with mice. IEEE Trans Sonics Ultrasonics Su-17:158

83. Edmonds PD (1979) Effects of ultrasound on biological structures. In: Hinselmann M, Anliker M, Mendt R (eds) Ultraschalldiagnostik in der Medizin. Thieme, Stuttgart, p 2

84. Brown N, Galloway WD, Henton WW (1981) Reflex development following in-utero exposure to ultrasound. In: Proceedings of the 26th Annual Meeting of American Institute of Ultrasound Medicine and 10th Annual Meeting of the Society of Diagnostic Medical Sonographers, Bethesda, MD, p 119

85. Salvesen KA, Eik-Nes SH (1995) Is ultrasound unsound? A review of epidemiological studies of human exposure to ultrasound. Ultrasound Obstet Gynecol 6:293–298

86. European Committee for Medical Ultrasound (1996) ECMUS Safety Committee Tutorial: Epidemiology of diagnostic ultrasound exposure during human pregnancy. EJU 4:69–73

87. Bernstein RL (1969) Safety studies with ultrasonic Doppler technique. Obstet Gynecol 34:707–709

88. Hellman LM, Duffus GM, Donald I et al (1970) Safety of diagnostic ultrasound in obstetrics. Lancet 1:1133–1134

89. Falus M, Koranyi G, Sobel M, Pesti E, van Bao T (1972) Follow-up studies on infants examined by ultrasound during the fetal age. Orv Hetil 13:2119–2121

90. Ziskin MC (1972) Survey of patient exposure to diagnostic ultrasound. In: Reid JM, Sikov MR (eds) Interaction of ultrasound and biological tissues. DHEW (FDA) 78-8008. Government Printing Office, Washington DC

91. Scheidt PC, Stanley F, Bryla DA (1978) One year follow-up of infants exposed to ultrasound in utero. Am J Obstet Gynecol 131:743–748

92. Environmental Health Directorate (1981) Safety Code 23: Guidelines for the safe use of Ultrasound. Part I. Medical and paramedical applications, Report 8-EHD-59. Ottawa Environmental Health Directorate, Health Protection Branch, Ottawa

93. Bakketeig L, Eik-Nes SH, Jacobsen G et al (1984) Randomised controlled trial of ultrasonographic screening in pregnancy. Lancet 2:207–211

94. Eik-Nes S, Okland O, Aure JC, Ulstein M (1984) Ultrasound screening in pregnancy: a randomised controlled trial. Lancet 2:1347

95. David H, Weaver JB, Pearson JF (1975) Doppler ultrasound and fetal activity. BMJ 2:62–64

96. Hertz RH, Timor-Tritsch I, Dierker LJ Jr et al (1979) Continuous ultrasound and fetal movement. Am J Obstet Gynecol 135:152–154

97. Powell-Phillips WD, Towell ME (1979) Doppler ultrasound and subjective assessment of fetal activity. BMJ 2:101–102

98. Murrills AJ, Barrington P, Harris PD, Wheeler T (1983) Influence of Doppler ultrasound on fetal activity. BMJ (Clin Res Ed) 286:1009–1012

99. Stark CR, Orleans M, Haverkamp AD et al (1984) Short and long term risks after exposure to diagnostic ultrasound in-utero. Obstet Gynecol 63:194–200

100. Lyons EA, Dyke C, Toms M, Cheang M (1988) In utero exposure to diagnostic ultrasound: a 6 year follow up. Radiology 166: 687–690

101. Moore RM Jr, Diamond EL, Cavalieri RL (1988) The relationship of birth weight and intrauterine diagnostic ultrasound exposure. Obstet Gynecol 71:513–517

102. Waldenstrom U, Axelsson O, Nilsson S et al (1988) Effects of routine one-stage ultrasound screening in pregnancy: a randomised controlled trial. Lancet 2:585–588

103. Newnham JP, Evans SF, Michael CA et al (1993) Effects of frequent ultrasound during pregnancy: a randomised controlled trial. Lancet 342:887–891

104. Ewigman B, Crane JP, Frigoletto FD et al (1993) Effect of prenatal ultrasound screening on perinatal outcome. N Engl J Med 329:821–827

105. Salvesen KA, Jacobsen G, Vatten LJ et al (1993) Routine ultrasonography in utero and subsequent growth during childhood. Ultrasound Obstet Gynecol 3:6–10

106. Grisso JA, Strom BL, Cosmatos I et al (1994) Diagnostic ultrasound in pregnancy and low birthweight. Am J Perinatol 11:297–301

107. Macdonald W, Newnham J, Gurrin L, Evans S (1996) Effect of frequent prenatal ultrasound on birthweight: follow up at 1 year of age. Western Australian Pregnancy Cohort (Raine) Working Group. Lancet 348:482

108. Neilson JP (2004) Ultrasound for fetal assessment in early pregnancy (Cochrane Review). In: The Cochrane Library, Issue 2. John Wiley & Sons, Ltd, Chichester, UK

109. Kinnier-Wilson LM, Waterhouse J (1984) Obstetric ultrasound and childhood malignancies. Lancet 2:997–999

110. Sorahan T, Lancashire R, Stewart A, Peck I (1995) Pregnancy ultrasound and childhood cancer: a second report from the Oxford Survey of Childhood Cancers. Br J Obstet Gynaecol 102: 831–832

111. Cartwright R, McKinney PA, Hopton PA et al (1984) Ultrasound examination in pregnancy and childhood cancer. Lancet 2:999–1000

112. Shu X, Jin F, Linet MS et al (1994) Diagnostic x-ray and ultrasound exposure and risk of childhood cancer. Br J Cancer 70: 531–536

113. Naumburg E, Bellocco R, Cnattingius S et al (2000) Prenatal ultrasound examinations and risk of childhood leukaemia: case–control study. BMJ 320:282–283

114. Salvesen KA, Bakketeig LS, Eik-nes SH et al (1992) Routine ultrasonography in utero and school performance at age 8-9 years. Lancet 339:85–89

115. Campbell JD, Elford RW, Brant RF (1993) Case-control study of prenatal ultrasonography exposure in children with delayed speech. CMAJ 149:1435–1440

116. Salvesen KA, Vatten LJ, Bakketeig LS, Eik-Nes SH (1994) Routine ultrasonography in utero and speech development. Ultrasound Obstet Gynecol 4:101–103

117. Kieler H, Ahlsten G, Haglund B et al (1998) Routine ultrasound screening in pregnancy and the children's subsequent neurologic development. Obstet Gynecol 91:750–756

118. Salvesen KA, Vatten LJ, Eik-Nes SH, Hugdahl K, Bakketeig LS (1993) Routine ultrasonography in utero and subsequent handedness and neurological development. BMJ 307:159–164

119. Kieler H, Axelsson O, Haglund B, Nilsson S, Salvesen KA (1998) Routine ultrasound screening in pregnancy and the children's subsequent handedness. Early Hum Dev 50:233–245

120. Kieler H, Cnattingius S, Haglund B, Palmgren J, Axelsson O (2001) Sinistrality – a side-effect of prenatal sonography: a comparative study of young men. Epidemiology 12:618–623

121. AIUM (1995) Conclusions Regarding Epidemiology

122. Haar GT (1997) Commentary: Safety of diagnostic ultrasound. Br J Radiol 69:1083–1085

123. Suslick K (1989) The Chemical Effects of Ultrasound. Sci Am 260:80–86

Chapter 9

Fetal and Maternal Cardiovascular Physiology

Joseph Itskovitz-Eldor, Israel Thaler

Pregnancy is a high-flow, low-resistance state of cardiovascular homeostasis associated with remarkable hemodynamic changes. In the human and most other mammalian species, cardiac output increases during early pregnancy, reaching a peak of 30%–50% above nonpregnant values at 20–24 weeks' gestation. It remains unchanged or falls slightly thereafter [1, 2]. This increment in maternal cardiac output is accounted for by the dramatic increase in uterine blood flow needed to satisfy the metabolic demands of the conceptus and by the significant increase in blood flow to certain nonreproductive organs that are involved in the physiologic adjustments to pregnancy (e.g., kidneys, skin, gastrointestinal tract) [3]. There is also a 20% increase in maternal heart rate, a slight fall in mean arterial pressure, and a significant decrease in systemic vascular resistance – hence the need for the 40% expansion in maternal blood volume during normal pregnancy [4].

In addition to these alterations, there is the development of attenuated pressor responses to several vasoactive agents during normal pregnancy. These agents include angiotensin II, α-agonists, and arginine vasopressin [5–7].

The hemodynamic changes described above are mandatory for the continuous growth and development of the uteroplacental and fetoplacental circulations. Interference with the normal growth and development of the uteroplacental and fetoplacental circulations may result in disruption of the oxygen and nutrient supply to the fetus, leading to reprogramming of fetal development. It ultimately may result in intrauterine growth retardation, one of the leading causes of perinatal mortality and morbidity. Thus assessment of uteroplacental and fetal hemodynamics is of primary clinical importance. Until recently, fetal heart rate monitoring and the biophysical profile have been useful routine surveillance techniques for detecting the fetus that is either already asphyxiated or soon likely to become so. Despite three decades of experience in this field, controversies still exist regarding the effectiveness of these tests for reducing perinatal mortality and morbidity.

The use of Doppler ultrasound technology for investigating human fetal and uteroplacental hemodynamics offers a novel approach to the identification of a wide variety of disorders related to pregnancy. Knowledge of the normal physiology of maternal and fetal hemodynamics is a prerequisite for the development of pathophysiologic hypotheses that can lead to the establishment of clinical principles for investigating the fetomaternal circulatory status. Most of the present knowledge of fetal and maternal cardiovascular physiology is derived from animal experiments, particularly in the pregnant sheep; there is a paucity of comparable information relating to human pregnancy. Although the general course of the fetal and maternal circulations are similar in various mammalian species, it is important to appreciate that significant variations are known to exist among species. This chapter briefly reviews the basic hemodynamic concepts of the fetal and maternal circulations relevant to the potential clinical application of Doppler ultrasound technology for the assessment of fetal well-being.

Uterine Circulation

Functional Anatomy of the Uteroplacental Circulation

The main uterine artery branches off the internal iliac artery. At the level of the internal cervical os it bifurcates into the descending (cervical) and ascending (corporal) branches. At the uterine tubal junction the ascending branch turns toward the ovary and anastomoses with the ovarian artery to form an arterial arcade that perfuses the internal genital organs. The tortuous ascending uterine artery gives off approximately eight branches – the arcuate arteries-which extend inward for about one-third the thickness of the myometrium and envelope the anterior and posterior walls of the uterus [8, 9]. The origin of these branches is asymmetric; some are large and thick and supply a large area of the uterus, whereas others are thin and supply smaller areas of the uterine wall. These arteries have a tortuous course and anastomose with the corresponding arteries from the other side closer to the midline [9, 10]. From this network arise the radial arteries, which are directed toward the uterine mucosa. The spinal arteries undergo cyclical changes that are synchronous with the ovarian cycle. During normal pregnancy, trophoblastic cells enter the lumen of the spiral arteries, partially replacing the endothelium and progressing down the inner wall of the arteries up to the level of the endometrium. At the end of the third month of pregnancy the invading trophoblast begins to destroy the elastic lamina, and at 16–22 weeks' gestation it replaces the smooth muscle elements of the intramyometrial portion of the spiral arteries and then degenerates [11, 12]. This transformation eventually leads to formation of a low-resistance vascular system in which relatively large maternal arteries pump blood directly into the intervillous spaces (Fig. 9.1). Failure or impairment of the trophoblastic cells to invade the spiral arteries has been associated with pregnancy-induced hypertension and intrauterine growth restriction [14, 15].

Anatomic and radiographic studies and uterine perfusion have demonstrated the richness of the arterial anastomosis of the human uterine circulation [8–10, 16, 17]. These anastomoses include ipsilateral connections between uterine and ovarian arteries, ipsilateral anastomosis of vessels of differing diameter of the uterine branches (arcuate and radial arteries), contralateral anastomosis between the right and left uterine arteries and their branches, and extrauterine connections between the uterine circulation and the systemic circulation (e.g., inferior mesenteric, middle sacral, and inferior epigastric arteries). This vast ipsilateral and contralateral anastomotic network ensures ample uteroplacental perfusion and may be activated to provide alternative routes of blood supply to the placenta. Data from human pregnancy indicate that anastomotic connections increase in size and are of

functional significance after occlusion of major vessels [16, 17]. In the rhesus monkey the contribution of the ovarian artery to uterine blood flow in the nonpregnant state and during early pregnancy is negligible. During late pregnancy it contributes about half of the flow to the upper third of the uterus [18]. Studies in sheep have shown that the uterine arteries contribute approximately 80% of the total uterine flow [19, 20], and that functional arterial anastomoses are present between the right and left sides of the uterine vasculature. Short-term changes in flow on one side are accompanied by compensatory changes in the flow rate on the contralateral side [21]. The venous drainage of the placenta usually follows its arterial supply, but it has also been demonstrated that in some instances the drainage of placental blood shifts rapidly between the two uteroovarian veins [22]. Thus the uteroplacental circulation is a dynamic system in which the magnitude of blood flow through a single vessel may vary considerably over a short time, making single vessel measurements of blood flow sometimes difficult to interpret.

Alterations in Uterine Blood Flow

Only limited information is available regarding the changes in uteroplacental blood flow throughout human pregnancy. Total uterine blood flow is estimated to increase from approximately 50 ml/min during early pregnancy to 500 ml/min near term. However, these figures were derived from studies that employed a diffusion-equilibrium technique [23, 24] or radioisotope-dilution methods [25–29], the accuracy of which is questionable [30].

Our most complete knowledge of uterine vascular changes have been obtained in farm animals (sheep, pigs), which have been shown to develop some hemo-

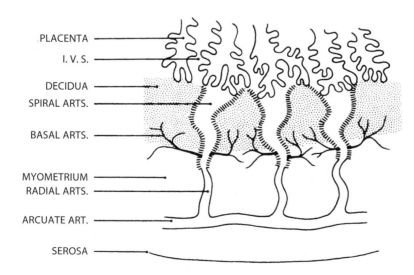

PLACENTA
I. V. S.
DECIDUA
SPIRAL ARTS.
BASAL ARTS.
MYOMETRIUM
RADIAL ARTS.
ARCUATE ART.
SEROSA

Fig. 9.1. Fully developed changes in the uteroplacental arteries of normal pregnancy. The *hatched portions* of the wall of spiral arteries indicate the extent of the physiological changes. *IVS* intervillous space. (Reprinted from [13] with permission)

dynamic alterations during pregnancy similar to those observed in humans. Although these animal experiments allow us to emphasize some common fundamental control mechanisms in both the development and control of the uteroplacental circulation, it should be appreciated that significant variations (e.g., type of placentation) are known to exist among species.

Blood flow to the uterus during early pregnancy has been most comprehensively studied in the pig [31]. In this species, a sharp peak of uterine blood flow to the pregnant horn is observed on days 12 and 13 after mating, before definite attachment of the embryo occurs, suggesting an early, local effect of the blastocyst on uterine blood flow. This phase is followed by a progressive and dynamic increase beginning on day 18 or 19, which corresponds to the day of implantation and the initiation of placentation.

Studies in sheep have correlated the changes in uteroplacental blood flow to the growth and development of the placenta of the fetus and have provided some insight into the long-term regulatory mechanisms controlling the development of the uteroplacental circulation. In the nonpregnant ovariectomized sheep, uterine blood flow is approximately 25 ml/min and increases to 400 ml/min at midpregnancy when definite placentation is complete. Absolute uterine blood flow increases beginning at midpregnancy until term to reach a level of 1,500 ml/min (term is at approximately 146 days), although uterine blood flow per gram of total uterine (and fetal) weight remains constant. These values of uterine blood flows represent approximately 0.5%, 8.0%, and 20.0% of cardiac output, respectively [19, 32].

The distribution of blood flow within the gravid uterus was measured using the radiolabeled microsphere technique [33]. At an early stage of gestation (second month) the myometrium and endometrium receive approximately 70% of total uterine blood flow. During the third month of pregnancy the placenta attains its maximum size and becomes the major component of uterine weight, and placental blood flow represents approximately 60% of the total. During the final 2 months there is no further placental growth, but fetal weight increases exponentially; during this stage of gestation there is a three- to fourfold increase in placental blood flow, and near term it accounts for 80%–90% of total uterine blood flow [19, 33].

These observations suggest that the longitudinal hemodynamic changes in the uteroplacental circulation are directly related to the growth rate of the tissue it supplies. There are two stages in the growth and development of the uteroplacental circulation. The first stage extends from the time of implantation through 80–90 days' gestation and is reflective of the period of placental growth and development of new blood vessels [34]. The second stage extends over the last 2 months of pregnancy. During this period there is no further growth of the placenta and no formation of new blood vessels, as reflected by the number of maternal and endothelial cells [34]. There is an increase in the cross-sectional area of the uterine vascular bed, however, and placental perfusion continues to increase until term to accommodate fetal growth. The progressive increment in uteroplacental perfusion and the progressive decline in uterine vascular resistance during the second stage of pregnancy are secondary not only to vasodilation of the uteroplacental vascular bed (inasmuch as studies in unanesthetized sheep have shown that the vasculature is nearly maximally dilated [35–38]) but also to the gradual increase in the luminal diameter of the resistance vessels. Indeed, there is rapid, active growth in the uterine arterial wall. The threefold increase in the internal radius of the uterine artery is not merely the result of passive dilatation, as wall thickness is unchanged; there is hypertrophy of its vascular smooth muscle and a decrease in its collagen fraction [39].

Regulation of Uteroplacental Circulation

The regulatory mechanisms that promote the described sequence of changes in uteroplacental blood flow by influencing the formation and growth of the uteroplacental blood flow are poorly understood. Putative regulatory agents include steroid hormones, angiogenic factors, growth factors, and other unknown substances of fetal or maternal origin.

Steroid Hormones and Vasoactive Agents

The uterine vasculature is sensitive to estrogens [37, 40, 41]. Estradiol is a potent uterine vasodilator in nonpregnant sheep, and the magnitude of increase of uterine blood flow at early gestation can be produced by injecting estradiol into nonpregnant sheep. Exogenously administered estradiol also increased placental blood flow, although the observed percentage increase from baseline is not striking as it is in the nonpregnant state. Furthermore, the response to estradiol appears to be more pronounced during early pregnancy than at later pregnancy [37], suggesting that during later pregnancy the placental vasculature is almost maximally dilated. Uterine blood flow response to estrogen is probably mediated largely by nitric oxide (NO), which can stimulate production of vascular endothelial growth factor (VEGF) and basic fibroblast growth factor (bFGF) [42, 43].

The role of progesterone in regulating the development of uteroplacental circulation and the rate of uterine blood flow is even more complex. In the sheep, progesterone given in pharmacologic doses induces overgrowth of caruncles (highly vascularized areas of the uterine mucosa that become the sites of implantation and the formation of placental cotyledons) [44] and growth of uterine blood vessels [45]. Its role in regulating uterine blood flow is controversial [46].

The uteroplacental vasculature is sensitive to the constrictive effect of catecholamines. Systemic infusion of suppressor doses of norepinephrine has been shown to reduce placental perfusion in the absence of significant changes in arterial pressure [47]. It is also sensitive to other endogenous vasoactive substances (e.g., angiotensin II, prostanoids), which have the potential to either increase or decrease uterine blood flow by acting directly on the blood vessels or indirectly by modifying the intrauterine pressure. Changes in partial pressures of oxygen and carbon dioxide have little direct effect on the uteroplacental circulation. However, severe disruption of oxygenation and acid-base balance (and maternal stress in general) may increase uterine vascular resistance secondary to the constrictive effect of catecholamines released into the circulation and activation of the sympathetic vasomotor nerves [30].

Pressure-Flow Relations

Data from animal experiments in which the pressure-flow relations in the uterine circulation were examined have demonstrated a negative correlation between amniotic pressure and uterine blood flow [48] and a linear relation between flow and perfusion pressure [20, 35, 49, 50]. In rhesus monkeys confined to restraining chairs, the highest blood flows tended to occur during the period of darkness when arterial and intraamniotic fluid pressures were low [48]. These observations suggest that the uteroplacental circulation is pressure-passive, is fully dilated, and has no tendency toward autoregulation. Meschia [30] compared the placenta and its venous outlets to a collapsible tube (Starling resistor) [51] contained within a cavity in which the pressure can increase above atmospheric pressure in this system, and flow through the placental bed depends on arterial perfusion pressure, the external pressure exerted by the amniotic fluid, and the pressure in the uterine venous outlet. Although these relations have been demonstrated experimentally, disparities were observed in the chronology and amplitude of the 24-h periodic functions for arterial blood pressure, intraamniotic pressure, and uterine blood flow recorded continuously in rhesus monkeys, indicating that uteroplacental perfusion is modulated by factors in addition to those imposed by pressure-flow relations [52].

The high basal rate of uterine perfusion provides a margin of safety for the fetus because the uteropla-

cental vasculature does not dilate in response to maternal hypotension or hypoxia but is sensitive to the constrictive effect of catecholamines. In the sheep, oxygen supply to the fetus is approximately twice the level necessary to maintain adequate fetal oxygen uptake and normal oxidative metabolism. Fetal oxidative metabolism can be sustained despite reductions in uterine blood flow of about 50% [53–55]. However, long-term reductions of even small magnitude have cumulative metabolic effects that ultimately affect fetal growth. It has been clearly demonstrated that fetal growth is directly related to the normal incremental increases in uterine blood flow throughout pregnancy [21]. When reduced uterine flow is prolonged, fetal and placental growth are slowed [21, 56]. Under these circumstances uterine blood flow per unit weight of the fetus and placenta may remain constant and does not significantly differ from that of normally growing fetuses [57, 58].

Fetal Circulation

During fetal life oxygenation is carried out in the placenta. A large gradient of oxygen partial pressure (PO_2), of about 60 mmHg, has been found between maternal arterial blood and fetal umbilical venous blood. The admixture of the oxygenated umbilical venous blood from the placenta and systemic venous blood from the fetal body further reduces the PO_2 of blood distributed to the fetal body. The PO_2 of arterial blood is 20–30 mmHg (considerably lower than the adult value of close to 100 mmHg); it is somewhat higher in the blood distributed to the brain and the upper body from the ascending aorta than in blood distributed from the descending aorta to the lower body and the placenta. Despite the existence of a low arterial concentration of oxygen, the fetus has adequate oxygen delivery because, similar to the adult, it does not extract more than one third of delivered oxygen [59].

The presence of ductus arteriosus, the large communication between the pulmonary trunk and the aorta (Fig. 9.2), accounts for the almost identical pressures in the aorta and the pulmonary artery in the fetus. Similarly, because of the presence of the foramen ovale, atrial pressures are almost identical, and so the right and left ventricles are subjected to the same filling pressure. Hence, unlike those in the adult, fetal cardiac ventricles work in parallel rather than in series. The output of the left ventricle is directed through the ascending aorta to upper body organs, thus preferentially perfusing the brain, whereas the right ventricle mainly perfuses the lower body and placenta through ductus arteriosus and the descending aorta.

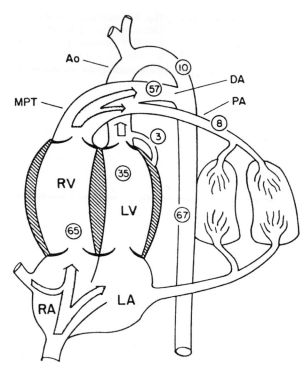

Fig. 9.2. Fetal heart showing the percentages of combined ventricular output by each ventricle and traversing the major vascular pathways. *Ao* aorta; *MPT* main pulmonary trunk; *DA* ductus arteriosus; *PA* pulmonary artery; *RV* right ventricle; *LV* left ventricle; *RA* right atrium; *LA* left atrium. (Reprinted from [60] with permission)

Before birth both ventricles contribute to fetal systemic flow in parallel, and the term "combined ventricular output" is commonly used to represent fetal cardiac output. After birth the ventricles are arranged in series, and each ventricle ejects a similar volume of blood.

Fetal Cardiac Output and Distribution

Much of today's knowledge of fetal cardiac output and distribution is derived from studies of fetal sheep. Fetal cardiac output and its distribution have been measured employing the radionuclide-labeled microsphere method or by electromagnetic flow transducers applied around the ascending aorta and the pulmonary trunk. In the near-term fetus, combined ventricular output is 450–500 ml·min⁻¹·kg⁻¹ of fetal body weight and appears to be consistent throughout the last half of gestation [61–63]. Doppler echocardiographic measurements of the combined cardiac output in the human fetus have yielded similar values [64–67], which far exceed the level of about 100 ml·min⁻¹·kg⁻¹ body weight for each of the adult ventricles.

In the fetal lamb, the right ventricle ejects two-thirds and the left ventricle ejects one-third of the combined ventricular output. The dominance of the right ventricle is also present in the human fetus [64, 68], but in the human the ratio is smaller (1.2–1.5) than in the fetal lamb (1.8). The larger brain mass of humans with respect to sheep may explain the higher left ventricular output and therefore the lower ratio between the right and left ventricular outputs. Reference ranges were established in the human fetus for cardiac output (Fig. 9.3) and ductus arteriosus blood flow (Fig. 9.4) [68]. Central blood flow distribution in the second and third trimesters of pregnancy was measured, confirming the conception of right heart dominance. Estimated pulmonary flow was 11% of biventricular output, higher than in the fetal lamb (6%–8%) [60].

Nearly 90% of the right ventricular output bypasses the pulmonary circulation via the ductus arteriosus to reach the descending aorta, whereas only 30% of the left ventricular output passes the aortic arch (isthmus) to the descending aorta (Fig. 9.2). Thus flow in the thoracic portion of the descending aorta represents about 65% of fetal combined ventricular output. The placenta receives 40% (180–200 ml·min⁻¹·kg⁻¹ fetal weight) of fetal cardiac output, or about 65% of the flow in the thoracic descending aorta and about 75% of the flow in the abdominal aorta distal to the origin of the renal arteries. In the human fetus, umbilical-placental blood flow measured by the Doppler ultrasound technique is approximately 120 ml·min⁻¹·kg⁻¹ fetal weight [69, 70], which represents about 25% of human fetal cardiac output and 50%–60% of the flow in the thoracic descending aorta.

The distribution of cardiac output in the fetal sheep is shown in Table 9.1. Only limited information is available regarding the distribution of fetal cardiac output in human and nonhuman primates. The distribution of blood flow expressed as percent of combined cardiac output in fetal lambs and in human fetuses is demonstrated in Table 9.2 [68]. The distribution of cardiac output was measured in acute studies of monkeys and previable human fetuses, and in general it is similar to that seen in the fetal lamb. In the human and the monkey, the brain, being proportionately larger than that of the sheep, receives a higher percentage of the cardiac output. In the fetal rhesus monkey, brain flow represents approximately 16% of the cardiac output [71] compared with 3%–4% in the sheep [63].

Regulation of Cardiac Function

As mentioned above, the right and left ventricles are subjected to the same filling pressures due to the presence of the foramen ovale. The resistances against which the ventricles eject are evidently different [60, 62]. Studies in fetal lambs have suggested that the

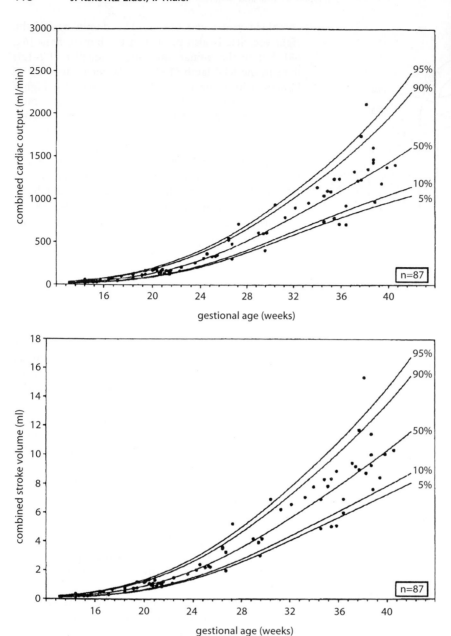

Fig. 9.3. Individual values and calculated 5th, 10th, 50th, 90th and 95th centiles of biventricular output per minute (upper trace) and stroke volume (lower trace). (Reprinted from [68])

aortic isthmus, the narrowest segment of the aorta between the origin of the brachiocephalic trunk and the ductus arteriosus, represents a site of functional separation between the two ventricles. As a result, the right ventricle is subjected to the afterload of the lower body, including the low resistance of the umbilical-placental circulation through the wide channel of the ductus arteriosus, whereas the left ventricle is presented with the resistance of the upper body and that of the aortic isthmus [60].

The differences in outflow resistance and ejection characteristics to the left and right ventricles are evident in the blood velocity profiles of the ascending aorta and the pulmonary trunk (Fig. 9.5). There is a much steeper rise in velocity in the pulmonary trunk compared to that of the aorta. After reaching a peak the aortic flow decreases rapidly, and there is a sharp incisura with some backflow at the end of systole. The peak velocity in the pulmonary trunk is greater than that in the ascending aorta. There is a characteristic sharp incisura in the descending limb of the pulmonary trunk velocity curve that may be related to the aortic valve wave reaching the ductus arteriosus and modifying right ventricular ejection [72].

As the ventricular output and velocity profiles are determined primarily by afterload or changes in the

Fig. 9.4. Individual values and calculated 5th, 10th, 50th, 90th and 95th centiles of blood flow per cycle (upper trace) and blood flow per minute (lower trace) in ductus arteriosus. (Reprinted from [68])

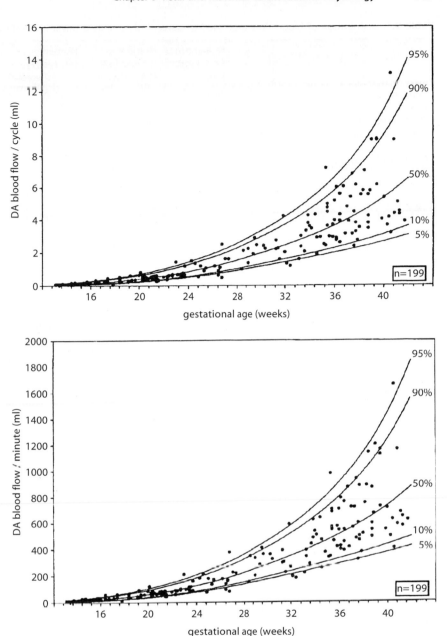

vascular resistances of the upper and lower circulations, it may be possible to define circulatory changes during fetal distress by examining the relative outputs of the two ventricles by echocardiography or by assessing the velocity profiles in the aorta and the pulmonary trunk by the Doppler technique [73–75]. The acceleration of the aortic flow (dV/dt) is one of the most reliable indices of myocardial contractility. Measurement of acceleration time (time to peak velocity) of both the aorta and the pulmonary artery can be used as a good index of ventricular performance [76–78].

During fetal hypoxemia resulting from reduced oxygen delivery across the placenta (uterine blood flow reduction, maternal hypoxemia), blood flow to the fetal body is reduced owing to peripheral vasoconstriction, but umbilical blood flow does not change. Under these circumstances the relative output of the right ventricle, compared to that of the left, may be expected to increase. However, if fetal hypoxemia results from umbilical blood flow reduction (partial cord compression), vascular resistance across the umbilical-placental circulation is increased; and it may be expected to be associated with a reduction of right, relative to left, ventricular output.

Table 9.1. Distribution of blood flow expressed as percent of combined (biventricular) cardiac output

	Near-term fetal lambs [24]	Human fetuses [68] (13–41 weeks)	Human fetuses [7] (19–39 weeks)	Human fetuses [4] (18–37 weeks)	Human fetuses [39] (age unknown)
Right cardiac output, %	60	59	53–60		
Left cardiac output, %	40	41	47–40		
Ductus arteriosus blood flow, %	54	46	32–40		
Pulmonary blood flow, %	6	11	13–25	22	6
Foramen ovale blood flow, %	34	33	34–18	17–31	36
Biventricular output, ml·min^{-1}·kg^{-1}	462	425	470-503		

Table 9.2. Combined ventricular output (450–500 ml·min^{-1}·kg^{-1}) and its distribution in fetal lambs

Anatomic site	%
Placenta	40
Carcass[a]	33
Lungs	7
Gastrointestinal tract	4
Brain	4
Myocardium	3
Kidneys	3
Spleen	1
Liver (hepatic artery)	1
Adrenals	0.1

[a] Skin, muscle and bone.

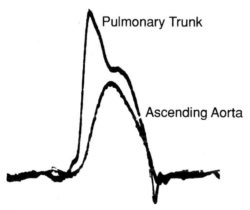

Fig. 9.5. Velocity tracings in the pulmonary trunk and ascending aorta obtained by electromagnetic flow transducer implantation. Note the rapid rise of velocity in the pulmonary trunk compared with that in the aorta. There is a characteristic notch in the descending limb of the velocity curve. The ascending aortic tracing also shows a sharp incisura at the end of ejection caused by backflow. The area under each curve reflects stroke volume; flow in the pulmonary trunk is about twice that in the aorta. (Reprinted from [72] with permission)

The factors regulating cardiac output in the fetus and the mechanisms responsible for the increase in output after birth have attracted considerable attention. Cardiac function and the volume of blood ejected by the heart are, in general, determined by cardiac and circulatory factors [79]. Early studies suggested that the normal fetal heart at rest operates close to the top of its ventricular function curve (Frank-Starling curve), with little reserve available to further increase the output [60, 80–82].

In these studies little attention was directed to the changes in arterial pressure that occur with volume loading or withdrawal. It is well known that the fetal heart is sensitive to an increase in afterload, and so the cardiac output falls dramatically as arterial pressure increases. In early studies the arterial pressure (afterload) was not controlled, and therefore left ventricular stroke volume showed little increase above the left atrial mean pressures of about 6 mmHg (slightly higher than normal atrial pressure at rest). However, when the left ventricular stroke volume was related to left atrial pressure at the same levels of mean arterial pressure, the stroke volume continued to increase above the atrial mean pressure of about 10 mmHg [83], suggesting that the fetal heart rate is able to increase its output provided the preload is increased and the afterload is maintained or if the preload is maintained but the afterload is decreased. However, because a large proportion of the fetal blood volume is sequestered in the highly compliant umbilical-placental circulation, the fetus is unable to increase venous return readily and therefore has limited ability to increase its cardiac output acutely [84].

While the plateau observed in the fetal cardiac function curve was related to arterial pressure and increasing afterload, it has been demonstrated that the maximal stroke volume in the fetus is largely determined by the constraining effect that the pericardium and the chest wall-lung combination (i.e., extracardiac constraint) has on ventricular filling [85]. When ventricular transmural pressure, a more appropriate measure of ventricular preload than ventricular filling pressure, is used in ventricular function curve analysis, stroke volume is linearly related to preload and the plateau is absent [85]. The major limitation upon left ventricular function in the near-term fetal lamb results from extracardiac constraint limiting ventricular filling while, at the same time, a much smaller limitation arises from increasing arterial pressure [86].

Patterns of Venous Returns

The combined ventricular output represents total venous return to the fetal heart. In the fetal sheep about 70% of the venous return to the heart is derived from the thoracic inferior vena cava (IVC), about 20% from the superior vena cava (SVC), 7% from the lungs, and the remaining 3% from heart muscle [61, 63].

Umbilical Vein and Ductus Venosus

The umbilical venous return with its well oxygenated blood is either distributed to the hepatic microcirculation or bypasses the liver through the ductus venosus (Fig. 9.6). The ductus venosus is a funnel-like vessel with a narrow lumen at its beginning in the umbilical sinus [87]. This bottleneck at the orifice should contribute most to the flow resistance between the umbilical vein and the caval vein. The resistance is in parallel to the resistance of the hepatic vascular bed. The ratio of conductances between the ductus venosus and the hepatic vascular bed defines the ratio of ductus venosus flow to hepatic flow. In the fetal lamb this ratio approximates 1, with about half the umbilical venous blood passing through the ductus venous, and the rest of the blood entering the hepatic circulation [88–94]. Doppler measurements in the human fetus have provided similar values [95]. The left lobe of the fetal liver receives only umbilical venous blood, whereas the right lobe receives both umbilical venous blood and portal venous blood. The hepatic arterial blood supply to the liver is small (3%–4%) in the fetus [88]. As a result of these flow patterns, right hepatic venous blood has a lower oxygen saturation than does the left hepatic venous blood [91]. The large blood flow through the ductus venosus and the liver (which together represent about 50% of total venous return to the heart) makes them important organs for regulating venous return to the heart. Streaming patterns in the IVC and right atrium preferentially distribute the highly oxygenated blood that passes through the ductus venosus to the fetal heart and brain [96]. During umbilical cord compression [94], increasing proportions of the blood returning in the umbilical vein from the placenta pass through the ductus venosus. A 50% decrease in umbilical blood flow is associated with a 75% decrease in hepatic blood flow [94]. During acute fetal hypoxemia induced by maternal hypoxia [93] or by uterine blood flow reduction [97], umbilical blood flow is maintained. The proportion of umbilical venous blood that passes through the ductus venosus increases, whereas the percentage to the liver falls. These observations

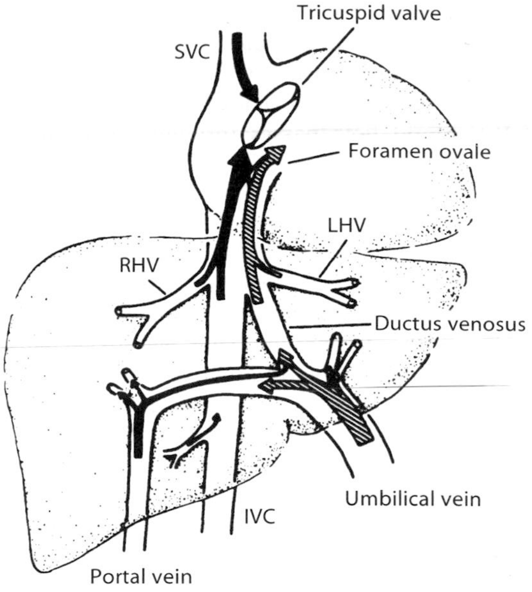

Fig. 9.6. Venous flow patterns in the fetal lamb. Umbilical venous blood is distributed to the left lobe of the liver, through the ductus venosus, and to the right lobe of the liver. Portal venous blood passes almost exclusively to the right lobe, but a small proportion enters the ductus venosus. Ductus venosus and left hepatic venous blood preferentially passes through the foramen ovale, whereas right hepatic venous and distal inferior vena caval blood is preferentially directed through the tricuspid valve. Superior vena caval blood almost all passes through the tricuspid valve. *SVC* superior vena cava; *IVC* inferior vena cava; *LHV* left hepatic vein; *RHV* right hepatic vein. (Reprinted from [84] with permission)

suggest that the ductus venosus (or actually the blood flow passing through the common orifice of the ductus venosus and left hepatic vein into the IVC [98]) facilitates the preferential distribution of highly oxygenated blood to the fetal brain and heart. The mechanisms responsible for the changes in flow patterns in the liver microcirculation and the ductus venosus have not been clearly delineated. These alterations in distribution can be accounted for by active relaxation of the ductus venosus or by vasoconstriction in the hepatic circulation [60, 99, 100]. The use of Doppler ultrasound techniques to monitor flow patterns and velocity profiles in the intraabdominal portion of the umbilical vein and in the ductus venosus carries the potential of evaluating changes in distribution of umbilical venous return to the liver and to the ductus venosus under conditions associated with fetal stress.

IVC and SVC

Using the microsphere method it has been demonstrated that almost all SVC blood is directed across the tricuspid valve into the right ventricle and is dis-

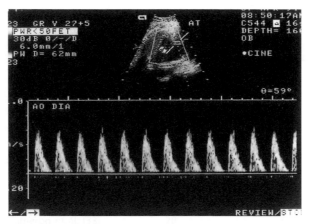

Fig. 11.11. Absence of end-diastolic velocity in the descending aorta of a growth-retarded fetus at 27 weeks' gestation

lated to the increased neonatal nucleated red blood cell counts that are considered a sign of intrauterine hypoxia [58]. Doppler results from the fetal descending aorta, umbilical artery, and maternal uterine arteries were independent determinants of neonatal nucleated red blood cell count.

In an experimental study on the fetal lamb, increasing the placental and hind limb resistance by embolization with microspheres caused a progressive increase in the aortic flow PI [59]. In another study on pigs, the aortic PI, recorded by Doppler ultrasonography, was shown to correlate with the total peripheral resistance calculated from the invasively measured blood flow and pressure ($r = 0.64–0.87$) [60]. In the study by Adamson and Langille [59] the aortic PI reflected not only the vascular resistance but also the pulsatile flow and pressure pulsatility (Fig. 11.12). Thus an increasing fetal aortic PI should not be interpreted solely as an expression of increasing placental vascular resistance.

When studying the aortic blood velocity waveforms of lamb fetuses during experimental asphyxia, Malcus et al. [61] found a loss of aortic end-diastolic flow velocities, a significant increase in the PI, and a decrease in mean velocity. Concomitantly, increases in the diameter and mean velocity were recorded in the fetal common carotid artery [62], and there was a slight decrease in the carotid artery PI. These changes indicate a redistribution of flow, although the changes occurred as relatively late phenomena in the development of acute asphyxia.

An interesting observation on fetal aortic isthmus has been reported, based on animal experiments [63] and human studies [64]. With increased resistance to flow in the placenta and fetal lower body, changes in the diastolic flow velocity occurred earlier in the aortic isthmus than in the descending aorta and umbili-

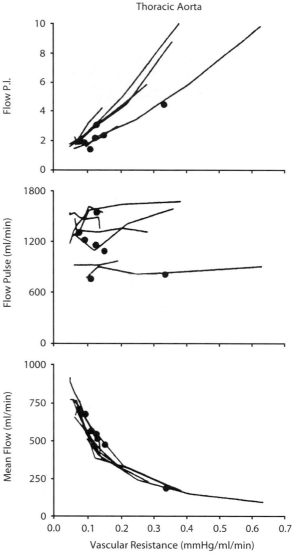

Fig. 11.12. Flow pulsatility index (*P.I.*), flow pulse amplitude, and mean blood flow measured with an electromagnetic flowmeter in the descending thoracic aorta of sheep fetuses versus the vascular resistance of the lower body circulation during progressive embolization of the hind limbs and placenta. *Solid circles* show values obtained during angiotensin II infusion. (Reprinted from [59], with permission)

cal artery. In the sheep fetus during an acute increase in placental vascular resistance, delivery of oxygen to the brain was preserved despite a significant decrease in arterial oxygen content as long as net flow through the aortic isthmus was antegrade [65]. These reports offer an interesting possibility of closely following the process of centralization of flow. The suggested concept awaits evaluation in prospective clinical studies.

Clinical Studies

Fetal Cardiac Arrhythmias

Doppler recording of fetal aortic velocities provides important information of the hemodynamic consequences of fetal cardiac arrhythmias. Simultaneous detection of Doppler signals from the fetal abdominal aorta, reflecting ventricular contractions, and the inferior vena cava, reflecting atrial contractions, can facilitate the classification of arrhythmias [66–68]. In most cases of fetal arrhythmia, the estimated aortic volume flow remains within normal limits, indicating the ability of the fetal heart to maintain cardiac output [67, 69]. Subnormally low values of aortic flow were found in fetuses with severe arrhythmias that caused heart failure [67]. In cases of bradyarrhythmias and tachyarrhythmias, a decrease in the aortic flow was observed when the fetal heart rate exceeded the limits of 50 or 230 bpm, respectively [69].

In fetuses with premature heartbeats, an increase in peak aortic velocities was observed with the first postextrasystolic beats [70]. Similarly, the peak systolic velocities are higher in fetuses with complete atrioventricular block than in those with regular sinus rhythm [67]. This finding, together with the above-described compensation for negative effects of cardiac arrhythmias on fetal cardiac output, indicates that the Frank-Starling mechanism is valid for fetal myocardium.

Fetuses with congestive heart failure caused by a cardiac arrhythmia sometimes require transplacental treatment with digoxin or antiarrhythmic drugs. In addition to the effect of treatment on heart rhythm, the improved performance of the fetal heart can be followed by serial measurements of fetal aortic volume blood flow [71].

Fetal Anemia

In isoimmunized pregnancies the degree of fetal anemia can be determined by analyzing fetal blood samples obtained by cordocentesis. It would facilitate their clinical management if these anemic fetuses could be identified with a noninvasive method. One of the early reports suggested that there was an inverse correlation between the cord hemoglobin at birth and the time-averaged mean velocity and volume blood flow recorded antenatally in the intraabdominal portion of the umbilical vein using Doppler ultrasonography [72]. In the descending aorta of previously untransfused isoimmunized fetuses, Rightmire et al. [73] reported an increased mean blood velocity and a negative correlation with the hematocrit of umbilical cord blood obtained by cord puncture under fetoscopic control. Their finding was confirmed by Nicolaides et al. [74], who related the values of mean aortic velocity to the hemoglobin deficit in blood samples obtained by cordocentesis. The findings of increased fetal aortic velocities in anemic fetuses (Fig. 11.13) are in accord with an increase in their cardiac output as a consequence of lowered blood viscosity, increased venous return, and cardiac preload. Doppler cardiac studies of anemic fetuses showed indications of increased cardiac output [76, 77]. After intrauterine transfusion, a decrease or even normalization of the mean velocity in the fetal aorta was observed [78]. In contrast to the changes in aortic time-averaged mean velocity seen with fetal anemia, there were no changes in the waveform indices.

Recently, it has been shown by Mari et al. [79] that Doppler examination of the fetal middle cerebral artery can be used for clinical management of pregnancies with red-cell alloimmunization. The sensitivity of the middle cerebral artery velocimetry for detection of fetal anemia seems to be superior to that of the velocimetry of fetal descending aorta.

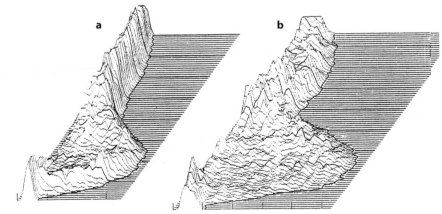

Fig. 11.13. Three-dimensional presentation of Doppler signals recorded from the descending aorta of a normal fetus (**a**) and an anemic fetus (**b**). Note the increase of velocity amplitudes and the right shift of the velocity power in the anemic fetus. (Reprinted from [75] with permission)

Diabetes Mellitus

Serial Doppler examinations were performed in a group of 40 pregnant women with diabetes mellitus [80]. A high-volume blood flow in the fetal descending aorta was found during the early third trimester; near term, blood flow approached normal values. The PI in the umbilical artery and fetal aorta was within the normal range, so long as there were no signs of fetal growth retardation or hypoxia. Otherwise no flow variations specific for diabetic pregnancies were seen. Similar findings were also reported for pregnant women with gestational diabetes [81].

Intrauterine Growth Restriction

Intrauterine growth restriction (IUGR) can have various etiologies, restricted flow through the placental vasculature being the most common cause of this relatively frequent complication of pregnancy. As described above, the increased vascular impedance in the placenta is reflected in a changed blood velocity waveform in the descending fetal aorta, with a reduction of diastolic velocities and a corresponding increase in PI [6, 19, 35]. These findings are similar to those reported for the umbilical artery of growth-retarded fetuses [82].

In a study that evaluated placental morphology in relation to intrauterine flow in IUGR fetuses, only the presence of placental infarction was significantly associated with abnormal flow velocity findings in the fetal descending aorta (high PI, BFC I–III, low mean velocity) [83].

In the descending aorta of growth-retarded fetuses, low values were obtained for the time-averaged mean velocity and volume flow, though they did not differ significantly from those of controls [19]. This similarity was probably due to the already mentioned methodologic difficulty of precisely estimating volume flow. Using an improved technique combining an ultrasonic phase-locked echo-tracking system for diameter measurement synchronized with a pulsed Doppler velocimeter [16], Gardiner et al. [84] found both the relative pulse amplitude, mean blood velocity, and volume flow to be significantly lower in the descending aorta of growth-restricted fetuses than in the controls. Also, the aortic pulse waves of growth-restricted fetuses showed values significantly different from those in controls, reflecting the chronic ventriculovascular responses to increased placental impedance [85].

In severely growth-restricted fetuses developing signs of intrauterine distress, the aortic end-diastolic velocity disappears or even becomes reversed (BFC II and III; Fig. 11.7) [18]. An association has been found to exist between the degree of fetal hypoxia, hypercapnia, acidosis, and hyperlactemia, as diagnosed in blood samples obtained by cordocentesis from growth-restricted fetuses and changes in the mean fetal aortic velocity [86] and the velocity waveform [87]. The aortic velocity waveform changes have been observed to precede the cardiotocographic changes, the median time lag being 2–3 days [19, 88], though the interval between the first blood velocity changes and the first changes in cardiotocographic tracings may be as much as several weeks [19, 89].

The finding of ARED flow in the fetal aorta is associated with an adverse outcome of the pregnancy [19, 90] and increased neonatal morbidity [91, 92]. Reverse flow during diastole identifies fetuses in danger of intrauterine death. Perinatal mortality in cases with reverse flow is reported to be high – in some series as high as 100% [93]. The combination of ARED flow in the fetal descending aorta and pulsations in the umbilical vein seems to indicate a fetus with severe hypoxia and iminent heart failure [18].

Aortic Doppler Velocimetry as a Diagnostic Test of IUGR and Fetal Hypoxia

Several prospective studies on IUGR pregnancies have been performed to evaluate the predictive capacity of fetal aortic velocity waveforms with regard to birth weight, occurrence of fetal distress, and perinatal outcome. Tables 11.3 and 11.4 summarize results of some of the studies in terms of sensitivity, specificity, and positive and negative predictive values. For the RI ratios between the common carotid artery and descending thoracic aorta of small-for-gestational-age (SGA) fetuses redistributing their flow, a sensitivity of 94% was reported for prediction of cesarean section for fetal distress [96]. It is obvious that in IUGR fetuses fetal aortic velocimetry is a better predictor of fetal health than fetal size, which is not surprising in view of the multiplicity of determinants of fetal growth.

The accumulated evidence suggests that, as is also the case for umbilical artery velocimetry, Doppler fetal aortic examination is better suited for use as a secondary diagnostic test in preselected high-risk pregnancies than as a primary screening test in a whole pregnant population [97]. In a prospective study of growth-retarded fetuses, Gudmundsson and Maršál [90] compared the predictive value of aortic versus umbilical artery velocity waveforms: The PI in the umbilical artery was found to be a slightly better predictor of fetal outcome than the aortic PI, though the BFC was similarly predictive in the two vessels. Two longitudinal studies confirmed that the changes in the umbilical artery PI preceded changes in the

Table 11.3. Diagnostic capacity of fetal aortic Doppler velocimetry with regard to the prediction of intrauterine growth restriction

Study	No. of pregnancies	Prev (%)	Sens (%)	Spec (%)	PPV (%)	NPV (%)	Kappa value
Aortic PI							
Gudmundsson and Maršál [90]	139	52	40	87	76	57	0.26
ARED flow							
Laurin et al. [94]	159	47	50	97	67	93	0.48
Chaoui et al. [89]	954	?	87	82	67	94	–
Gudmundsson and Maršál [90]	139	52	87	61	46	93	0.38

Prev, prevalence; Sens, sensitivity; Spec, specificity; PPV, positive predictive value; NPV, negative predictive value; PI, pulsatility index; *ARED flow*, absent or reversed end-diastolic flow.
Definition of intrauterine growth retardation: reference 89: birth weight <5th percentile; references 90 and 94: birth weight ≤mean −2 SD.

Table 11.4. Diagnostic capacity of fetal aortic Doppler velocimetry with regard to the prediction of operative delivery for fetal distress

Study	No. of pregnancies	Prev (%)	Sens (%)	Spec (%)	PPV (%)	NPV (%)	Kappa value
Aortic PI							
Arabin et al. [95]	171	?	68	88	58	93	–
Gudmundsson and Maršál [90]	139	34	62	87	71	81	0.50
ARED flow							
Laurin et al. [94]	159	19	83	90	66	96	0.66
Chaoui et al. [89]	954	?	88	82	85	95	–
Gudmundsson and Maršál [90]	139	34	91	88	74	96	0.74

For explanation of abbreviations see Table 11.3.

thoracic aorta of IUGR fetuses [98, 99]. Doppler examination of the umbilical artery is technically easier and can be done with less sophisticated and less expensive instruments. Therefore for simple monitoring of fetal health in suspected cases of IUGR, umbilical artery Doppler velocimetry seems preferable. The investigation of fetal aortic arterial waveforms might provide more detailed information on the circulatory adaptation and pathophysiologic mechanisms in the process of IUGR. It should be validated, however, in randomized clinical trials comprising management protocols based on the results from Doppler examinations of several vessel areas: uteroplacental circulation, umbilical artery, fetal aorta, and fetal cerebral vessels. Possibly such a concept can improve clinical decision making for preterm growth-restricted fetuses, a group usually posing a difficult problem for the clinician.

Follow-up Studies

It is of interest to follow the postnatal development of infants who suffered growth restriction and hypoxia in utero and to evaluate the possible predictive value

of Doppler fetal velocimetry with regard to long-term prognosis. The Malmö group performed extensive somatic, neurologic, and psychological investigations of 149 children at 7 years of age. All of them had been subjects for Doppler velocimetry of the descending aorta in utero and about half were SGA at birth. A univariate analysis showed that infants with abnormal intrauterine aortic blood flow had an increased frequency of minor neurologic abnormalities [100] and lower mean intelligence quotient [101] than infants with normal intrauterine hemodynamics. Logistic regression analysis revealed a statistically significant association between the aortic BFC and the neurologic [102] and intellectual [101] status at age 7 years (Table 11.5).

The above findings invite speculation as to whether an early intervention in cases of growth-restricted fetuses with an abnormal BFC might prevent not only fetal mortality but also some minor development deficits. Such management policy, however, engenders the danger of iatrogenic prematurity. Therefore a protocol for management of preterm babies, based on the results of fetal velocimetry, should be tested in randomized clinical trials before adopting it in clinical practice.

analysis included independent ante- and postnatal variables and an evaluation of the effect of socio-economic variables and interval complications occurring during postnatal life. In multivariate analysis, MND-1 was best predicted by the combination of increasing birth-weight deviation and male sex, whereas the best combination of variables contributing significantly to MND-2 was abnormal BFC and male sex. Global IQ≤85 was best predicted by abnormal BFC, fetal gestational age at measurement, and social group. Fetal gestational age at measurement was present as an additional risk factor, due to interaction with BFC. When the last BFC measurement was normal and performed after 37 gestational weeks of pregnancy, only one child of 40 had a global IQ<85. The dichotomous variable SGA/AGA showed no association with any of the intellectual outcome variables. The association of fetal growth restriction to both short-term and long-term outcome will generally be more powerfully expressed when using a continuous variable, such as birth-weight deviation, as compared with birth-weight categories.

A reduction in mean fetal aortic blood flow velocity has been correlated to hypoxia in the IUGR fetus, blood–gas values being obtained by cordocentesis [70]. The association found between an abnormal fetal aortic waveform and unfavorable neurodevelopmental outcome, which remained after adjustment for other confounding variables, may be attributed to fetal hypoxia. The fetal aortic velocity waveform reflects conditions both in the peripheral fetal circulation and in the placental circulation. The hemodynamic mechanism responsible for the abnormal waveform may therefore be both reduced peripheral blood supply due to hypoxia or increased impedance of the placental circulation, or both.

Cognitive Outcome at 18 Years of Age

We continued the prospective follow-up study on a subgroup of the previously described cohort. A total of 51 subjects were examined at a median age of 18.2 years [71]. Twenty-eight of the subjects, 18 women and 10 men, were SGA at birth with a median deviation of weight at birth of –31% (range –42 to –22%) from the gestational age-related mean, at a median gestational age of 38.7 completed weeks (35–41 weeks). Nine subjects had BFC III, 10 subjects had BFC II, 2 subjects had BFC I, and 7 subjects had a normal BFC. The remaining 23 subjects, 13 women and 10 men, had a normal estimated fetal weight, normal aortic BFC, and an AGA weight at birth with median weight deviation –2% (–10 to 22%) at a median gestational age of 39.7 weeks (36–42 weeks).

At 18 years of age, a psychologist evaluated the cognitive capacity using the Wechsler Adult Intelli-gence Scale (WAIS) that, similarly to the WIPPSI test performed at 6 years of age, consists of several subtests resulting in a performance IQ and a verbal IQ. The SGA subjects had a lower performance IQ as compared with those with birth-weight AGA, but did not differ significantly in verbal IQ. Fetal aortic blood flow class was not related to global IQ; however, the subjects with BFC II and III had a lower processing speed index (PSI) as compared with those with BFC 0 and I. The PSI measures fine motor ability, visual and working memory, and psychomotor speed. We found a high correlation between cognitive test results at 6 years and those at 18 years of age. Interestingly, the correlation between test results at the respective ages was higher for the SGA group. The results suggest that cognitive level at 6 years of age as determined by a standardized IQ test is more predictive of cognitive level at 18 years of age in subjects with IUGR than in those with normal fetal growth and birth weight. A retrospective assessment of attention deficit hyperactivity disorder (ADHD), the Wender Utah Rating scale, showed that the rate of ADHD was increased in the group with birth-weight SGA. These subjects had low IQ scores at both 6 and 18 years of age and also reported more psychiatric symptoms at 18 years. Although the majority of subjects with IUGR had IQ score within the normal range at 18 years of age, we found an increased rate of individuals with multiple impairments, i.e., ADHD, decreased cognitive capacity, and emotional disturbance.

Retinal Neural Morphology and Function

At 18 years of age, all subjects had an eye examination, including fundus photography after cycloplegia. Quantitative analysis of fundus photographs, utilizing a computer-assisted digital mapping system, evaluated two outcome measures: (a) the neuroretinal rim area (obtained by subtraction of the cup area from the optic disc area) as a measure of the optic nerve central nervous tissue; and (b) the number of branching points of retinal arterioles and venules as a measure of vascularization. The mean of the measurements from the two eyes in one subject represented the value of each ocular fundus variable. Visual function was assessed by using Rarebit perimetry which is a recently developed method for measuring central field vision [72].

We found that a more pronounced negative birth-weight deviation was associated with a decrease in neuroretinal rim area ($p = 0.0001$) [73]. The subjects with fetal aortic BFC III had a reduced neuroretinal rim area, median 1.59 mm^2 (range 1.33–1.86 mm^2) as compared with those with fetal aortic BFC II (1.85 mm^2; range 1.37–2.13 mm^2) and to those with normal fetal aortic BFC (2.22 mm^2; range 1.70–

2.71 mm²; $p < 0.05$ and $p < 0.0001$, respectively; Figs. 12.3, 12.4). These findings indicate that IUGR is associated with a reduced axonal area in the optic nerve at young adult age. Degree of deviation in weight at birth and extent of fetal blood flow velocity abnormality were both associated with an increased reduction of the axonal area of the optic nerve. The observed reduction in axonal area may reflect either reduced axonal growth with a reduction of axonal volume or a decrease in the number of axons, i.e., in the number of neurons.

It can be speculated as to whether the observed reduction in axonal area is restricted to the optic nerve tract or represents a more global affection of neuronal growth within the brain. We found a strong association between MND at 6 years of age and a reduced axonal area suggesting that other regions of the central nervous system might be affected. The subjects with severe MND at 6 years of age had among other deviations consistent abnormalities in test items measuring coordination and balance suggestive of changes in the cerebellum or basal ganglia [63]. Experimental studies on induced fetal growth restriction during late pregnancy in guinea pigs and fetal sheep have shown a reduction in volume of cerebellar layers and in the number of Purkinje neurons in the cerebellum [74, 75]. Neuroradiological studies on humans following IUGR with volumetric quantification of the cerebellar region have, to our knowledge, not yet been performed.

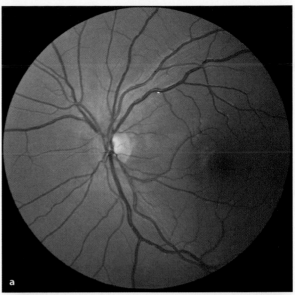

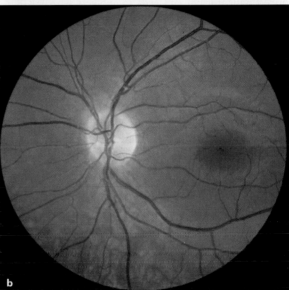

Fig. 12.4. a Ocular fundus photography showing a reduced neuroretinal rim area of the optic nerve in a 18-year-old male subject with an SGA birth weight and reverse diastolic flow in fetal descending aorta (BFC III). **b** Neuroretinal rim area of the optic nerve in an 18-year-old male subject with normal fetal growth and normal fetal aortic blood flow. (From Ley et al. [73])

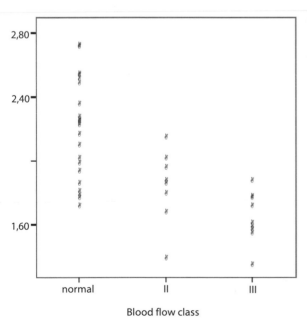

Fig. 12.3. Relationship between neuroretinal rim area of the optic nerve examined at 18 years of age and fetal aortic blood flow class (BFC). BFC III corresponds to absent or reverse flow in diastole. (From Ley et al. [72])

Fetal hypoxia as well as fetal malnutrition may be considered as plausible causes for the observed reduction in axonal area of the optic nerve. Fetal malnutrition during IUGR may be an important factor in disturbing cellular growth and differentiation in the central nervous system. Trophic factors, such as IGF-I, are essential for cellular growth and differentiation as well as for tissue repair after a damaging insult. Undernutrition in humans and in experimental animals decreases IGF-I expression in many tissues and in the circulation [76, 77]. Circulatory levels of IGF-I have been shown to be decreased in SGA fetuses and in fetuses with abnormal blood flow velocity [78, 79].

In our study at 18 years of age, the central field vision, as represented by the Rarebit mean hit rate [72], ranged from 93 to 100% in subjects with birthweight AGA and from 48 to 100% in those with birth-weight SGA with the median hit rate being significantly lower in the SGA group as compared with that in the AGA group ($p = 0.03$). Eight of the SGA subjects and none of the controls had a hit rate below the normal range ($p = 0.006$). The deviant hit rates detected by the Rarebit microdot perimetry in some SGA subjects may reflect defects in the matrix of detectors, i.e., the neural channels, and may be caused by disturbed axonal growth or development. This finding of abnormal function lends support to the previously mentioned morphological finding of reduced neuroretinal rim area in subjects with IUGR.

Fetal Aortic Blood Flow and Postnatal Cardiovascular Function

Aortic Vessel Wall Characteristics and Blood Pressure at 9 Years of Age

We used an electronic phase-locked echo-tracking system DIAMOVE (Teltec, Lund, Sweden) for non-invasive monitoring of pulsatile diameter changes in the descending aorta [81, 82] of a subgroup of 68 children from the original Malmö cohort. Neither abnormal fetal aortic blood flow nor birth-weight deviation were reflected in any significant changes in elastic modulus or stiffness of the abdominal aorta at 9 years of age [80]. Within the examined group, the subjects with the highest body weight at the time of examination had the highest levels of systolic blood pressure. These results support the hypothesis that the link between fetal growth failure and high blood pressure in adult life may mainly be expressed among those with obesity.

Children born SGA had significantly lower vessel diameters than those born AGA and these differences remained significant after adjustment for body surface area. These findings resemble in part those of Stale et al. [83] who found lower values of end-diastolic diameters in SGA fetuses than in AGA fetuses of the same gestational age using an identical technique for aortic measurements; however, when the fetal aortic diameters were adjusted for estimated fetal weight, the relationship was reversed. The larger weight-related diastolic diameter taken together with the finding of a lower relative pulse amplitude in the SGA fetuses suggested an increase in diastolic blood pressure, possibly as a response to the increased peripheral resistance, namely that of the placental circulation, found in pregnancies complicated by IUGR. The present findings obtained at 9 years of age [80] showed no evidence of an increase in diastolic blood pressure related to restricted fetal growth. On the contrary, IUGR was associated with lower diastolic blood pressure. As the influence of the increased resistance to fetal blood flow caused by the abnormal placenta in fetal growth restriction will cease to exist after birth, it would seem plausible that the postulated compensatory increase in blood pressure during the fetal period would no longer be present in childhood.

Pulse pressure was significantly higher within the group of children born SGA than in those born AGA [80]. An increase in pulse pressure has previously been described in SGA infants at 6 weeks of age [84] and has been associated with signs of low arterial compliance and hypertensive disease in adults [85, 86]; however, we were unable to detect any corresponding changes in aortic compliance in association with either abnormal fetal aortic blood flow or SGA birth weight. A previous study of human aortic compliance and its normal variation with age found a profound increase in compliance between 4 and 11 years of age [87]. Aortic compliance thereafter exhibited a gradual decrease with values beyond 16 years being similar to those of healthy adults. This may imply that changes in aortic vessel compliance due to fetal causes may be detectable at a later age when aortic compliance decreases due to the normal ageing process. The increase in pulse pressure observed in the SGA group [80] might suggest, in the absence of changes in elastic modulus and stiffness of the abdominal aorta, the possibility of corresponding changes in more peripheral segments of the arterial tree.

Size and Function of Large Arteries at 18 Years of Age

At 18 years of age [88], vascular mechanical properties of the common carotid artery (CCA), abdominal aorta (AO), and popliteal artery (PA) were assessed by echo-tracking sonography in 21 adolescents with IUGR and abnormal fetal aortic blood flow, and in 23 adolescents with normal fetal growth and normal fetal aortic blood flow, all belonging to the Malmö-Lund follow-up cohort [71–73, 89]. Endothelium-dependent and endothelium-independent vasodilatation of the brachial artery was measured by high-resolution ultrasound.

The IUGR group had significantly smaller mean vessel diameters compared with controls in the AO and PA in proportion to the body size, with a similar trend in the CCA. Stiffness in all three vascular regions was comparable between the two groups. Men from the IUGR group had a lower compliance coefficient in the AO (corrected for body surface area) than men from the control group. The time course of vasodilatation in the IUGR group appeared to be different from the control group with higher values of flow-mediated vasodilatation at 2 min after cuff deflation in the IUGR group. Smaller aortic dimensions and the lower aortic compliance coefficient seen in male adolescents with previous IUGR may influence the future cardiovascular health of these individuals. Sustained flow-mediated vasodilatation may indicate an increased synthesis of nitric oxide in response to forearm occlusion.

Retinal Vascular Morphology at 18 Years of Age [89]

In the cohort of young adults, followed by us, we found that increasing negative birth-weight deviation was associated with a decrease in the number of retinal vascular branching points ($p = 0.02$; Fig. 12.5). Neither age at examination, gender, nor the degree of abnormal fetal blood flow were associated with the number of retinal vessel-branching points. It is unclear whether the finding of reduced vessel-branching points in IUGR subjects is restricted to the retina or whether it reflects a more general affection of vascular growth within the body. A previous study in IUGR rats induced by protein restriction has shown reduced vasculature in the cerebral cortex [90]. Our findings of a reduced size of large arteries in subjects with IUGR detected at 9 and 19 years of age, and that of a reduced number of branches in the retinal vasculature, support a general affection of angiogenesis. Others have shown signs of impaired endothelial function in small and large arteries in school children born SGA [91]. We found that aortic compliance appeared unaffected at 9 years of age [80], whereas men at 19 years of age had signs of decreased compliance [88]. These findings of functional and morphological deficits may contribute to a better understanding of the link between restricted fetal growth and cardiovascular disease.

Conclusion

In conclusion, several studies have shown abnormal fetal hemodynamics in the growth-restricted fetus, especially umbilical AREDF, to be associated with a clear increase in perinatal mortality and neonatal morbidity. The long-term follow-up studies performed until now did not show clear evidence of major neurological handicap being associated with abnormal fetal hemodynamics. This is not surprising as

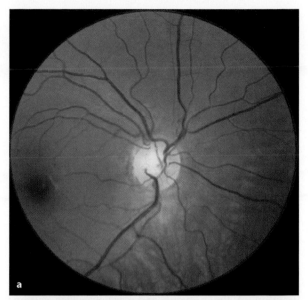

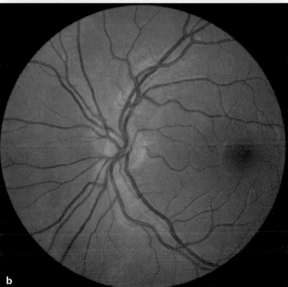

Fig. 12.5. a Ocular fundus photography demonstrating a reduced number of retinal vessel-branching points in an 18-year-old female with an SGA birth weight and abnormal fetal aortic blood flow (BFC III). **b** Ocular fundus photography with a normal number of retinal vessel-branching points in an 18-year old female with normal fetal growth and normal fetal aortic blood flow. (From Hellström et al. [89])

the much larger body of prospective follow-up studies on IUGR, in terms of birth-weight SGA, seldom showed an increase in major neurological impairment associated with fetal growth impairment. Minor neurological dysfunction, behavioral abnormality, and learning problems at school age, all frequently reported as overrepresented in perinatal risk groups, would probably be more adequate as outcome variables when assessing the effects of fetal hemodynamics on postnatal neurodevelopment.

Hemodynamic evaluation of the fetus has increased our understanding of the physiological mechanisms involved in fetal growth restriction and is of proven clinical value in the management of high-risk pregnancies. Knowledge of changes in umbilical and fetal blood flow has also been of great value in the definition of true IUGR in subjects with deviation in weight during fetal life or at birth; thus, follow-up studies in subjects with abnormal fetal blood flow with varying degrees of deviation in weight have supplied valuable information on effects of IUGR on different aspects of postnatal development. Abnormal fetal blood flow reflects changes in the feto-placental unit associated with a reduced fetal supply of oxygen and nutrients. Other authors, in addition to us, have shown that such fetal deprivation may lead to long-standing disturbances in morphology and subsequent function of the nervous and cardiovascular system. This information, coupled with insights derived from experimental and clinical studies allowing for interaction with genetic differences, will increase understanding of mechanisms leading to postnatal morbidity due to restricted fetal growth. Furthermore, this knowledge will make it possible to design clinical trials evaluating management protocols aiming not only to prevent perinatal mortality, but also to improve the postnatal development and health later in life of individuals with abnormal intrauterine blood flow.

References

1. Dobbing J (1981) The later development of the brain and its vulnerability. In: Davis JA, Dobbing J (eds) Scientific foundation of pediatrics, 2nd edn. William Heinemann Medical Books Ltd., London, pp 744–759
2. Dobbing J (1979) Nutrition and brain development. In: Thalhammer O, Baumgarten K, Pollak A (eds) Perinatal medicine. Sixth European Congress. Thieme, Stuttgart
3. Chase HP, Welch NN, Dabiere CS, Vasan NS, Butterfield LJ (1972) Alterations in human brain biochemistry following intrauterine growth retardation. Pediatrics 50:403–411
4. Sarma MKJ, Rao KS (1974) Biochemical compositions of different regions in brains of small-for-date infants. J Neurochem 22:671–677
5. Breart G (1988) Available evidence relating intrauterine growth retardation to neuromotor dysfunction and mental handicap. In Kubli F, Patel N, Scmidt W (eds) Perinatal events and brain damage in surviving infants. Springer, Berlin Heidelberg New York, pp 92–98
6. Fitzhardinge PM, Stevens EM (1972) The small for date infant. II. Neurological and intellectual sequelae. Pediatrics 50:50–57
7. Hagberg G, Hagberg B, Olow I (1976) The changing panorama of cerebral palsy in Sweden 1954–1970. III. The importance of fetal deprivation of supply. Acta Paediatr Scand 65:403–408
8. Hadders-Algra M, Huisjes HJ, Touwen BCL (1988) Preterm or small-for-gestational age infants. Neurological and behavioural development at the age of 6 years. Eur J Pediatr 147:460–467
9. Walther FJ, Raemakers LHJ (1990) Developmental aspects of subacute fetal distress: behaviour problems and neurological dysfunction. Early Hum Dev 6:1–10
10. Hawdon JM, Hey E, Kolvin I, Fundudis T (1990) Born too small. Is outcome still affected? Dev Med Child Neurol 32:943–953
11. Ounsted M, Moar VA, Scott WA (1988) Neurological development of small-for-gestational age babies during the first year of life. Early Hum Dev 16:163–172
12. Villar J, Smerigilo V, Martorell R, Brown CH, Klein RE (1984) Heterogenous growth and mental development of intrauterine growth retarded infants during the first 3 years of life. 74:783–791
13. Berg AT (1989) Indices of fetal growth retardation, perinatal hypoxia-related factors and childhood neurological morbidity. Early Hum Dev 19:271–283
14. Westwood M, Kramer MS, Muntz D, Locett JM, Watters GV (1983) Growth and development of full-term non-asphyxiated small for gestational age newborns: follow up through adolescence. Pediatrics 71:367–382
15. Lou HC (1996) Etiology and pathogenesis of Attention-Deficit Hyperactivity Disorder (ADHD): significance of prematurity and perinatal hypoxic-haemodynamic encephalopathy. Acta Paediatr 85:1266–1271
16. Mallard EC, Williams CE, Johnston BM, Gunning MI, Davis S, Gluckman PD (1995) Repeated asphyxia causes loss of striatal projection neurons in the fetal sheep brain. Neuroscience 65:827–836
17. Gennser G, Rymark P, Isberg PE (1988) Low birth weight and risk of high blood pressure in adulthood. Br Med J 296:1498–1500
18. Barker DJP, Bull AR, Osmond O, Simmons SJ (1990) Fetal and placental size and risk of hypertension in adult life. Br Med J 301:259–262
19. Barker DJP, Osmond C, Golding J, Kuh D, Wadsworth MEJ (1989) Growth in utero, blood pressure in childhood and adult life, and mortality from cardiovascular disease. Br Med J 298:564–567
20. Hales CN, Barker DJP, Clark PMS (1991) Fetal and infant growth and impaired glucose tolerance at age 64. Br Med J 303:259–262
21. Barker DJP, Hales CN, Fall CHD, Osmond C, Phipps K, Clark PMS (1993) Type 2 (non-insulin dependent) diabetes mellitus, hypertension and hyperlipidaemia (syndrome X): relation to reduced fetal growth. Diabetologia 36:62–67
22. Edwards C, Benediktsson R, Lindsay R, Seckl J (1993) Dysfunction of placental glucocorticoid barrier: link between fetal environment and adult hypertension? Lancet 341:355–357
23. Morley R, Lister G, Leeson-Payne C, Lucas A (1994) Size at birth and later blood pressure. Arch Dis Child 70:536–537
24. Williams S, St George IM, Silva PA (1992) Intrauterine growth retardation and blood pressure at age seven and eighteen. J Clin Epidemiol 45:1257–1263

25. Launer LJ, Hofman A, Grobbee DE (1993) Relation between birth weight and blood pressure: longitudinal study of infants and children. Br Med J 307:1451–1454

26. Montenegro N, Santos F, Tavares E, Matias A, Barros H, Leite LP (1998) Outcome of 88 pregnancies with absent or reversed end-diastolic blood flow (ARED flow) in the umbilical arteries. Eur J Obstet Gynecol Reprod Biol 79:43–46

27. El Bishy G, Sturgiss SN (2003) Absent-end-diastolic flow velocity in the umbilical artery. Fetal Maternal Med Rev 143:251–271

28. Karsdorp VHM, van Vugt JMG, van Geijn HP, Kostense PJ, Arduini D, Montenegro N, Todros T (1994) Clinical significance of absent or reversed end diastolic velocity waveforms in umbilical artery. Lancet 344:1664–1668

29. Westergaard HB, Langhoff-Roos J et al. (2001) A critical appraisal of the use of umbilical artery Doppler ultrasound in high risk pregnancies: use of meta-analyses in evidence-based obstetrics. Ultrasound Obstet Gynecol 17:466–476

30. Gudmundsson S, Maršál K (1991) Blood velocity waveforms in the fetal aorta and umbilical artery as predictors of fetal outcome: a comparison. Am J Perinatol 8:1–6

31. Hackett GA, Campbell S, Gamsu H, Cohen-Overbeek T, Pearce JMF (1987) Doppler studies in the growth retarded fetus and prediction of neonatal necrotising enterocolitis, haemorrhage and neonatal morbidity. Br Med J 294:13–15

32. Brar HS, Platt LD (1988) Reverse end-diastolic flow velocity and umbilical artery velocimetry in high-risk pregnancies; an ominous finding with adverse pregnancy outcome. Am J Obstet Gynecol 159:559–561

33. Malcolm G, Ellwood D, Devonald K, Beilby R, Henderson-Smart D (1991) Absent or reversed end diastolic flow velocity in the umbilical artery and necrotising enterocolitis. Arch Dis Child 66:805–807

34. Wilson DC, Harper A, McClure G (1991) Absent or reversed end diastolic flow velocity in the umbilical artery and necrotising enterocolitis. Arch Dis Child 66:1467

35. Kempley ST, Gamsu HR, Vyas S, Nicolaides K (1991) Effects of intrauterine growth retardation on postnatal visceral and cerebral blood flow velocity. Arch Dis Child 66:1151–1158

36. McDonnell M, Serra-Serra V, Gaffney G, Redman CW, Hope PL (1994) Neonatal outcome after pregnancy complicated by abnormal velocity waveforms in the umbilical artery. Arch Dis Child 70:F84–F89

37. Adiotomre P, Johnstone FD, Laing IA (1997) Effect of absent end diastolic flow velocity in the fetal umbilical artery on subsequent outcome. Arch Dis Child 76:35–38

38. Eronen M, Kari A, Pesonen E, Kaaja R, Wallgren EI, Hallman M (1993) Value of absent or retrograde end-diastolic flow in fetal aorta and umbilical artery as a predictor of perinatal outcome in pregnancy-induced hypertension. Acta Paediatr 82:919–924

39. Vossbeck S, Kraus de Camargo O, Grab D, Bode H, Pohlandt F (2001) Neonatal and neurodevelopmental outcome in infants born before 30 weeks of gestation with absent or reversed end-diastolic flow velocities in the umbilical artery. Eur J Pediatr 160:128–134

40. Weiss E, Ulrich S, Berle P (1992) Condition at birth of infants with previously absent or reverse umbilical artery end-diastolic flow velocities. Arch Gynecol Obstet 252:37–43

41. Weiss E, Ulrich S, Berle P, Picard-Maureau A (1994) CK-BB as indicator of prenatal brain-cell injury in fetuses with absent or reverse end-diastolic flow velocities of the umbilical arteries. J Perinat Med 22:219–226

42. Rizzo G, Arduini D, Luciano R, Rizzo C, Tortorolo G, Romanini C, Mancuso S (1989) Prenatal cerebral Doppler ultrasonography and neonatal neurologic outcome. J Ultrasound Med 8:237–240

43. Scherjon SA, Smolders-DeHaas H, Kok JH, Zondervan HA (1993) The "brain-sparing" effect: antenatal cerebral Doppler findings in relation to neurologic outcome in very preterm infants. Am J Obstet Gynecol 169:169–175

44. Ley D, Maršál K (1992) Doppler velocimetry in cerebral vessels of small for gestational age infants. Early Hum Dev 31:171–180

45. Scherjon SA, Smolders-DeHaas H, Oosting H, Kok JH, Zondervan HA (1994) Neonatal cerebral circulation in relation to neurosonography and neurological outcome: a pulsed Doppler study. Neuropediatrics 25:208–213

46. Weiss E, Ulrich S, Berle P (1992) Blood flow velocity waveforms of the middle cerebral artery and abnormal neurological evaluations in live-born fetuses with absent or reverse end-diastolic flow velocities of the umbilical arteries. Eur J Obstet Gynecol Reprod Biol 45: 93–100

47. Valcamonico A, Danti L, Frusca T, Soregaroli M, Zucca S, Abrami F, Tiberti A (1994) Absent end-diastolic velocity in umbilical artery: risk of neonatal morbidity and brain damage. Am J Obstet Gynecol 170:796–801

48. Todd AL, Trudinger BJ, Cole MJ, Cooney GH (1992) Antenatal tests of fetal wellfare and development at age 2 years. Am J Obstet Gynecol 167:66–71

49. Wilson DC, Harper A, McClure G, Halliday H, Reid M (1992) Long term predictive value of Doppler studies in high risk fetuses. Br J Obstet Gynecol 99:575–578

50. Kirsten GF, Van Zyl JI, Van Zijl F, Maritz JS, Odendaal HJ (2000) Infants of women with severe early pre-eclampsia: the effect of absent end-diastolic umbilical artery doppler flow velocities on neurodevelopmental outcome. Acta Paediatr 89:566–570

51. Wienerroither H, Steiner H, Tomaselli J, Lobendanz M, Thun-Hohenstein L (2001) Intrauterine blood flow and long-term intellectual, neurologic and social development. Obstet Gynecol 97:449–453

52. Scherjon S, Oosting H, Ongerboer de Visser BW, de Wilde T, Zondervan HA, Kok JH (1996) Fetal brain sparing is associated with accelerated shortening of visual evoked potential latencies during early infancy. Am J Obstet Gynecol 175:1569–1575

53. Hempel MS (1993) Neurological development during toddling age in normal children and children at risk of developmental disorders. Early Hum Dev 34:47–57

54. Scherjon SA, Oosting H, Smolders-DeHaas H, Zondervan HA, Kok JH (1998) Neurodevelopmental outcome at three years of age after fetal "brain-sparing". Early Hum Dev 52:67–79

55. Scherjon S, Briet J, Oosting H, Kok J (2000) The discrepancy between maturation of visual-evoked poten-

Chapter 13

Cerebral and Umbilical Doppler in the Prediction of Fetal Outcome

Philippe Arbeille, Gabriel Carles, Murielle Chevillot, Alain Locatelli, Philippe Herve, Frank Perrotin, Dev Maulik

Fetal Cerebral Flow Adaptation to Hypoxia

Hypoxia is present in most of the chronic or acute fetal patency stages. In severely growth-restricted fetuses pO_2 is about 15 mmHg, whereas in normal fetuses it is about 23 mmHg. Fetal adaptation to hypoxia consists mainly of a humoral process and a cardiovascular process. Severe hypoxia is generally associated with a pCO_2 increase and pH decrease. Erythropoiesis is stimulated, leading to polyglobulia, and polycythemia. The fetus protects against hypoxia by using the glucose reserves and the acid–base buffers. The initial cardiovascular response includes a redistribution of the main fetal flows and later blood pressure increase, bradycardia, and modification of the cardiac (left and right) hemodynamics. It is generally accepted that there is a significant vasoconstriction of most of the fetal territories (pulmonary, splanchnic, skeletal, and muscular areas) and an increased perfusion of the brain, the heart, and the adrenal glands [1–4]. This phenomenon, called the "brain-sparing effect", attempts to compensate for fetal hypoxia by providing more oxygen to the brain via a cerebral vasodilation. Nevertheless, in the case of hypoxia blood oxygen saturation may not be normal [5, 6], and the increased brain perfusion may be responsible for brain edema with tissue deterioration. Finally, although the adapted response to hypoxia (brain vasodilation) is observed, it is difficult to evaluate if the brain tissue is protected against the deleterious effects of hypoxia and to what extent.

It was demonstrated that in cases of transient or chronic placental insufficiency (malaria, hypertension, drug abuse) abnormal fetal heart rate (FHR) occurs after some days and brain damage can develop after some weeks despite flow redistribution [7–10]. These observations suggest that the occurrence of functional (abnormal FHR) or organic fetal damage may depend on the amplitude of the pO_2 decrease as already suggested and on the duration of the exposure to hypoxia [8]. Severe maternal anemia, which induces acute but reversible hypoxia without placental insufficiency, is frequently associated with prematur-ity, reduced neonatal weight, and infant iron deficiency [11–14]. In this condition, oxygen supply to the fetus might be reduced and result in blood flow redistribution with similar consequences (abnormal FHR) as previously described, despite no evidence of placental insufficiency. On the other hand, several studies have suggested that decelerations in the FHR are a late sign of fetal deterioration before which the fetus might be delivered [15–18]; thus, anticipation of FHR abnormality by Doppler monitoring of the fetal flow redistribution occurring before worsening hypoxia could provide opportunity for early intervention [19–21].

Animal studies have demonstrated that fetal cerebral circulation is also affected by vasoconstrictive drugs administered during pregnancy. For example, nicotine induces in fetal lambs a reduction of the flow toward the brain, and affects the cerebral flow response to the CO_2 test. Even drugs considered necessary to treat a mother's pathology (hypertension) may have, after long-term treatment, unsuitable effects on the fetus by blocking or reducing the fetal adaptation to hypoxia.

Examination Technique

Human Investigations (Duplex B, Pulsed Wave Doppler, and Color Doppler)

The first studies were based on the exploration of the anterior and middle cerebral arteries [22–24] or of the intracranial portion of the internal carotid artery [25]. Due to the generally poor resolution of the ultrasound images, it was necessary to visualize well-known cerebral structures (cerebral peduncles, middle cerebral line) and use them as anatomical references to identify the intracerebral vessels. The significant improvement in ultrasound technology has facilitated this examination. It is now easy to detect the arterial pulsation of the cerebral vessels and to localize correctly the Doppler sample volume (Figs. 13.1, 13.2). On the biparietal image plane the middle cerebral arteries are found on a transverse line passing

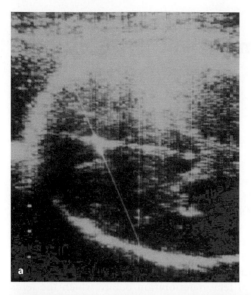

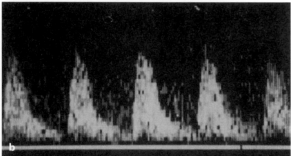

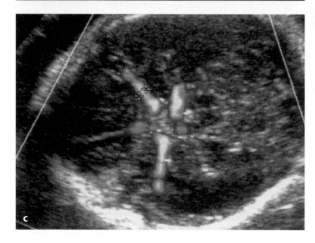

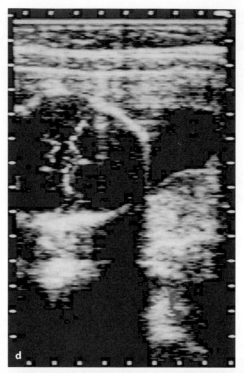

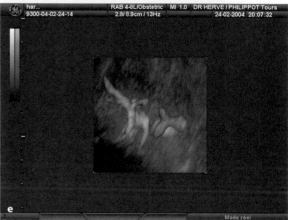

Fig. 13.1. Investigation of the fetal cerebral arteries (**a, b**). Fetal cranial cross section with the cerebral peduncle and the Doppler sample volume on the anterior cerebral arteries and the corresponding Doppler spectrum. **c, d** Color Doppler of the circle of Willis. **e** Three-dimensional color Doppler

anterior to the cerebral peduncles, and the anterior arteries are found on a line perpendicular to the previous line approximately 2 cm in front of the peduncles' anterior limit.

With color Doppler technology it became possible to visualize and investigate the main cerebral arteries and to evaluate vascular resistance in various vascular areas of the brain supplied by these arteries [26]. In Figure 13.1 the two anterior, middle, and posterior ce-

rebral arteries, and the posterior communicating arteries, can be easily identified. The incidence displaying these vessels is similar to the "biparietal incidence" used for measuring the fetal head diameter. The vessels most easily investigated by this incidence are the middle cerebral arteries, because they are oriented toward the Doppler transducer. In this case the angle between the vessel axis and the Doppler beam is close to zero and the Doppler frequency is maximum.

Fig. 13.2. Umbilical and cerebral velocity waveform in normal pregnancies at 22, 30, and 37 weeks of gestation. Note that the cerebral end-diastolic flow velocity is always lower than the umbilical flow velocity; thus, the cerebral to umbilical index is always higher than the umbilical to cerebral index.

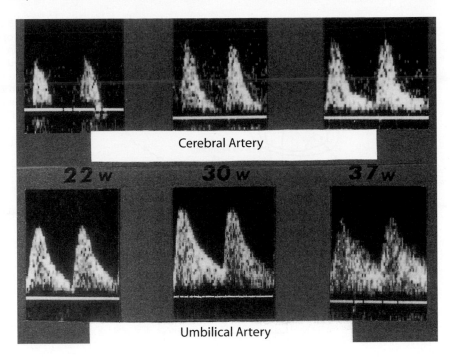

Animal Investigations (Implanted Doppler Sensors)

Although fetal Doppler examinations in the human pregnancy provide useful information to the obstetrician, it is not possible to collect all the biological and hemodynamic data required to understand the physiopathological mechanisms involved in the development of the intrauterine growth restriction (IUGR) and the hypoxia.

With the animal model it is possible to measure blood pressure, blood velocity and blood volume, to collect blood samples, to perform pharmacological tests, and to simulate some human pathologies.

Several studies have been carried out on lamb fetuses using electromagnetic flow meters placed around the umbilical cord and catheters with pressure sensors inserted into the fetal aorta. Mostly, only the umbilical flow was assessed on the fetal side. Flat Doppler probes were developed to be implanted in the fetus and the mother, making it possible to assess atraumatically the fetal (cerebral/umbilical) and maternal flows in real time over a period of approximately 20 days' gestation. The 4-MHz continuous wave (CW) or pulsed wave (PW) Doppler probe consists of two rectangular piezoelectric transducers, pre-oriented at 45° from the surface of the probe, and placed in a plastic case (6 mm high, 2 cm² area) with small holes on the edges to sew the probe to the fetal skin. The sensors are affixed to the fetal skin, facing the umbilical cord, the fetal cerebral arteries and in front of the uterine arteries. The output wires and the fetal catheter connectors are stowed in a pocket affixed to the back of the ewe, and at each measurement session the fetus is simply connected for 1 or 2 h (without any anesthesia) to the Doppler and pressure system (Fig. 13.3).

On the Doppler waveforms the blood flow volume and the vascular resistance changes in the area supplied by the vessel (placenta, brain, uterus) and the fetal heart rate are calculated. This system has been tested on normal gestations, during simulated fetal hypoxia, and during pharmacological treatments (Fig. 13.3) [7, 27, 28].

Cerebral Hemodynamics and Doppler Indices

Cerebral Resistance to Flow

Accessibility to the main fetal cerebral arteries by Doppler has led to the development of various hemodynamic indices. The amplitude of the end-diastolic flow in the fetal vessels is directly related to the vascular resistances in the area supplied by these vessels [29–31]. In order to quantify the vascular resistances, various indices, which measure the proportion of systolic flow within the total forward flow (M) during one cardiac cycle, or the relative amplitude of systolic (S) to diastolic (D) flow, have been proposed: $PI=(S-D)/M$ [32]; $R=D/S$ [30]; $RI=(S-D)/S$ [33]; $R=S/D$ [34]. Most of these parameters change according to the resistance to flow into the vascular territory un-

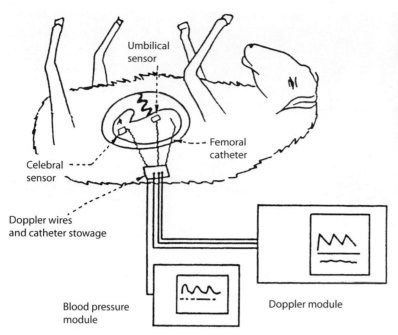

Fig. 13.3. Instrumentation of the fetus. Flat Doppler sensors are sewn on the fetal skin in front of the artery to be investigated (on the abdomen for the umbilical arteries, on the neck for the internal carotid artery, on the maternal abdomen for the uterine artery). A catheter is inserted into the fetal femoral artery, for blood pressure measurements and blood sampling (blood gases)

der investigation; therefore, any increase of these indices above the upper limit of the normal range corresponds to an increase of the vascular resistances (Fig. 13.4). In contrast, the D/S index decreases as the resistance to flow increases. The vascular resistance increase may be due to vascular disease (placental infarction or fibrosis) or to distal arteriolar vasoconstriction (brain response to increased pO_2 or to vasoactive drugs). Conversely, abnormally decreased resistance to flow values are displayed below the lower limit of the normal range of the index for S-D/M, S-D/S, S/D (Fig. 13.4) and above the upper limit for the D/S index. The decreased resistance to flow may be due to the existence of arterio-venous shunts, or to an arteriolar vasodilation (brain adaptation to hypoxia or to drugs).

Cerebral–Umbilical Ratio for Evaluating pO_2 Changes

The cerebral–umbilical (C/U) ratio (also known as the cerebral/placental ratio (CPR)) changes are indicators of peripheral fetal flow distribution. These parameters, based on the comparison of the brain (cerebral to umbilical index, CRI) and the placental (umbilical to cerebral index, URI) resistances, are expressed as either CRI/URI [22, 23] or URI/CRI [2], the cerebral vascular resistances being measured from one of the intracerebral arteries (anterior or middle) or from the intracranial part of the carotid artery. By measuring the flow redistribution between the placenta and brain, these C/U ratios (in cases of pathologic pregnancies) take into account the placental dis-

turbances due to vascular disease at this level, and the cerebral response (vasodilation) to the hypoxia induced by placental dysfunction.

In normal pregnancies the diastolic component in the cerebral arteries is lower than in the umbilical arteries at any gestational age (Fig. 13.2); therefore, the cerebral vascular resistances remain higher than the placental resistances and the C/U ratio (C/U = CRI/URI) is >1.1 (Figs. 13.4, 13.5). The C/U ratio (CRI/URI) becomes <1.1 if any flow redistribution in favor of the brain occurs (Figs. 13.6–13.8). In such case the cerebral diastolic flow amplitude is higher than normal, and the umbilical flow amplitude is lower. Animal and human studies have demonstrated that the C/U changes in proportion to fetal pO_2 [35, 36]. The URI/CRI ratio used by other authors to detect fetal flow redistribution varies in the opposite direction.

Effect of Fetal Heart Rate on Doppler Vascular Resistance Indices

It is well known that an elevation of the fetal heart rate increases the end-diastolic velocity and therefore decreases the resistance index (Fig. 13.9). On the other hand, diminution of the heart rate increases the index value. This effect of the heart rate is eliminated by the use of the C/U ratios because both indices, CRI and URI, are measured on the same fetus with the same heart rate. The two C/U ratios mentioned above are not heart rate dependent, because the cerebral as well as the umbilical index are equally affected by the heart rate changes. Figure 13.5 shows the fluctuations of both the placental and the umbilical in-

Fig. 13.4. Resistance index [R=(S-D/S)] and cerebral–umbilical ratio (C/U=CRI/URI) in a population of 90 hypertensive pregnancies, with 17 (19%) having moderate IUGR (S=systolic peak, D=end-diastolic velocity). Normal range delimited from a population of 100 normal pregnancies. **a** Evolution of the umbilical vascular resistance index (URI) in normal (open symbols), and in growth-restricted (closed symbols) fetuses. The URI is abnormal when higher than the upper limit of the normal range. The sensitivity of these indices for the detection of IUGR is about 60%. **b** Evolution of the cerebral (CRI) vascular resistance in normal (open symbols), and in growth-restricted (closed symbols) fetuses. The CRI is abnormal when it is lower than the lower limit of the normal range. **c** Cerebral–umbilical ratio in normal (open symbols) and growth-restricted (closed symbols) fetuses. The sensitivity of this index for the detection of IUGR is about 85%

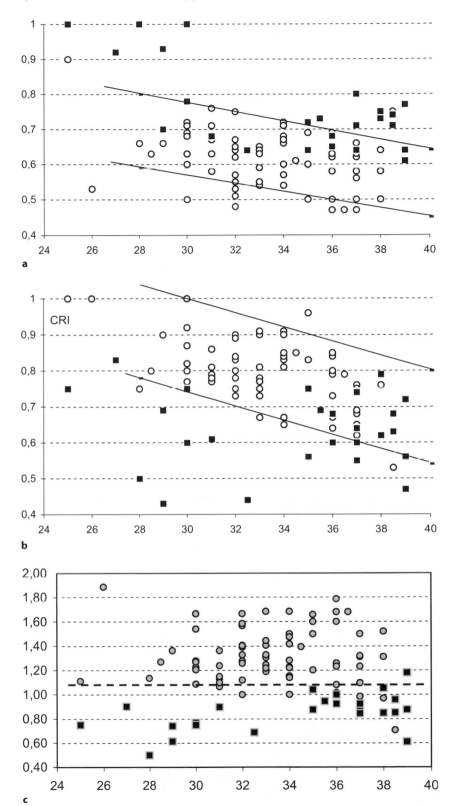

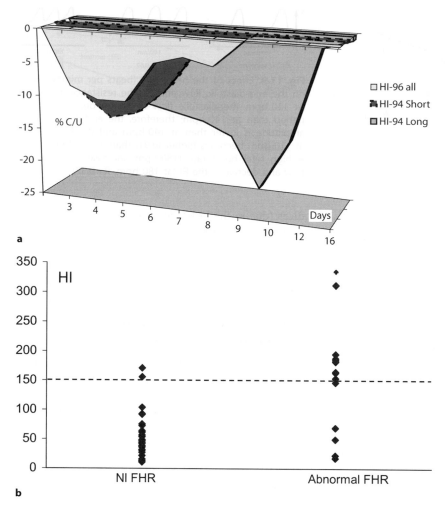

Fig. 13.10. a Mean variations of the ratio (C/U=cerebral resistance/umbilical resistance) during the malaria crises in group 1 (1994 short and long crisis) and in group 2 (1996 crisis). The C/U change is expressed in percentage from cut-off limit 1.1. In group 1 C/U decreased significantly more during long crisis than during short ones ($p<0.05$). The area between the C/U ratio curve and the time axis is the hypoxic index (*HI*). As the C/U ratio changes proportionately to the fetal pO_2, this area represents the cumulated deficit in pO_2 over the crisis. **b** Correlation between occurrence of abnormal fetal heart rate (*FHR*) vs HI. The HI is abnormal when >150% → PPV=80%, NPV=85%

In normal pregnancies the HI remains equal to zero as only C/U values lower than 1.1 which indicate a flow redistribution are taken into account. A flow redistribution characterized by a C/U ratio equal to 0.77 (–20% below 1.1) means that it could correspond to a 20% pO_2 reduction. If this situation remains stable for 10 days, the HI will be equal to $20\% \times 10 = 200\%$.

Cerebral Circulation in Normal Pregnancy

Cerebral Flow Changes with Gestational Age

The diastolic flow in the cerebral vessels is reduced at the beginning of the second half of pregnancy (20–25 weeks) but continues developing progressively. The increase in the diastolic component with the gestational age is interpreted as a decrease in the cerebral resistance due to brain development. The cerebral vascular resistance changes are measured using the same Doppler indices as for the placenta (Figs. 13.2, 13.4, 13.5).

The increase in the diastolic component begins later in the cerebral arteries (at approximately 25 weeks) than in the umbilical arteries (at approximately 15 weeks). The amplitude of the diastolic flow in the cerebral arteries is always lower than in the umbilical arteries, meaning that in normal pregnancy the cerebral vascular resistances are higher than the umbilical resistances. In other words, the umbilical flow volume is higher than the cerebral flow volume. This led to the definition of the C/U ratio (cerebral resistance/umbilical resistances), which is inversely proportional to cardiac output distribution between brain and placenta, and which is higher than 1.1 in normal pregnancies.

Variations According to the Site of Examination

In normal fetuses the resistance index is significantly higher in the middle cerebral artery ($p < 0.01$) [26] than in the anterior and posterior cerebral arteries. In pathological pregnancies with cerebral vasodilation (decreased cerebral index) the sensitivity of cerebral Doppler examination is not dependent on the choice of the cerebral artery explored. Since the Doppler indices measured on two different vessels will not differ by more than 5–10%, the conclusions of the Doppler investigation will not be changed. Nevertheless, during assessment of the fetal circulation over several days or weeks, successive examinations must be performed on the same vessel.

Cerebral Flow Changes with Behavioral States

Fetal behavioral states are defined according to the fetal heart rate pattern and the body and eye movements [40, 41]. In normal pregnancies at 37–38 weeks' gestation, blood flow velocity waveforms in the descending aorta and the internal carotid artery are affected by fetal behavioral states. In both vessels a significant reduction in the pulsatility index was established during behavioral state 2F (active sleep), compared with behavioral state 1F (quiet sleep) [41–43]. The decreased peripheral vascular resistance induces increased perfusion to the musculature and brain required by the increased energy demand during active sleep. In addition, peak flow velocity decrease in the fetal ductus arteriosus during active sleep has been demonstrated [43]. This observation confirms the existence of a redistribution of flow between the two ventricles with increased left cardiac output, which may contribute to the increased brain perfusion.

Clinical Significance of Cerebral and Cerebral/Umbilical Indices

Cerebral Flow in Growth-restricted and Hypoxic Human Fetuses

The Doppler indices measured in the main fetal cerebral arteries are sensitive to any vasoconstriction or vasodilatation of the brain vessels. An increase in the diastolic cerebral flow is interpreted as a vasomotor response (vasodilation) to hypoxia [25, 26, 44]. Comparisons between the cerebral Doppler index and the measurement of pO_2, pCO_2, pH, and O_2 content by cordocentesis have demonstrated a good correlation between pO_2 and the cerebral Doppler index in cases of severe hypoxia (the cerebral index decreases with the pO_2). Nevertheless, when acidosis appears there is sometimes an increase in the cerebral vascular resistance index due to a decrease in the diastolic flow [36, 45].

At first it appears difficult to quantify hypoxia using the CRI, but if it is measured every day in fetuses with abnormally decreased CRI, the evolution of the hypoxia can be followed through the brain's vascular resistance changes as illustrated in the following scenarios:

- Scenario 1: The cerebral vascular index is abnormal (lower than normal) but decreases progressively, as in normal fetuses. This can be related to high HR values, or to a hypoxic stable stage, but no reliable answer can be provided.
- Scenario 2: The abnormal cerebral index continues to decrease significantly and becomes more and more pathological. Hypoxia develops but the fetus is probably not acidemic.
- Scenario 3: A cerebral RI below the normal range but not changing over 2–3 days means that the small vessels beyond the measuring point can no longer change their diameters. Such a pattern was observed in pre-mortem fetuses in which brain edema and neuronal deterioration were observed at post-mortem anatomical examination [10].
- Scenario 4: Lastly, the cerebral index, already much lower than the normal limit, increases and enters the normal range again. In this case the capability of the brain vessels to vasodilate has been overwhelmed. Hypoxia is decompensated and the fetus becomes acidemic.

In all these circumstances it is hazardous to use only one absolute value of the cerebral Doppler index for the assessment of hypoxia and for making a decision about delivery. Only the evolution of the cerebral index or the C/U ratio over several days may provide information on the development of fetal hypoxia. Nevertheless, a good correlation has been found between the existence of significantly decreased (< 2 SD) cerebral resistance and the development of postasphyxial encephalopathy in the neonate [46]. In this study, the specificity and the sensitivity of fetal cerebral Doppler as a predictor of neonatal outcome were about 75 and 87%, respectively; however, it is emphasized that the vasodilation compensates only partially for the hypoxia, and its persistence over a long period of time does not guarantee the absence of brain tissue damage.

moglobin content lower than 5 g/100 ml was closely associated with fetal flow redistribution and abnormal FHR. On the other hand, the occurrence of abnormal FHR was associated with C/U < 1.1, which indicates that fetal flow redistribution plays a role in the development of cardiac dysfunction. Sixty-seven percent of the fetuses with abnormal FHR had a C/U < 1.1. Nevertheless, the modest values of the sensitivity (73%), specificity (33%), positive predictive value (PPV; 50%), and negative predictive value (NPV; 57%) confirm that the amplitude of the flow redistribution (C/U ratio) is not sufficient to predict the effects of this hemodynamic adaptation over time.

Other studies demonstrated that fetal cerebral vasodilation during a period of several weeks does not protect against cerebral organic damages [7, 9, 10]; thus, as the severe maternal anemia triggers a marked fetal cerebral vasodilation, the hemoglobin content has to be recovered as soon as possible in order to suppress the cerebral vasodilation. Moderate maternal anemia (Hb > 6 g/100 ml) did not trigger fetal flow redistribution or abnormal FHR which suggest that fetal oxygenation was still satisfactory.

With Placenta Insufficiency (Malaria)

During a malaria crisis destruction of red blood cells and inflammatory processes probably affect the placental microcirculation and thus the fetal-maternal exchanges. The fetus triggers a flow redistribution in favor of the brain, most likely in response to hypoxia, but this redistribution disappears at the end of the crisis.

A 1994 study of fetal hemodynamic changes investigated cerebral and umbilical responses to short- and long-term malaria crises [8]. In the short crisis group (< 7 days) 61% of the fetuses were premature, 23% had abnormal FHR at delivery (several weeks later), C/U decreased by –8 ± 6%, and the mean HI was equal to –62 ± 54. In the long crisis group (> 7 days) 70% of the fetuses were premature, 70% had abnormal FHR at delivery (several weeks later), C/U decreased by –14 ± 6%, and the mean HI was equal to –187 ± 54. (Fig. 13.10).

A second similar study performed in 1996 in the same area and using the same protocol showed only a short crisis (< 7 days). In this group, 35% of the fetuses were premature, 17.5% had abnormal FHR at delivery (several weeks later), C/U decreased by –7 ± 4%, and the mean HI was equal to –49 ± 26. In both studies a HI > 150% was predictive of abnormal FHR at delivery with a sensitivity of 80% and specificity of 85%.

The HI allowed prediction of abnormal FHR at delivery several weeks in advance. Moreover, the lower amplitude of the hemodynamic response (lower HI) in the second group associated with a lower rate of abnormal FHR was likely related to an improvement in pregnancy recruitment and management or with the acquisition of an adapted immunity by the mother.

C/U Ratio in Non-Reversible Hypoxia (Pregnancy-Induced Hypertension) Prediction of Abnormal FHR at Delivery

In a study of fetal cerebral and umbilical flow adaptation in pregnancies complicated by hypertension, which included 82% with IUGR, the fetal hemodynamics were monitored every 2 days by Doppler over several days from admission until delivery [59]. As flow redistribution was identified at its early stage both the intensity and the duration of the flow redistribution period (hypoxic period) were considered for predicting the occurrence of abnormal FHR. By the end of the study the limit for the HI was 160%. Figure 13.12 shows a graphic representation of HI (area between the C/U curve and the C/U=1.1 cut-off line). This area represents the total oxygen deficit during the period of observation.

A HI higher than 160% was much more powerful (PPV: 87%; NPV: 88%) than the final URI, CRI, or C/U value measured for predicting abnormal FHR at delivery [URI (PPV: 63%; NPV: 74%) – CRI (PPV: 59%; NPV: 70%) – C/U (PPV: 57%; NPV: 92%)]. Moreover, as shown on Fig. 13.12, the C/U may change from one day to another; thus, a single Doppler measurement is not sufficient to identify the real hemodynamic stage induced by hypoxia. On the other hand, the HI increase is associated with an increase in the degree of fetal growth restriction as expressed in percentile. This suggests that the HI, by measuring the cumulated oxygen deficit during the observation period, also likely expresses the deficit in the nutrition supply responsible for the fetal growth restriction.

Finally, it should be noted that this study addressed high-risk pregnancy but not very poor fetal outcomes: 22% of all fetuses required intensive care assistance (but < 2 days and two-thirds of them < 33 weeks) and all survived in good health; only one fetus died at delivery. Thus, HI is a very early predictor of poor fetal outcome. In contrast, absent end-diastolic flow in the umbilical arteries was found in 9 cases (13% of the whole population), but all delivered before 33 weeks; all presented abnormal FHR; all were severely growth restricted (centile: 6+2); 8 (88%) delivered by Cesarean section; and 5 (56%) required intensive care assistance. These fetuses presented the lowest C/U ratio (0.7 ± 0.1) and umbilical cord pO_2 value at delivery (16 ± 6) and the highest HI values (387 ± 173%) in the population.

Fig. 13.12. Evolution of C/U reduction (in percentage from 1.1 cut-off value). The HI is represented as the area between the C/U (%) *bold curve* and the 0% *horizontal dotted line* (corresponding to C/U = 1.1). **a** IUGR fetus, delivered at 34 weeks, normal FHR, HI = 81% (approx.: mean C/U decrease of −5% × 17 days]. **b** IUGR fetus, delivered at 34 weeks, abnormal FHR, HI = 183% (approx.: mean C/U decrease of − 18% × 10 days). **c** Correlation between occurrence of abnormal FHR vs C/U ratio (C/U abnormal when >1.1 → PPV = 57%, NPV = 92%). **d** Correlation between occurrence of abnormal FHR vs hypoxic index. The HI is abnormal when >160% → PPV = 87%, NPV = 88%

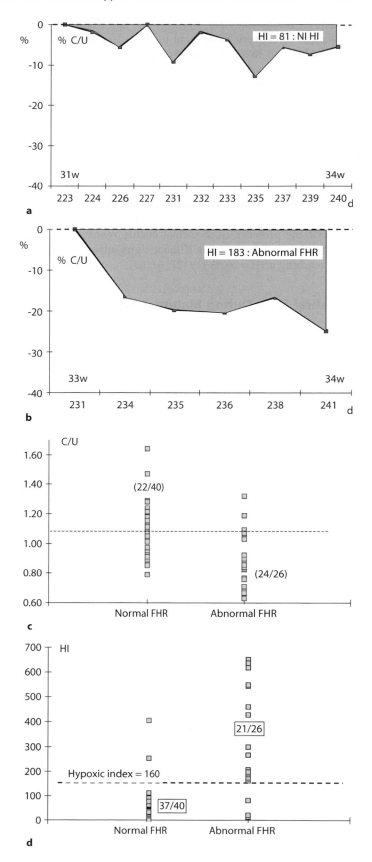

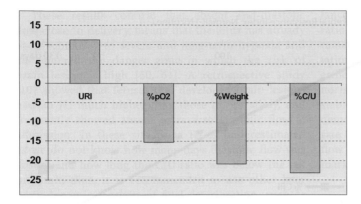

Fig. 13.15. Chronic cocaine administration. Fetal umbilical resistance (*URI*), cerebral resistance (CRI), cerebral–umbilical (*C/U*) ratio, fetal weight, and pO$_2$ (in the "70 mg/kg day^{-1}", and "140 mg/kg day^{-1}" cocaine groups), expressed in percentage of the control group value. Data collected at the end of the gestation (134 days). The C/U and pO$_2$ are significantly decreased (in parallel) in the cocaine groups (20–25% for C/U and 10–15% for pO$_2$). The C/U is decreased in response to the development of a chronic fetal hypoxia.

Cerebral–Umbilical Ratio and Mechanically Induced Hypoxia

Induced hypoxia (Fig. 13.16) in lamb fetuses has demonstrated a sensitive and rapid brain vasodilation. The fetal cerebral and umbilical flows were assessed by Doppler sensors implanted on the fetus during fetal hypoxia induced by umbilical cord compression, aortic compression, and drug injection [27, 35].

Umbilical cord compression ($n = 8$) decreases the venous return and the umbilical arterial flow, which induces hypoxia instantaneously and simulates fetal central hypovolemia. During a 10-min compression the cerebral vascular resistance decreased and the cerebral flow was maintained or only slightly decreased. Simultaneous recordings of the cerebral and umbilical Doppler waveforms together with the pO$_2$ showed that the C/U ratio decreased proportionately with the pO$_2$. The umbilical flow (Q$_p$) decreased together with the C/U (Fig. 13.16a,c). The pH and the heart rate remained normal. In the case of progressive cord compression (progressive changes of the umbilical resistance), the C/U closely followed the changes in fetal pO$_2$.

Aortic compression ($n = 8$) reduced the uterine flow and induced fetal hypoxia after about 30 s. After 1 min of compression, the heart rate dropped and the compression was interrupted. The heart rate recovered 30 s after the end of the compression. The pH did not change during the test and the umbilical flow remained stable; however, the umbilical resistance increased and the cerebral resistance decreased. As with umbilical cord compression, the C/U follows the variations of the fetal pO$_2$ (Fig. 13.16b).

Simultaneous measurements of the fetal pO$_2$ and the C/U during these compression tests showed a good correlation between the two parameters (Fig. 13.16c). Nevertheless, the amplitude of the C/U variations were higher during umbilical cord compression than during the aortic compression. In fact,

cord compression induces a central hypovolemia, which does not exist with aortic compression; therefore, one can speculate that during cord compression the C/U drop may be related to the hypoxia and the hypovolemia, which may stimulate the baroreflex.

Cerebral–Umbilical Ratio and Acute Drug Effect

Propranolol (4 μg/kg) was injected intravenously into pregnant ewes ($n = 3$), which were instrumented 24 h before (Fig. 13.3). The umbilical resistance increased and the cerebral resistance decreased beginning 1 min after injection leading to a significantly decreased C/U [27]. In this study, pO$_2$ was not measured but the fetal flow redistribution detected by C/U after each injection leads us to suspect that repeated injections of this drug may induce repeated hypoxic stresses for the fetus; hence, the beneficial effects of any drug (for the mother) and its deleterious effects (i.e., hypoxia) on the fetus must be evaluated before its use.

Conclusion

The objective of fetal Doppler is to detect at an early stage any hemodynamic changes that allow us to identify and quantify a placental dysfunction (with associated fetal malnutrition and low oxygenation). Fetal Doppler studies also allow us to determine the consequences of this abnormality on fetal growth and well-being.

The URI has been used to confirm the existence of placental hemodynamic disorders in the case of IUGR, but the sensitivity of this parameter for the follow-up of fetal growth remains at only 60%. Nevertheless, the absence of end-diastolic flow in the umbilical or aortic Doppler waveform is an indicator of severe fetal distress and neonatal cerebral complications [60, 64–70].

Fig. 13.16. a Umbilical cord compression. Variations in percentage from the pre-test value of the: Heart rate (*HR*), umbilical vascular resistances (*URI*), umbilical flow (*UBF*), cerebral–umbilical ratio (*C/U*), fetal pO$_2$, and cerebral flow (*CBF*) during a period of chord compression. The C/U decreases in proportion with the fetal pO$_2$ and the UBF, whereas CBF remains unchanged. **b** Aortic compression. Variations in percentage from the pre-test value of the HR, URI, UBF, C/U, fetal pO$_2$, and CBF during a period of chord compression. The C/U decreases in proportion with the fetal pO$_2$, whereas the UBF and CBF remain unchanged. **c** Relationship between absolute values of the C/U ratio and the pO$_2$ during induced hypoxia

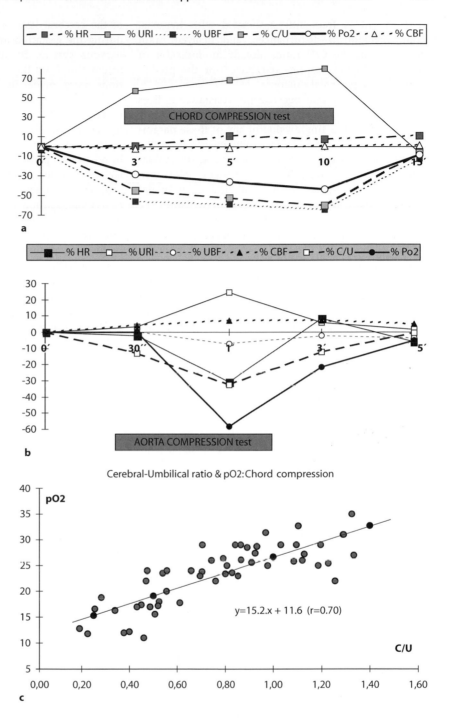

Cerebral flow changes in relation to hypoxia and fetal distress continues to be one of the most interesting areas of investigation. Even though many studies have already demonstrated positive correlations between cerebral Doppler data and fetal hypoxia or fetal well-being, it is too early to draw a conclusion as to how to use cerebral Doppler studies in routine practice for the management of fetal distress and for making the decision to interrupt a gestation.

The C/U, which measures the proportion of flow supplying the brain and the placenta, is now the most widely used parameter for the assessment of IUGR and hypoxia. Firstly, it takes into account the causes and consequences of the placental insufficiency responsible for IUGR and hypoxia. Secondly, it is not heart-rate dependent. Thirdly, it has a single cut-off value (C/U is normal if > 1.1), at least during the second half of the pregnancy. On the other hand, because IUGR is frequently associated with hypoxia, brain metabolism disturbances, and delayed brain development, the C/U ratio, already an indicator of IUGR, is also an accurate parameter for the prediction of poor perinatal outcome.

It is also clear that because the resistance indices are heart-rate dependent, it is hazardous to draw any conclusion from a single value of any of these parameters. Only several successive daily measures of the Doppler indices can lead to a more realistic evaluation of cerebral hemodynamic changes. Moreover, any significant increase in the umbilical index or decrease in the cerebral or C/U index, even within the normal range, must be considered pathological; however, in such cases the C/U ratio may approach the lowest normal limit (1.1) or pass into the abnormal range (<1.1).

On the other hand, the amplitude of C/U change was in the same range at any of the gestational ages investigated in cases of maternal anemia and hypertension. Such observations suggest that the capacity

of the cerebral vessels to vasodilate does not change during the gestation and thus is not mediated by the nervous system. It may be a biochemical reaction originating from the cerebral vessels. Similar observations were made in animal (fetal lamb: gestation 145 days) studies, the flow redistribution amplitude in response to a calibrated reduction in pO_2 being the same at 80 days or at 134 days (personal data).

In all the acute or chronic fetal hypoxic conditions in relation to placental insufficiency (i.e., anemia, malaria, hypertension) the C/U ratio was the most appropriate parameter to detect and quantify the fetal flow redistribution [3, 8, 70]. The assessment of the flow redistribution amplitude (C/U change) and the duration of the flow redistribution period allowed prediction of the consequences of the exposure to hypoxia (HI).

Finally, even though Doppler measurements increasingly help the obstetrician, the objectives for the near future must be (a) to test the true possibilities of Doppler indices in large randomized clinical stud-

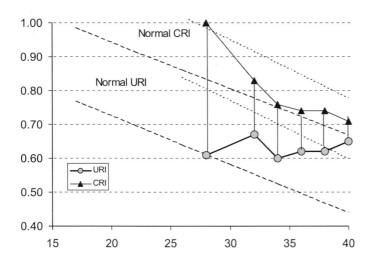

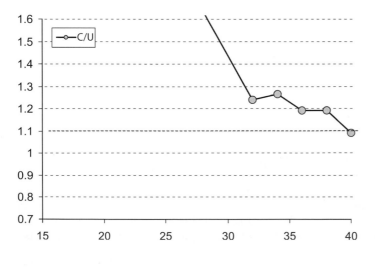

Fig. 13.17. a Evolution of the umbilical and the cerebral resistance indices during the early phase of development of moderate IUGR (normal delivery, fetal weight 10 centile). **b** Evolution of the C/U ratio. Note that the two resistance indices show large fluctuations even within or at the limit of their normal range; however, the C/U decreases regularly toward its cut-off line of normality (1.1)

ies, and (b) to point out the physiopathological phenomena responsible for fetal flow disturbances. For the latter aims, animal experimentation will be of great interest.

Figure 13.17 shows the evolution of URI and CRI in a pregnancy without evident complication but in which the fetal weight at term was at the tenth centile; however, the C/U ratio was at the limit of its normal range, demonstrating that even in the absence of any fetal or maternal clinical signs, the fetal circulation can change with consequent alterations in the oxygen and nutrient supply.

References

1. Cohn HE, Sacks EJ, Heymann MA, Rudolph AM (1974) Cardiovascular responses to hypoxemia and acidemia in fetal lambs. Am J Obstet Gynecol 120:817–824
2. Wladimiroff JW, van de Wijngaard JA, Degani S, Stewart PA (1987) Cerebral and umbilical arterial blood flow velocity waveform in normal and growth retarded pregnancies. Obstet Gynecol 69:705–709
3. Arbeille P, Maulik D, Laurini R (eds) (1999) Fetal hypoxia. Parthenon, London
4. Itskovitz J, LaGamma EF, Bristow J, Rudolph AM (1991) Cardiovascular responses to hypoxemia in sino-aortic-denervated fetal sheep. Pediatr Res 30:381–385
5. Fouron JC, Teyssier G, Maroto E, Lessart M, Marquette G (1991) Diastolic circulatory dynamics in the presence of elevated placental resistance and retrograde diastolic flow in the umbilical artery: Doppler echographic study in lambs. Am J Obstet Gynecol 164:195–203
6. Kjellmer I, Thordstein M, Wennergren M (1992) Cerebral function in the growth-retarded fetus and neonate. Biol Neonate 62:265–270
7. Arbeille Ph, Maulik D, Salihagic A, Locatelli A, Lansac J, Platt LD (1997) Effect of long term cocaine administration to pregnant ewes on the utero-placental flows, fetal pO$_2$, and growth. Obstet Gynecol 90:795–802
8. Arbeille P, Carles G, Tobal N, Herault S, Georgescus M, Bousquet F, Perrotin F (2002) Fetal flow redistribution to the brain in response to malaria infection. Does protection of the fetus against malaria develops across time. J Ultrasound Med 21:739–746
9. Laurini R, Arbeille B, Genberg C, Akoka S, Locatelli A, Lansac J, Arbeille P (1999) Brain damage and hypoxia in an ovine fetal chronic cocaine model. Eur J Obstet Gynecol Reprod Biol 86:15–22
10. Salihagic A, Georgescus M, Perrotin F, Laurini R, Arbeille B, Fignon A, Zudenogo D, Kurjak A, Arbeille P (2000) Daily Doppler assessment of the fetal hemodynamic response to chronic hypoxia: a five case report. Prenat Neonat Med 5:35–41
11. Lindsay H (1997) Pregnancy and iron deficiency. Nutr Rev 4:91–101
12. Steep P, Ash A, Wadsworth J, Welch A (1995) Relation between material haemoglobin concentration and birth weight in different ethnic group. Br Med J 310:489–491
13. Allen LH (2000) Anemia and iron deficiency effects on pregnancy outcome. Am J Clin Nutr Suppl 71:1280–1284
14. Colomer J, Colomer C, Gutierrez D, Jubert A, Nolasco A, Donat J, Fernandez-Delgado R, Donat F, Alvarez-Dardet C (1990) Anaemia during pregnancy as a risk factor for infant iron deficiency: report from the Valencia Infant Anaemia Cohort (VIAC) study. Paediatr Perinat Epidemiol 4:196–204
15. Ribbert LS, Snijders RJ, Nicolaides KH, Visser GH (1991) Relation of fetal blood gases and data from computer-assisted analysis of fetal heart rate patterns in small for gestation fetuses. Br J Obstet Gynaecol 98:820–823
16. Dawes GS, Moulden M, Redman CW (1996) Improvements in computerized fetal heart rate analysis antepartum. J Perinat Med 24:25–36
17. Lenstrup C, Haase N (1985) Predictive value of antepartum fetal heart rate non-stress test in high risk pregnancy. Acta Obstet Gynecol Scand 64:133–138
18. Weiner Z, Farmakides G, Schulman H, Lopresti S, Schneider E (1996) Surveillance of growth-retarded fetuses with computerized fetal heart rate monitoring combined with Doppler velocimetry of the umbilical and uterine arteries. J Reprod Med 41:112–118
19. Hecher K, Bilardo CM, Stigter RH, Ville Y, Hackeloer BJ, Kok HJ, Senat MV, Visser GH (2001) Monitoring of fetuses with intrauterine growth restriction: a longitudinal study. Ultrasound Obstet Gynecol 18:564–570
20. Baschat A, Gembruch U, Harman CR (2001) The sequence of changes in Doppler and biophysical parameters as severe fetal growth restriction worsens. Ultrasound Obstet Gynecol 18:571–577
21. Ferrazzi E, Bozzo M, Rigano S, Bellotti M, Morabito A, Pardi G, Battaglia FC, Galan HL (2002) Temporal sequence of abnormal Doppler changes in the peripheral and central circulatory systems of the severely growth-restricted fetus. Ultrasound Obstet Gynecol 19:140–146
22. Arbeille P, Tranquart F, Body G (1986) Evolution de la circulation artérielle ombilicale et cérébrale du foetus au cours de la grossesse. Progrès en néonatologie. Karger Edit 6:30–37
23. Arbeille P, Roncin A, Berson M (1987) Exploration of the fetal cerebral blood flow by Doppler ultrasound in normal and pathological pregnancies. Ultrasound Med Biol 13:329–333
24. Woo JSK, Liang ST, Lo RLS, Chang FY (1987) Middle cerebral artery Doppler flow velocity waveform. Obstet Gynecol 70:613–616
25. Wladimiroff JW, Tonge HM, Stewart PA (1986) Doppler ultrasound assessment of cerebral blood flow in the human fetus. Br J Obstet Gynaecol 93:471–475
26. Arbeille P, Montenegro N, Tranquart F, Berson M (1990) Assessment of the fetal cerebrovascular areas by color coded Doppler. J Echocardiogr 7:629–634
27. Arbeille P, Berson M, Maulik D, Bodard S, Locatelli A (1992) New implanted Doppler sensors for the assessment of the main fetal hemodynamics. Ultrasound Med Biol 18:97–103
28. Arbeille P, Bosc M, Vaillant M, Bodart S (1992) Nicotine-induced changes in cerebral circulation in ovine fetuses. Am J Perinatol 9:268–272
29. Adamson SL, Morrow RJ, Languille BL (1990) Side dependent effects of increases in placental vascular resistance on the umbilical arterial velocity waveform in fetal sheep. Ultrasound Med Biol 6:19–27
30. Maulik D, Yarlagada P, Nathanielsz LP (1989) Hemodynamic validation of Doppler assessment of fetoplacental

circulation in a sheep model system. J Ultrasound Med 8:177

31. Maulik D, Arbeille P, Kadado T (1992) Hemodynamic foundation of umbilical arterial Doppler waveform analysis. Biol Neonate 62:280–289

32. Gosling RG (1976) Extraction of physiological information from spectrum analysed Doppler-shifted continuous ultrasound signals obtained non-invasively from the arterial tree. In: Hull DW, Watson BW (eds) IEE medical electronics monographs (13–22). Peregranns, London, pp 73–125

33. Pourcelot L (1974) Applications cliniques de l'eamen Doppler transcutané vélocimétrie ultrasonore Doppler. Semin INSERM 34:213–240

34. Stuart B, Drumm J, Fitzgerald DE, Duignan NM (1980) Fetal blood velocity waveforms in normal pregnancies. Br J Obstet Gynaecol 87:780–785

35. Arbeille P, Maulik D, Fignon A, Stale H, Berson M, Bodard S, Locatelli A (1995) Assessment of the fetal pO_2 changes by cerebral and umbilical Doppler on lamb fetuses during acute hypoxia. Ultrasound Med Biol 21:861–870

36. Bonnin P, Guyot O, Blot P (1992) Relationship between umbilical and fetal cerebral flow velocity waveforms and umbilical venous blood gases. Ultrasound Obstet Gynecol 2:18–22

37. Brar HS, Horenstein J, Medearis AL, Platt LD, Phelan JP, Paul JH (1989) Cerebral, umbilical and uterine resistance using Doppler velocimetry in postterm pregnancy. J Ultrasound Med 8:187–191

38. Gramellini D, Folli MC, Raboni S, Vadora E, Merialdi A (1992) Cerebral–Umbilical Doppler ratio as a predictor of adverse perinatal outcome. Obstet Gynecol 79:416–420

39. Bahado-Singh RO, Kovanci E, Jeffres A, Oz U, Deren O, Copel J, Mari G (1999) The Doppler cerebro-placental ratio and perinatal outcome in intrauterine growth restriction. Am J Obstet Gynecol 180:750–756

40. Groome LJ, Watson JE (1992) Assessment of in utero neurobehavioral development. J Matern Fetal Invest 2:183–194

41. van Eyck J, Wladimiroff J, Van den Wijngaard J, Noordam M, Prechtl H (1987) The blood flow velocity waveform in the fetal internal carotid and umbilical artery: its relationship to fetal behavioral states in normal pregnancy. Br J Obstet Gynaecol 94:736

42. Maršál K, Lindblad A, Lingman G, Eik-Nes S (1984) Blood flow on the fetal descending aorta: intrinsic factors affecting fetal flow, i.e fetal breathing movements and cardiac arrhythmia. Ultrasound Med Biol 10:330

43. van der Mooren K, van Eyck J, Wladimiroff J (1989) Human fetal ductal flow velocity waveforms relative to behavioral states in normal pregnancy. Am J Obstet Gynecol 160:371–374

44. Archer L, Levene MI, Evans DH (1986) Cerebral artery Doppler ultrasonography and prediction of outcome after perinatal asphyxia. Lancet 2:1116–1118

45. Bilardo CM, Nicolaides KH, Campbell S (1990) Doppler measurements of fetal and uteroplacental circulations: relationship with umbilical venous blood gases measured at cordocentesis. Am J Obstet Gynecol 162:115–120

46. Rizzo G, Arduini D, Luciano R et al. (1989) Prenatal cerebral Doppler ultrasonography and neonatal neurologic outcome. J Ultrasound Med 8:237–240

47. Gaziano E, Gaziano C, Brandt D (1998) Doppler velocimetry determined redistribution of fetal blood flow: correlation with growth restriction in diamniotic monochorionic and dizygotic twins. Am J Obstet Gynecol 178:1359–1367

48. Arbeille P, Henrion C, Paillet C (1988) Hemodynamique cerebrale et placentaire dans les grossesses gemellaires. Progrès en néonatologie. Karger Edit 7:223–229

49. Arbeille P, Maulik D, Stree JL, Fignon A, Amyel C, Deufel M (1994) Fetal renal and cerebral Doppler in small for gestational age fetuses in hypertensive pregnancies. Eur J Obstet Gynecol Reprod Biol 56:111–116

50. Carles G, Tobal N, Raynal P, Herault S, Beucher G, Marret H, Arbeille P (2003) Doppler assessment of the fetal cerebral hemodynamic response to moderate or severe maternal anemia. Am J Obstet Gynecol 188:794–799

51. Arduini D, Rizzo G, Romanini C, Mancuso S (1989) Hemodynamic changes in growth retarded fetuses during maternal oxygen administration as predictors of fetal outcome. J Ultrasound Med 8:193–196

52. Edelstone DI, Peticca BB, Goldblum LJ (1985) Effects of maternal oxygen administration on fetal oxygenation during reductions in umbilical blood flow in fetal lambs. Am J Obstet Gynecol 152:351–358

53. Mori A, Iwashita M, Nakabyashi M, Takeda Y (1992) Effect of maternal oxygen inhalation on fetal hemodynamics in chronic hypoxia with IUGR. J Matern Fetal Invest 2:93–99

54. Nicolaides KH, Bradley RJ, Soothill PW et al. (1987) Maternal oxygen therapy for intrauterine growth retardation. Lancet 1:942

55. Veille JC, Penry M (1992) Effect of maternal administration of 3% carbon dioxide on umbilical artery and fetal renal and middle cerebral artery Doppler waveforms. Am J Obstet Gynecol 167:1668–1671

56. Texeira JMA, Duncan K, Letsky E, Fisk NM (2000) Middle cerebral artery peak systolic velocity in the prediction of fetal anemia. Ultrasound Obstet Gynecol 15:205–208

57. Mari G, Moise KJ, Deter RL, Kirshon B, Stefos T, Carpenter RJ Jr (1990) Flow velocity waveforms of the vascular system in the anemic fetus before and after intravascular transfusion for severe red cell alloimmunization. Am J Obstet Gynecol 162:1060–1064

58. Vyas S, Nicolaides KH, Campbell S (1990) Doppler examination of the middle cerebral artery in anemic fetuses. Am J Obstet Gynecol 162:1060–1064

59. Arbeille P, Perrotin F, Salihagic A, Stale H, Lansac J, Platt LD (2004) Fetal Doppler hypoxic index for the prediction of abnormal fetal heart rate at delivery in chronic fetal distress. Eur J Obstet Gynecol Reprod Biol

60. Brar HS, Platt LD (1988) Reverse end-diastolic flow on umbilical artery velocimetry in high-risk pregnancies: an ominous finding with adverse pregnancy outcome. Am J Obstet Gynecol 159:559–561

61. Fleischer A, Schulmann M, Farmakides G (1995) Umbilical artery velocity waveform and intrauterine growth retardation. Am J Obstet Gynecol 151:502–505

62. Hofstaetter C, Gudmundsson S, Dubiel M, Maršál K (1996) Ductus venosus velocimetry in high-risk pregnancies. Eur J Obstet Gynecol Reprod Biol 70:135–140

63. Kiserud T (2000) Fetal venous circulation: an update on hemodynamics. J Perinatol Med 28:90–96

64. Arbeille P, Asquier E, Moxhon E, Berson M, Pourcelot L (1983) Nouvelle technique dans la surveillance de la grossesse: l'étude de la circulation foetale et placentaire pour les ultrasons. J Gynécol Obst Biol Reprod 12:851–859

65. Divon MY, Girz BA, Lieblich R, Langer O (1989) Clinical management of the fetus with markedly diminished umbilical artery end-diastolic flow. Am J Obstet Gynecol 161:1523–1527

66. Nicolaides KH, Bilardo CM, Soothill PW, Campbell S (1988) Absence of end diastolic frequencies in umbilical artery: a sign of fetal hypoxia and acidosis. Br Med J 297:1026–1027

67. Rochelson B, Schulman H, Farmakides G et al. (1987) The significance of absent end-diastolic velocity in umbilical artery velocity waveforms. Am J Obstet Gynecol 156:1213–1218

68. Schulman H, Fleischer A, Stern W, Farmakides G, Jagani N, Blattner P (1984) Umbilical velocity wave ratios in human pregnancy. Am J Obstet Gynecol 148:985–990

69. Trudinger B, Giles W, Cook C, Connelly A (1985) Fetal umbilical artery flow waveforms and placental resistance: clinical significance. Br J Obstet Gynaecol 92:20–23

70. Arbeille P, Leguyader P, Fignon A, Locatelli A, Maulik D (1994) Fetal hemodynamics and flow velocity indices. In: Copel JA, Reed KL (eds) Doppler ultrasound in obstetrics and gynecology. Raven Press, New York, pp 19–29

Chapter 14

Cerebral Blood Flow Velocity Waveforms: Clinical Application

Laura Detti, Maria Segata, Giancarlo Mari

This chapter reviews the clinical application of Doppler ultrasound velocimetry of the cerebral blood flow in the fetus. There are two main clinical applications of the fetal Doppler cerebral blood flow velocity waveforms:

1. Intrauterine growth restriction (IUGR) pregnancies
2. Diagnosis of fetal anemia

Which Is the Cerebral Vessel to Assess in the Fetus?

The circle of Willis is composed anteriorly of the anterior cerebral arteries (branches of the internal carotid artery that are interconnected by the anterior communicating artery) and posteriorly of the two posterior cerebral arteries (which are branches of the basilar artery and are interconnected on either side with the internal carotid artery by the posterior communicating artery). These two trunks and the middle cerebral artery (MCA), another branch of the internal carotid artery, supply the cerebral hemispheres on each side. These arteries have different flow velocity waveforms (FVWs) [1, 2] and, therefore, it is important to know which artery is being studied (Fig. 14.1). The MCA is the vessel of choice to assess the fetal cerebral circulation because it is easy to identify, has a high reproducibility, and provides in-

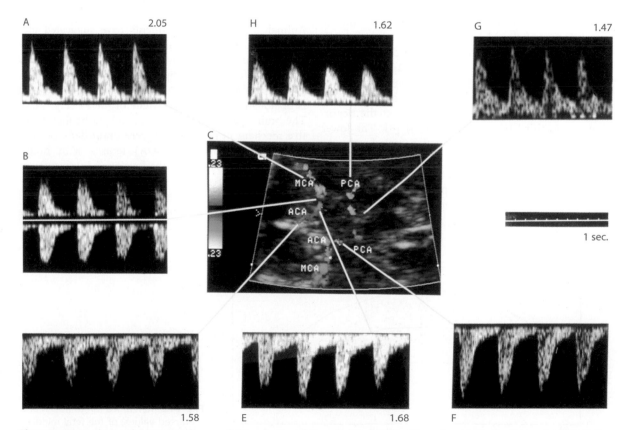

Fig. 14.1 A–H. Flow velocity waveforms of the arteries of the circle of Willis. The values indicate the pulsatility index. (From [2])

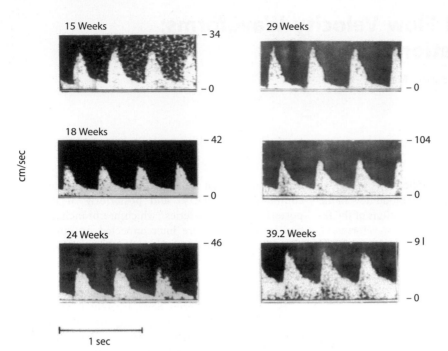

Fig. 14.2. Flow velocity waveforms of the middle cerebral artery in appropriate-for-gestational-age (AGA) fetuses at different gestational ages. (From [4])

formation on the brain-sparing effect [3, 4]. Additionally, it can be studied easily with an angle of zero degrees between the ultrasound beam and the direction of blood flow and, therefore, information on the true velocity of the blood flow can be obtained [5]. Flow velocity waveforms of the middle cerebral artery change with advancing gestation (Fig. 14.2). The pulsatility index (PI) of the MCA is lower between 15 and 20 weeks' gestation, whereas it has a higher value at the end of the second trimester and at the beginning of the third trimester (Fig. 14.3) [3]. The lower PI values early and late in gestation may be due to the increased metabolic requirements of the brain in these two periods of gestation [6].

Middle cerebral artery peak systolic velocity (MCA-PSV) increases exponentially with advancing gestation (Fig. 14.4) [5].

Cerebral Blood Flow Velocity Waveforms in the IUGR Fetus

Animal and human experiments have suggested that in the IUGR fetus there is an increase of blood flow to the brain [3, 4, 7–10]. This increase of blood flow can be evidenced by Doppler ultrasound of the MCA [3]. This effect is called the brain-sparing effect and is demonstrated by a lower value of the PI (Fig. 14.5). The brain-sparing effect appears to be a benign adaptive mechanism preventing severe brain damage [11]. Small-for-gestational-age (SGA) fetuses with brain-sparing effect less frequently developed intraventricular hemorrhage (IVH) than appropriate-for-gestational-age (AGA) premature fetuses with normal pulsatility index value of the MCA [12]. Following

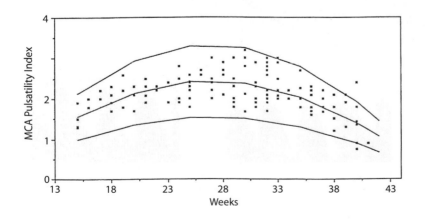

Fig. 14.3. Reference range (mean and predicted values) of the fetal middle cerebral artery pulsatility index with advancing gestation. (From [4])

Fig. 14.4. Reference range of the fetal middle cerebral artery (*MCA*) peak systolic velocity during gestation. (From [5])

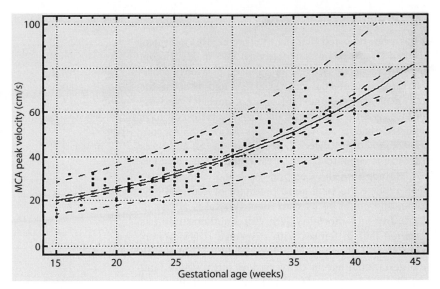

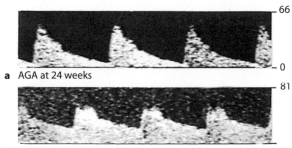

a AGA at 24 weeks

b IUGR fetus at 24 weeks

Fig. 14.5. Flow velocity waveform of the MCA obtained in AGA (**a**) and IUGR fetuses studied at the same gestational age (**b**)

35 weeks' gestation a low PI is physiologically present in the AGA fetus (unpublished data). In IUGR fetuses with a PI below the normal range there is a greater incidence of adverse perinatal outcome [3]. It has also been reported that in SGA fetuses with normal umbilical artery PI and abnormal MCA there is an increased risk of developing distress and being delivered by emergency cesarean delivery. The risk is increased by the presence of abnormal maternal uterine arteries [13]. The brain-sparing effect may be transient, as reported during prolonged hypoxemia in animal experiments, and the overstressed human fetus can also lose the brain-sparing effect [8]. It has been reported that the MCA PI is below the normal range when the pO_2 is reduced [14]. Maximum reduction in PI is reached when the fetal pO_2 is 2–4 SD below normal for gestation. When the oxygen deficit is greater there is a tendency for the PI to rise, this presumably reflects the development of brain edema.

In IUGR fetuses, the disappearance of the brain-sparing effect is a very critical event for the fetus, and appears to precede fetal death [15–17]. This has been confirmed in a few fetuses in situations where obstetrical interventions were refused by the parents. Unfortunately, to demonstrate this concept, it is necessary to perform a longitudinal study on severely IUGR fetuses up to the point of fetal demise; therefore, presently we cannot rely on the disappearance of the brain-sparing effect for timing the delivery. It is noted that reversed flow of the MCA velocity waveforms, although it has been reported in pathological situations [16, 18–20], can be observed in the normal fetus and appears to be a consequence of head compression in normal pregnancies (Fig. 14.6) [21]. A number of longitudinal studies have assessed several fetal vessels with Doppler ultrasonography and have reported that the cerebral circulation is one of the first blood flows to become abnormal in IUGR [22–25].

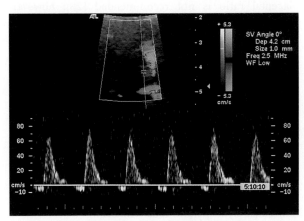

Fig. 14.6. Flow velocity waveforms of the MCA in an AGA fetus. The reversed flow is due to head compression

Cerebral–Placental Ratio

It has been reported that the internal carotid/umbilical artery PI ratio has a sensitivity of 70% in identifying growth-restricted fetuses, as opposed to a 60% sensitivity for the internal carotid artery and 48% for the umbilical artery alone [26]. Others have selected the middle cerebral artery/umbilical artery ratio and have reported that in AGA fetuses this ratio remains constant following 30 weeks' gestation. In AGA fetuses the ratio is equal to 1 [27]. A ratio above 1 is considered pathological. The Cerebral–Placental ratio has also been reported to be a good predictor of neonatal outcome, and could be used to identify fetuses at risk of morbidity and mortality [28, 29]. Another study has reported that in fetuses with suspected IUGR, abnormal Cerebral–Placental ratio is strongly associated with low gestational age at delivery, low birth weight, and low umbilical artery pH. Abnormal Cerebral–Placental ratio is also significantly associated with a shorter interval to delivery and the need for emergent delivery [30]. A question that arises is: Does the Cerebral–Placental ratio make any difference when compared with the umbilical artery? The answer is that the ratio is useful on those conditions characterized by a borderline umbilical artery. If there is absent/reversed flow of the umbilical artery, the ratio is not helpful.

What to Do in Presence of an Abnormal Cerebral–Placental Ratio?

The management of a pregnancy in the presence of an abnormal cerebral–placental ratio depends on the gestational age. Prior to 34 weeks, steroids and close monitoring with non-stress test (NST) and biophysical profile (BPP) twice a week, and assessment of fetal growth every 2 weeks, is a good management option. Following 34 weeks' gestation the cerebral–placental ratio does not appear very helpful and, therefore, a clinical decision based on the results of the cerebral–placental ratio is not recommended [28]; however, others have reported that cerebral–placental ratio continues to be useful [31, 32]; therefore, this requires further investigations.

Finally, maternal hyperoxygenation could improve fetal hemodynamics in IUGR fetuses [33].

Prediction of Fetal Hematocrit

Fetal hemoglobin increases with advancing gestation (Table 14.1) [34]. Fetal anemia is categorized as mild, moderate, or severe, based on the degree of deviation from the median for gestational age. Severe anemia may cause hydrops and fetal demise.

There are many causes of fetal anemia (Table 14.2), the most common being red cell alloimmunization in

Table 14.1. Increase of fetal hemoglobin with advancing gestation

Weeks	Mean	95	5	0.55 MoM	0.65 MoM
18	10.6	11.8	9.4	5.8	6.9
19	10.9	12.2	9.6	6.0	7.1
20	11.1	12.5	9.8	6.1	7.2
21	11.4	12.8	9.9	6.2	7.4
22	11.6	13.0	10.1	6.4	7.5
23	11.8	13.3	10.2	6.5	7.6
24	12.0	13.6	10.3	6.6	7.8
25	12.1	13.8	10.4	6.7	7.9
26	12.3	14.0	10.5	6.8	8.0
27	12.4	14.3	10.6	6.8	8.1
28	12.6	14.5	10.7	6.9	8.2
29	12.7	14.7	10.7	7.0	8.3
30	12.8	14.9	10.8	7.1	8.3
31	13.0	15.1	10.8	7.1	8.4
32	13.1	15.3	10.9	7.2	8.5
33	13.2	15.5	10.9	7.2	8.6
34	13.3	15.7	10.9	7.3	8.6
35	13.4	15.8	10.9	7.4	8.7
36	13.5	16.0	10.9	7.4	8.7
37	13.5	16.2	10.9	7.5	8.8
38	13.6	16.4	10.9	7.5	8.9
39	13.7	16.5	10.9	7.5	8.9
40	13.8	16.7	10.9	7.6	9.0

Table 14.2. Causes of fetal anemia

Red cell alloimmunization
Alpha-thalassemia
Enzyme disorder
  Pyruvate kinase deficiency
  Glucose phosphate isomerase deficiency
  G6PD deficiency
Kasabach-Merritt sequence
Fetomaternal hemorrhage
Intracranial hemorrhage
Parvovirus B19 infection
Twin-to-twin transfusion
Blackfan-Diamond syndrome
Transient myeloproliferative disorder
Congenital leukemia

the United States. The primary cause of red cell alloimmunization is maternal sensitization to D antigen of the rhesus blood group system; however, many other antigens, the so-called irregular antigens, may be responsible for maternal sensitization. Prophylaxis with rhesus immunoglobulins has decreased the incidence of Rh-hemolytic disease; however, this phenomenon is still present.

Several other conditions can lead to fetal anemia. Hematological disorders can lead to fetal anemia and they are implicated in approximately 10–27% of cases of nonimmune hydrops [35–37]. Fetal anemia may also result from excessive erythrocyte loss by hemolysis or hemorrhage, or erythrocyte underproduction [36].

In Southeast Asia homozygous alpha-thalassemia-1 (hemoglobin Bart's) is the most common cause of fetal hydrops, accounting for 60–90% of cases [38]. This condition, however, has become more frequent in Canada and in North America due to an increased number of immigrants from Southeast Asia [39, 40].

Massive fetomaternal hemorrhage, defined as loss of more than 150 ml, is a rare condition that may result in severe fetal anemia with or without hydrops, and fetal death [41–43]. Red blood cell enzymopathies, such as autosomal-recessive inherited deficiencies of pyruvate kinase and glucose phosphate isomerase, and G6PD deficiency, are rare conditions that may cause fetal anemia and hydrops [36, 44–46].

Parvovirus infection can lead to severe fetal anemia and consequently hydrops because of virus tropism for immature erythrocytes in the bone marrow or fetal liver [47]. Conditions such as large placental chorioangioma, twin–twin transfusion syndrome, transient myeloproliferative disorder, congenital leukemia, intracranial hemorrhage, and Blackfan-Diamond syndrome, may also cause fetal anemia [48–50].

Noninvasive diagnosis of fetal anemia has been the goal of many investigators for more than 20 years. The pulsatility index of fetal cerebral vessels does not have good parameters to diagnose fetal anemia [51]. The PI of the cerebral arteries can become abnormal when the hematocrit is close to 10%. In such a condition, the pulsatility index of the middle cerebral artery decreases, suggesting hypoxemia in the severely anemic fetus. The MCA PI in 101 cases of fetal anemia was below 2 SD in 7 anemic fetuses (unpublished data). In these fetuses the hematocrit was <15%.

When the anemia is severe, there is an increase of blood flow to the brain, which is reflected by a low MCA PI; however, this phenomenon is not always present and it allows recognition of only a small number of anemic fetuses. The assessment of the MCA plays the most important role in the noninvasive diagnosis of fetal anemia [5, 34].

Red Cell Alloimmunization and MCA Peak Systolic Velocity

Amniocentesis and cordocentesis are invasive tools for diagnosis and management of fetal anemia due to red cell alloimmunization. They are associated with significant complications. Both invasive procedures could worsen maternal alloimmunization due to secondary fetal hemorrhage. It has been reported that more than 70% of fetuses that underwent invasive procedures, because they were defined as severely anemic based on traditional criteria, were found to be either non-anemic or mildly anemic [34]. The use of MCA-PSV could have detected all the cases of significant fetal anemia requiring transfusion and would have avoided approximately 70% of the unnecessary invasive procedures [34].

In a multicenter study, the sensitivity of MCA-PSV for prediction of moderate and severe anemia prior to the first cordocentesis was 100%, with false-positive rates of 12% at 1.50 multiples of the median (Fig. 14.7) [34].

Other robust data for the use of MCA-PSV have been reported in a multicenter trial with intention to treat. In this study, the authors monitored pregnancies complicated by red cell alloimmunization by studying MCA-PSV longitudinally. The MCA-PSV was used for timing cordocentesis [52]. This prospective

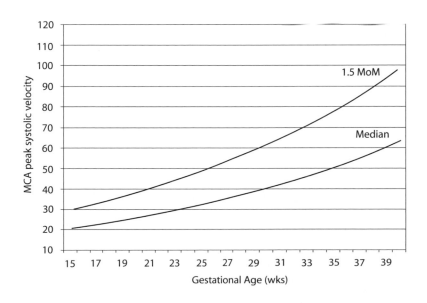

Fig. 14.7. Middle cerebral artery peak systolic velocity values used for detection of anemia. Fetuses with a MCA-PSV value above 1.5 multiples of the median are likely to be anemic. (From [34])

study confirmed that MCA-PSV is an accurate method of monitoring pregnancies complicated by red cell antibodies. In this study two anemic fetuses were missed in a group of 125 fetuses at risk of anemia. The interval between the last assessment of MCA-PSV and the delivery in those two fetuses was 3.5 and 2.5 weeks. This suggested that a closer assessment of MCA-PSV is necessary. This study also demonstrated that the number of false positives increased following 35 weeks' gestation. A recent prospective study compared MCA-PSV with Delta OD 450 in the prediction of moderately and severely anemic fetuses [53]. The authors concluded that both procedures are useful in the prediction of fetal anemia, but Doppler ultrasound assessment remains a method that has the advantage of being less expensive and noninvasive than amniocentesis. The MCA-PSV represents a more suitable tool in the diagnosis and management of pregnancy complicated by alloimmunizations than Delta OD 450 [24, 54, 55].

The MCA-PSV performed prior to the first transfusion has been used to estimate the real value of fetal hemoglobin [56]. The difference between the observed and calculated hemoglobin was lower in fetuses that exhibited moderate to severe anemia compared with cases when the fetus was mildly anemic (Fig. 14.8); therefore, MCA-PSV performs better in cases of clinically significant anemia. The explanation is that initial small decreases in fetal hemoglobin only slightly change cardiac output and blood viscosity. When the anemia becomes more severe, these compensatory

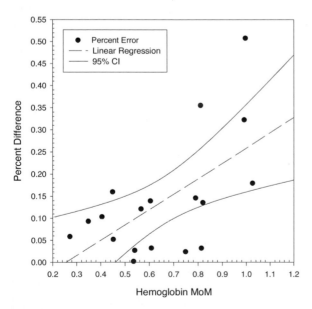

Fig. 14.8. Quadratic function expressing the correlation of percentage difference between the predicted and the actual hemoglobin value and the hemoglobin multiples of the median. (From [56]) $Y = 0.2876 - 0.922 \times 0.9498 \times 2$

mechanisms operate more to maintain the oxygen and metabolic equilibrium in the various organs.

Intrauterine transfusion decreases fetal anemia significantly and normalizes the value of fetal MCA-PSV (Figs. 14.9, 14.10) due to an increased blood viscosity and an increased oxygen concentration in fetal blood [57]. The MCA-PSV may also be used for timing the second fetal transfusion and the cut-off point to detect severe anemia is higher than that used for never-transfused fetuses [58]. This is probably the consequence of the different blood viscosity of the adult blood when compared with the fetal blood.

Several other studies have confirmed the utility of MCA-PSV for diagnosing fetal anemia [59–62]. This parameter may also diagnose fetal anemia in dichorionic twin pregnancies complicated by red blood cell alloimmunization [63].

The above studies have used only one value of MCA-PSV, which indicates whether the fetus is anemic or not at the time of the evaluation; however, it does not predict whether the fetus will become anemic. In a longitudinal study, it has been shown that the MCA slope is an excellent tool for identifying those fetuses that will become severely anemic and, therefore, need to be followed up more closely during the pregnancy (Fig. 14.11) [64]. The same author suggested the following protocol for monitoring pregnancies at risk for fetal anemia due to red cell alloimmunization [65]:

1. MCA-PSV should be performed in fetuses at risk of fetal anemia on a weekly basis for three consecutive weeks.
2. Cordocentesis is indicated when the MCA-PSV value is over 1.5 MoM.
3. If the MCA-PSV remains below 1.5 MoM a regression line has to be obtained from the following three values.

If the plotted regression line is to the right of the dotted line shown in Fig. 14.11, the examination has to be repeated every 2 or 4 weeks based on the initial risk of the patient – with a lower initial risk (e.g., a Coombs titer between 1:16 and 1:32) the examination can be repeated every 4 weeks, but with a higher initial risk it should be repeated every 2 weeks. If the plotted regression line is between the dotted and the thin line (Fig. 14.11), the examination has to be repeated every 1–2 weeks based on the initial risk to the patient. If the plotted regression line is to the left of the thin line and the MCA-PSV value is below 1.50 MoM, the examination has to be repeated in 1 week. Figure 14.12 represents the algorithm we use for the management of pregnancies at risk of fetal anemia because of red cell alloimmunization.

Centers with minimal experience with the assessment of MCA-PSV should initially perform these

Fig. 14.9. Middle cerebral artery peak systolic velocity before and after transfusion in a group of fetuses never transfused. The values are compared to the reference range for gestational age. (From [57])

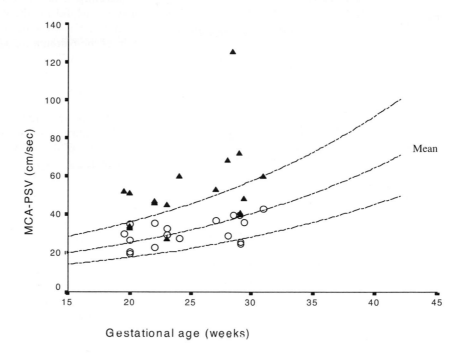

Fig. 14.10. Middle cerebral artery peak systolic velocity before and after transfusion in a group of fetuses previously transfused. (From [57])

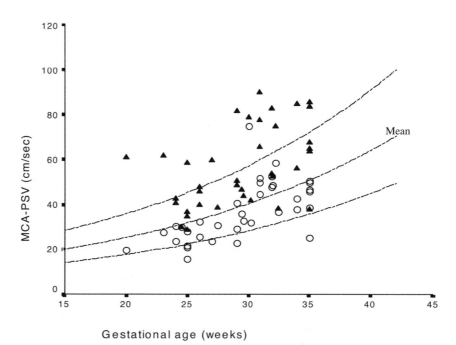

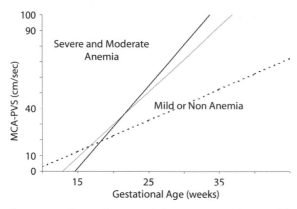

Fig. 14.11. Slopes for normal fetuses (*dotted line*), mildly anemic fetuses (*thin line*), and severely anemic fetuses (*thick line*). (From [64])

measurements in conjunction with serial amniocentesis for Delta OD 450 because of the learning curve associated with performing MCA Doppler [66].

Alloimmunization is also discussed in Chap. 22.

MCA-PSV in Other Causes of Fetal Anemia

Delle Chiaie et al. [59] found an inverse correlation between MCA-PSV measurements and hemoglobin values in fetuses at risk for fetal anemia due to red cell alloimmunization and fetal parvovirus infection. In a longitudinal multicenter study on fetuses at risk for anemia resulting from parvovirus infection, the measurement of MCA-PSV predicted fetal anemia with a sensitivity of 94.1%. All cases with moderate and severe anemia were detected either by MCA-PSV alone or in combination with real-time ultrasonography [67].

MCA-PSV may also be a useful test in cases of severely anemic fetuses due to fetomaternal hemorrhages [43]. An increased peak blood flow velocity has been reported in cases of acute severe fetomaternal hemorrhage [68].

Recently, it has also been reported that MCA-PSV may be helpful for the diagnosis of anemia in twin–twin transfusion syndrome following laser coagulation of the placental vessels [69].

The MCA-PSV appears to be the best test for the noninvasive diagnosis of fetal anemia. It is important to emphasize that training sonographers and sonologists is the "conditio sine qua non" for the correct sampling of MCA-PSV.

The following steps are necessary for the correct assessment of the MCA.

1. The fetus needs to be in a period of rest (no breathing or movements).
2. The circle of Willis is imaged with color Doppler.
3. The sonographer zooms the area of the MCA so that it occupies more than 50% of the screen. The MCA should be visualized for its entire length (Fig. 14.13).
4. The sample volume (1 mm) is placed soon after the origin of the MCA from the internal carotid artery (1–2 mm).
5. The angle between the direction of blood flow and the ultrasound beam is as close as possible to zero degrees. The angle corrector should not be used.
6. The waveforms (between 15 and 30) should be similar to each other. The highest PSV is measured (Fig. 14.14).
7. Repeat the above steps at least three times.

The MCA distal to the transducer can be an alternative to the MCA proximal to the transducer [70]; however, the latter is preferable because it has the lowest intra- and interobserver variability [71].

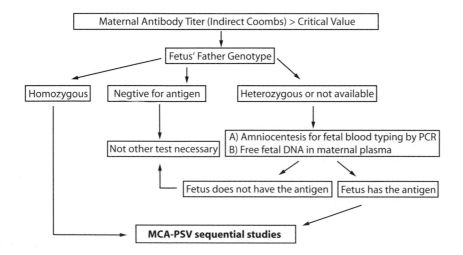

Fig. 14.12. Management algorithm in pregnancies at risk of having an anemic fetus because of red cell alloimmunization

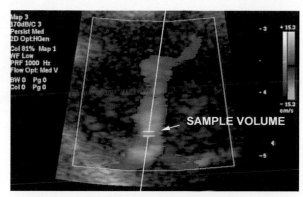

Fig. 14.13. Middle cerebral artery imaged by color Doppler. The sample volume is positioned soon after the origin of the MCA from the internal carotid artery (*arrow*). Note the angle between the ultrasound beam and the direction of the blood flow

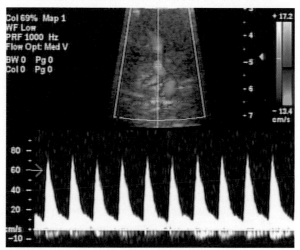

Fig. 14.14. Flow velocity waveforms of the MCA in a fetus that underwent cordocentesis following this study. MCA-PSV was above 1.50 MoM (*arrow*). The hematocrit was 26%

References

1. Mari G, Moise KJ Jr, Deter RL et al. (1989) Doppler assessment of the pulsatility index in the cerebral circulation of the human fetus. Am J Obstet Gynecol 160:698–703

2. Mari G (1994) Regional cerebral flow velocity waveforms in the human fetus. J Ultrasound Med 13:343–346

3. Woo JK, Liang ST, Lo RS, Chan FY (1987) Middle cerebral artery Doppler flow velocity waveforms. Obstet Gynecol 70:613–616

4. Mari G, Deter RL (1992) Middle cerebral artery flow velocity waveforms in normal and small-for-gestational-age fetuses. Am J Obstet Gynecol 166:1262–1270

5. Mari G, Adrignolo A, Abuhamad AZ, Pirhonen J, Jones DC, Ludomirsky A, Copel JA (1995) Diagnosis of fetal anemia with Doppler ultrasound in the pregnancy complicated by maternal blood group immunization. Ultrasound Obstet Gynecol 5:400–405

6. Dobbing J, Sands J (1970) Timing of neuroblast multiplication in developing human brain. Nature 226:639–640

7. Cohn HE, Sacks EJ, Heymann MA, Rudolph AM (1974) Cardiovascular responses to hypoxemia and academia in fetal lambs. Am J Obstet Gynecol 120:817–824

8. Richardson BS, Rurak D, Patrick JE, Homan J, Carmichael L (1989) Cerebral oxidative metabolism during sustained hypoxaemia in fetal sheep. J Dev Physiol 11:37–43

9. Wladimiroff JW, Tonge HM, Stewart PA (1986) Doppler ultrasound assessment of cerebral blood flow in the human fetus. Br J Obstet Gynaecol 93:471–475

10. Veille JC, Cohen I (1990) Middle cerebral artery blood flow in normal and growth-retarded fetuses. Am J Obstet Gynecol 162:391–396

11. Scherjon SA, Smolders-DeHaas H, Kok JH, Zondervan HA (1993) The "brain-sparing" effect: antenatal cerebral Doppler findings in relation to neurologic outcome in very preterm infants. Am J Obstet Gynecol 169:169–175

12. Mari G, Abuhamad AZ, Keller M et al. (1996) Is the fetal brain-sparing effect a risk factor for the development of intraventricular hemorrhage in the preterm infant? Ultrasound Obstet Gynecol 8:329–332

13. Severi FM, Bocchi C, Visentin A et al. (2002) Uterine and fetal cerebral Doppler predict the outcome of third-trimester small-for-gestational age fetuses with normal umbilical artery Doppler. Ultrasound Obstet Gynecol 19:225–228

14. Vyas S, Nicolaides KH, Bower S, Campbell S (1990) Middle cerebral artery flow velocity waveforms in fetal hypoxemia. Br J Obstet Gynaecol 97:797–803

15. Mari G, Wasserstrum N (1991) Flow velocity waveforms of the fetal circulation preceedings fetal demise in a case of lupus anticoagulant. Am J Obstet Gynecol 164:776–778

16. Sepulveda W, Peek MJ (1996) Reverse end-diastolic flow in the middle cerebral artery: an agonal pattern in the human fetus. Am J Obstet Gynecol 174:1645–1647

17. Konje JC, Bell SC, Taylor DJ (2001) Abnormal Doppler velocimetry and blood flow volume in the middle cerebral artery in very severe intrauterine growth restriction: Is the occurrence of reversal of compensatory flow too late? Br J Obstet Gynaecol 108:973–979

18. Respondek M, Woch A, Kaczmarek P, Borowski D (1997) Reversal of diastolic flow in the middle cerebral artery of the fetus during the second half of pregnancy. Ultrasound Obstet Gynecol 9:324–329

19. Zeki S, Mehmet U, Hakan P (2003) Reversed diastolic flow in the middle cerebral artery: its clinical value in fetal growth restriction. Prenat Diagn 23:861–868

20. Leung WC, Tse KY, Tang MHY, Lao TT (2003) Reversed diastolic flow in the middle cerebral artery: Is it a terminal sign in a growth-retarded fetus? Prenat Diagn 23:265–267

21. Vyas S, Campbell S, Bower S, Nicolaides KH (1990) Maternal abdominal pressure alters fetal cerebral blood flow. Br J Obstet Gynaecol 97:740–747

22. Ozcan T, Sbracia M, d'Ancona RL et al. (1998) Arterial and venous Doppler velocimetry in the severely growth

restricted fetus and associations with adverse perinatal outcome. Ultrasound Obstet Gynecol 12:39–44

23. Hecher K, Bilardo CM, Stigter RH et al. (2001) Monitoring of fetuses with intrauterine growth restriction: a longitudinal study. Ultrasound Obstet Gynecol 18:564–570

24. Baschat AA, Gembruch U, Harman CR (2001) The sequence of changes in Doppler and biophysical parameters as severe fetal growth restriction worsens. Ultrasound Obstet Gynecol 18:571–577

25. Ferrazzi E, Bozzo M, Rigano S et al. (2002) Temporal sequence of abnormal Doppler changes in the peripheral and central circulatory systems of the severely growth-restricted fetus. Ultrasound Obstet Gynecol 19:140–146

26. Wladimiroff JW, van den Wijngaard JAC, Degani S et al. (1987) Cerebral and umbilical arterial blood flow velocity waveforms in normal and growth retarded pregnancies: a comparative study. Obstet Gynecol 69:705–709

27. Gramellini D, Folli MC, Raboni S et al. (1992) Cerebral–umbilical Doppler ratio as a predictor of adverse perinatal outcome. Obstet Gynecol 79:416–420

28. Bahado-Singh R, Kovanci E, Jeffres A et al. (1999) The Doppler cerebroplacental ratio and perinatal outcome in intrauterine growth. Am J Obstet Gynecol 180:750–756

29. Makhseed M, Jirous J, Ahmed MA, Viswanathan DL (2000) Middle cerebral artery to umbilical artery resistance index ratio in the prediction of neonatal outcome. Int J Gynecol Obstet 71:119–125

30. Sterne G, Shields LE, Dubinsky TJ (2001) Abnormal fetal cerebral and umbilical Doppler measurements in fetuses with intrauterine growth restriction predicts the severity of perinatal morbidity. J Clin Ultrasound 29:146–151

31. Hershkovitz R, Kingdom JCP, Geary M, Rodeck CH (2000) Fetal cerebral blood flow redistribution in late gestation: identification of compromise in small fetuses with normal umbilical artery Doppler. Ultrasound Obstet Gynecol 15:209–212

32. Harrington K, Thompson MO, Carpenter RG, Nguyen M, Campbell S (1999) Doppler fetal circulation in pregnancies complicated by pre-eclampsia or delivery of a small for gestational age baby: longitudinal analysis. Br J Obstet Gynaecol 106:453–466

33. Arduini D, Rizzo G, Romanini C, Mancuso S (1989) Fetal haemodynamic response to acute maternal hyperoxygenation as predictor of fetal distress in intrauterine growth retardation. Br Med J 298:1561–1562

34. Mari G, Deter RL, Carpenter RL et al. (2000) Non-invasive diagnosis by Doppler ultrasonography of fetal anemia due to maternal red-cell alloimmunization. Collaborative group for Doppler assessment of the blood velocity in anemic fetuses. N Engl J Med 342:9–14

35. Jauniaux E, Van Maldergem L, De Munter C et al. (1990) Nonimmune hydrops fetalis associated with genetic abnormalities. Obstet Gynecol 75:568–572

36. Murat OA, Gallagher PG (1995) Hematologic disorders and nonimmune hydrops fetalis. Semin Perinatol 19:502–515

37. Norton ME (1994) Nonimmune hydrops fetalis. Semin Perinatol 18:321–332

38. Chui DH, Waye JS (1998) Hydrops fetalis caused by alpha-thalassemia: an emerging health care problem. Blood 91:2213–2222

39. Old J (1996) Haemoglobinopathies. Prenat Diagn 16:1181–1186

40. Leung WC, Oepkes D, Seaward G, Ryan G (2002) Serial sonographic findings of four fetuses with homozygous alpha-thalassemia-1 from 21 weeks onwards. Ultrasound Obstet Gynecol 19:56–59

41. Owen J, Stedman CM, Tucker TL (1989) Comparison of predelivery versus postdelivery Kleihauer-Betke stains in cases of fetal death. Am J Obstet Gynecol 161:663–666

42. Giacoia GP (1997) Severe fetomaternal hemorrhage: a review. Obstet Gynecol Surv 52:372–380

43. Sueters M, Arabin B, Oepkes D (2003) Doppler sonography for predicting fetal anemia caused by massive fetomaternal hemorrhage. Ultrasound Obstet Gynecol 22:186–189

44. Tercanli S, Gembruch U, Holzgreve W (2000) Nonimmune hydrops fetalis in diagnosis and management. In: Callen PW (ed) Ultrasonography in obstetrics and gynecology, 4th edn. Saunders, Philadelphia, pp 563–566

45. Mentzer WC, Collier E (1975) Hydrops fetalis associated with erythrocyte G-6-PD deficiency and maternal ingestion of fava beans and ascorbic acid. J Pediatr 86:565–567

46. Perkins RP (1971) Hydrops fetalis and stillbirth in a male glucose-6-phosphate dehydrogenase-deficient fetus possibly due to maternal ingestion of sulfisoxazole: a case report. Am J Obstet Gynecol 111:379–381

47. Brown KE, Anderson SM, Young NS (1993) Erythrocyte P antigen: cellular receptor for B19 parvovirus. Science 262:114–117

48. Haak MC, Oosterhof H, Mouw RJ et al. (1999) Pathophysiology and treatment of fetal anemia due to placental chorioangioma. Ultrasound Obstet Gynecol 14:68–70

49. Rogers BB, Bloom SL, Buchanan GR (1997) Autosomal dominantly inherited Diamond-Blackfan anemia resulting in nonimmune hydrops. Obstet Gynecol 89:805–807

50. McLennan AC, Chitty LS, Rissik J, Maxwell DJ (1996) Prenatal diagnosis of Blackfan-Diamond syndrome: case report and review of the literature. Prenat Diagn 16:349–353

51. Mari G, Deter RL, Carpenter R et al. (1990) The peak systolic velocity of the middle cerebral artery is a better indicator of fetal anemia than the pulsatility index. Proc Soc Gynecologic Investigation, St. Louis, Missouri

52. Zimmerman R, Durig P, Carpenter RJ Jr, Mari G (2002) Longitudinal measurement of peak systolic velocity in the fetal middle cerebral artery for monitoring pregnancies complicated by red cell alloimmunisation: a prospective multicenter trial with intention-to-treat. Br J Obstet Gynaecol 109:746–752

53. Nishie EN, Brizot ML, Liao AW et al. (2003) A comparison between middle cerebral artery peak systolic velocity and amniotic fluid optical density at 450 nm in the prediction of fetal anemia. Am J Obstet Gynecol 188:214–219

54. Mari G, Penso C, Sbracia M et al. (1997) Delta OD 450 and Doppler velocimetry of the middle cerebral artery peak velocity in the evaluation for fetal alloimmune

hemolytic disease. Which is best? Am J Obstet Gynecol 176:S18

55. Pereira L, Jenkins TM, Berghella V (2003) Conventional management of maternal red cell alloimmunization compared with management by Doppler assessment of middle cerebral artery peak systolic velocity. Am J Obstet Gynecol 189:1002–1006

56. Mari G, Detti L, Oz U et al. (2002) Accurate prediction of fetal hemoglobin by Doppler ultrasonography: a preliminary study. Obstet Gynecol 99:589–593

57. Stefos T, Cosmi E, Detti L, Mari G (2002) Correction of fetal anemia and the middle cerebral artery peak systolic velocity. Obstet Gynecol 99:211–215

58. Detti L, Oz U, Guney I et al. (2001) Doppler ultrasound velocimetry for timing the second intrauterine transfusion in fetuses with anemia from red cell alloimmunization. Am J Obstet Gynecol 185:1048–1051

59. Delle Chiaie LD, Buck G, Grab D, Terinde R (2001) Prediction of fetal anemia with Doppler measurement of the middle cerebral artery peak systolic velocity in pregnancies complicated by maternal blood group alloimmunization or parvovirus B19 infection. Ultrasound Obstet Gynecol 18:232–236

60. Teixeira JM, Duncan K, Letsky E, Fisk NM (2000) Middle cerebral artery peak systolic velocity in the prediction of fetal anemia. Ultrasound Obstet Gynecol 15: 205–208

61. Deren O, Onderoglu L (2002) The value of middle cerebral artery systolic velocity for initial and subsequent management in fetal anemia. Eur J Obstet Gynecol Reprod Biol 101:26–30

62. Abdel-Fattah SA, Soothill PW, Carroll SG, Kyle PM (2002) Middle cerebral artery Doppler for the prediction of fetal anemia in cases without hydrops: a practical approach. Br J Radiol 75:726–730

63. Chmait RH, Hull AD (2002) Doppler ultrasonographic evaluation of twins discordant for Rh alloimmunization. Am J Obstet Gynecol 187:250–251

64. Detti L, Mari G, Akiyama M et al. (2002) Longitudinal assessment of the middle cerebral artery peak systolic velocity in healthy fetuses and in fetuses at risk for anemia. Am J Obstet Gynecol 187:937–939

65. Detti L, Mari G (2003) Noninvasive diagnosis of fetal anemia. Clin Obstet Gynecol 46:923–930

66. Moise KJ Jr (2002) Management of rhesus alloimmunization in pregnancy. Obstet Gynecol 100:600–611

67. Cosmi E, Mari G, Delle Chiaie L et al. (2002) Noninvasive diagnosis by Doppler ultrasonography of fetal anemia resulting from parvovirus infection. Am J Obstet Gynecol 187:1290–1293

68. Mari G, Detti L (2001) Doppler ultrasound: application to fetal medicine. In: Fleischer AC, Manning AF, Jeanty P, Romero R (eds) Sonography in obstetrics and gynecology: principles and practice, 6th edn. McGraw-Hill, New York, pp 274–276

69. Senat MV, Loizeau S, Couderc S, Bernard JP, Ville Y (2003) The value of middle cerebral artery peak systolic velocity in the diagnosis of fetal anemia after intrauterine death of one monochorionic twin. Am J Obstet Gynecol 189:1320–1324

70. Abel DE, Grambow SC, Brancazio LR, Hertzberg BS (2003) Ultrasound assessment of the fetal middle cerebral artery peak systolic velocity: a comparison of the near-field versus the far-field vessel. Am J Obstet Gynecol 189:986–989

71. Akiyama M, Detti L, Abuhamad A, Bahado-Singh R, Mari G (2002) Is the middle cerebral artery peak systolic velocity measurement affected by the site of vessel sampling? Am J Obstet Gynecol 187:S164

Chapter 15

Pulsed Doppler Ultrasonography of the Human Fetal Renal Artery

Jean-Claude Veille

The renal arteries arise directly from the aorta just below the projection of the 12th rib and below the superior mesenteric artery. The left renal artery is usually a little higher and longer than that on the right (Fig. 15.1). Close to the renal hilum the renal arteries divide into multiple branches with large anterior and posterior branches. These branches in turn divide into large segment arteries, which eventually terminate in arcuate arteries. The best way to assess the renal arteries is to find the abdominal aorta and the renal hilum using a coronal axis view. The renal arteries are usually seen arising from the lateral aspect of the abdominal aorta. The superior artery is often difficult to visualize in the fetus compared to that in the adult, but the renal artery can be seen using a multipurpose midfrequency scanhead (3–5 MHz). Respiratory or total body movement make it difficult to obtain an adequate duplex signal. With patience, experience, and perseverance, a Doppler examination of the renal artery can be performed successfully in about 90% of patients.

The abdominal aorta and fetal kidney should be localized first using a two-dimensional examination (Fig. 15.2). The Doppler cursor is placed in the area where the ultrasonographer suspects the renal artery to be, with the Doppler sample volume and Doppler

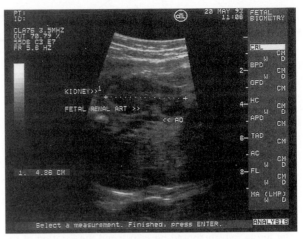

Fig. 15.2. Two-dimensional examination of a fetus at 30 weeks' gestation. The fetal abdominal aorta is easily seen at the level of the left kidney. On careful inspection, the fetal renal artery is seen at its bifurcation with the aorta

angle adjusted *prior* to turning on the Doppler instrument (Fig. 15.3) so Doppler ultrasound exposure is minimized. The power output should be decreased to about 50%–75% of its spatial peak temporal average (SPTA) specification. Even at this lower power output the Doppler signal is adequate to obtain echoes from the fetal renal artery. Color mapping is used last to confirm the two-dimensional impression that the Doppler signal is indeed coming from the renal artery and not from the fetal aorta (Fig. 15.4). The renal artery Doppler waveform has a characteristically high peak forward velocity and low but continuous forward flow during diastole that is easily differentiated from the adjacent fetal abdominal aorta.

Like any other Doppler examination, the renal velocity waveforms should be obtained during a period of fetal quiescence. The velocity waveforms should be recorded at a fast speed, with the lowest pass filter. Using these guidelines, most ultrasonographers are able to obtain adequate Doppler waveforms from these small renal vessels. It is of the utmost importance to minimize Doppler and color exposure, as the safety of such techniques on human fetuses has not been fully evaluated [1].

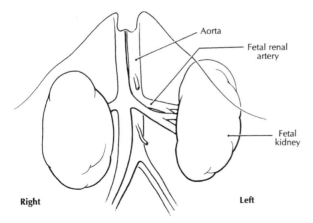

Fig. 15.1. Fetal renal arteries. Note that the left renal artery is behind the renal vein and is longer than the right renal artery

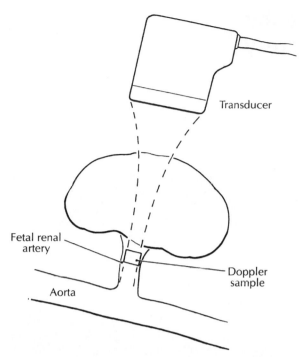

Fig. 15.3. Doppler sample is placed on the area of the fetal renal artery without turning the Doppler apparatus. It allows adjustment of the Doppler sample volume, the Doppler angle (which should be <30°), and the location of the Doppler sample within the lumen of the "presumed" location of the fetal renal artery

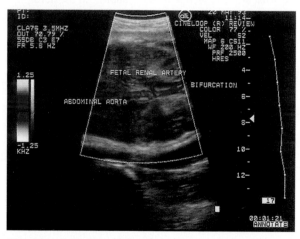

Fig. 15.4. Color should be the last part of the fetal renal artery localization, not the first. Note the abdominal aorta and its bifurcation as it enters the pelvis. The fetal renal artery is seen bifurcating from the abdominal aorta and entering the renal parenchyma. The Doppler is finally turned on to display the returning signals either on the video monitor or recorded to allow analysis at a later time

Doppler Principles and Hints

Flow is determined by a pressure difference between two points and by the resistance to flow within that structure. This relation is known as Poiseuille's law and has been mathematically described:

$$Q = \Delta P/R,$$

where ΔP is the flow difference, and R is the flow resistance. The heart (pump) is the driving force behind generating the pressure difference, which in turn is the force behind fluid flow. The flow resistance is mostly determined by the length and radius of the vessel of interest, in this case the renal artery. Increasing the length of the vessel increases the resistance, whereas doubling the radius of the vessel decreases resistance to blood flow by one-sixteenth of the original value [1]. Other than vessel size and pressure differences, the pulsatile nature of blood flow in the fetus results in expansion and contraction of the vessel, which in turn affects the Doppler waveform profile. Thus pulsatile flow in compliant vessels affects forward flow during systole and flow reversal during diastole.

When assessing Doppler flow of the fetal renal artery, attention must be given to whether flow is best described as plug flow or laminar flow [1]. At the immediate bifurcation of the renal artery with the abdominal aorta (i.e., at the entrance of the renal vessel), the flow of the blood is essentially constant across the vessel. Closer to the renal parenchyma, flow becomes more laminar and assumes a parabolic profile (i.e., maximum flow velocity is at the center of the vessel, whereas flow is almost zero at or close to the walls of the vessel). Hence depending on the position of the Doppler sample, the Doppler velocity pattern is affected.

The acute angle between the bifurcation of the abdominal aorta and the renal artery can significantly affect the renal blood flow profile. Theoretically, flow is turbulent at such sites and can result in a random, chaotic flow pattern of red blood cells [1]. Because these aberrant flow patterns can affect the final Doppler waveform profile, the fetal renal artery is sampled close to the renal parenchyma, keeping the Doppler sample within the lumen of the vessel (Fig. 15.3). A Doppler sample size of 1.5 mm is used and is adequate for most studies done on fetuses beyond 20–24 weeks.

Doppler measurement is angle-dependent. Thus it is important to keep the angle at or less 30° when obtaining Doppler signals from the fetal renal artery. Doppler angles of more than 30° could significantly affect the Doppler shift and thus the Doppler waveform signals. This point is even more important when using color-flow studies of the fetal renal artery. An angle of 80°–90°, for example, results in no Doppler shift, which in turn results in an inability to visualize color flow of the fetal renal artery. The Doppler angle is not critical, however, when assessing qualitative spectral indices, such as the pulsatility index (PI), resistance index (RI), or systolic/diastolic (S/D) ratio as the angle does not change the relation between the peak systolic and end-diastolic flows. To optimize visualization of the fetal renal artery, Duplex ultrasound is used in order to combine real-time cross-sectional ultrasound images of the fetal renal artery and precisely locate the Doppler sample (Fig. 15.3). These expansive duplex systems are difficult to operate, as data acquisition is machine- and operator-dependent.

Although the diastolic flow of the fetal renal artery is a low-impedance/low-resistance flow, the diastolic flows are not as high as those observed in the umbilical artery. Diastolic flow of this vascular bed has always been present in normal fetuses at gestational ages of less than 16 weeks. Absent or reverse diastolic flows of this vascular bed in the fetus should be considered abnormal. It is imperative to keep the wall filter at a minimum to avoid causing artifacts that may have serious clinical implications. We elect to reduce the wall filter to 50 Hz during the Doppler acquisition in order to avoid this problem.

When this circulation is quantitatively assessed, in addition to the problems associated with signal acquisition it is important to understand the Doppler waveform. The Doppler spectrum is composed of a range of scattered velocities derived electronically using fast Fourier transformation. When tracing the Doppler curve for quantitative flow assessment, it is important to trace the sharpest part of the ascending and the descending part of the curve in order to avoid the inclusion of contaminated signals. This point is particularly important because quantitative determination of blood flow of such a small vessel as the fetal renal artery may easily be over- or underestimated. Consistency when tracing the curve is therefore essential. To make analysis of the Doppler curve consistent, the returning Doppler signals should be as sharp and pure as possible.

Clinical Application: Fetal Renal Artery Doppler Assessment

The first report on noninvasive measurement of human circulation using ultrasound was published in 1977 by FitzGerald and Drumm [2]. Since then numerous papers have emerged in the literature describing application of the technique to the study of maternal, placen-

tal, and fetal circulations [3–8]. With the introduction of duplex ultrasonography, fetal intracardiac [9] and regional [10–17] circulations have been assessed. Pulsed-wave (PW) Doppler ultrasound is particularly well suited for studying the hemodynamics of the human fetus, as the associated techniques are noninvasive, well accepted by the patients, easily reproducible, and relatively safe for the human fetus.

Fetal Renal Doppler Imaging

Since the introduction of pulsed Doppler ultrasound to obstetrics, volume flow measurement of the central and the peripheral fetal circulation has been possible (Table 15.1). Previously most of the data on the actual measurement of the fetal circulation were acquired using invasive techniques, which obviously was not possible in human fetuses. Although volume flow measurements are not widely acceptable and are done only in high-risk pregnancies, a few investigators have given some insight on the normal and abnormal human fetal circulation. Pulsed Doppler requires expensive equipment, is usually cumbersome, and has some inherent errors in volume flow [18]. Color flow imaging allows the operator to interrogate most of the fetal vascular beds including the fetal renal artery. This vascular bed is usually easy to identify at its origin, which is at a 90° angle from the abdominal aorta (Fig. 15.3) [11]. The pulsed Doppler range gate is placed in the renal artery with an angle close to zero. This methodology is powerful but needs to be validated. Using such technology, we were able to longitudinally follow normal fetuses in order to determine fetal vascular changes across gestation (Fig. 15.5). Although these values changed with advancing gestation, the changes were not significant.

In one study, using color and pulsed Doppler ultrasonography, interobserver reliability of measurements in the fetal circulation was evaluated in 41 pregnancies of 25–39 weeks' gestation. Two observers recorded flow velocity waveforms from the middle cerebral and renal arteries for measurement of peak systolic, minimum diastolic, and mean velocities, PI, and RI. Intraclass correlation coefficient of reliability was calculated by analysis of variance. Substantial interobserver agreement was found for the pulsatility index and minimum diastolic velocity in both arteries. Therefore, these measurements have the greatest clinical applicability [19].

Renal Artery Doppler Studies in the Normal Fetus

Vyas et al. established reference ranges for the PI of the fetal renal artery in a cross-sectional study done on 114 human fetuses [11] between weeks 17 and 43

Table 15.2. Resistance index (RI) of the renal artery in normal fetuses and children

Age group	Number	RI
Fetuses (3rd trimester)	32	0.67–0.88
0–1 month	30	0.57–0.90
1–3 months	20	0.60–0.84
3–6 months	11	0.65–0.75

creased significantly after maternal meal ingestion in normally grown fetuses during late pregnancy ($n=14$) (fasting $= 2.36 \pm 0.16$ versus fed $= 2.09 \pm 0.33$; $P = 0.021$). These authors postulated that the decrease in the resistance may be associated with increased fetal urine production after maternal meals [25].

Renal Artery Doppler Studies in IUGR Fetuses

Using duplex Doppler ultrasound and a low wall filter (50 Hz), Veille and Kanaan could not demonstrate absent end-diastolic flow of the fetal renal artery in a group of asymmetric fetuses who were suffering intrauterine growth restriction (IUGR) [13]. The PI in the IUGR fetuses was significantly higher than in normally grown fetuses. Among the IUGR group, fetuses with signs of hypoxia had an even higher S/D ratio than the fetuses without signs of hypoxia [13]. These investigators suggested that local mechanisms are operational in the fetal kidneys that may in turn influence renal blood flow.

Vyas and Campbell found that 64% of small-for-gestational-age (SGA) human fetuses had a PI higher than the 90th percentile confidence interval of the reference range for gestation (Fig. 15.6) [15]. They found no association between the change in PI and a

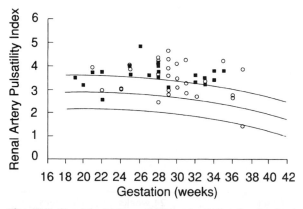

Fig. 15.6. The 5th, 50th, and 90th percentiles for the fetal renal artery pulsatility index (PI) and gestational age. Sixty-four percent of small-for-gestational age fetuses had a PI above the 90th percentile. (Reprinted from [15] with permission)

change in umbilical cord PO_2 concentration. In this group of SGA fetuses, 20 of 48 (42%) had oligohydramnios. The PI of 16 of 20 fetuses with oligohydramnios (80%) were above the 95th percentile of their normal reference range [15]. The authors concluded that as the impedance to fetal renal blood flow increases, which indicates a higher PI, it is associated with a decrease in fetal urine production.

In a prospective longitudinal study, the changes within the fetal renal circulation were assessed by Doppler sonography in preterm severely growth-restricted fetuses during the period of gradual deterioration prior to delivery; the relationship between Doppler measurements, amniotic fluid index, birth weight, and fetal condition at birth were examined. Sixteen preterm growth-restricted fetuses between 26 and 35 weeks of gestational age were studied. Serial Doppler measurements were made of the renal artery, umbilical artery, middle cerebral artery, and ductus venosus. The PI in the renal artery did not show any correlation with cord blood pH, birth weight, or amniotic fluid index corrected for gestational age (Delta/SDAFI). Peak systolic velocities in the renal artery showed a significant reduction with time ($n=7$, $P < 0.05$) and a significant correlation with venous cord pH at delivery ($n=12$, $r=0.84$, $P < 0.001$), Delta/SDAFI ($n=16$, $r=0.67$, $P < 0.01$), and birth weight ($n=16$, $r=0.61$, $P < 0.02$). Birth weight correlated significantly with Delta/SDAFI ($n=15$, $r=0.57$, $P < 0.05$), PI values of the middle cerebral artery ($n=15$, $r=-0.61$, $P < 0.02$), and PI values of the ductus venosus ($n=16$, $r=0.55$, $P < 0.05$). Delta/SDAFI correlated significantly with pulsatility index values of the ductus venosus ($n=15$, $r=0.51$, $P < 0.05$) and arterial cord pH values at delivery ($n=8$, $r=0.78$, $P < 0.05$). These authors concluded that a progressive redistribution of the circulation occurs with deterioration of the fetal condition in the growth-restricted preterm fetus as reflected by changes in peak systolic velocities, but not by changes in pulsatility values of the fetal renal artery waveforms [26].

Doppler has been used to test the hypothesis that infants exhibiting catch-up growth as an indicator of IUGR have a higher incidence of predelivery abnormal Doppler results. In total, 196 women with singleton pregnancies at high risk of IUGR were followed up for postnatal catch-up growth during the first 7 months. Forty-six of the 196 infants demonstrated catch-up growth and were therefore classified as growth restricted; 85% of this group had had abnormal Doppler results prior to delivery, compared with 14% of the normal growth group. The authors concluded that Doppler appears to distinguish IUGR (as defined by catch-up growth) from normal growth more successfully in infants with an average birth weight ratio than in infants with a low birth weight ratio and is a better predictor of IUGR than SGA [27].

In another study, the renal volume in fetuses with IUGR fetuses was 31% (95% CI, 20%–40%), which was less than the renal volume obtained in the group of non-IUGR fetuses after adjusting for gestational age. The ratio of renal volume to estimated fetal weight was 15% (95% CI, 1%–26%), which was less than the same ratio in the non-IUGR fetuses. No differences were seen in the renal artery Doppler measurements. These authors concluded that IUGR appears to be associated with a decrease in fetal renal volume. Because renal volume is a likely proxy for nephron number, this study supports the hypothesis that IUGR may be linked to congenital oligonephropathy and potentially to hypertension in later life and other related vascular diseases [28].

Some authors have determined the fetal blood flow redistribution and the amount of amniotic fluid in appropriate-for-gestational-age (AGA) fetuses and growth-restricted fetuses. In one study, Yoshimura determined the blood flow velocity waveforms of the umbilical artery, descending aorta, middle cerebral artery, renal artery, and uterine artery using pulsed Doppler ultrasonography in 100 AGA fetuses and 39 growth-restricted fetuses. The PI values and the amount of amniotic fluid were compared between the two groups. The PI values of the umbilical artery and renal artery were significantly higher in AGA fetuses with oligohydramnios than in fetuses with an adequate amount of amniotic fluid. The PI values of the umbilical artery and renal artery were significantly higher and the PI of the middle cerebral artery was significantly lower in growth-restricted fetuses with oligohydramnios than in fetuses with an adequate amount of amniotic fluid. Furthermore, there was a significant negative correlation between the PI value of the renal artery and the vertical diameter of amniotic fluid, and between the PI value of the renal artery and the amniotic fluid index. The PI value of the renal artery was related to the amount of amniotic fluid in growth-restricted fetuses, and the same relationship was demonstrated in AGA fetuses [29].

Arduini and Rizzo reported on the renal blood flow velocity waveforms of 114 IUGR fetuses and 97 postterm fetuses [16]. They found that the IUGR fetuses had a higher PI than a group of normally grown fetuses especially if there was oligohydramnios. Interestingly, postterm fetuses had PIs similar to those of normal term fetuses. In the postterm fetuses there was no correlation between the amount of amniotic fluid and the fetal renal PI values. To explain these apparent discrepancies, the authors suggested that the etiology of the oligohydramnios could have different mechanisms in these two subsets of fetuses. They speculated that the oligohydramnios in the

IUGR fetuses was related to changes in intrarenal vascular resistance [16], and in postterm fetuses it was related to changes in tubular reabsorption.

Mari et al. [17] found that among four human fetuses affected by asymmetric IUGR who had oligohydramnios and abnormal fetal renal artery velocimetry the perinatal mortality was high (three of four), confirming the findings of Veille and Kanaan [13].

Thus most of the published studies on fetal renal artery waveforms support the concept that IUGR fetuses with oligohydramnios have a PI above the established values for the 95th percentile (Fig. 15.7). The combination of IUGR, oligohydramnios, and elevated PI of the fetal renal artery seems to be associated with an increase in perinatal morbidity and mortality. These Doppler studies support an intrarenal increase in impedance, which in turn affects renal perfusion and urine production.

Akita et al. evaluated renal blood flow in 102 normal human fetuses between weeks 20 and 40 of gestation and compared these normative results to those of 11 IUGR fetuses with normal amniotic fluid, 15 fetuses with oligohydramnios, and 10 IUGR fetuses with oligohydramnios [30]. Color duplex PW Doppler ultrasound was used to evaluate the fetal renal artery. The ascending aorta and pulmonary arteries were evaluated at the same time. Akita et al. concluded that the kidneys of IUGR fetuses with oligohydramnios were poorly perfused because of a decrease in stroke volume, which was found to be associated with these fetuses [30].

Although a prerenal etiology for oligohydramnios is always possible, human and animal data strongly suggest that the human kidney is capable of modifying intrarenal resistances according to alterations in the in utero environment. Evidence obtained from fetal renal arteries of guinea pigs, for example, suggests that the fetal circulation exhibits heterogeneity in

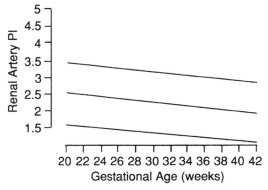

Fig. 15.7. Confidence intervals for a group of normal fetuses. This graph and the one in Fig. 15.6 are comparable and point to an elevated pulsatility index (PI) of the fetal renal artery. (Reprinted from [16] with permission)

28. Silver LE, Descamps PJ, Korst LM, Platt LD, Castro LC (2003) Intrauterine growth restriction is accompanied by decreased renal blood volume in the human fetus. Am J Obstet Gynecol 188:1320–1325

29. Yoshimura S, Masuzaki H, Gotoh H, Ishimaru T (1997) Fetal redistribution of blood flow and amniotic fluid volume in growth-retarded fetuses. Early Hum Dev 47:297–304

30. Akita A, Okada O, Saito T, Koresawa M, Kato H (1991) Evaluation of the renal artery in the fetuses with growth retardation and oligohydramnios by two dimensional Doppler ultrasonography. Acta Obstet Gynaecol Jpn 43:1554–1560

31. Thompson LP, Weiner CP (1993) Effect of nitro-L-arginine on contractile responses of carotid and renal arteries of fetal guinea pigs during hypoxia. In: Proceedings from the Society for Gynecologic Investigation 40th Annual Meeting, Toronto, abstract 106

32. Veille JC, Penry M (1992) Effects of maternal administration of 3% carbon dioxide on umbilical artery and fetal renal and middle cerebral artery Doppler waveforms. Am J Obstet Gynecol 167:1668–1671

33. Suranyi A, Streitman K, Pal A, Nyari T, Retz C, Foidart JM, Schaaps JP, Kovacs L (2000) Fetal renal artery flow and renal echogenicity in the chronically hypoxic state. Pediatr Nephrol 14:393–399

34. Veille JC, Penry M, Mueller-Heubach E (1993) Fetal renal pulsed Doppler waveform in prolonged pregnancies. Am J Obstet Gynecol 169:882–884

35. Schroder H, Gilbert RD, Power GG (1984) Urinary and hemodynamic responses to blood volume changes in fetal sheep. J Dev Physiol 6:131–141

36. Mari G, Moise KJ, Deter MD, Carpenter RJ (1991) Doppler assessment of renal blood flow velocity waveforms in the anemic fetus before and after intravascular transfusion for severe red cell alloimmunization. J Clin Ultrasound 19:15–19

37. Oz AU, Holub B, Mendilcioglu I, Mari G, Bahado-Singh RO (2002) Renal artery Doppler investigation of the etiology of oligohydramnios in postterm pregnancy. Obstet Gynecol 100:715–718

38. Veille JC, Penry M, Mueller-Heubach E (1993) Fetal renal pulsed Doppler waveform in prolonged pregnancies. Am J Obstet Gynecol 169:882–884

39. Scott L, Casey BM, Roberts S et al. (2000) Predictive value of Serial Middle Cerebral and Renal Artery Pulsatility Indices in Fetuses with Oligohydramnios. J Maternal-Fetal Medicine 9:105–109

40. Keirse MJNC (1981) Potential hazards of prostaglandin synthetase inhibitors for the management of pre-term labour. J Drug Res 6:915

41. Huhta JC, Moise KJ, Fisher DI et al. (1987) Detection and quantitation of constriction of the fetal ductus arteriosus by Doppler echocardiography. Circulation 75:406–412

42. Matson JR, Stokes JB, Robillard JE (1981) Effects of inhibition of prostaglandin synthesis on fetal renal function. Kidney Int 20:621–627

43. Mari G, Moise KJ, Deter RL, Kirshon B, Carpenter RJ (1990) Doppler assessment of the renal blood flow velocity waveform during indomethacin therapy for preterm labor and polyhydramnios. Obstet Gynecol 75:199–201

44. Van Bel F, Guit GL, Schiooer J, van de Bor M, Baan J (1991) Indomethacin-induced changes in renal blood flow velocity waveform in premature infants investigated with color Doppler imaging. J Pediatr 118:621–626

45. Beaufils M, Donsimoni R, Uzam S, Colan JC (1985) Prevention of preeclampsia by early antiplatelets therapy. Lancet 1:840–842

46. Wallenburg HCS, Makovitz JW, Dekker GA, Rotmans O (1986) Low-dose aspirin prevents pregnancy-induced hypertension and preeclampsia in angiotensin sensitive primigravidae. Lancet 1:1–3

47. Veille JC, Hanson R, Sivakoff M, Swain M, Henderson L (1993) The effects of maternal low dose aspirin on the fetal cardiovascular system. Am J Obstet Gynecol 168:1430–1442

48. Rasanen J (1990) The effects of ritodrine infusion on fetal myocardial function and fetal hemodynamics. Acta Obstet Gynecol Scand 69:487–492

49. Guignard JP, Gouyon JB (1988) Adverse effects of drugs on the immature kidney. Biol Neonate 53:243–252

50. Martin RA, Jones KL, Mendoza A, Barr M Jr, Benirschke K (1992) The effect of ACE inhibition on the fetal kidney: decreased renal blood flow. Teratology 46:317–321

51. Edwards A, Baker LS, Wallace EM (2002) Changes in fetoplacental vessel flow velocity waveforms following maternal administration of betamethasone. Ultrasound Obstet Gynecol 20:240–244

52. Holmes RP, Stone PR (2000) Severe oligohydramnios induced by cyclooxygenase-2 inhibitor nimesulide. Obstet Gynecol 96:810–811

53. Romagnoli C, De Carolis MP, Papacci P, Polimeni V, Luciano R, Piersigilli F, Delogu AB, Tortorolo G (2000) Effects of prophylactic ibuprofen on cerebral and renal hemodynamics in very preterm neonates. Clin Pharmacol Ther 67:676–683

54. Kang NS, Yoo KH, Cheon H, Choi BM, Hong YS, Lee JW, Kim SK (1999) Indomethacin treatment decreases renal blood flow velocity in human neonates. Biol Neonate 76:261–265

55. Wang Z, Li W, Ouyang W, Ding Y, Wang F, Xu L, Su X (1998) Cervical ripening in the third trimester of pregnancy with intravaginal misoprostol: a double-blind, randomized, placebo-controlled study. J Tongji Med Univ 18:183–186

56. Kramer WB, Saade GR, Belfort M, Dorman K, Mayes M, Moise KJ Jr (1999) A randomized double-blind study comparing the fetal effects of sulindac to terbutaline during the management of preterm labor. Am J Obstet Gynecol 180:396–401

57. Maršál K, Nicolaides K, Kaminpetros P, Hackett G (1992) The clinical value of waveforms from the descending aorta. In: Pearce JM (ed) Doppler ultrasound in perinatal medicine. Oxford University Press, New York, pp 239–267

58. Kara SA, Noyan V, Karadeniz Y, Yucel A, Altinok D, Bayram M (2003) Resistance index in fetal interlobar renal artery with renal pelvic dilatation up to 10 mm. J Clin Ultrasound 31:75–79

59. Bates JA, Irving HC (1992) Inability of color and spectral Doppler to identify fetal renal obstruction. J Ultrasound Med 11:469–472

Fig. 16.3. Fully
changes in the
during normal
tions of the wa
cate the extent
changes. *I. V. S.*
[113] with perm

changes. In
spiral arteries
that these uter
to respond to v

The questic
small muscula
entirely respor
100 ml/min to
the pregnant t
ply the placen
pertrophy [17]
area leads to a
velopment of t
luminal diame
counts for the
the third trime
mones estroge
blood volume
blood viscosity
influence uterir

60. Rooks VJ, Lebowitz RL (2001) Extrinsic ureteropelvic junction obstruction from a crossing renal vessel: demography and imaging. Pediatr Radiol 31:120–124

61. Gill B, Bennett RT, Barnhard Y, Bar-Hava I, Girz B, Divon M (1996) Can fetal renal artery Doppler studies predict postnatal renal function in morphologically abnormal kidneys? A preliminary report. J Urol 156:190–192

62. Hata T, Mari G, Reiter AA (1991) Doppler velocity waveforms of blood flow in the fetal renal artery in a case of Meckel syndrome. Am J Roentgenol 156:408

63. Alverson DC, Eldridge M, Dillon T et al. (1989) Noninvasive pulsed Doppler determination of cardiac output in neonate and children. J Pediatr 7:265–297

64. Claflin KS, Alverson DC, Patak D et al. (1988) Cardiac output determinations in the newborn: reproducibility of pulsed Doppler velocity measurement. J Ultrasound Med 7:311–315

65. Lewis JF, Kuo LC, Nelson JG, Linager MC, Quinones MA (1984) Pulsed Doppler echocardiographic determination of stroke volume and cardiac output: clinical validation of two new methods using the apical window. Circulation 70:425–431

66. Silverman NH, Schmidt KG (1989) The current role of Doppler echocardiography in the diagnosis of heart disease in children. Cardiol Clin 7:265–297

67. Visser MO, Leighton JO, van de Bor M, Walter FJ (1992) Renal blood flow in neonates: quantification with color flow and pulsed Doppler ultrasound. Radiology 183:441–444

68. Rudolph AM, Heyman MA (1970) Circulatory changes during growth in the fetal lamb. Circ Res 26:289–299

69. Veille JC, Figueroa JP, Mueller-Heubach E (1992) Validation of noninvasive fetal renal artery measurement by pulsed Doppler in the lamb. Am J Obstet Gynecol 167:1663–1667

70. Veille JC, Hanson R, Tatum K (1994) Renal hemodynamics: longitudinal study from the late fetal life to one year of age. 7th Congress of International Perinatal Doppler Society, Toronto, Canada, Sept 21–24 (abstract 36)

71. Rosnes J, Penry M, Veille JC (1996) Fetal cardiac and renal Doppler evaluation in pregnancies with idiopathic polyhydramnios (abstract 246). Am J Obstet Gynecol 174:379

Fig. 16.4. Differei
and preeclamptic
ing the extent of
in the uteroplacei
preeclampsia thes
extent beyond the
junction. (From [1

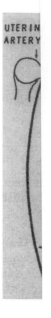

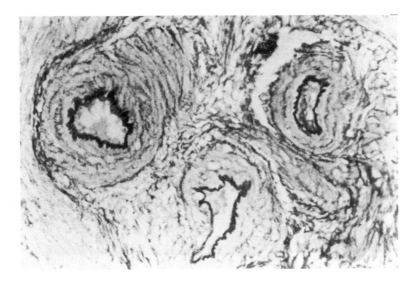

Fig. 16.5. Preeclampsia. Myometrial spiral artery is unaffected by physiologic changes and retains a normal internal elastic lamina. (Reprinted from [15] with permission)

Norm
of Ut
Durir

During
blasts i
and re
with a
fibrous
comple
uents p
trophob
station
the sec
move ir

cies. What has not been studied is whether the large vessels in the uterine artery circulation in the presence of preeclampsia undergo the same degree of hyperplasia as is seen in normotensive pregnancies.

Another placental bed lesion seen with preclampsia is an acute arteriopathy, termed acute atherosis by Zeek and Assali [20]. Here the wall of the spiral artery shows fibrinoid necrosis with lipophages, and there is a mononuclear cellular infiltrate around the artery (Fig. 16.6). This lesion is seen in the decidual and myometrial segments of the placental bed spiral arteries that have not undergone physiologic changes.

In pregnancies complicated by essential hypertension, hyperplastic arteriosclerosis of the myometrial segments of the placental bed spiral arteries can be seen [15, 16]. Here there is proliferation of all coats of the vessel wall, collagenous sclerosis, and stenosis of the lumen. The breadth and severity of the lesions

correlate with the severity and duration of the hypertension. This lesion is not seen with preeclampsia unless there is a history of essential hypertension (Fig. 16.7). When essential hypertension is complicated by superimposed preeclampsia, both acute atherosis and hyperplastic arteriosclerosis are seen [15, 16].

In normotensive pregnancies resulting in intrauterine growth-restricted (IUGR) fetuses, acute artherosis has been seen in the decidual spiral arteries, with the myometrial spiral arteries retaining their muscular coats [18, 19]. This finding implies that these lesions are not particular to preeclampsia.

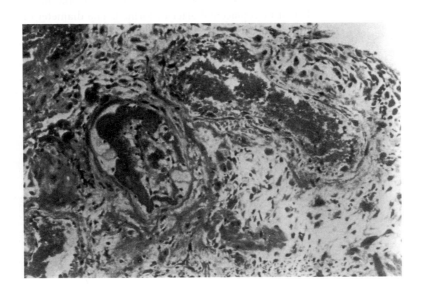

Fig. 16.6. Preeclampsia. Decidual portion of a spiral artery shows acute atherosis characterized by fibrinoid necrosis and infiltration of lipophages into the damaged vessel wall. (Reprinted from [15] with permission)

Fig. 16.7. Preeclampsia complicating essential hypertension. Myometrial spiral artery is unaffected by physiologic changes but shows hyperplastic changes in all layers of the vessel. (Reprinted from [15], with permission)

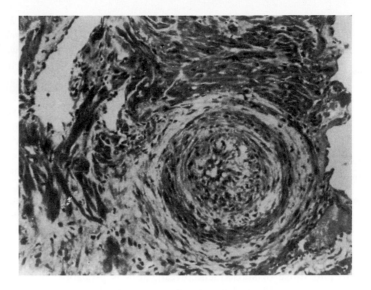

Indices of Uterine Artery Waveform Analysis

Uterine artery Doppler waveforms are most commonly analyzed by simple semiquantitative techniques based on analysis of the maximum Doppler shift frequencies of the time-velocity waveform, which varies during the cardiac cycle. Evaluation of the change in maximal Doppler shifts over time provides information on the impedance of the circulatory bed being fed. Time-velocity waveforms with high diastolic flow are seen when downstream resistance is low, and those with low or reverse diastolic flow are found when downstream resistance is high. The heart rate can significantly modify the waveform: high heart rates shorten the diastolic runoff time, producing high end-diastolic frequency shifts; low heart rates have an opposite effect. The Doppler shift frequencies are proportional to flow velocity. If the angle of insonation is kept constant over the course of the cardiac cycle, comparisons of Doppler frequency shifts from any point of the waveform are angle-independent.

There are three widely used semiquantitative techniques for analysis of uterine artery waveforms. The pulsatility index (PI) is the most complex of the three. The PI is equal to peak systole minus end diastole divided by the mean value of the area under the curve over one cardiac cycle: (S-D)/mean velocity. This index has an advantage when analyzing complex waveforms that have absent or reverse flow during parts of the diastole. However, it requires a computer program that can calculate the area under the curve. Whether the computer outlines the maximum frequency envelope or whether it is done manually, some degree of error is involved that is probably greater than that for other techniques. When uterine circulation resistance is high, the uterine artery waveform has shorter upstroke and downstroke times and an early diastolic notch. Infrequently, there is absent early diastolic flow or reverse flow of the main uterine artery. These characteristics can be incorporated in the waveform analysis if one uses the PI but not when other, simpler methods are utilized.

The other, simpler forms of uterine waveform analysis are the S/D ratio (or A/B ratio) and the resistance index (RI), or Pourcelot ratio [(S-D)/S]. All that is required here is measurements of peak systole and end diastole. The main problem with the S/D (A/B) ratio is that it becomes infinity when there is no or reversed end-diastolic velocity. The other obstacle is its nonparametric distribution at high values, which could be a problem because there are many occasions in the presence of severe preeclampsia where uterine artery S/D ratios are greater than 5.0. Nonparametric analysis is required when using the S/D (A/B) ratio [21]. To reiterate, these simple techniques would not be affected by the presence of a waveform early diastolic notch. Regardless of any peculiarities inherent in each type of waveform index, none has been proved to offer a clinical advantage over the other.

The general principles of Doppler indices are discussed in depth in Chap. 4.

Normal and Abnormal Development of Uterine Artery Doppler Waveform

In the nonpregnant state the uterine artery waveform exhibits high pulsatility with a rapid rise and fall in frequency shifts during systole, an early diastolic notch, and low diastolic shifts. Schulman et al. [22], using transvaginal continuous-wave Doppler revealed high S/D ratios during the proliferative phase of the menstrual cycle (12.9±4.4, mean±standard deviation) that dropped significantly during the secretory phase (7.2±3.2; *p*=0.003) (Fig. 16.8). Scholtes et al. [23], using transvaginal pulsed Doppler found no significant difference in the PIs between the two uterine arteries, with mean PI values between 2.9 and 3.2. They found no correlation between the PI and stage of menstrual cycle. Long et al. [24], using transabdominal pulsed Doppler found similar results, with PI values of 3.25±0.83. They also reported no difference between the uterine arteries and no correlation with the menstrual cycle. Thaler and colleagues [25], using transvaginal pulsed Doppler, obtained S/D ratios of 5.3±1.1 in a group of 27 nonpregnant women (Fig. 16.9). The difference in the data of Schulman et al. and those of subsequent investigators is probably due to the problem of using continuous-wave Doppler sonography when trying to determine if a waveform showing the characteristics of high resistance is from the uterine artery.

Pregnancy results in marked changes in the uterine artery waveform. Schulman et al., using abdominal and vaginal continuous-wave Doppler ultrasonography, showed striking increases in uterine artery compliance between weeks 8 and 16 of gestation (Fig. 16.8) [22]. Increases in compliance continued

until 26 weeks but in a less dramatic fashion. From 26 weeks onward the S/D ratios were similar, whether they were obtained abdominally or vaginally, and did not change in value throughout the remainder of pregnancy. The diastolic notch disappeared by 20–26 weeks' gestation. Thus the full evolution of the uterine artery waveform may not be complete until 26 weeks. These investigators defined abnormal uterine artery waveforms as those with S/D ratios greater than or equal to 2.7 (the average of the right and left uterine arteries) or persistence of the early diastolic notch.

Deutinger et al. [26] repeated Schulman's work using transvaginal pulsed Doppler ultrasonography and reported similar results except for a more gradual, smoother drop in S/D ratios during the first 14–16 weeks of gestation. Their mean averaged S/D values for each trimester were 5.5, 2.9, and 2.1. Deutinger et al. believed the S/D ratios plateaued at 24 weeks.

Thaler et al. [25] followed up using transvaginal pulsed Doppler (Fig. 16.9). Again, during the first 14–16 weeks the drop in S/D ratios was not as rapid as those obtained with continuous-wave Doppler ultrasound. During the first 26 weeks' gestation the S/D ratios were lower and had narrower standard deviations than did the continuous-wave data of Schulman et al. Thaler et al. also showed that the S/D values do

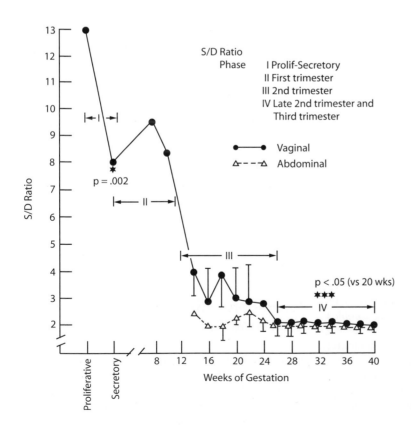

Fig. 16.8. Uterine artery complicance during the menstrual cycle and throughout pregnancy (means±SD). *Circles* represent measurements through the vaginal fornices; *triangles* represent measurements across the abdomen. Each value represents the average between the left and right arteries. *S/D* systolic/diastolic. (Reprinted from [44] with permission)

Fig. 16.9. Systolic/diastolic (*S/D*) flow velocity ratios in the uterine artery in the nonpregnant state and during weeks of gestation. (Reprinted from [28], with permission)

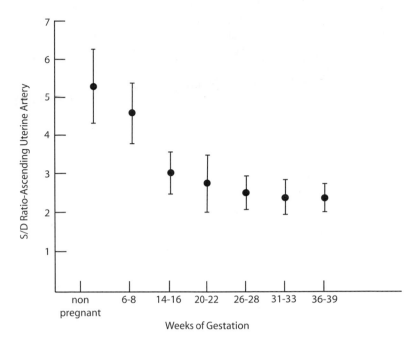

not plateau until 26 weeks. Thus the uterine artery waveform transforms rapidly to one of lower pulsatility during the first 16 weeks and shows continual but less dramatic increases in compliance until 26 weeks' gestation, by which time it should lose its diastolic notch. From 26 weeks onward the waveform has a stable appearance.

Pearce et al. [27], using a pulsed duplex Doppler technique, portrayed similar evolutions in the RI from 16 weeks onward. They noted that there was increased compliance in the placental (versus nonplacental) uterine artery. Trudinger et al. [28] studied the subplacental vascular bed with continuous-wave Doppler ultrasound. They were probably insonating the arcuate and radial arteries, and they reported a progressive drop in S/D ratios. Their values were lower than those of other investigators, however, because they were interrogating distal branches of the uterine circulation whereas the configuration of the main uterine artery waveform is affected by the summation of resistances of the entire vascular tree. They did not report a notch in any subplacental waveform.

A lesson learned from these studies is that continuous-wave Doppler ultrasound is probably unreliable for studying the uterine artery in the nonpregnant state and up to 14–16 weeks' pregnancy, as pattern recognition is used to identify the uterine artery. It is not until 14–16 weeks' gestation that there is a generous diastolic component to the waveform, thereby clearly distinguishing it from waveforms of other pelvic vessels.

A number of other investigators have looked at the early development of the uterine artery (during the first 18 weeks' gestation) using continuous-wave, pulsed-wave, and color Doppler techniques [29–32]. Regardless of the equipment or waveform index used, all showed a significant, smooth, progressive decrease in waveform indices (Fig. 16.10). Using transvaginal color Doppler sonography, Jurkovic et al. [30] and Juaniaux et al. [31] showed uterine artery mean RIs decreasing from 0.80 at 8 weeks to around 0.63 at 17 weeks; and the mean PI of 2.0 at 8 weeks dropped to nearly 1.3 at 18 weeks' gestation. Their variation around the mean was narrower than those of other investigators, probably because they used color Doppler ultrasonography as the method of vessel identification.

Uterine Artery Diameter and Volume Flow

Estimations of volume flow of the uterine arteries would be an ideal method to determine the state of this circulation. However, to determine volume flow, knowledge of the angle of incidence and vessel diameter is required. Any error when estimating vessel diameter becomes squared, and small errors when determining the angle of incidence result in even larger errors in the velocity calculations. Estimates of volume flow are accurate when the angle of incidence is zero and the vessel of interest is straight. Such conditions are difficult to achieve when studying the main uterine arteries. Volume flow assessments of the uterine artery are confounded further by the abundant collateral circulation.

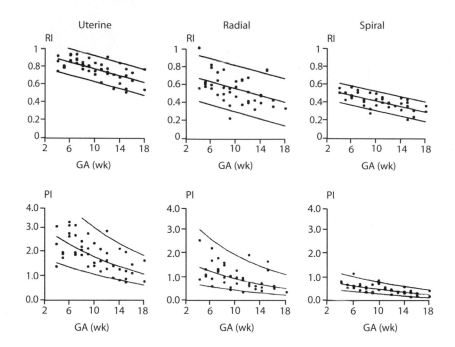

Fig. 16.10. Individual values and reference ranges (mean and 90% confidence interval) of the resistance index (*RI*) and pulsatility index (*PI*) in the utero-placental circulation with gestational age (*GA*). Both indices decreased significantly with gestation in all three arteries. (Reprinted from [30] with permission)

Three investigative groups have reported their data on uterine volume flow. Thaler et al. [25] used the transvaginal approach to study the left ascending uterine artery. They reported a mean volume flow rate of 94.5 ml/min before pregnancy, which increased to a mean of 342 ml/min during late pregnancy (Fig. 16.11); it represented a 3.5-fold increase. The standard deviation about the mean volume flow during the last trimester was reasonable at ±50 ml/min. The mean diameter was 1.6 mm before pregnancy and increased to 3.7 mm at term, which represented more than a twofold increase (Fig. 16.12). Thaler et al. did not see a significant difference in volume flow between the two uterine arteries in a group of 32 women who were studied up to 26 weeks' gestation.

Palmer et al. [33], with transabdominal pulsed Doppler ultrasonography and without the color Doppler technique, reported remarkably similar results for vessel diameter and volume flow measurements. The uterine artery diameter doubled by week 21 (from 1.4±0.1 to 2.8±0.2 mm; $p < 0.05$), did not change between weeks 21 and 30 (2.9±0.1 mm), and increased between weeks 30 and 36 (to 3.4±0.2 mm). Uterine artery volume flow was approximately 312 ml/min by 36 weeks' gestation. These investigations showed that increases in uterine artery flow during the first 21 weeks of pregnancy were due equally to changes in uterine artery diameter and mean velocity, whereas the rise during late pregnancy (30–36 weeks) was mainly due to increases in mean flow velocity. Their use of two pulsed Doppler devices to separately measure uterine artery diameter and

mean velocity and then combine the measurements to determine volume flow is not technically sound.

Bower and Campbell [34] estimated uterine volume flow using the transabdominal approach. They found marked differences in volume flow between the placental and nonplacental uterine arteries, with values of approximately 400 ml/min and 290 ml/min, respectively, at 42 weeks' gestation. Although their

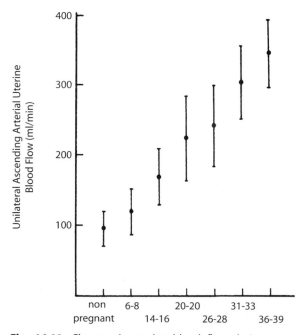

Fig. 16.11. Changes in uterine blood flow during pregnancy. (Reprinted from [28] with permission)

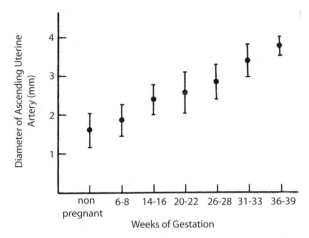

Fig. 16.12. Diameter of ascending uterine artery at various gestational ages. (Reprinted from [28] with permission)

mean volume flow values were similar to those of Thaler et al. and Palmer et al., there was great variation around the mean, and their measurements were skewed. Some of their volume recordings of the placental uterine were greater than or equal to 1 l/min – readings that were not seen in the studies of Thaler et al. or Palmer et al.

These data show that changes in the placental spiral arteries do not solely explain the development of the uterine circulation, and that the increase in flow is in part due to hypertrophy of the larger uterine vessels. Moreover, the preliminary data show that volume flow estimates of the uterine artery may be more reproducible with the transvaginal approach. Additional work is requested to assess its association with perinatal outcome and the potential for clinical usefulness.

Uterine Artery Maximum and Mean Flow Velocity

Maximum and mean velocities of the uterine artery in the nonpregnant and pregnant state have been studied. Jurkovic et al. [30], using transvaginal color Doppler sonography, showed a significant increase in maximum peak systolic velocity, from approximately 53 cm/s at 6 weeks' to 140 cm/s at 18 weeks' gestation. Jauniaux et al. [31], using the same technique, found almost identical changes in peak systolic velocities. At 10 weeks' the peak velocity of 68.0 ± 8.5 cm/s increased to 74.0 ± 6.5 cm/s at 13 weeks' gestation. At 14 weeks gestation there was an abrupt significant increase to 117 ± 7 cm/s ($p = 0.005$). A slow increase continued until 17 weeks (127.0 ± 9.3 cm/s). During these time periods both investigators noted decreasing impedance in the uterine, radial, and spiral ar-

teries (Fig. 16.10). They believed that it supported the hypothesis that endovascular trophoblastic invasion of the spiral arteries reduces resistance. Also, the progressive fall in resistance from the uterine artery to the radial and spiral arteries was due to an increase in branching and cross-sectional area of the circulation.

Palmer et al. [33], using transabdominal pulsed Doppler sonography without color flow mapping, was able to insonate the uterine artery as it branched off the internal iliac artery. They recorded a mean flow velocity of 8.4 ± 2.2 cm/s in the nonpregnant state. At 21 weeks of pregnancy the mean flow velocity rose to 38.5 ± 4.9 cm/s and continued to increase to 46.6 ± 3.4 cm/s at 30 weeks and 61.4 ± 3.0 cm/s at 36 weeks of pregnancy. Bower and Campbell [34], using transabdominal pulsed Doppler sonography with color flow mapping, obtained signals from the uterine artery as it crossed medially to the external iliac artery. Their measurements of mean flow velocity at similar gestational ages were lower, with large variation around the means. Mean velocities in the placental uterine artery were greater than those in the nonplacental uterine artery. Their data were also markedly skewed.

These data show that maximal and mean flow velocities of the uterine artery increase throughout gestation. The velocity data during early pregnancy [30, 31] were remarkably similar, showed reasonable variation, and were obtained by the technique that should be best suited for these measurements (transvaginal pulsed Doppler sonography with color flow mapping). However, the data need to be reproduced by others. Mean and maximal velocities from midpregnancy onward must be studied with the same technique. The method Palmer et al. used to detect signals from the uterine artery as it branches off the internal iliac artery deep in the pelvis (transabdominal approach with color flow mapping) is difficult, and the transabdominal approach of Bower and Campbell results in considerable variation. The clinical usefulness of such data must also be explored.

Uterine Artery Waveform Notch

The uterine artery Doppler waveform has an early diastolic notch in the nonpregnant state, and it often persists in the pregnant state until weeks 20–26. What constitutes an early diastolic notch during pregnancy has never been defined. Campbell et al. [35] defined a "true" abnormal notch during pregnancy as a deceleration of at least 50 Hz below the maximum diastolic velocities after 20 weeks. They believed that it is rarely seen on the placental side beyond that point of pregnancy. Fleischer et al. [36] thought that it is a normal finding until week 26 of gestation. Later, Thaler et al. [37] identified a group of women who had both systolic and diastolic notches in the uterine artery waveform and demonstrated that perinatal outcome was worse than when there was a diastolic notch only (Fig. 16.13). Retention of the early diastolic notch is thought to represent persistence of the inherent total high impedance of the uterine artery circulation. It has been identified in waveforms of the main uterine artery and its most proximal branches.

Fleischer et al. [36] were the first to note the importance of the uterine notch in their study of 71 women with hypertensive disorders of pregnancy. Ninety percent (27 of 30) of women who developed preeclampsia or chronic hypertension with superimposed preeclampsia had a uterine waveform notch. When normal pregnancy outcome was defined as delivery at 37 weeks or later or a birth weight of 2500 g or more, the uterine artery notch had better sensitivity (93%), specificity (91%), positive predictive value (87%), and negative predictive value (95%) compared to the mean arterial blood pressure, creatine clearance, uric acid level, and uterine S/D ratios.

Thaler et al. [37] evaluated a group of 140 hypertensive pregnant women. Of 39 women with diastolic or systolic notches (or both) in the uterine artery waveform, 82% (32 of 39) had pregnancy-related hypertensive complications. Hypertensive women with uterine systolic and diastolic notches had higher waveform indices of both uterine and umbilical arteries, higher diastolic and systolic blood pressures, and worse perinatal outcomes than those without notches (Tables 16.1 and 16.2). When umbilical artery resistance was normal and both uterine arteries had elevated resistance indices, the group with the uterine waveform notch had worse perinatal outcomes (Table 16.3). When the uterine artery and umbilical artery waveforms were abnormal, the presence of the

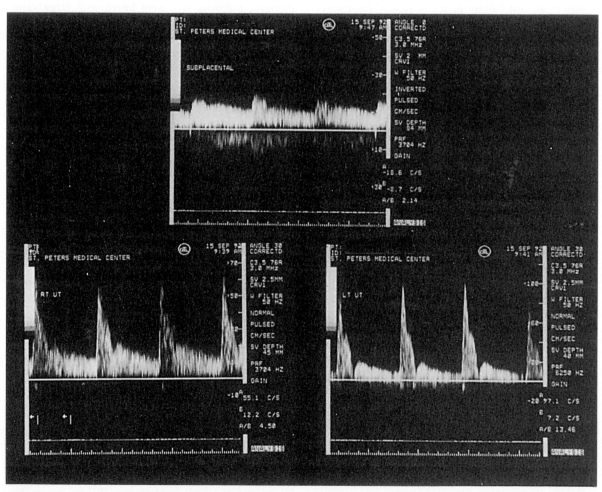

Fig. 16.13. Subplacental (*top*), right uterine (*bottom left*), and left uterine (*bottom right*) waveforms in a chronically hypertensive pregnant woman at 22 weeks' gestation. Both uterine arteries have systolic and diastolic notches. The placenta was central and posterior. At 26 weeks' gestation she presented with a fetal demise after an arrest of fetal growth at 19 weeks

Table 16.1. Resistance indexes and blood pressures in hypertensive pregnant patients with and without a systolic or diastolic notch (from [37] with permission)

Parameter	Notch absent (n=101)	Diastolic notch (n=25)	p	Systolic notch (n=14)	p
Resistance index					
Left uterine artery	0.64±0.1	0.77±0.1	<0.0001	0.78±0.07	<0.0001
Right uterine artery	0.65±0.1	0.75±0.09	<0.01	0.78±0.07	<0.0001
Umbilical artery	0.66±0.1	0.74±0.1	<0.01	0.78±0.1	<0.0001
Blood pressure (mmHg)					
Systolic	140.3±14.8	146±17.7	NS	153±20	<0.003
Diastolic	91.4±9.3	99.0±8.9	<0.006	98±7.9	<0.004

NS, not significant. Data are presented as means±SD.

Table 16.2. Pregnancy outcomes in hypertensive pregnant patients with and without a systolic or diastolic notch in the uterine artery flow velocity waveform (from [37] with permission)

Parameter	Notch absent (n=101)	Diastolic notch (n=25)	p	Systolic notch (n=14)	p
Delivery (weeks)	37.6±2.48	34±3.5	<0.001	33.4±2.8	<0.001
Perinatal mortality (%)	5	12		14.3	
Fetal growth retardation (%)	12.9	64	<0.00001	64.3	<0.00003
Abnormal FHR in labor (%)	13.9	28		42.9	<0.025
Cesarean for fetal distress (%)	29.7	56	<0.03	64.3	<0.025
Apgar score <7 at 5 min (%)	6.9	16		25.6	<0.04
NICU >48 h (%)	16.8	52	<0.0006	71.5	<0.00003

FHR, fetal heart rate; NICU, neonatal intensive care unit.

Table 16.3. Pregnancy outcomes in hypertensive pregnant patients with an abnormally elevated resistance index in both uterine arteries[a] (from [37], with permission)

Parameter	Normal umbilical artery RI		Abnormal umbilical artery RI	
	Notch absent (n=11)	Notch present (n=8)	Notch absent (n=13)	Notch present (n=19)
Delivery (weeks)	38.2±1.4	35.7±2	36.3±3	33.4±2.8
Perinatal mortality (%)	0	12.5	0	21.1
Fetal growth retardation (%)	0	62.5*	15.4	73.7**
Abnormal FHR during labor (%)	0	37.5	23.1	36.8
Cesarean for fetal distress (%)	27.3	50	46.2	52.6
Apgar score <7 at 5 min (%)	0	37.5	7.7	21.2
NICU >48 h (%)	0	62.5*	30.8	63.2
Resistance index				
Left uterine artery	0.72±0.05	0.76±0.09	0.72±0.08	0.79±0.07
Right uterine artery	0.72±0.04	0.78±0.07	0.72±0.04	0.76±0.06
Umbilical artery	0.57±0.06	0.60±0.04	0.75±0.06	0.78±0.09

FHR, fetal heart rate; NICU, neonatal intensive care unit; RI, resistance index.
[a] Based on resistance index in the umbilical artery and presence or absence of notch in the uterine artery.
* p<0.005; ** p<0.002.

uterine notch portended a worse perinatal outcome (Table 16.3). When the umbilical RI was normal and there was no notch in the uterine artery waveform, perinatal outcome was similar whether the uterine artery RI was normal or abnormal (Table 16.4). Thaler et al. clearly showed that the uterine artery systolic and diastolic notches were the better predictor of perinatal outcome than the RI alone. Aristidou et al. [38] undertook uterine artery screening in women with elevated maternal serum α-fetoprotein levels, and they too noted that the uterine artery notch was a good predictor of poor perinatal outcome.

Kofinas et al. [41] believed that they could define placental location by ultrasonography. They found that in both normal and hypertensive pregnancies with unilateral placentas the S/D ratio of the placental uterine artery was significantly lower than that of the contralateral artery (1.73 ± 0.35 versus 2.46 ± 0.73; $p < 0.001$, and 2.38 ± 1.01 versus 4.04 ± 1.77, $p = 0.0012$). Ito et al. [42] and Oosterhof and Aarnoudse [43] found the same placental effect on the ipsilateral uterine artery, but in addition Ito et al. [41] observed that the lower the placental site, the lower the uterine waveform index.

Kofinas et al. [45] reexamined the relation between placental location and uterine artery velocimetry and found that perinatal outcome correlated best with the placental uterine artery; the mean index using both uterine arteries had the next best condition, and the nonplacental uterine artery was the poorest predictor. As they pointed out, the placental uterine artery perfuses most of the placental bed and the nonplacental uterine artery primarily perfuses nonplacental myometrial vessels.

It is clear from these studies that the unilateral placenta results in greater erosion and recruitment of the subplacental spiral arteries of the ipsilateral uterine circulation. The question is whether placental location is essential when evaluating uterine artery Doppler waveforms.

Doppler Waveforms of the Arcuate, Radial, and Spiral Arteries

Color flow mapping has allowed us to interrogate specific sites of the uterine circulation. Several investigators have demonstrated a progressive drop in impedance in all aspects of the uterine circulation, from the main uterine arteries to the spiral arteries, as pregnancy advances (Fig. 16.10) [30–32, 46]. Also, there is a drop in resistance from the proximal to the distal branches of the uterine circulation, the uterine artery having the highest impedance and the spiral arteries the least (Fig. 16.18). These studies are important physiologic observations whose clinical value has yet to be realized.

If one considers the subplacental spiral artery lesions identified in the presence of preeclampsia, essential hypertension, or fetal intrauterine growth restriction (IUGR), the subplacental vessels seem to be the ideal site of Doppler sampling to detect abnormal resistance in the uteroplacental circulation. Trudinger et al. [28], using continuous-wave Doppler sonography, was the first to obtain signals from the arcuate and radial arteries. However, they detected increases in the S/D (A/B) ratios in some but not all high-risk pregnancies. Some subplacental radial and arcuate arteries are normal in the face of significant pathology in others.

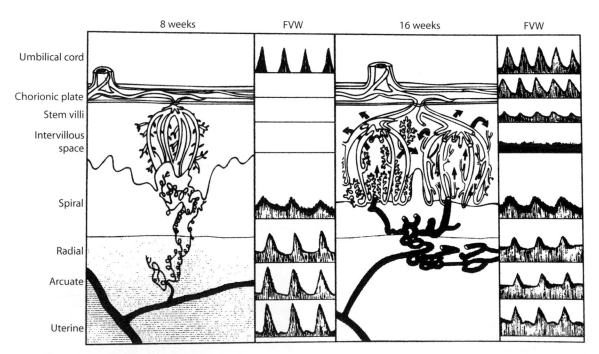

Fig. 16.18. Flow velocity waveforms (*FVW*) obtained from both placental circulations at 8 and 16 weeks' gestation, respectively. Note the progressive increase in diastolic flow of the uteroplacental waveforms from the uterine artery to the spiral artery and as gestational age advances. (From [31] with permission)

Voigt and Becker [47] studied 58 women with pregnancy-induced hypertension ($n = 49$) or fetal IUGR using pulsed Doppler sonography of the subplacental arcuate arteries. They correlated the arcuate artery PI with placental bed biopsy findings. There were marked increases in the subplacental arcuate artery PI when the placental bed biopsies were pathologic.

Judging from these studies it appears that using information from sites other than the main uterine artery for clinical purposes requires color and pulsed Doppler sonography. Even with this technology it remains difficult to differentiate the radial, arcuate, and spiral artery waveforms. The difference in the main uterine waveform indices between normal and pathologic pregnancies is probably greater than at other sites. This difference allows clearer distinction between normal and abnormal waveform index values. Measurement of the main uterine artery may be more reproducible and allow standardized longitudinal follow-up. It seems that studying the main uterine artery waveform, a reflector of total subplacental resistance, remains the most clinically important parameter.

Effect of Pharmacologic Agents and Epidural Anesthesia on Uterine Artery Waveforms

Uterine Doppler velocimetry has been used to study the effects of drugs on the uterine circulation. Nifedipine [48], dihydralazine [49], indomethacin [50], oxymetazoline [51], pseudoephedrine [52], smoking [53], and nicotine gum [53] have not been shown to alter uterine waveform indices during pregnancy. Estrogen and progesterone hormonal replacement therapy after 6–10 weeks or on a chronic basis and magnesium sulfate therapy for tocolysis have been shown to lower uterine artery resistance [54]. Magnesium sulfate was found either to have no effect [55] or to lower [56] resistance. Methyldopa had no effect on the uterine artery PI [57]. The effects of several β-blockers have been looked at with varying results. In one study propranolol had no effect, but pindolol decreased resistance [58]. Atenolol was found to increase the arcuate artery PI [59]. The latter study must be reproduced, as it has important implications for management of the pregnant hypertensive woman.

There is evidence that preeclampsia is associated with a deficiency of prostacyclin, which could lead to generalized vasoconstriction. Therefore prostacyclin infusion seems to be a potential form of treatment for preeclampsia. Jouppila et al. [60] intravenously infused prostacyclin in 13 preeclamptic women. It resulted in significant decreases in maternal blood pressure and a rise in maternal plasma 6-ketoprostaglandin $F_{1\alpha}$. However, there was no effect on uterine artery flow when studied with the intravenous xenon 133 isotope clearance method. This study would be worth repeating using Doppler technology.

Uterine artery waveforms have been studied after infusion of angiotensin II. Erkkola and Pirhonen [61] used color and pulsed Doppler sonography to study the uterine artery between 24 and 26 weeks' gestation and found increases in the S/D ratio after angiotensin II infusion (1.6 ± 0.1 versus 2.09 ± 0.29, $p < 0.001$). This increase was not affected by placental location. Interestingly, the increases in uterine artery resistance followed the increases in blood pressure, providing evidence of a differential response in the uterine circulation versus the systemic vasculature. In a follow-up report they compared the uterine artery response to angiotensin II infusion in normotensive and hypertensive pregnant women [62]. The uterine S/D ratios increased equally in the two groups but the increase was faster and recovery slower in the hypertensive group. Jones and Sanchez-Ramos [63] reported no changes in uterine artery S/D ratios using continuous-wave Doppler ultrasonography in nine normotensive pregnant women.

The effects of epidural anesthesia on uterine artery resistance have been studied using Doppler velocimetry. Four studies using anesthetic agents with and without epinephrine showed no change in uterine artery resistance in normal, term, laboring patients or in those prior to elective cesarean section [64–67].

Ramos-Santos et al. [68] evaluated the effects of epidural anesthesia in normal and hypertensive patients in active term labor. The mean uterine artery S/D ratios did not change in normotensive and chronically hypertensive patients but fell significantly in the term mildly preeclamptic patients – to values similar to those of the normotensive group. Both placental and nonplacental uterine artery S/D ratios fell to values seen in the normotensive group. The uterine S/D ratios in the chronic hypertensive group, which were similar to those of the preeclamptic group, did not change after administration of epidural anesthesia. The authors accepted this finding as evidence of underlying vascular disease. This study demonstrates the benefits of epidural anesthesia in the presence of mild preeclampsia at term. The study must be reproduced and involve women with preeclampsia of varying severity.

uterine artery notching which may result in the highest positive predictive value for early-onset preeclampsia. However, as pointed out by Harrington et al., these trials may have to await further refinements in uterine artery Doppler waveform analysis or combining uterine artery Doppler results with biochemical testing to improve screening efficacy. Other variables were differences in patient medical background, parity, socio-economic background, race, prior hypertensive medication use, and timing of screening and initiation of aspirin therapy.

We propose that studies performed in the immediate future should involve multiple centers, to achieve appropriate numbers of outcome events, with screening performed at 18–20 weeks' gestation and bilateral uterine artery notching as the definition of abnormal testing. Doppler reevaluation at 22–24 weeks' gestation should be performed and as in the Harrington et al. trial, aspirin therapy should be terminated if the results are normal. This would leave us with four groups to analyze based on the Doppler results at 22–24 weeks' gestation: aspirin therapy terminated secondary to normal Doppler results, aspirin with abnormal Doppler studies, and placebo with normal and abnormal Doppler studies. Proposed outcomes would be the early onset of preeclampsia (<34 weeks), gestational age at delivery when preeclampsia was the indication for delivery, the degree of severity of preeclampsia, and the incidence and severity (<10th percentile or <3rd percentile) of IUGR. Survival analysis of gestational age at birth would be interesting to determine whether, regardless of indications for delivery, aspirin therapy results in significantly greater pregnancy duration.

Part of the pathophysiology of preeclampsia is endothelial dysfunction, which increases the sensitivity to vasoconstricting agents leading to vasospasm [95]. Free radicals are thought to injure the maternal vascular endothelium and promote endothelial cell dysfunction. Therefore, antioxidant therapy has the potential to prevent and/or modify preeclampsia. Chambers et al. [96] recently showed *in vivo* reversal of endothelial dysfunction in preeclampsia with ascorbic acid. These results require confirmation from larger randomized clinical trials.

Nitric oxide is produced by the endothelium of vessels and is a well-known vasodilator and platelet aggregation inhibitor. In preeclamptic women, inhibition of nitric oxide synthase and cyclooxygenase attenuates endothelial-derived relaxation. It has been suggested by several investigators that since preeclampsia is associated with decreased function of nitric oxide, introducing a nitric oxide agent, such as glyceryl dinitrate, would reduce the severity or prevalence of preeclampsia. Grunewald et al. [97] performed intravenous infusions of nitroglycerin in 12 severe preeclamptics. This resulted in a significant reduction in maternal blood pressure; however, the PI of the uterine arteries did not change significantly [1.23 (95% CI 1.01–1.61) versus 1.30 (95% CI 1.01–1.88)]. Thaler et al. [98] studied 18 women with low-risk pregnancy at 17–24 weeks' gestation, who were given a single 5 mg dose of sublingual isosorbide dinitrate. Blood flow velocity waveforms in the ascending uterine artery were measured by pulsed color Doppler ultrasound before and after the medication was administered. Maternal blood pressure and heart rate were also monitored. The S/D ratio in the uterine artery decreased from 4.83 (95% CI 3.99–5.56) to a nadir of 4.02 at 10 min (95% CI 3.41–4.63, $p < 0.001$). This study suggests a potential benefit of nitric oxide therapy.

Lees et al. [99] identified 40 healthy normotensive women with bilateral uterine artery Doppler waveform notching at 24–26 weeks' gestation and randomized them to transdermal glyceryl trinitrate (GTN) 5 mg/day patch versus placebo patch for 10 weeks or until delivery. There was no statistically significant difference in maternal systolic and diastolic blood pressure, mean uteine artery RI, or the rates of preeclampsia or IUGR. However, there was a significant increase in women who delivered at term an AGA infant without evidence of preeclampsia in the GTN group in comparison to the placebo group [15/21 (71%) vs 5/19 (26%), $p = 0.004$, hazard ratio 0.267 (95% CI 0.102, 0.701), 73% reduction in hazard]. Taken collectively these studies suggest that nitric oxide donor therapy needs further investigation.

Medical Conditions and Uterine Artery Doppler Velocimetry

Uterine Artery Doppler Velocimetry in IUGR Fetuses and Hypertensive Disorders of Pregnancy

The findings reported in the original article of Campbell et al. [10] in 1983 on uteroplacental Doppler velocimetry – that women with abnormal uterine waveforms had a higher frequency of proteinuric hypertension, poor fetal growth, and fetal hypoxia – inspired a wave of observational studies [28, 35–37, 39, 44, 45, 87, 100–107]. In addition to confirming the work of Campbell et al., these studies found that a significant number of women with hypertension or IUGR fetuses could also have abnormal umbilical artery Doppler waveforms alone or in combination with abnormal uterine artery waveforms. It became clear that a thorough investigation of hypertension during pregnancy and IUGR would require analysis of both uterine and umbilical circulations.

The results of these studies are best summarized by the work of Ducey and colleagues [86], who classified hypertension according to four vascular patterns (Table 16.9). The most common vascular pattern in hypertensive pregnancies is defined by normal uterine and umbilical velocimetry. Although most of these women had chronic hypertension, preeclampsia and pregnancy-induced hypertension also occurred with this pattern. Regardless of the clinical diagnosis, the perinatal outcome was similar to that of a normal obstetric population. These data support optimal medical management of hypertensive women who display this velocimetry pattern rather than aggressive intervention for fear of fetal risk.

The next most common category was abnormal uterine and umbilical artery velocimetry. The authors hypothesized that this group lacks endovascular trophoblastic invasion of the myometrial portion of the subplacental spiral arteries. The women had the worst perinatal outcome and accounted for all the perinatal deaths in the study. They and their fetuses experienced severe early disease. Most of the preeclamptic women and a significant number of the women with pregnancy-induced hypertension had this vasculopathy. For optimal outcome these patients must be identified early, and both mother and fetus require intensive surveillance. The potential for early delivery is great, with many requiring operative delivery. Consideration should be given to using preventive or modifying medication, such as aspirin.

The next two categories consisted of women with isolated deficiencies of either the uterine arteries or umbilical arteries. Surprisingly, the less common of the two was abnormal uterine artery flow only. The Doppler pattern of abnormal umbilical flow belies the popular concept that the placental ischemia seen with pregnancy hypertension is the result of poor maternal perfusion. The perinatal outcome is poorer than when there is abnormal uterine flow only. The fetus is protected by the umbilical artery circulation, and it adapts well to reductions in uterine artery flow. Guzman et al. [108] also described pregnancy-induced hypertension associated with abnormal umbilical flow, only with greater consequences to the fetus than the mother.

When viewing the results of all the observational studies, a pattern emerges wherein abnormalities in uterine artery flow correlate best with maternal complications. Moreover, the state of the umbilical artery circulation is more predictive than that of the uterine artery circulation in terms of fetal-neonatal outcome.

Uterine artery Doppler velocimetry has been shown to correlate very well with pregnancy outcome in women with chronic hypertension. Caruso et al. [109] studied 42 women with chronic hypertension and showed increased incidences of preeclampsia

Table 16.9. Velocimetry for hypertension and pregnancy (reproduced from [86] with permission)

Parameter	Normal flow velocity in uterine artery		Abnormal flow velocity in uterine arery	
	Nl. umb. (n=66)	Abnl. umb. (n=27)	Nl. umb. (n=12)	Abnl. umb. (m=31
Maternal data				
Age (years)	29±7	27±6	24±7	27±6
Nullipara (%)	57	52	80	63
MAP, 2nd trimester (mmHg)	97±12	95±13	105±21	96±21
Abnormal platelets (%)	0	26*	13	0
Uric acid (mg/dl)	5.6±1.1	6.5±2.2	6.0±1.4	6.5±1.5*
Proteinuria (%)	24	71**	75**	86***
Uterine artery S/D ratio	2±0.3	2.1±0.3	3.4±9.0***	4.1±1.5***
Fetal/neonatal data				
Birth weight (g)	3,261±522	2,098±811***	2,464±722***	1,627±697***
Gestational age (weeks)	39±2	35.7±3.2***	36.3±3.0**	33.3±2.7***
Delivery <37 weeks (%)	11	61***	67***	84***
SGA (%)	2	29**	17	51***
C/S fetal distress (%)	8	39**	8	62***
NICU (%)	12	68***	50*	89***
Umbilical artery S/D ratio	2.4±0.3	4.2±1.1***	2.5±0.3	4.6±1.1***
Clinical diagnosis (%)				
Chronic hypertension (n=43)	65***	23	5	7
PIH (n=34)	59***	15	6	21
Preeclampsia (n=51)	20	24	16	41

MAP, mean arterial pressure; Nl. umb., normal flow velocity in umbilical artery; Abnl. umb., abnormal flow velocity in umbilical artery; S/D, systolic/diastolic; SGA, small for gestational age; C/S, cesarean section; NICU, neonatal intensive care unit; PIH, pregnancy-induced hypertension.
* $p < 0.05$; ** $p < 0.01$; *** $p < 0.001$.

are limited to the decidual portion of the spiral arteries during the first trimester. During the early second trimester a new wave of endovascular trophoblast migration penetrates as far as the myometrial portion of the spiral arteries [2]. The second wave of trophoblastic migration is complete in most women by 20 weeks' gestation [3]. Normal uterine blood supply to the placenta is shown in Fig. 17.1. The physiological changes are functionally complete by 17 weeks as was demonstrated by measuring spiral artery blood flow using color Doppler ultrasound in the second trimester [4].

By 19 weeks' gestation the coiling of the spiral arteries disappears [5]. This event is probably due to stretching of the uterine wall, as the shape of the uterus changes from spheroidal to cylindrical as it grows [6].

The disappearance of musculoelastic tissue from the decidual and myometrial spiral arteries allows them to attain a substantial increase in diameter. A 30-fold increase in diameter, compared to that of the nonpregnant state, has been described [7]. The physiologic correlate of these structural alterations is a reduction in vascular resistance in the spiral arteries and increased uteroplacental flow rates throughout gestation [8]. This change has also been verified by radioisotopic techniques [9–11] and Doppler flow studies [12–14].

In normal pregnancy the trophoblast invades all spiral arteries in both the decidual endometrium and the myometrium. A defective maternal vascular response at the time of placentation is found in pregnancies complicated by preeclampsia and in a proportion of those with small-for-gestational-age (SGA) fetuses [15, 16]. In those pregnancies the vascular changes in the spiral arteries are restricted to the de-

cidual segments or are totally absent. The arterial vascular response may be partial, so only a portion of the spiral arteries undergo normal "physiologic changes", whereas others are not affected by endovascular trophoblast and remain in the same state as in the nonpregnant uterus. It is believed that a defective maternal response to placentation is due to failure of the second wave of intravascular trophoblastic migration [17]. The myometrial segments of the spiral arteries are unaltered in their musculoelastic architecture and so are responsive to vasomotor influences (e.g., vasoactive peptides). Figure 17.2 demonstrates abnormal uterine blood supply to the placenta secondary to abnormal placentation.

Intraluminal trophoblast is a normal finding, then, during the first and second trimesters of normal pregnancy, where it plays a role in establishing placentation [18]. A defective interaction of trophoblast and uterine tissue, well established in preeclampsia and some forms of fetal growth restriction, may be due to immunologic maladaptation [18, 19]. Disturbance of trophoblastic invasion during early pregnancy is frequently associated with renewed trophoblastic migration during the third trimester [16, 20]. The luminal lining in the uteroplacental arteries remains trophoblastic and not endothelial [20]. The disrupted endothelium may be responsible for endothelial cell dysfunction, thought to be of pathogenetic importance in preeclampsia [21]. In addition, many of the affected vessels demonstrate necrotizing vascular lesions – deposition of fibrinoid material and adjacent foam cell invasion – a process also termed atherosis [22].

Hemodynamic studies using radioisotope clearance values [10, 11], dynamic placental scintigraphy [23],

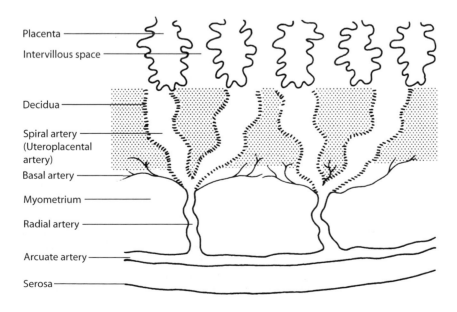

Placenta
Intervillous space

Decidua

Spiral artery
(Uteroplacental
artery)
Basal artery

Myometrium

Radial artery

Arcuate artery

Serosa

Fig. 17.1. Normal blood supply to the placenta. Note the termination of radial arteries each into two spiral arteries that have been physiologically converted to uteroplacental arteries (*dotted areas*). (Reprinted from [16] with permission)

Fig. 17.2. Abnormal blood supply to the placenta. Physiologic changes (*dotted areas*) in some decidual segments of spiral arteries are absent. Myometrial segments are shown without physiologic changes as in preeclampsia or some cases of fetal growth retardation. (Reprinted from [16] with permission)

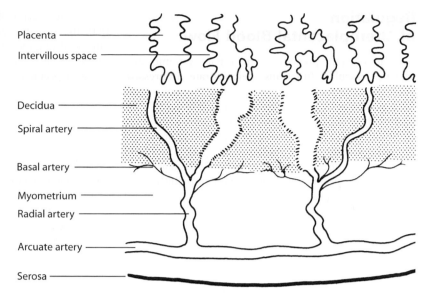

Fig. 17.3. Pulsatility indices (PI) of uteroplacental arteries prior to delivery plotted against the normal reference curve (3rd, 50th, and 90th percentiles). Cases with normal placental bed biopsies are marked by *open* and *closed circles*, and those with pathologic findings are marked by *stars* and *crosses*. The PI values in the group with uteroplacental insufficiency but no hypertension are marked by *encircled stars* and *crosses*. (Reprinted from [28] with permission)

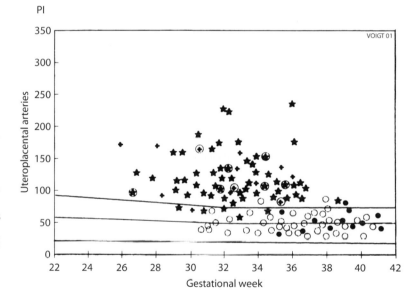

and Doppler flow measurements [12, 24, 25] demonstrated reduced uterine blood flow in cases of preeclampsia and fetal growth restriction. Although these studies were performed during late gestation, it should be recalled that abnormal placentation begins during the early second trimester (with the second wave of trophoblastic invasion) or even during the first trimester. For example, acute atherosis in the decidua, usually found during the third trimester in cases of preeclampsia, has also been observed during the first trimester, from as early as 8 weeks (R. Laurini, personal communication). It is not surprising therefore that abnormal flow patterns (using Doppler flow measurements) can be detected as early as the second trimester [26, 27]. An association between ab-

normal Doppler flow patterns in the uterine artery and histomorphologic changes in the placental bed has been demonstrated [28–30] (Fig. 17.3). However, all studies reported a considerable overlap in the degree of physiologic changes between normal and complicated pregnancies. The association between pregnancy complications and increased uteroplacental resistance as indicated by abnormal Doppler flow cannot then be solely explained by abnormal uteroplacental vessel histopathology [29]. Impaired physiological adaptation of the spiral arteries may not be the single causal factor in preeclampsia and the concept of heterogeneous causes of preeclampsia as was recently suggested [31].

temic vascular resistance [40]. The difference between the uterine and systemic vascular beds may reflect an adaptive mechanism necessary for the maintenance of uteroplacental perfusion and fetal well-being, as angiotensin II normally increases during pregnancy and likely increases even more, although intermittently, during the course of normal daily activities. The systemic concentrations of the stable metabolite of prostacyclin, 6-ketoprostaglandin $PGF_{1\alpha}$, is increased during pregnancy [56]. Furthermore, the synthesis of prostacyclin by ovine uterine artery is increased during pregnancy [57] (Fig. 17.7). This increased synthesis by the uterine artery cannot by itself explain the blunted response to vasoconstrictors, as indomethacin-treated vessels from pregnant animals are still less sensitive to vasoconstrictors than untreated vessels from nonpregnant animals [55]. Other vascular factors, such as EDRF, may compensate for the loss of endothelial PGI_2 in the uterine vascular bed.

Prostacyclin has been demonstrated in trophoblastic tissues at 6 weeks' gestation and is known to increase during the first trimester [58]. Both villous core cells and cytotrophoblasts produce thromboxane A_2 and prostacyclin during the first trimester [59]. It has been hypothesized that successful invasion of trophoblast into the spiral arteries may be dependent on a delicate balance between thromboxane A_2 and PGI_2 [59].

While prostanoids have been proposed to play a major role in the regulation of uteroplacental blood flow, studies on the effect of hypoxia on the produc-

tion of prostaglandin E(2)(PGE(2)), thromboxane B(2)(TXB(2)), and prostacyclin (measured as 6-keto-PGF(1alpha)) by human term trophoblast cells and villous placental explants have shown that hypoxia could be responsible for abnormal profiles of prostanoid production commonly observed in women with preeclampsia [60]. The results indicate a putative link between hypoxia and compromised placental perfusion.

Endothelium-Derived Relaxing Factor

Endothelium-derived relaxing factor, thought to be mainly nitric oxide, originates from endothelial cell metabolism of L-arginine [44]. The vasodilating effects of EDRF and nitric oxide are ultimately mediated by stimulation of soluble guanylate cyclase (cGMP) [44]. Competitive inhibitors of nitric oxide synthetase such as N-monomethyl-L-arginine (L-NMMA) or L-nitroarginine methylester (L-NEMA) reduce the production of nitric oxide (Fig. 17.8). The relation between EDRF and cardiovascular changes during pregnancy is being extensively investigated; in the meantime, experimental data have accumulated demonstrating that EDRF is elevated during normal pregnancy and that the uterine vasculature has a greater ability to release endogenous EDRF. The EDRF-mediated decrease in the uterine artery contractile response to norepinephrine during pregnancy has been described [55, 61] and could result from either increased basal or stimulated release of EDRF.

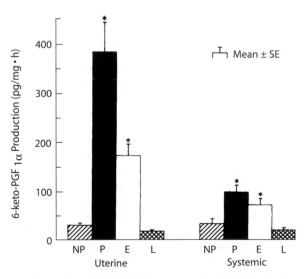

Fig. 17.7. In vitro basal production of 6-keto-prostaglandin $F_{1\alpha}$ ($PGF_{1\alpha}$) by nonpregnant (*NP*), pregnant (*P*), early postpartum (*E*), and late postpartum (*L*) uterine and omental (*systemic*) arteries, *$p < 0.05$, values different from NP and L. (Reprinted from [57] with permission)

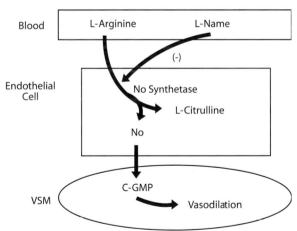

Fig. 17.8. Nitric oxide synthetase pathway in which L–arginine is converted to L-citrulline, giving off nitric oxide in endothelial cells, which leads to stimulation of cyclic guanosine monophosphate (*c-GMP*) in vascular smooth muscle and vasodilation. L-Nitroarginine methyl ester (*L-NAME*) competes with L-arginine as substrate for nitric oxide (*NO*) synthetase and is able to block the synthesis of nitric oxide. VSM, vascular smooth muscle. (Reprinted from [64] with permission)

Fig. 17.9. Increases in uterine blood flow as percent of maximum response to estradiol-17β (E_2) 1μg/kg plotted against time. Beginning at 120 min after E_2, L-nitroarginine methylester (*L-NAME*), a nitric oxide synthetase inhibitor, was administered as an intraarterial bolus injection of increasing doses. UBF, uterine blood flow. (Reprinted from [64] with permission)

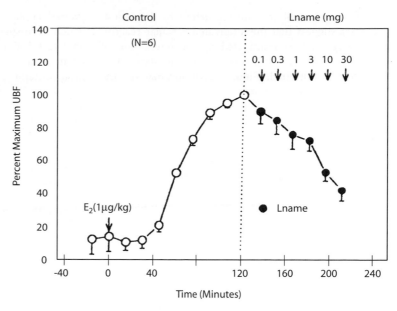

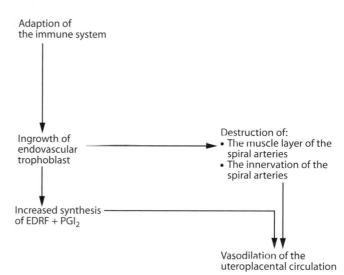

Fig. 17.10. Factors leading to vasodilation of the uteroplacental circulation in normotensive pregnancy. (From [130] with permission)

Indirect evidence supports both mechanisms. Compounds that are known to release EDRF (e.g., acetylcholine, bradykinin, histamine) increase uterine blood flow when infused directly into the uterine vascular bed of chronically instrumented sheep [62, 63]. Acetylcholine increases uterine vascular conductance in nonpregnant and pregnant sheep [63]. Also, local injection of L-arginine analogs causes local decreases in uterine blood flow while avoiding alterations in blood pressure that could directly influence uterine blood flow [69].

An important observation in this regard was the finding that estradiol-17β-induced increases in uterine blood flow are mediated by nitric oxide [64]. Moreover, L-NEMA antagonizes the vasodilating effects of estradiol-17β on the uterine vasculature in a

dose-dependent manner [64] (Fig. 17.9). This antagonism of estrogen-induced vasodilation demonstrates that nitric oxide is important for mediating the vasodilating effect of estradiol-17β, and it could play a role in regulating uterine and possibly uteroplacental blood flow during pregnancy.

When administered systemically, L-arginine analogs increase blood pressure and reverse pregnancy-induced refractoriness to vasopressor agents [65]. These observations support the notion that blunted pressor responsiveness during normal gestation is due largely to increased elaboration of endothelium-derived nitric oxide, which also plays a key role in regulating blood pressure during pregnancy. It has been demonstrated that endothelium-derived relaxing factors (e.g., prostacyclin and EDRF) reduce the contractile response of the uterine artery to thromboxane. Data suggest that the attenuated vascular reactivity of pregnancy is modulated by the interaction of EDRF and PGI_2, and that one system can adapt when the other is inhibited. Figure 17.10 summarizes the various factors leading to vasodilation of the uteroplacental arteries.

Endothelin

Control of uterine vascular function by the endothelium is more complex than anticipated because the cells not only release various vasodilator substances but also mediate contractions of the underlying smooth muscle with diffusible endothelium-derived contracting factors [66]. Endothelium-dependent contractions are elicited by thromboxane [56] or by the release of endothelin [67] and superoxide anion [68]. Endothelin-1, a 21-amino-acid peptide, is the most potent natural pressor substance known [67]. It is a vasoconstrictor in the human uterine artery, and the effect is mediated by receptors on smooth muscle cells [69, 70]. This peptide may play an important role in the regulation of vascular resistance on the maternal side of the uteroplacental unit [71].

More studies are needed to evaluate the relation between these (and perhaps other) endothelial mediators of vascular function during pregnancy. Such information can increase our understanding of the physiologic factors that regulate uterine blood flow during normal pregnancy and the pathophysiologic mechanisms involved in disease states where uteroplacental blood flow may be deranged.

Doppler Velocimetry of the Uteroplacental Circulation

Methodology

The Doppler devices commonly used for clinical or investigational measurements during early pregnancy are the continuous-wave and pulsed-wave systems. The former consists of a simple transducer that continuously sends ultrasonic sound waves; it is attached to a second transducer, which continuously receives the reflected echoes returning from the sound's beam path. The main advantages of this system are its ease of operation, portability, low output sound intensity (<25 mW/cm^2), and relatively low price. In addition it permits high-frequency shifts (i.e., high blood flow velocities) to be measured, even in deep vessels. It does not, however, permit visualization of the sound beam as it crosses the tissues or of the blood vessels themselves. Moreover, it is not range-specific, and the rather large volume of overlap between the two probes' crystals may contribute to the Doppler shift, which is displayed after spectrum analysis. In fact, any vessel that happens to lie across the sound's beam path is sampled and "contaminates" the sonogram obtained. These limitations make the continuous-wave Doppler system unsuitable for sampling small, specific vessels or for obtaining flow measurements from vascular segments at a particular location (e.g., the main branch of the ascending uterine artery or the umbilical artery adjacent to its placental location) [72].

Early Doppler studies of uterine arteries were performed with a continuous-wave Doppler apparatus using either the abdominal [12, 13] or the transvaginal [14] approach. Subplacental vessels [12] and uterine vessels [13] can be studied with this method. Flow velocity waveforms in the uterine vessels were captured by pointing the probe into the paracervical area via the lower abdomen [13]. The vaginal route has the advantage of being close to the main branch of the uterine artery as it enters the lower part of the uterus [13]. Vaginal studies are performed by inserting the transducer (covered by a rubber condom and lubricated with coupling jelly) into the vaginal fornix and directing it along the paracervical area. During the first trimester the failure rate was reported to be 10%. The mean intraobserver and interobserver error between examinations was 4%, with a standard deviation of 2.3% [13].

With pulsed-wave Doppler systems, the transducer sends short pulses of high-frequency sound waves repetitively. The same transducer is used to receive the reflected echoes during the intervals between sending the pulses. With such pulse-echo systems the range (or depth) of the target can be estimated from the corresponding time delay in the reception of echoes following transmission of the ultrasonic pulse, assuming a constant value for the speed of ultrasound (1,540 cm/s). This range-gated detection permits selection of Doppler frequency shift signals from moving targets according to their distance from the ultrasonic probe.

This principle is implemented in duplex scanning, where a pulsed-wave Doppler transducer is integrated into a two-dimensional ultrasound imaging unit to permit accurate identification of the volume in space from which Doppler-shifted frequencies are to be received. This volume is commonly termed the sample volume, and both its width and distance from the transducer can be controlled by the user. This orientation in space and the depth selectivity make the pulsed duplex systems much superior to the continuous-wave Doppler systems [72, 73].

A significant limitation when using pulsed Doppler systems is the maximum range limitation, or the range-velocity limitation [72, 73]. Analog signals (such as Doppler shift signals) can be unambiguously represented by samples only if they are sampled at a rate that exceeds twice the highest frequency in the signal itself (also known as the Nyquist limit). It means that when high flow velocities are encountered, the pulse repetition frequency must be increased sufficiently to accommodate this limitation. If the vessel is situated far from the transducer (e.g., when performing Doppler studies on deep pelvic vessels using an abdominal probe), the potential increase in pulse repetition frequency is limited by the pulse-echo round-trip delay time. Under such conditions false signals are displayed, a phenomenon termed aliasing [72, 73]. One way to partially overcome this problem is to use a lower-frequency transducer when operating in the Doppler mode on duplex systems. The Doppler shift frequency would then be lower for any given velocity of the target, and the range-velocity ambiguity problem would be less likely to arise [72, 73].

The optimal method for performing pelvic Doppler flow measurements during early pregnancy is the transvaginal image-directed pulsed Doppler system [74]. With such a duplex Doppler system, two-dimensional real-time scanning enables appropriate placement of the ultrasonic Doppler beam. Using real-time imaging, pelvic anatomic structures can be scanned, and particular vessels can be identified (Fig. 17.11). As the female pelvis contains various soft tissue structures that have similar acoustic properties (and are therefore poor reflectors) the transvaginal ultrasonic probe offers the most suitable approach. The close proximity of the transducer probe to the pelvic organs makes it possible to increase its frequency (typically 5–7 MHz). At this range attenuation is still acceptable, and images resolution is greatly improved. As the vagina is a rather elastic organ, the probe can be manipulated so as to bring it as close to a specific structure as possible, thereby placing it within the focal region of the transducer. With the probe situated close to the vessel, the range-velocity ambiguity problem is largely overcome [73, 74]. This technique also makes it possible to use a higher-frequency Doppler transducer and obtain a higher-frequency shift at any angle of insonation, thereby increasing the accuracy of the measurement. Moreover, the examination is performed with an empty bladder, preventing distortion of normal anatomy and vessel displacement. Using this approach, one can study patterns of blood flow in uterine vessels (including spiral arteries and decidual vessels), ovarian vessels, and embryonal and fetal vessels (e.g., umbilical artery, intracranial vessels, aorta) [75].

The introduction of color flow mapping has made vessel localization much simpler. The user can identify the required vessel with certainty, and the duration

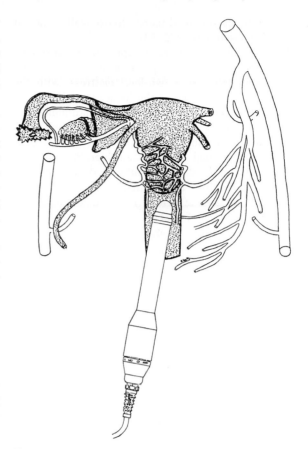

Fig. 17.11. Transvaginal probe in relation to the female pelvic vessels. (From [131] with permission)

of the examination is considerably shortened [76]. The main application of duplex scanning is the detailed study of well-defined anatomic regions. Such systems do not readily convey information about blood flow throughout the entire scan plane. Doppler color flow mapping is particularly helpful, as it produces real-time two-dimensional images that are color coded according to flow conditions and superimposed on real-time two-dimensional gray-scale pulse-echo images of anatomic structures. It facilitates evaluation of vessels within organs or those that are not readily delineated by conventional scanning. Color Doppler sonography is based on the Doppler autocorrelation flow detector, which rapidly extracts Doppler signals line by line as the ultrasonic beam is scanned through the image plane. The resulting display image is a combination of Doppler and anatomic information. The output from the autocorrelation detector consists of directional real-time velocity (or Doppler frequency) signals. These signals are arranged to color code the real-time gray-scale image. Forward flow is usually presented in red and reverse flow in blue. The degree of turbulence is color coded in green.

Best results are obtained using electronically scanned linear or phased array [72, 73].

During the transvaginal Doppler examination the patient lies in the supine position on a gynecologic examination table or a two-level mattress, with the upper part of the body on the higher level [77]. This positioning enables the examiner to manipulate the probe at various angles, applying the push-pull technique, and locate the vessel of interest [77]. A coupling gel is applied to the vaginal probe, which is subsequently covered with a lubricated rubber glove and is inserted into the vaginal fornix. A real-time image of the uterine artery is obtained employing color flow imaging if practical, and the line of insonation of the Doppler beam is adjusted so it crosses the vessel at the smallest possible angle. Several measurements of vessel diameter are obtained at this stage, and the mean diameter is calculated. The sample volume is then placed to cover the entire cross-sectional area of the vessel (Fig. 17.12). Once achieved, the system is switched to the dual-mode operation, where both the two-dimensional scanning and the range-gated pulsed Doppler operate in a quasisimultaneous mode. The flow velocity waveforms are displayed after spectral analysis in real time. Once a good-quality signal is obtained based on audio recognition, visual waveform recognition, and maximum measured velocity, the image is frozen, including good-quality waveform signals. Figure 17.13 demonstrates flow velocity waveforms in the main uterine artery obtained by transvaginal pulsed Doppler ultrasonography before and during pregnancy. Once

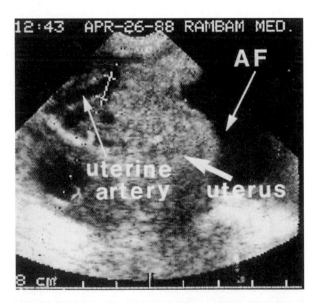

Fig. 17.12. Transvaginal sonographic scan demonstrating a short segment of the uterine artery, sample volume (situated between the *two short parallel lines*), uterine wall, and amniotic sac (*AF*). (Reprinted from [75] with permission)

the vessel is located and displayed, the angle of insonation is determined by aligning a linear cursor parallel to the long axis of the vessel itself. All the flow parameters are calculated at this stage, and the results are displayed on a separate video display unit. The images and values obtained can be recorded on a video tape for subsequent review. An immediate hard copy can also be obtained using video printer. A high-pass filter of 100 Hz is activated to remove low-frequency/high-intensity echoes originating from vessel wall movements [77].

Some investigators use a combination of continuous-wave Doppler ultrasound and color flow imaging of the uterine artery to calculate the resistance to flow as well as the mean velocity and volume flow [78]. By placing the transducer in the lower lateral quadrant of the uterus and angling it medially, an apparent crossover of the external iliac artery and vein and the main uterine artery can be identified. This "crossover" is used as a reference point to identify the main uterine artery and is easily reproducible. A clear image of a length of the artery can be obtained and the diameter of the artery measured. Direct visualization of the artery and knowledge of the angle of insonation of the vessel enable the calculation of resistance, mean velocity of flow, and total volume of flow to the uterus in both uterine arteries [78].

Anatomic Considerations

Because investigators use different methodologies it is not surprising that the reported flow impedance values in the uterine arteries for normal pregnancy vary considerably [12, 13, 79–81]. In early studies a large uteroplacental vessel was sampled in the lateral uterine wall by duplex equipment close to the bifurcation of the common iliac artery [24, 80]. The investigators called these vessels the "arcuate arteries". Other groups obtained signals from subplacental vessels using a continuous-wave Doppler apparatus [12, 79]. Another group of investigators used a continuous-wave Doppler system to locate the uterine artery in the lower uterine segment on both sides and averaged the readings [13]. Other groups studied the main branches of the ascending uterine arteries at the level of the internal os [14, 82] using a transvaginal pulsed Doppler system. Figure 17.14 demonstrates the various insonation sites used to study the uteroplacental circulation.

Investigators may then use different Doppler ultrasound equipment and insonate different parts of the uteroplacental circulation. Moreover, different indices of impedance to flow have been used, with each group defining their own normal range, often constructed from measurements obtained in small numbers of retrospectively defined, normal women fol-

Fig. 17.13. Flow velocity waveforms in the ascending uterine artery and arcuate vessels obtained by transvaginal pulsed Doppler transducer before and during various stages of pregnancy. (Reprinted from [75] with permission)

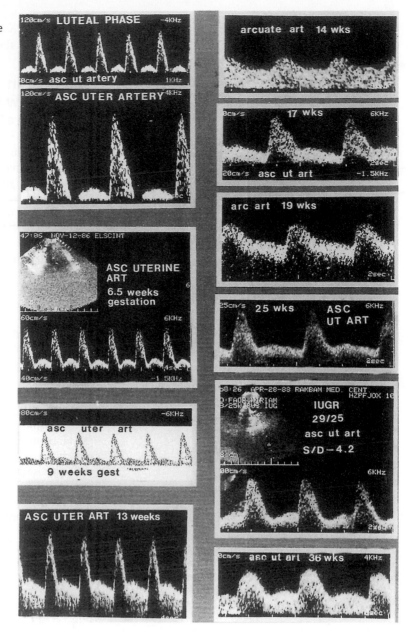

lowed longitudinally. Some groups also include a description of flow velocity waveforms, particularly the presence of a dicrotic or early diastolic notch as an indicator of high resistance to flow [24, 25, 83]. With so many techniques, the results obtained are hardly comparable. For example, the mean resistance index (RI) at 20 weeks' gestation has been reported as ranging between 0.31 [80] and 0.57 [13].

These methodologic problems were highlighted in a large cross-sectional study in which reference ranges for uteroplacental waveforms during the second trimester were established [84]. A 4-MHz continuous-wave Doppler system was used to insonate the uteroplacental vessels of an unselected group of 977 women. The uterine artery was investigated near its origin ('U'terine site, Fig. 17.14) and in the anterolateral uterine wall halfway between the fundus and the most lateral point, parallel to the abdominal surface insonating only the uterine wall ('A'rcuate site, Fig. 17.14). The placental site was also noted. The RI was always higher at the uterine site than at the arcuate site regardless of placental location [84] (Fig. 17.15). At each site the RI was always lower on the placental side (Fig. 17.15). The fall in resistance with placental site and with distance from the origin of the uterine artery can be explained by the increasing

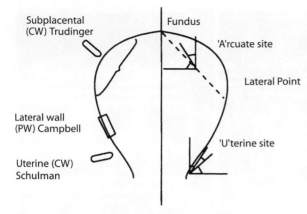

Fig. 17.14. Insonation sites used to study the uteroplacental circulation. (Reprinted from [84] with permission)

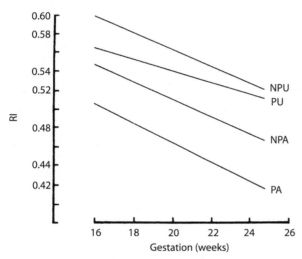

Fig. 17.15. Mean resistance index (*RI*) at four insonation sites: nonplacental uterine (*NPU*), placental uterine (*PU*), nonplacental arcuate (*NPA*), and placental arcuate (*PA*) sites. It shows the difference between uterine and arcuate sites and the effect of placental location. (Reprinted from [84] with permission)

cross-sectional area as the uterine artery branches from its origin, and pressure and impedance fall continuously from the uterine artery to the intervillous space. These facts can be summarized to indicate that it is not possible to study the uteroplacental circulation without having clear definition of the site studied and the position of the placenta. It is likely that Doppler measurements should be obtained from the main uterine vessels. Such measurements should provide more predictive information on impaired uteroplacental perfusion as the major vessels reflect the sum of resistances of the placental bed and therefore are more likely to provide an overall picture of placental perfusion [79, 83]. Moreover, measurements of

the main uterine artery are more reproducible [83], and the likelihood of demonstrating a systolic or diastolic notch in flow velocity waveforms increases [83].

Changes in Uteroplacental Blood Flow During Early Normal Pregnancy

The development of uterine artery compliance throughout pregnancy was studied by continuous-wave Doppler sonography [13]. Although no significant changes were observed during the first trimester, there was a rapid decline in the systolic/diastolic flow velocity ratio (S/D ratio) starting early in the second trimester. These changes plateaued at 22–24 weeks. When a transvaginal image-directed pulsed Doppler system was used, the resistance to flow (expressed by the S/D ratio or the pulsatility index, or PI) rapidly declined in the ascending branch of the uterine artery from as early as 5 weeks and continued to 22 weeks' gestation [14, 85].

Figure 17.16 demonstrates the decline in S/D ratio from 5 to 28 weeks. During this period the vessel diameter increased linearly (Fig. 17.17), and the volume of blood flow to the uterus increased by more than 50% [14] (Fig. 17.18). At 20–22 weeks the second wave of trophoblastic migration is mostly complete [3], and any further increase in volume flow rates may be attributed to an increase in vessel diameter and cross-sectional area of the entire uterine vascular bed [14]. The rate of increase of uterine blood flow was found to be maximal between 20–24 weeks (39 ml/min/week) as was the increase in uterine artery diameter, in a study where uterine blood flow was measured between 20 and 38 weeks' gestation [86]. The rate of increase in mean quantified volume

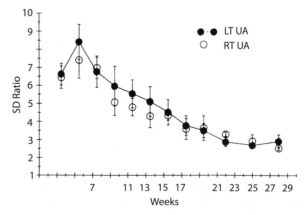

Fig. 17.16. Changes in S/D ratio in the uterine arteries (*UA*) during the first and second trimesters of pregnancy

Fig. 17.17. Changes in diameter of the main uterine artery at various gestational ages. (Reprinted from [14] with permission)

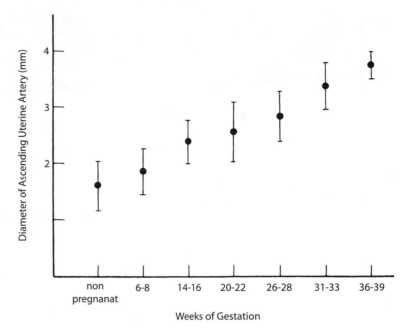

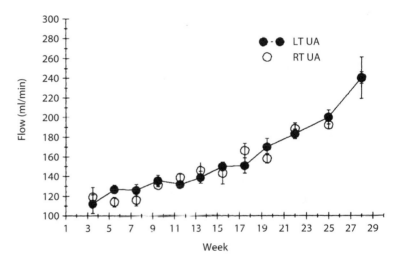

Fig. 17.18. Changes in blood flow in the uterine arteries (*UA*) during the first and second trimesters of pregnancy

flow per week declined to 14 ml/min/week between 36–38 weeks' gestation [86].

During the first and early second trimesters the decline in resistance to flow occurs not only in the main uterine artery [14, 86] but also in the arcuate [87], radial [88], spiral [88], and trophoblastic [87, 89] vessels. Trophoblastic Doppler signals are obtained by placing the sample volume in the hyperechoic area adjacent to the gestational sac. As could be expected, the resistance to flow was progressively lower as one moved from the main branch of the uterine artery through the arcuate, radial, spiral, and trophoblastic vessels. This phenomenon is demonstrated in Fig. 17.19. When these measurements are performed

in a twin pregnancy, the resistance to flow is consistently lower and volume flow rates are consistently higher than those of singleton pregnancies (Tables 17.1 and 17.2, respectively). Values are presented as the mean ± SEM. These changes in the resistance to flow during the early second trimester are consistent with endovascular trophoblastic invasion of the decidual portion of the spiral arteries, as previously described [1–3].

Many investigators described a difference in blood flow velocity between the left and right uterine arteries during the first trimester [85, 90, 91] (Table 17.3). In the latter study [91] there appeared to be no essential difference in frequency or magnitude be-

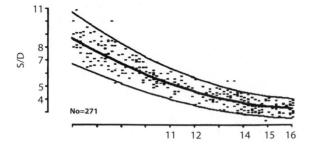

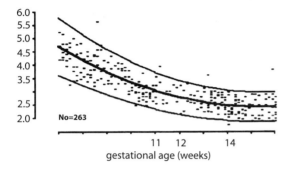

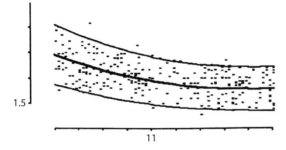

Fig. 17.19. Reference ranges (mean±2 SD) and individual values of systolic/diastolic (*S/D*) ratio from both main uterine arteries (*top*), arcuate arteries (*middle*), trophoblastic vessels (*bottom*). (Reprinted from [27] with permission)

Table 17.1. S/D ratio in uterine arteries during the first and early second trimesters for singleton and twin pregnancies

Gestational age (weeks)	S/D ratio (mean±SEM)		
	Singleton	Twins	*p*
4–7	7.63±0.45	6.77±0.34	NS
8–11	5.56±0.36	4.37±0.26	<0.01
12–15	4.60±0.33	2.84±0.16	<0.0001
16–19	3.23±0.15	2.38±0.10	<0.0001

NS, not significant; SEM, standard error of the mean.

Table 17.2. Total blood flow to the uterus[a] during the first and early second trimester for singleton and twin pregnancies

Gestational age (weeks)	Total blood flow (ml/min) (mean±SEM)		
	Singleton	Twins	*p*
4–7	237.6±6.15	242.8±7.19	NS
8–11	251.2±7.12	300.0±8.96	<0.0001
12–15	279.0±7.19	343.4±7.73	<0.0009
16–19	323.4±8.07	391.4±8.69	<0.0002

NS, not significant; SEM, standard error of the mean.
[a] Sum of flows in both uterine arteries.

Table 17.3. Frequency and magnitude of difference of PI between left and right uterine arteries of normal pregnancies at 8–13 weeks' gestation (from [91] with permission)

Gestation (weeks)	Differences in PI				
	No.	L>R	No.	R>L	R=L (No.)
8	7	0.64±0.37	6	0.86±0.67	–
9	3	0.27±0.24	4	0.35±0.23	2
10	5	0.50±0.39	4	0.60±0.32	1
11	5	0.54±0.31	5	0.53±0.33	–
12	12	0.48±0.59	12	0.51±0.30	2
13	8	0.60±0.24	9	0.43±0.40	2

Results are means±SD of the differences between the left uterine artery (L) and right uterine artery (R).
L>R, left predominance; R>L, right predominance; R, L indicates no predominance.

tween left (L>R) and right (R>L) predominance for both PI and RI values. On average there appeared to be no difference between the left and right uterine arteries. The most likely explanation for the difference in the PI or RI between the left and right uterine arteries is that changes in down-stream impedance in the uterine artery supplying the placenta precede those in the uterine artery on the nonplacental side of the uterus. As clear delineation of the placenta is often impossible during early gestation, one can only assume about the relation between the resistance to flow and placental location at this stage of gestation [91]. Some investigators prefer to calculate the mean RI or PI of both sides of the uterus, which would indicate the total downstream impedance [85, 90, 91].

When using the transvaginal pulsed Doppler technique the intraobserver coefficient of variation ranged between 7.6% [84] and 9.0% [14]. The reported range for the continuous-wave Doppler method was between 4.0% [13] and 5.6% [91].

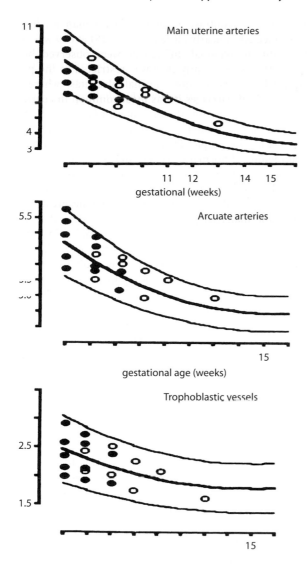

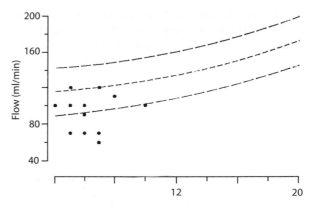

Fig. 17.21. Uterine blood flow in women who aborted (*closed circles*) plotted on normal reference ranges (5th, 59th, and 90th percentiles). Fifty percent were below the 5th percentile, and another 33% were below the 50th percentile

Fig. 17.20. Systolic/diastolic (*S/D*) ratios of 19 patients with anembryonic pregnancy (*closed circles*) and missed abortion (*open circles*), plotted on reference ranges for normal gestations. (Reprinted from [27] with permission)

Doppler Velocimetry During Early Pregnancy and Pregnancy Outcome

Normal Early Pregnancy and Early Pregnancy Failure

Few investigations have been conducted to study the relation between Doppler velocimetry in the uteroplacental circulation and pregnancy failure; and of those undertaken, most investigators found no association. In one study, no significant modifications were observed in the velocity waveforms obtained from sub-placental vessels of seven pregnancies with early failure [92]. In another study [87] flow velocity waveforms were recorded from different points of the uterine circulation in 19 patients with early pregnancy failure. The S/D ratio always fell within the normal range, in both anembryonic pregnancies and in cases of missed abortion (Fig. 17.20). Trophoblastic flow was observed in all cases studied. In another study [93], 77 pregnant women were followed longitudinally by Doppler flow measurements of the ascending uterine arteries, starting from as early as 4–5 weeks' gestation. Twelve patients subsequently aborted. The S/D ratio obtained prior to pregnancy loss fell within the normal range. Howerver, when volume flow rates were measured prior to pregnancy loss, the mean flow was significantly lower in women who aborted (95.8 ± 6.9 ml/min) than in those who did not abort (118.8 ± 3.16 ml/min, $p < 0.002$) (Fig. 17.21).

One group [94] reported lower RI values in the uterine artery in patients with blighted ovum ($n = 41$, RI $= 0.77 \pm 0.11$) or missed abortion ($n = 6$, RI $= 0.69 \pm 0.13$) than in those with normal pregnancies ($n = 6$, RI $= 0.81 \pm 0.06$). The mean RI in the trophoblastic region was 0.48 ± 0.08 in normal pregnancies compared to 0.42 ± 0.15 in cases of blighted ovum. In several patients with missed abortion and blighted ovum no trophoblastic flow could be detected. Vaginal bleeding with or without subchorionic hematoma was associated with increased radial artery impedance at 7 weeks of pregnancy [95]. Time-average velocity and peak systolic velocity did not change significantly and spiral artery blood flow remained unaffected. In another study, patients with threatened miscarriage also had significantly higher radial artery PI values compared to normal gestations [96]. PI, RI, and peak systolic velocity were measured in patients affected

Table 17.4. Resistance index above the 95th percentile or the presence of a diastolic notch for prediction of severe proteinuric pregnancy-induced hypertension (from [79] with permission)

Gestation (weeks)	Sensitivity (%)	Specificity (%)	PPV (%)	HPV (%)
20	79	85	7.6	99.6
24	79	96	25.9	99.7
26	79	98	36.6	99.7

PPV, positive predictive value; NPV, negative predictive value.

Studies of the uterine artery were performed in 1,300 pregnant women using continuous-wave Doppler ultrasonography to screen at 20 weeks and color flow imaging for follow-up at 24 and 26 weeks.

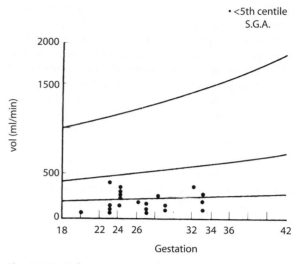

Fig. 17.23. Reference ranges of the total volume of flow in the uterine arteries and the total volume of flow in 21 women whose pregnancies were complicated by growth restriction. *S.G.A.* small for gestational age. (Reprinted from [78] with permission)

nography and color flow imaging of the uterine artery was used to calculate the resistance to flow as well as the mean velocity and volume flow. The women were recruited from the routine antenatal clinic and had a continuous-wave Doppler ultrasound examination of both uterine arteries at the 20-week admission scan. It the flow velocity waveforms obtained were found to have a high RI (>2 standard deviations from the mean of the normal range), an early diastolic notch, or both, the patient was asked to return for follow-up with color flow imaging initially at 24 weeks and then at 26 weeks if the results were still abnormal. Of the 1,300 women studied, 19 subsequently had severe proteinuric pregnancy-induced hypertension, and 15 of the 19 had abnormal findings on the uterine artery Doppler studies. The results are summarized in Table 17.4. A total of 206 women were identified as having an abnormal waveform at the admission scan; 95% of these women had an early diastolic notch (68% without and 27% with increased RI), and only 5% had an increased RI alone. These findings demonstrate that a notch is a much better predictor that a notch is a much better predictor of poor outcome than the RI alone.

The same investigators [78] also found that the total volume of flow in the uterine arteries in 21 women whose pregnancies were complicated by fetal growth restriction (most of whom were found to be hypoxemic at cordocentesis), was below the 50th percentile; 62% were below the 5th percentile (Fig. 17.23). What needs to be determined is whether patients with low volume of flow at or before 24 weeks have increased risk of having a pregnancy complicated by fetal growth restriction.

More recently a multicenter, cohort study was conducted to determine the utility of transvaginal color Doppler assessment of uterine arteries at 23 weeks' gestation in the prediction of preeclampsia and fetal growth restriction [125]. A mean PI of 1.63 (the 95th percentile) or more or bilateral notching was considered abnormal. In 932 of the 7,851 study patients (i.e., 11.9%) at least one of these abnormalities was present. The sensitivity, specificity, and positive and negative predictive values of an abnormal test were 83.3%, 88.5%, 3.8%, 99.9%, respectively, with a likelihood ratio of 7.3. The sensitivities in predicting either preeclampsia without fetal growth restriction or fetal growth restriction without preeclampsia were much lower, however (40.8% and 24.4%, respectively). The sensitivities in the prediction of either one of the two outcomes further decreased when only one of the uterine artery Doppler patterns was abnormal. The investigators concluded that Doppler screening at 23 weeks is valuable at identifying the more severe cases of preeclampsia and fetal growth restriction (and therefore the most clinically relevant cases).

Recently a metaanalysis was performed to examine how useful uterine artery Doppler flow velocimetry is in the prediction of preeclampsia, fetal growth restriction, and perinatal death [126]. Twenty-seven published and unpublished observational studies involving 12,994 pregnancies were analyzed. These pregnancies were classified into high-risk and low-risk for developing preeclampsia and its associated complications. Based on the results obtained the authors concluded that uterine artery Doppler flow velocimetry has limited diagnostic accuracy in predicting preeclampsia, fetal growth restriction, and perinatal death.

The second wave of trophoblastic migration is completed in most women by 20 weeks' gestation [3].

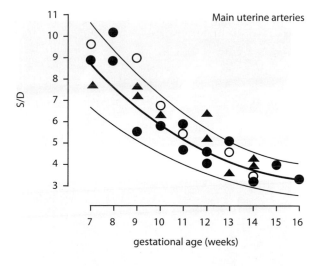

Main uterine arteries

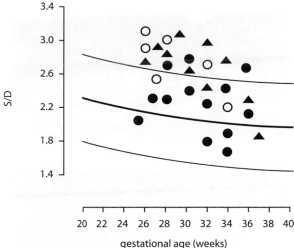

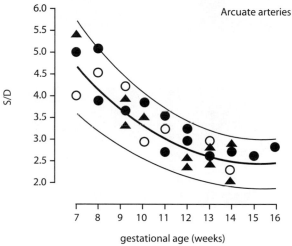

Arcuate arteries

Fig. 17.24. Systolic/diastolic (*S/D*) ratio in the uterine and arcuate arteries of 29 women who developed gestational hypertension (*triangles*), intrauterine growth restriction (*closed circles*), or both complications (*open circles*), plotted on reference ranges. (Reprinted from [27] with permission)

Fig. 17.25. Uterine artery systolic/diastolic (*S/D*) ratio during the second and third trimesters in 29 women who developed gestational hypertension (*triangles*), intrauterine growth restriction (*closed circles*), or both complications (*open circles*), plotted on reference ranges. (Reprinted from [28] with permission)

It seems logical that screening studies should be conducted at this period of gestation. By screening too early, the false-positive rate may be too high, leading to lower specificity because the process of physiologic changes is not completed. On the other hand, screening too late during the second trimester may mean that the pathologic process is already well developed and that preventive treatment may be less effective.

It should be recalled that the first wave of trophoblastic migration may also demonstrate abnormal features (R. Laurini, personal communication), which may be reflected in Doppler measurements of the uteroplacental circulation. One group investigated whether Doppler measurements during early pregnancy can predict adverse pregnancy outcome [27]. Reference ranges of uteroplacental waveform indices

were constructed from a cross-sectional study of 282 women with retrospectively defined normal singleton pregnancies. This group of women was selected from a population with 330 low-risk pregnancies and was followed longitudinally throughout gestation. In the remaining 48 cases, pregnancy complications were evident either at the time of the study or later with advancing gestation. Of the 48 patients, 19 had an abortion and 29 subsequently had intrauterine growth restriction (IUGR), gestational hypertension, or both. The S/D ratio was measured in the main uterine arteries, the arcuate arteries, and in trophoblastic vessels using an image-directed transvaginal color Doppler system. Measurements were started from as early as 7 weeks' gestation. In the 29 women who subsequently had PIH/PET, IUGR, or both, all S/D ratio values were within the normal range in all vessels studied (Fig. 17.24). Fourteen patients had an increased S/D ratio (>2 standard deviations) in the main uterine artery during late second and third trimester of pregnancy (Fig. 17.25). The presence or absence of a notch in the uterine artery flow velocity waveforms was not reported in this study.

Another group [93] investigated the association between abnormal blood flow velocity waveforms and subsequent complications of pregnancy (PIH/PET or IUGR). Serial Doppler examinations of the uterine arteries were performed in 77 pregnant patients. The Doppler studies commenced at 5–6 weeks' gestation and were repeated every 2–3 weeks during the first trimester and every 4–6 weeks thereafter. A transvaginal image-directed pulsed Doppler ultrasound system

pregnancy. IV. Circulatory homeostasis by preferential perfusion of the placenta. Am J Obstet Gynecol 1034: 10–31

8. Pinjeborg R, Robertson WB, Brosens I et al (1981) Trophoblast invasion and the establishment of haemochorial placentation in man and laboratory animals. Placenta 2:71–92

9. Browne JCM, Veall N (1953) The maternal placental blood flow in normotensive and hypertensive women. J Obstet Gynaecol Br Emp 60:141–147

10. Dixon HG, Browne JCM, Davey D (1963) Choriodecidual and myometrial blood flow. Lancet 1:369–373

11. Maini CL, Rosati P, Galli G et al (1985) Noninvasive radioisotopic evaluation of placental blood flow. Gynecol Obstet Invest 19:196–206

12. Trudinger BJ, Giles WB, Cook CM (1985) Uteroplacental blood flow velocity-time waveforms in normal and complicated pregnancy. Br J Obstet Gynaecol 92:39–45

13. Schulman H, Fleischer A, Farmakides G et al (1986) Development of uterine artery compliance in pregnancy as detected by Doppler ultrasound. Am J Obstet Gynecol 155:1031–1036

14. Thaler I, Manor D, Itskovitz J et al (1990) Changes in uterine blood flow during human pregnancy. Am J Obstet Gynecol 162:121–125

15. Brosens I, Robertson WB, Dixon HG (1972) The role of the spiral arteries in the pathogenesis of preeclampsia. Obstet Gynecol Annu 1:177

16. Khong TY, De Wolf F, Robertson WB et al (1986) Inadequate maternal vascular response to placentation in pregnancies complicated by pre-eclampsia and by small-for-gestational age infants. Br J Obstet Gynaecol 93:1049–1059

17. Robertson WB (1976) Uteroplacental vasculature. J Clin Pathol 29[Suppl 10]:9–17

18. Khong TY, Robertson WB (1992) Spiral artery disease. In: Coulam CB, Faulk WP, McIntyre JA (eds) Immunologic obstetrics. Norton, New York

19. Stirrat GM (1987) The immunology of hypertension in pregnancy. In: Sharp F, Symonds EM (eds) Hypertension in pregnancy. Perinatology Press, Ithaca, NY, p 249

20. Khong TY, Sawyer H, Heryet AR (1992) An immunohistologic study of endothelialization of uteroplacental vessels in human pregnancy: evidence that endothelium is focally disrupted by trophoblast in preeclampsia. Am J Obstet Gynecol 167:751–756

21. Sibai BM (1990) Preeclampsia-eclampsia. Curr Probl Obstet Gynecol Infertil 13:6

22. DeWolf F, Robertson WB, Brosens I (1975) The ultrastructure of acute atherosis in hypertensive pregnancy. Am J Obstet Gynecol 123:164–174

23. Lunell NO, Nylund L, Lewander R et al (1982) Uteroplacental blood flow in preeclampsia: measurements with indium-113 and a computer-linked gamma camera. Clin Exp Hypertens 11:105–117

24. Campbell S, Griffin DR, Pearce JMF et al (1983) New Doppler technique for assessing uteroplacental blood flow. Lancet 1:675–677

25. Fleischer A, Schulman H, Farmakides G et al (1986) Uterine artery Doppler velocimetry in pregnant women with hypertension. Am J Obstet Gynecol 154:806–813

26. Campbell S, Pearce JMF, Hackett G et al (1986) Qualitative assessment of uteroplacental blood flow: early screening test for high risk pregnancies. Obstet Gynecol 68:649–653

27. Arduini D, Rizzo G, Romanini C et al (1987) Uteroplacental blood flow velocity waveforms as predictors of pregnancy-induced hypertension. Eur J Obstet Gynecol Reprod Biol 26:335–341

28. Voigt J, Becker V (1992) Uteroplacental insufficiency: comparison of uteroplacental blood flow velocimetry and histomorphology of placental bed. J Matern Fetal Invest 2:251–255

29. Aardema MW, Oosterhof H, Timmer A, Van Rooy I, Aarnoudse JG (2001) Uterine artery Doppler flow and uteroplacental vascular pathology in normal pregnancies and pregnancies complicated by preeclampsia and small for gestational age fetuses. Placenta 22:405–411

30. Lin S, Shimuzu I, Suehara N, Nakayama M, Aono T (1995) Uterine artery Doppler velocimetry in relation to trophoblast migration into the myometrium of the placental bed. Obstet Gynecol 85:760–765

31. Ness RB, Roberts JM (1996) Heterogeneous causes constituting the single syndrome of preeclampsia; a hypothesis and its implications. Am J Obstet Gynecol 175:1365–1370

32. Walters WAW, Lim YL (1975) Blood volume and haemodynamics in pregnancy. Clin Obstet Gynecol 2:301–320

33. Christianson RE (1976) Studies of blood pressure during pregnancy. I. Influence of parity and age. Am J Obstet Gynecol 125:509–513

34. Clark SL, Cotton DB, Lee W et al (1989) Central hemodynamics of normal term pregnancy. Am J Obstet Gynecol 161:1439–1442

35. Weir RJ, Brown JJ, Fraser R et al (1975) Relationship between plasma renin, renin-substrate, angiotensin II, aldosterone and electrolytes in normal pregnancy. J Clin Endocrinol Metab 40:108–115

36. Taufield PA, Mueller FB, Edersheim TG et al (1988) Blood pressure regulation in normal pregnancy: unmasking the role of renin angiotensin system with captopril (abstract). Clin Res 36:433A

37. Gant NF, Daley GL, Chand S et al (1973) A study of angiotensin II pressor response throughout primigravid pregnancy. J Clin Invest 52:2682–2689

38. Rosenfeld CR (1989) Changes in uterine blood flow during pregnancy. In: Rosenfeld CR (ed) The uterine circulation. Perinatology Press, Ithaca, NY, pp 135–156

39. Massicotte G, St Louis T, Parent A et al (1987) Decreased in vitro response to vasoconstrictors during pregnancy in normotensive and spontaneously hypertensive pregnant rats. Can J Physiol Pharmacol 65: 2466–2471

40. Naden RP, Rosenfeld CR (1981) Effect of angiotensin II on uterine and systemic vasculature in pregnant sheep. J Clin Invest 68:468–474

41. Moncada S, Gryglewski R, Bunting S et al (1976) An enzyme isolated from arteries transforms prostaglandin endoperoxides to an unstable substance that inhibit platelet aggregation. Nature 263:663–665

42. Furchgott RF, Zawadzki JV (1980) The obligatory role of endothelial cells in the relaxation of arterial smooth muscle by acetylcholine. Nature 288:373–376

43. Furchgott RF, Vanhoutta PM (1989) Endothelium-derived relaxing and contracting factors. FASEB J 3:2007–2018

44. Palmer RMJ, Ferrig AG, Moncada S (1987) Nitric oxide release accounts for the biological activity of endothelium-derived relaxing factor. Nature 327:524–526

45. Ignarro LJ (1989) Biological actions and properties of endothelium-derived nitric oxide formed and released from artery and vein. Circ Res 65:1–21

46. Gardiner SM, Compton AM, Bennett T et al (1990) Control of regional blood flow by endothelium-derived nitric oxide. Hypertension 15:486–492

47. Ahokas RA, Sibai BM, Mabie MD et al (1988) Nifedipine does not adversely affect uteroplacental blood flow in the hypertensive term-pregnant rat. Am J Obstet Gynecol 159:1440–1445

48. Greiss FC (1966) Pressure-flow relationship in the gravid uterine vascular bed. Am J Obstet Gynecol 96:41–47

49. Venuto RC, Cox JW, Stein JH et al (1976) The effect of changes in perfusion pressure on uteroplacental blood flow in the pregnant rabbit. J Clin Invest 57:938–944

50. Lindow SW, Davies N, Davey DA et al (1988) The effects of sublingual nifedipine on uteroplacental blood flow in hypertensive pregnancy. Br J Obstet Gynaecol 95:1276–1281

51. Thaler I, Weiner Z, Manor D et al (1991) Effect of calcium channel blocker nifedipine on uterine artery flow velocity waveforms. J Ultrasound Med 10:301–304

52. Landauer M, Phernetton TM, Parisi VM et al (1985) Ovine placental vascular response to the local application of prostacyclin. Am J Obstet Gynecol 151:460–464

53. Husslein P, Gitch E, Pateisky N et al (1985) Prostacyclin does not influence placental blood flow in vivo. Gynecol Obstet Invest 19:78–81

54. Speroff L, Haning RV Jr, Levin RM (1977) The effect of angiotensin II and indomethacin on uterine artery blood flow in pregnant monkey. Obstet Gynecol 50:611–614

55. Weiner CP, Liu KZ, Thompson L et al (1991) Effect of pregnancy on endothelium and smooth muscle: their role in reduced adrenergic sensitivity. Am J Physiol 261:H1275–H1283

56. Ylikorkala O, Makila UM (1985) Prostacyclin and thromboxane in gynecology and obstetrics. Am J Obstet Gynecol 152:318–329

57. Magness RR, Osei-Boaten K, Mitchell MD et al (1985) In vitro prostacyclin production by ovine uterine and systemic arteries. J Clin Invest 76:2206–2212

58. Rakoczi I, Tihanyi K, Gero G et al (1988) Release of prostacyclin (PGI_2) from trophoblast in tissue culture: the effect of glucose concentration. Acta Physiol Hung 71:545–549

59. Diss EM, Gabbe GS, Moore JW et al (1992) Study of thromboxane and prostacyclin metabolism in an in vitro model of first-trimester human trophoblast. Am J Obstet Gynecol 167:1046–1052

60. Blumenstein M, Keelan JA, Mitchell MD (2001) Hypoxia attenuates PGE(2) but increases prostacyclin and thromboxane production in human term villous trophoblast. Placenta 22:519–525

61. Weiner CP, Martinez E, Chestnut DH et al (1989) Effect of pregnancy upon the uterine and carotid artery response to norepinephrine, epinephrine and phenylephrine in vessels with documented functional endothelium. Am J Obstet Gynecol 161:1605–1610

62. Resnik R, Killman AP, Barton MD et al (1976) The effect of various vasoactive compounds upon the uterine vascular bed. Am J Obstet Gynecol 125:201–206

63. Greiss FC Jr, Gabbe FL Jr, Anderson SG et al (1967) Effect of acetylcholine on the uterine vascular bed. Am J Obstet Gynecol 99:1073–1077

64. Van Buren GA, Yang D, Clark KE (1992) Estrogen induced uterine vasodilation is antagonized by L-nitroarginine methyl ester, an inhibitor of nitric oxide synthesis. Am J Obstet Gynecol 167:828–833

65. Molnar M, Hertelendy F (1992) Nw-nitro-L-arginine, an inhibitor of nitric oxide synthesis, increases blood pressure in rats and reverses the pregnancy-induced refractoriness to vasopressor agents. Am J Obstet Gynecol 166:1560–1571

66. Luscher TF (1990) The endothelium: target and promoter of hypertension? Hypertension 15:482–485

67. Yanagisawa M, Kurihara H, Kimura S et al (1988) A novel potent vasoconstrictor-peptide produced by vascular endothelial cells. Nature 332:411–415

68. Katusie ZS, Vanhoutta PM (1989) Superoxide anion is an endothelium-derived contacting factor. Heart Circ Physiol 26:H33

69. Bodelsson G, Sjoberg NO, Stjernquist M (1992) Contactile effect of endothelium in human uterine artery and autoradiographic localization of its binding sites. Am J Obstet Gynecol 167:745–750

70. Svane D, Larsson B, Alm P et al (1993) Endothelin-1: immunocytochemistry, localization of binding sites, and contractile effects in human uteroplacental smooth muscle. Am J Obstet Gynecol 168:233–241

71. Taylor RN, Varma M, Nelson NHT et al (1990) Women with preeclampsia have higher plasma endothelin levels than women with normal pregnancies. J Clin Endocrinol Metab 71:1675–1677

72. Burns PN (1993) The physics of Doppler. In: Chervenak FA, Isaacson GC, Campbell S (eds) Ultrasound in obstetrics and gynecology. Little, Brown, Boston, pp 33–54

73. Thaler I, Bruck A (1991) Transvaginal sonography and Doppler measurements: physical considerations. In: Timor-Tritsch IE, Rottem S (eds) Transvaginal sonography. Elsevier, New York, pp 1–27

74. Thaler I, Manor D (1990) Transvaginal imaging: applied physical principles and terms. J Clin Ultrasound 18:235–238

75. Thaler I, Manor D, Rottem S et al (1990) Hemodynamic evaluation of the female pelvic vessels using a high-frequency transvaginal image-directed Doppler system. J Clin Ultrasound 18:364–369

76. Kurjak A, Jurkovic D, Alfirevic Z et al (1990) Transvaginal color Doppler imaging. J Clin Ultrasound 18:227–234

77. Thaler I, Manor D, Rottem S (1993) Transvaginal Doppler duplex system. In: Chervenak FA, Isaacson GC, Campbell S (eds) Ultrasound in obstetrics and gynecology. Little, Brown, Boston, pp 141–148

78. Bowere SJ, Campbell S (1993) Doppler velocimetry of the uterine artery as a screening test in pregnancy. In: Chervenak FA, Isaacson GC, Campbell S (eds) Ultrasound in obstetrics and gynecology. Little, Brown, Boston, pp 579–586

Doppler Ultrasound in the Diagnosis and Management of Intrauterine Growth Restriction

William J. Ott

Introduction

The antenatal recognition of fetal intrauterine growth restriction (IUGR) is an important goal for every obstetrician, since significant neonatal complications may be associated with altered fetal growth. Numerous studies have reported a 5%–27% incidence of congenital abnormalities associated with IUGR, as compared with a 0.1%–4% anomaly rate in control groups of normally grown neonates [1, 2]. The incidence of chromosomal abnormalities in IUGR infants is four to five times that of average-for-gestational-age (AGA) infants (2% vs 0.4%), and intrauterine infection, especially cytomegalovirus, has been reported in 0.3%–3.5% of IUGR infants [1, 2]. In addition, growth-restricted infants have up to an eight- to tenfold increase in stillbirth and neonatal mortality [3–8]. Other developmental problems, such as necrotizing enterocolitis or intraventricular hemorrhage, also can be related to IUGR. Those infants that survive the immediate perinatal period are still at risk for neonatal hypothermia, hypoglycemia, polycythemia, or other complications, and have increased risk for long-term neurological or developmental complications [1, 4, 9–11].

Although there is no uniform agreement as to an exact definition of IUGR, it is usually equated with the small-for-gestational-age (SGA) infant, and this is not necessarily the best definition to use. In addition, there is no agreement as to which weight cut-off point (i.e., the 10th, 5th, or 3rd percentile, or two or more standard deviations from the mean) should be used to define it [12–14]. Controversy also exists as to which growth curve should be used. Numerous birth weight curves exist, and there is no universally accepted national standard. It is also controversial as to whether birth-weight-for-gestational-age curves or fetal weight-for-gestational-age curves should be used. Work at our own institution and at other centers has shown that IUGR infants are over-represented in premature deliveries, and therefore the use of birth-weight curves will significantly under-estimate the incidence of IUGR in the premature infant [15–21]. Using fetal weight curves would seem to be more appropriate. Table 18.1 shows the combined fetal weight for gestational age curve that is used in the author's institution [20], whereas Fig. 18.1 shows a comparison of the 10th percentile birth-weight curve of Alexander et al. [22] to the 10th percentile fetal weight curve, illustrating the potential under-estimation of IUGR in premature infants (20–33 weeks' gestation) if the neonatal weight curve is used.

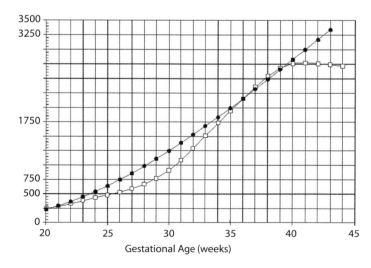

Fig. 18.1. Comparison of the 10th percentile curves of the birth weight (*open symbols*) to the fetal weight (*closed symbols*) for gestational age. Between 20 and 33 weeks' gestation the birth weight curve underestimated the incidence of intrauterine growth restriction (IUGR)

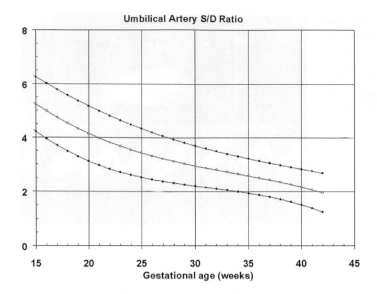

Fig. 18.4. Umbilical artery systolic/diastolic (*S/D*) ratio curve. Mean (*open symbols*) and 5th and 95th percentile values (*closed symbols*)

Table 18.3. Neonatal outcome based on weight and Doppler studies. *GA* gestational age, *NICU* neonatal intensive care, *NS* no significant difference between groups

	Group 1	Group 2	Group 3	Group 4	Significance
Number	231	215	37	95	
GA at delivery	33.9 (3.7)	34.1 (3.6)	33.6 (3.5)	34.0 (3.3)	NS
Birth weight (g)	2779 (757)	2543 (801)	1984 (635)	1916 (623)	1
Cesarean section for distress (%)	4.7	8.9	3.0	10.5	2
Days in the NICU	7.0 (14.8)	11.3 (20.5)	16.0 (25.1)	19.7 (29.7)	3

Group 1: average-for-gestational-age (AGA) fetuses with normal umbilical artery S/D ratios (normal Doppler); group 2: AGA fetuses with umbilical artery S/D ratios above the 90th percentile curve for gestational age (abnormal Doppler); group 3: small-for-gestational-age fetuses (SGA) with normal Doppler; group 4: SGA fetuses with abnormal Doppler Figures in parentheses are standard deviations.
1 No significant difference between categories 3 and 4; significant differences between categories 1–4 (combined); $p=0.0241$.
2 Abnormal Doppler (2 and 4) vs normal Doppler (1 and 3); $p=0.034$. No other differences were significant.
3 Significant differences between category 4 vs category 2 or category 1; $p=0.0001$. No significant differences between the other categories.

Table 18.3 lists the gestational age at delivery, birth weight, incidence of cesarean section for fetal distress, and length of stay in the NICU for the four study categories. There were no differences in gestational age at delivery between the four groups, and the expected differences in birth weight between the groups was seen. These findings did not change when the patients were analyzed by term or pre-term delivery. There were significant differences between the groups in cesarean section for fetal distress and in the length of stay in the NICU, both for the total patient population and when broken down into term or pre-term delivery. The presence of abnormal umbilical Doppler studies correlated better with cesarean section for distress or length of stay in the NICU than did fetal weight estimation.

There was a significant increase in neonatal morbidity in a combined group of patients with abnormal Doppler studies but not in the combined group of SGA infants. These differences became more apparent when the patients were analyzed by term or preterm delivery, with preterm infants having marked increased morbidity when Doppler studies were abnormal. Logistic regression analysis confirmed these findings. There were no differences in morbidity between AGA fetuses with normal blood flow studies or SGA fetuses with normal blood flow studies.

The results of this study suggest that categorizing fetuses at risk for poor perinatal outcome based on weight estimation and umbilical artery Doppler velocity flow studies has important prognostic significance. Neonatal outcome of SGA fetuses with normal Doppler studies was not significantly different from their AGA cohorts. Both AGA and SGA infants with abnormal Doppler studies had increased neonatal morbidity, with the SGA infants in this subgroup having the worst prognosis.

Recent studies by Soothill et al. [69], and Holme and Soothill [70], and a study by Craigo et al. [71], using similar ultrasonic techniques, came to the same conclusions: namely, the combined use of fetal weight estimation and Doppler velocity studies better defines true IUGR. The current study seems to indicate that both fetal weight estimation and Doppler evaluation of the umbilical artery are useful in the prediction of neonatal morbidity in high-risk patients. Doppler ultrasound, however, appears to be a more sensitive indicator of potential fetal compromise than does weight estimation. Combining weight estimation (or abdominal circumference) with Doppler ultrasound is currently the best method for diagnosing IUGR.

Uterine Arteries

Since utero-placental dysfunction is a major cause of IUGR, evaluation of blood flow through the uterine arteries would logically seem to be an excellent method of identifying patients at risk for IUGR; however, controversy does exist as to the value of Doppler velocity studies of the uterine arteries [76]. Steel et al. evaluated 200 primiparous patients at 24 weeks' gestation with Doppler studies of the uterine arteries and found a low sensitivity for the prediction of hypertensive disease of pregnancy, but a very high sensitivity for predicting the development of IUGR associated with hypertension [72]. Vergani et al. found that abnormal uterine artery Doppler wave forms in IUGR fetuses in the third trimester were associated with a fourfold increase in adverse perinatal outcome [75]. Studies by North et al. [73] and Atkinson et al. [74], however, found only slight correlation between abnormal Doppler indices in the uterine arteries at 24 weeks' gestation and the later development of hypertensive disease, with or without IUGR, and both groups felt that uterine artery Doppler velocity studies were not a good method of screening for these complications of pregnancy.

More recent studies by Nicolaides et al. found that a one-stage color Doppler screening of the uterine arteries at 23–24 weeks of gestation was a highly sensitive method of identifying those patients that subsequently developed serious complications of impaired placentation (pregnancy-induced hypertension and/or IUGR) [76–80]. Calculation of the uterine artery pulsatility indices (which can be done as early as 14 weeks) [81] and evaluation of the presence or absence of uterine artery notches were highly predictive for the development of complications later in gestation. Other investigators have confirmed these findings

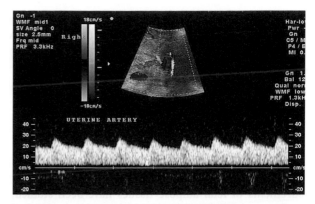

Fig. 18.5. Normal uterine Doppler wave form at 24 weeks' gestation

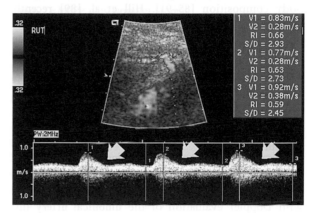

Fig. 18.6. An abnormal uterine artery Doppler wave form at 24 weeks' gestation in a hypertensive patient who later developed superimposed pregnancy-induced hypertension associated with IUGR. The *arrows* indicate uterine artery "notching"

Table 18.4. Predictive value of uterine artery Doppler studies for IUGR. *PPV* positive predictive value, *NPV* negative predictive value, *PI* pulsatility index

Criterion	Sensitivity (%)	Specificity (%)	PPV (%)	NPV (%)	Reference
Bilateral notching	50	84	40	89	[83]
PI >1.44 or bilateral notching	13	96	25	93	[77]
PI >1.6	13	96	23	92	[78]
bilateral notching	20	92	19	92	[78]

[82, 83]. Table 18.4 shows the sensitivity, specificity, and predictive values of uterine artery Doppler studies at 23 weeks in predicting IUGR. Figure 18.5 illustrates normal uterine artery flow at 24 weeks, and Fig. 18.6 shows abnormal uterine artery flow with

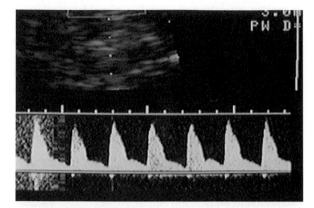

Fig. 18.8. Normal (high-resistance) Doppler wave form in the middle cerebral artery

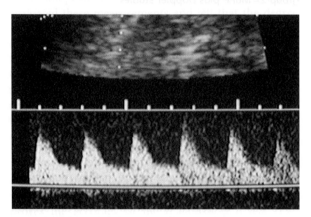

Fig. 18.9. Increased diastolic flow ("shunting") in the middle cerebral artery in a fetus with IUGR

circulation and a fall in resistance in the middle cerebral artery [120–122]. Figure 18.8 shows the normal, high-resistance flow in the fetal middle cerebral artery, whereas Fig. 18.9 shows increased diastolic flow ("shunting" or "brain sparing") in the middle cerebral artery of a fetus with significant IUGR. Serial Doppler flow studies of previable fetuses prior to fetal demise have shown progressive increased resistance in the umbilical artery with decreasing resistance in the middle cerebral artery until just prior to fetal demise, when resistance in the middle cerebral artery increases and signs of fetal heart failure (such as tricuspid regurgitation) develop [123, 124]. Of particular interest is the ratio of resistance indices of the middle cerebral artery and the umbilical artery. This ratio remains relatively constant throughout pregnancy but is significantly altered in fetuses with IUGR [125]. A number of studies involving fetal cerebral circulation suggest that there is an increase in cerebral flow in infants affected by uteroplacental insufficiency [126–129]. Studies at the author's institu-

tion of the ratio between carotid or middle cerebral and umbilical artery S/D ratio velocity waveforms (MC/UA) showed significant differences in neonatal outcome when these ratios were abnormal [130, 131]. A number of studies have shown the value of Doppler velocity flow studies in the diagnosis and management of IUGR, and have suggested that the MC/UA ratio may be more sensitive than other antenatal tests for the prediction of neonatal outcome in IUGR fetuses [130–134].

Growth-restricted fetuses, especially those that are delivered prematurely, are also at increased risk of intracranial hemorrhage or other CNS complications. The use of Doppler blood flow studies of the CNS in the fetus and neonate to identify those infants at increased risk for CNS complications may be an important tool; however, conflicting results have been obtained. Some investigators have shown a correlation between CNS complications and increased blood flow to the brain, whereas other investigators have shown a correlation between CNS complications and decreasing blood flow to the brain (increased resistance), or no correlation at all [135–140]. A recent study at the author's institution attempted to evaluate the ability of Doppler flow studies of the fetal CNS to predict CNS complications in the neonate.

Neonatal outcome of singleton pregnancies who delivered within 1 week of their final antenatal testing and had NST and fetal Doppler ultrasound (including measurements of blood flow in the fetal umbilical artery and middle cerebral artery [systolic/diastolic ratios (S/D)]) done at that time were studied. Since S/D ratios in both the umbilical and middle cerebral arteries decrease with advancing gestational age, these values were converted to multiples of the mean (MOM) derived from previously published norms [141, 142]. Both univariant and multivariant analyses were used to correlate the Doppler blood flow studies with the development of CNS complications. Correlations were also made for other tests of fetal wellbeing (NST and amniotic fluid volume), birth weight, and gestational age at delivery with the development of CNS complications.

Three hundred eighty-five patients were evaluated. The CNS complications occurred only in infants that were delivered at less than 37 weeks of gestation; therefore, the analysis was limited to the 131 patients that delivered at less than 37 weeks. Fourteen of the 131 patients (10.7%) developed CNS complications (IVH(1) 8; IVH(4) 1; encephalopathy 2; neonatal seizures 3), and Table 18.6 compares neonatal outcome parameters and results of antenatal testing between neonates with and without CNS complications. Univariant analysis showed that only birth weight, decreased amniotic fluid volume, and a non-reactive NST were statistically correlated with CNS complica-

Table 18.6. Central nervous system (*CNS*) complications: infants delivered at <37 weeks gestation. *SGA* small for gestational age (<10th percentile), *AFI* amniotic fluid index (sum of four-quadrant deepest pockets), *NST* non-reactive non-stress test, *Umb/MC ratio* ratio of the umbilical artery S/D to middle cerebral artery S/D, *MCmom* middle cerebral artery S/D ratio multiple of the mean, *UAmom* umbilical artery S/D ratio multiple of the mean, *High UA* umbilical artery S/D ratio multiple of the mean >1.5, *Low MC* middle cerebral artery S/D ratio multiple of the mean less than 0.7, *AbnUmb/MC* ratio of the umbilical artery S/D to middle cerebral artery S/D >1.0

	CNS complications	No CNS complications	P [OR][a]
Number	14	117	
Maternal age	28.6 (6.8)	29.6 (5.9)	6365
Days scan to delivery	2.5 (3.6)	2.8 (2.4)	7807
Gestational age at delivery	32.9 (2.9)	33.9 (2.8)	2505
Birth weight (g)	1639 (729)	2142 (715)	0264
SGA	57.1%	34.5%	1718 [2.33 (0.71–9.45)]
AFI (cm)	9.2 (3.7)	13.9 (7.2)	0039
NST	64.3%	24.8%	0041 [5.46 (1.48–22.16)]
Umb/MC ratio	1.39 (0.81)	1.17 (1.30)	8425
MCmom	0.62 (0.32)	0.70 (0.34)	3773
UAmom	1.34 (0.51)	1.71 (4.24)	7611
High UA	42.9%	31.6%	2869 [1.62 (0.43–5.75)]
Low MC	57.1%	63.2%	8777 [0.77 (0.22–2.73)]
AbnUmb/MC	35.7%	23.9%	2551 [1.77 (0.43–6.43)]

[a] Chi-square or Fisher's exact test for distributional data; two-sample *t*-test for parametric data.
Figures in brackets are odds ratios, with confidence intervals in parentheses.
Figures in parentheses are standard deviations.

tions. Neither abnormal blood flow in the fetal umbilical artery or in the middle cerebral artery, nor evidence of "brain-sparing" (elevated umbilical artery/middle cerebral artery ratios), were found to be associated with CNS complications. Multivariant logistic regression analysis showed that a non-reactive NST had the strongest correlation with CNS complications, whereas there was a trend towards decreased CNS complications with increasing middle cerebral flow.

A number of investigators have evaluated the relationship between middle cerebral artery Doppler blood flow and the development of CNS complications in the neonate with conflicting results. Mullaart et al. [143], studying flow in the internal carotid artery, found a correlation between increased diastolic flow and CNS complications, but determined that fluctuations in flow, rather than the flow itself, was the significant correlate. VanBel et al. [144] evaluated the flow in the anterior cerebral artery and found similar results. Bada et al. [135] and Mires et al. [136] performed similar studies but came to the opposite conclusion: a correlation between CNS complications and increased resistance to flow in the CNS (decreased diastolic flow). Other investigators, however [138–140], could find no association between alterations in middle cerebral artery flow and CNS complications, whereas Mari et al. [145] found a lower risk of CNS complications in fetuses with increased middle cerebral artery blood flow.

These conflicting findings might be partially explained by the complex mechanisms that regulate fe-

tal blood flow during developing uteroplacental insufficiency [144]. Akalin-Sel et al. studied Doppler flow in multiple fetal vessels and obtained umbilical venous blood gases in 32 severely growth-restricted fetuses [146]. They found that there are multiple mechanisms that regulate redistribution of blood flow in the fetus so that different clinical circumstances may result in difference changes in CNS blood flow. Investigators have also shown that just before fetal death, increased diastolic flow in the middle cerebral artery is lost, with a return to high resistance to flow, so that both the clinical cause of altered flow and the timing of the study may affect results [147].

In the author's study of CNS blood flow, neither abnormal umbilical artery nor middle cerebral artery blood flow were correlated with the development of CNS complications; but a non-reactive NST did show a strong correlation. Serial studies of high-risk patients with biophysical and Doppler tests have shown that the biophysical parameters (which include the NST) become abnormal only very late in the course of fetal deterioration, and this is consistent with the author's findings [148, 149]. This suggests that serial biophysical and Doppler studies could determine the time course of developing fetal anoxia and lead to a timely intervention.

Venous Doppler

Evaluation of the venous side of the circulation in fetuses suspected of IUGR also provides important in-

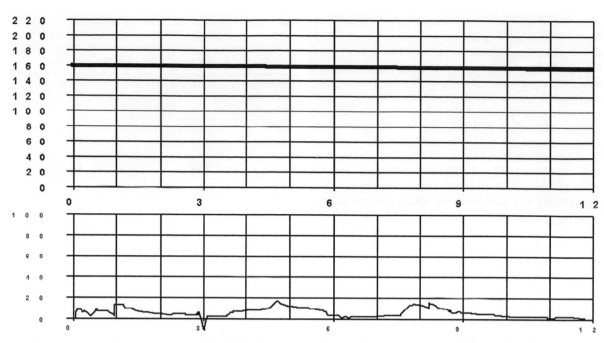

Fig. 18.14. Non-reactive non-stress testing with no acceleration and absent variability at 32 weeks' gestation

clinical situation [170]. In situations where the data is unclear, especially in the preterm fetus, the use of amniocentesis to determine lung maturity may be helpful. Growth-restricted fetuses will frequently have lungs that are more mature than would be expected for their gestational age. Fetal venous Doppler studies give additional information about the time frame and significance of the IUGR [134].

An aggressive approach to the management of IUGR would, hopefully, lead to a reduction in perinatal mortality and morbidity in these high-risk fetuses. A study from the UK showed that IUGR infants identified in the antenatal period (and managed aggressively) had a lower perinatal mortality and less severe 2-year neurodevelopmental, clinical, or growth morbidity than similar IUGR infants that were not identified antenatally [171].

Since approximately half of IUGR fetuses are found in otherwise low-risk pregnancies, a strong point could be made for routine screening for IUGR. At the author's institution it is recommended that an ultrasound examination to evaluate fetal growth in all patients be done at 32–34 weeks' gestation. If fetal weight estimation is below the 10th percentile of the fetal weight curve, additional evaluation is undertaken, which would include a detailed ultrasound examination to look for structural abnormalities and Doppler velocity flow studies of the fetal umbilical artery. If any abnormalities are found, then additional testing is done; if not, then the fetus is considered to be constitutionally SGA and not IUGR. A repeat scan

may be done in 2–3 weeks if the clinical condition warrants and IUGR is still suspected. In those patients with the diagnosis of IUGR weekly (or more frequent) evaluation of the fetus should include both biophysical testing and Doppler studies of the umbilical artery and middle cerebral artery, and in many clinical situations venous Doppler studies are extremely helpful [172–174].

Once the fetus reaches 34 completed weeks of gestation, little is to be gained by prolonging the pregnancy, although in situations where the biophysical testing is normal and the Doppler studies are only minimally abnormal, waiting until 36 weeks may be permissible. In premature fetuses (<32–34 weeks) with immature fetal lung studies, it may be difficult to determine the best time for delivery. Factors that might suggest the need for immediate delivery despite an early gestational age include:

1. Persistent non-reactive non-stress test; the presence of spontaneous late decelerations on the non-stress test; severe oligohydramnios
2. Evidence of "brain sparing" on Doppler ultrasound (lower resistance in the middle cerebral artery than in the umbilical artery)
3. Ominous Doppler studies: reverse diastolic flow in the umbilical artery; umbilical vein pulsatile flow
4. Maternal compromise.

Figures 18.14–18.16 illustrate the combined use of weight estimation, Doppler studies, and biophysical testing in a 32-week singleton gestation being evalu-

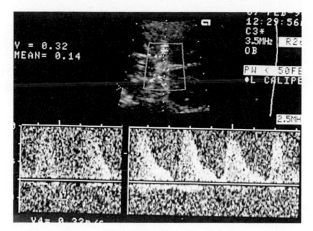

Fig. 18.15. Fetus from Fig. 18.14. High-resistance flow in the middle cerebral artery (loss of "shunting"?)

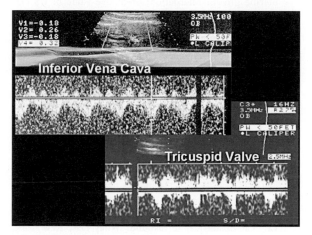

Fig. 18.16. Markedly increased A wave and tricuspid regurgitation in the fetus from Figs. 18.14 and 18.15

ated for IUGR. The estimated fetal weight was 1420 g (less than the 5th percentile) and there were no obvious anomalies seen on the ultrasound examination. The fetus had a non-reactive NST and received a score of 2 on the biophysical profile (only normal fluid). Doppler blood flow studies showed increased resistance in the umbilical artery but no CNS shunting, abnormal inferior vena cava flow, and tricuspid regurgitation. A viable male infant was delivered by cesarean section with Apgar scores of 2 and 6, an arterial pH of 7.15, and a pCO_2 of 61. Placental pathology showed hypoplasia with chronic infarction and decidual necrosis. No organisms were isolated. In this case significant uteroplacental dysfunction leading to IUGR and a compromised fetus was reflected in abnormal weight estimation, biophysical studies, and Doppler ultrasound. The combined use of these modalities enabled the clinicians to better evaluate the seriousness of the fetus' condition.

References

1. Hack M, Flannery DJ, Schluchter M, Cartar L, Borawski E et al (2002) Outcomes in young adulthood for very-low-birth infants. N Engl J Med 346:149–157
2. Taylor DJ (1984) Low birth weight and neurodevelopmental handicap. Clinics in Obstet Gynecol 11:525–531
3. Edouard L, Alberman E (1980) National trends in the identified causes of perinatal mortality 1960–1978. Br J Obstet Gynaecol 87:833–841
4. Simchen MJ, Beiner ME, Strauss-Livianthan N, Dulitsky M, Kuint J et al (2000) Neonatal outcome in growth-restricted versus appropriately grown preterm infants. Am J Perinatol 17:187–192
5. Tejani N, Mann LI (1977) Diagnosis and management of the small for gestational age fetus. Clin Obstet Gynecol 20:943–950
6. Hsieh HL, Lee KS, Khoshnood B et al (1997) Fetal death rate in the United States, 1979–1990: trend and racial disparity. Obstet Gynecol 89:33–39
7. Ahlenius I, Floberg J, Thomassen P (1995) Sixty-six cases of intrauterine fetal death: a prospective study with an extensive test protocol. Acta Obstet Gynecol Scand 74:109–117
8. Cefalo RC (1978) The hazards of labor and delivery for the intrauterine-growth-retarded fetus. J Reprod Med 21:300–314
9. Hediger ML, Overpeck MD, Ruan WJ, Troendle JF (2002) Birthweight and gestational age effects motor and social development. Paediatr Perinat Epidemiol 16:33–46
10. Doctor NA, O'Riordan MA, Kirchner HL, Shah D, Hack M (2001) Perinatal correlates and neonatal outcomes of small for gestational age infants born at term gestation. Am J Obstet Gynecol 185:652–659
11. Bernstein IM, Horbar JD, Badger GJ, Ohlsson A, Golan A (2000) Morbidity and mortality among very-low-birth-weight neonates with intrauterine growth restriction. Am J Obstet Gynecol 182:198–206
12. Keirse MJNC (1984) Epidemiology and aetiology of the growth retarded baby. Clin Obstet Gynaecol 11:415–422
13. Seeds JW (1984) Impaired fetal growth: definition and clinical diagnosis. Obstet Gynecol 64:303–330
14. Varma TR (1984) Low birth weight babies. The small for gestational age. A review of current management. Obstet Gynecol Surv 39:616–631
15. Ott WJ (1993) Intrauterine growth retardation and preterm delivery. Am J Obstet Gynecol 168:1710–1717
16. Zeitlin JA, Ancel P, Saurel-Cubizolles MJ, Papiernik E (2001) Are risk factors the same for small for gestational age versus other preterm births? Am J Obstet Gynecol 185:208–215
17. Ott WJ (1988) The diagnosis of altered fetal growth. Obstet Gynecol Clin North Am 15:237–263
18. Goldenberg AL, Cutter GR, Hoffman HJ et al (1989) Intrauterine growth retardation: standards for diagnosis. Am J Obstet Gynecol 161:271–277
19. Goldenberg RL, Nelson KG, Koski JF et al (1985) Low birth weight, intrauterine growth retardation, and preterm delivery. Am J Obstet Gynecol 152:980–984
20. Ott WJ (ed) (1999) Reference curves. Clinical obstetrical ultrasound. Wiley-Liss, New York, pp 353–384

21. Tamura RK, Sabbagha RE, Depp R et al (1984) Diminished growth in fetuses born preterm after spontaneous labor or rupture of membranes. Am J Obstet Gynecol 148:1105–1110

22. Alexander G, Himes JH, Kaufman RB et al (1997) A United States national reference for fetal growth. Obstet Gynecol 87:163–168

23. Anderson GD, Blidner IN, McClemont S et al (1984) Determinants of size at birth in a Canadian population. Am J Obstet Gynecol 150:236–245

24. Khoury MJ, Cohen BH (1987) Genetic heterogeneity of prematurity and intrauterine growth restriction: clues from the Old Order Amish. Am J Obstet Gynecol 157:400–409

25. Miller HC (1988) Prenatal factors affecting intrauterine growth retardation. Clin Perinatol 12:307–315

26. Peters TJ, Golding J, Butler NR et al (1983) Predictors of birth weight in two national studies. Br J Obstet Gynaecol 90:107–112

27. Raine T, Powell S, Krohn MA (1994) The rise of repeating low birth weight and the role of prenatal care. Obstet Gynecol 84:485–489

28. Hickey CA, Cliver SP, McNeal SF et al (1996) Prenatal weight gain patterns and birth weight among nonobese black and white women. Obstet Gynecol 88:490–496

29. Mittendorf R, Herschel M, Williams MA et al (1994) Reducing the frequency of low birth weight in the United States. Obstet Gynecol 83:1056–1059

30. Bakketeig LS, Hoffman HJ, Harley EE (1979) The tendency to repeat gestational age and birth weight in successive births. Am J Obstet Gynecol 135:1086–1099

31. Jones OW (1978) Genetic factors in the determination of fetal size. J Reprod Med 21:305–310

32. Bada HS, Das A, Bauer CR, Shankaran S, Lester B et al (2002) Gestational cocaine exposure and intrauterine growth: maternal lifestyle study. Obstet Gynecol 100: 916–924

33. Ounsted M, Moar VA, Scott A (1985) Risk factors associated with small-for-dates and large-for-dates infants. Br J Obstet Gynaecol 92:226–232

34. Visser GHA, Huisman A, Saathof PWF et al (1986) Early fetal growth retardation: obstetric background and recurrence rate. Obstet Gynecol 67:40–46

35. Wolfe HM, Gross TL, Sokol RJ (1987) Recurrent small for gestational age birth. Perinatal risks and outcomes. Am J Obstet Gynecol 157:288–297

36. Duverot JJ, Cheriex E, Pieters FAA et al (1995) Maternal volume homeostasis in early pregnancy in relation to fetal growth restriction. Obstet Gynecol 85:361–367

37. Salafia CM, Ernst LM, Pezzullo JC et al (1995) The very low birthweight infant: maternal complications leading to preterm birth, placental lesions, and intrauterine growth. Am J Perinatol 12:106–110

38. Benson CB, Doubilet PM, Saltzman DH (1986) Intrauterine growth retardation: predictive value of US criteria for antenatal diagnosis. Radiology 160:415–426

39. Brown HL, Miller JM, Gabert HA et al (1987) Ultrasonic recognition of the small-for-gestational-age fetus. Obstet Gynecol 69:631–647

40. Crane JP, Lopta MM, Welt SI et al (1977) Abnormal fetal growth patterns: ultrasonic diagnosis and management. Obstet Gynecol 50:205–209

41. Deter RL, Harrist RB, Hadlock FP et al (1982) The use of ultrasound in the detection of intrauterine growth retardation: a review. J Clin Ultrasound 10:9–22

42. Deter RL, Hadlock FP, Harrist RB (1983) Evaluation of normal fetal growth and the detection of intrauterine growth retardation. In: Callen PW (ed) Ultrasonography in obstetrics and gynecology. Saunders, Philadelphia, pp 113–140

43. Hadlock FP, Deter RL, Harrist RB et al (1983) Sonographic detection of fetal intrauterine growth retardation. Perinatol Neonatol 7:21–32

44. Little D, Campbell S (1982) Ultrasound evaluation of intrauterine growth retardation. Radiol Clin North Am 20:335–342

45. Ott WJ (1985) Fetal femur length, neonatal crown-heel length and screening for IUGR. Obstet Gynecol 65:460–465

46. Ott WJ (1985) The diagnosis of altered fetal growth. Obstet Gynecol Clin North Am 15:237–249

47. Benson CB, Doubilet PM, Saltzman DH (1986) Intrauterine growth retardation: predictive value of US criteria for antenatal diagnosis. Radiology 160:415–417

48. Schild RL, Fimmers R, Hansmann M (2000) Fetal weight estimation by three-dimensional ultrasound. Ultrasound Obstet Gynecol 16:445–452

49. Song TB, Moore TR, Lee JY, Kim YH, Kim EK (2000) Fetal weight prediction by thigh volume measurements with three-dimensional ultrasonography. Obstet Gynecol 69:157–161

50. Lee W, Comstock CH, Kirk JS, Smith RS, Monck JW et al (1997) Birthweight prediction by three-dimensional ultrasonographic volumes of the fetal thigh and abdomen. J Ultrasound Med 16:799–805

51. Ott WJ (2002) The diagnosis of intrauterine growth restriction: comparison of ultrasound parameters. Am J Perinatol 19:133–137

52. Ott WJ (1999) Altered fetal growth. In: Ott WJ (ed) Clinical obstetrical ultrasound. Wiley-Liss, New York, pp 229–262

53. Soothill PW, Bobrow CS, Holmes RP (1999) Small for gestational age is not a diagnosis. Ultrasound Obstet Gynecol 13:225–228

54. Craigo SD, Beach ML, Harvey-Wilkes KB, D'Alton ME (1996) Ultrasound predictors of neonatal outcome in intrauterine growth restriction. Am J Perinatol 13:465–471

55. Resnik R (2002) Intrauterine growth restriction. Obstet Gynecol 99:490–496

56. Krebs C, Macara LM, Leiser R et al (1996) Intrauterine growth restriction with absent end-diastolic flow velocity in the umbilical artery is associated with maldevelopment of the placental terminal villous tree. Am J Obstet Gynecol 175:1534–1542

57. Giles W, Ocallaghan S, Read M et al (1997) Placental nitric oxide synthase activity and abnormal umbilical artery flow velocity waveforms. Obstet Gynecol 89:49–52

58. Giles W, Falconer J, Read M et al (1997) Ovine fetal umbilical artery Doppler systolic diastolic ratios and nitric oxide synthase. Obstet Gynecol 89:53–56

59. MacLean M, Mathers A, Walker J et al (1992) The ultrasonic assessment of discordant growth in twin pregnancies. Ultrasound Obstet Gynecol 2:30–34

60. Reed K, Anderson C, Shenker L (1987) Changes in intracardiac Doppler blood flow velocities in fetuses with absent umbilical artery diastolic flow. Am J Obstet Gynecol 157:774–779

61. Chandran R, Serra-Serra V, Sellers S et al (1993) Fetal cerebral Doppler in the recognition of fetal compromise. Br J Obstet Gynaecol 100:139–144

62. Vyas S, Nicolaides K, Bower S et al (1990) Middle cerebral artery flow velocity waveforms in fetal hypoxemia. Br J Obstet Gynaecol 97:797–803

63. Trudinger BJ, Giles WB, Cook CM et al (1985) Fetal umbilical artery flow velocity waveforms and placental resistance: clinical significance. Br J Obstet Gynaecol 92:23–31

64. Erskin RLA, Ritchie JWK (1985) Umbilical artery blood flow characteristics in normal and growth-retarded fetuses. Br J Obstet Gynaecol 92:605–615

65. Giles WB, Trudinger BJ, Baird PJ (1985) Fetal umbilical artery flow velocity waveforms and placental resistance: pathological correlation. Br J Obstet Gynaecol 92:31–39

66. Hitschold T, Weiss E, Beck T et al (1993) Low target birth weight or growth retardation? Umbilical doppler flow velocity waveforms and histometric analysis of fetoplacental vascular tree. Am J Obstet Gynecol 168:1260–1264

67. Locci M, Nazzaro G, DePlacido G et al (1993) Correlation of Doppler and placental immunohistochemical features in normal and intrauterine growth-retarded fetuses. Ultrasound Obstet Gynecol 3:240–245

68. Ott WJ (2000) Intrauterine growth restriction and Doppler ultrasound. J Ultrasound Med 19:661–668

69. Soothill PW, Bobrow CS, Holmes RP (1999) Small for gestational age is not a diagnosis. Ultrasound Obstet Gynecol 13:225–228

70. Holmes RP, Soothill PW (1999) Small fetuses with normal Dopplers are appropriately grown with normal pregnancy outcomes. J Obstet Gynecol 19 (Suppl 1):23

71. Craigo SD, Beach ML, Harvey-Wilkes KB, D'Alton ME (1996) Ultrasound predictors of neonatal outcome in intrauterine growth restriction. Am J Perinatol 13:465–471

72. Steel SA, Pearce M, Chamberlain GV (1988) Doppler ultrasound of the uteroplacental circulation as a screening test for severe pre-eclampsia with intrauterine growth retardation. Eur J Obstet Gynecol Reprod Biol 28:279–287

73. North RA, Ferrier C, Long D et al (1994) Uterine artery Doppler flow velocity waveforms in the second trimester for the prediction of preeclampsia and fetal growth retardation. Obstet Gynecol 83:378–386

74. Atkinson MW, Maher JE, Owen J et al (1994) The predictive value of umbilical artery doppler studies for preeclampsia or fetal growth retardation in a preeclampsia prevention trial. Obstet Gynecol 83:609–612

75. Vergani P, Roncaglia N, Andreotti C, Arreghini A, Teruzzi M et al (2002) Prognostic value of uterine artery Doppler velocimetry in growth-restricted fetuses delivered near term. Am J Obstet Gynecol 187:932–936

76. Chien PF, Arnott N, Gordon A, Owen P, Khon K (2000) How useful is uterine artery Doppler flow velocimetry in the prediction of pre-eclampsia, intrauterine growth retardation and perinatal death? Br J Obstet Gynaecol 107:196–208

77. Albaiges G, Missfelder-Lobos H, Lees C, Parra M, Nicolaides KH (2000) One-stage screening for pregnancy complications by color Doppler assessment of the uterine arteries at 23 weeks' gestation. Obstet Gynecol 96:559–564

78. Papageorghiou AT, Yu CKH, Bindra R, Pandis G, Nicolaides KH (2001) Multicenter screening for pre-eclampsia and fetal growth restriction by transvaginal uterine artery Doppler at 23 weeks of gestation. Ultrasound Obstet Gynecol 18:441–449

79. Lees C, Parra M, Missfelder-Lobos H, Morgans A, Fletcher O, Nicolaides KH (2001) Individualized risk assessment for adverse pregnancy outcome by uterine artery Doppler at 23 weeks. Obstet Gynecol 98:369–373

80. Missfelder-Lobos H, Teran E, Lees C, Albaiges G, Nicolaides KH (2002) Platelet changes and subsequent development of pre-eclampsia and fetal growth restriction in women with abnormal uterine artery Doppler screening. Ultrasound Obstet Gynecol 19:443–448

81. Martin AM, Bindra R, Curcio P, Cicero S, Nicolaides KH (2001) Screening for pre-eclampsia and fetal growth restriction by uterine artery Doppler at 11–14 weeks of gestation. Ultrasound Obstet Gynecol 18:583–583

82. Hernandez-Andrade E, Brodszki J, Lingman G, Gudmundsson S, Molin J, Maršál K (2002) Uterine artery score and perinatal outcome. Ultrasound Obstet Gynecol 19:438–442

83. Venkat-Raman N, Backos M, Teoh TG, Lo WTS, Regan L (2001) Uterine artery Doppler in predicting pregnancy outcome in women with antiphospholipid syndrome. Obstet Gynecol 98:235–242

84. Abramowicz JS, Sherer DM, Bar-Tov E et al (1991) The cheek-to-cheek diameter in the ultrasonographic assessment of fetal growth. Am J Obstet Gynecol 165:846–852

85. Hill LM, Guzick D, Thomas ML et al (1989) Thigh circumference in the detection of intrauterine growth retardation. Am J Perinatol 6:349–352

86. Catalano PM, Tyzbir ED, Allen SR et al (1992) Evaluation of fetal growth by estimation of neonatal body composition. Obstet Gynecol 79:46–50

87. Sumners JE, Findley GM, Ferguson KA (1990) Evaluation methods for intrauterine growth using neonatal fat stores instead of birth weight as outcome measures: fetal and neonatal measurements correlated with neonatal skinfold thickness. J Clin Ultrasound 18:9–14

88. Berstein IM, Goran MI, Amini SB et al (1997) Differential growth of fetal tissues during the second half of pregnancy. Am J Obstet Gynecol 176:28–32

89. Hill IM, Guzick D, Doyles D et al (1992) Subcutaneous tissue thickness cannot be used to distinguish abnormalities of fetal growth. Obstet Gynecol 80:268–271

90. Gardeil F, Greene R, Stuart B et al (1999) Subcutaneous fat in the fetal abdomen as a predictor of growth restriction. Obstet Gynecol 94:209–212

91. Gimondo P, Mirk P, LaBella A et al (1995) Sonographic estimation of fetal liver weight: an additional biometric parameter for assessment of fetal growth. J Ultrasound Med 14:327–333

92. Alfrevic Z, Neilson JP (1995) Doppler ultrasonography in high-risk pregnancies: systematic review with meta-analysis. Am J Obstet Gynecol 172:1379–1387

93. Divon MY (1995) Randomized controlled trials of umbilical artery Doppler velocimetry: How many are too many? Ultrasound Obstet Gynecol 6:377–379

94. Divon MY (1996) Umbilical artery Doppler velocimetry: clinical utility in high-risk pregnancies. Am J Obstet Gynecol 174:10–14

95. Wienerroither H, Steiner H, Tomaselli J, Lobendanz M, Thuyn-Hohenstein L (2001) Intrauterine blood flow and long term intellectual, neurologic, and social development. Obstet Gynecol 97:449–453

96. Rochelson B, Schulman H, Farmakides G et al (1987) The significance of absent end-diastolic velocity in umbilical artery waveforms. Am J Obstet Gynecol 156:1213–1218

97. Divon MY, Girz BA, Lieblich R et al (1989) Clinical management of the fetus with markedly diminished umbilical artery end diastolic flow. Am J Obstet Gynecol 161:1523–1527

98. Karsdorp VHM, van Vugt JMG, van Geijn HP et al (1994) Clinical significance of absent or reverse end diastolic velocity waveforms in umbilical artery. Lancet 344:1664–1667

99. Valcomonico A, Danti L, Frusca T et al (1994) Absent end-diastolic velocity in umbilical artery: risk of neonatal morbidity and brain damage. Am J Obstet Gynecol 170:796–801

100. Gaziano EP, Knox H, Ferrera B et al (1994) Is it time to reassess the risk for the growth-retarded fetus with normal Doppler velocimetry of the umbilical artery? Am J Obstet Gynecol 170:1734–1743

101. Almstrom H, Axelsson O, Snattingius S et al (1992) Comparison of umbilical-artery velocimetry and cardiotocography for surveillance of small-for-gestational-age fetuses. Lance 340:936–941

102. DeVore GR (1994) The effect of an abnormal umbilical artery doppler on the management of fetal growth restriction: a survey of maternal-fetal medicine specialists who perform fetal ultrasound. Ultrasound Obstet Gynecol 4:294–303

103. Maršál K, Persson P (1988) Ultrasonic measurement of fetal blood velocity wave form as a secondary diagnostic test in screening for intrauterine growth retardation. J Clin Ultrasound 16:239–244

104. Yoon BH, Romero R, Roh CR et al (1993) Relationship between the fetal biophysical profile score, umbilical artery Doppler velocimetry, and fetal blood acid–base status determined by cordocentesis. Am J Obstet Gynecol 169:1586–1594

105. Johnstone FD, Prescott R, Hoskins P et al (1993) The effect of introduction of umbilical Doppler recordings to obstetric practice. Br J Obstet Gynaecol 100:733–741

106. Yoon BH, Lee CM, Kim SW (1994) An abnormal umbilical artery waveform: a strong and independent predictor of adverse perinatal outcome in patients with preeclampsia. Am J Obstet Gynecol 171:713–721

107. Wladimiroff JW, Wijngaard AGW, Degani S et al (1987) Cerebral and umbilical arterial blood flow velocity waveforms in normal and growth-retarded pregnancies. Obstet Gynecol 69:705–709

108. Gramellini D, Folli MC, Raboni S et al (1991) Cerebral–umbilical Doppler ratio as a predictor of adverse perinatal outcome. Obstet Gynecol 79:416–420

109. Devine PA, Bracero LA, Lysikiewicz A et al (1994) Middle cerebral to umbilical artery Doppler ratio in postdate pregnancies. Obstet Gynecol 84:856–860

110. Mari G (1994) Regional cerebral flow velocity waveforms in the human fetus. J Ultrasound Med 13:343–346

111. Arabin B, Snyjders R, Mohnhaupt A et al (1993) Evaluation of the fetal assessment score in pregnancies a risk for intrauterine hypoxia. Am J Obstet Gyneocl 169:549–554

112. Baschat AA, Gembruch U, Harman CR (2001) The sequence of changes in Doppler and biophysical parameters as severe fetal growth restriction worsens. Ultrasound Obstet Gynecol 18:571–577

113. Hecher K, Bilardo CM, Stigter RH et al (2002) Monitoring of fetuses with intrauterine growth restriction: a longitudinal study. Ultrasound Obstet Gynecol 19:564–570

114. Ott WJ (1999) Comparison of the non-stress test with the evaluation of centralization of blood flow by the prediction of neonatal compromise. Ultrasound Obstet Gynecol 14:38–41

115. Ott WJ, Mora G, Arias F et al (1998) Comparison of the modified biophysical profile to a "new" biophysical profile incorporating the middle cerebral artery to umbilical artery velocity flow systolic/diastolic ratio. Am J Obstet Gynecol 178:1346–1353

116. Rizzo G, Capponi A, Pietropolli A et al (1994) Fetal cardiac and extracardiac flows preceding intrauterine death. Ultrasound Obstet Gynecol 4:139–142

117. Akalin-Sel T, Nicolaides K, Peacock J et al (1994) Doppler dynamics and their complex interrelation with fetal oxygen pressure, carbon dioxide pressure, and pH in growth-retarded fetuses. Obstet Gynecol 84:439–444

118. Guzman E, Vintzileos A, Martins M (1995) Relationship between middle cerebral artery velocimetry, computer fetal heart rate assessment and degree of acidemia at birth in intrauterine growth restricted fetuses. Am J Obstet Gynecol 172:337

119. Detti L, Mari G, Akiyama M, Cosmi E, Moise KJ et al (2002) Longitudinal assessment of the middle cerebral artery peak systolic velocity in healthy fetuses and in fetuses at risk for anemia. Am J Obstet Gynecol 187:937–939

120. Woo JK, Liang ST, Chan FY (1987) Middle cerebral artery Doppler flow velocity waveforms. Obstet Gynecol 70:613–616

121. Wladimiroff JW, Tonge HM, Sewart PA (1986) Doppler ultrasound assessment of cerebral blood flow in the human fetus. Br J Obstet Gynaecol 93:471–475

122. Vyas S, Nicolaides KH, Bower S et al (1990) Middle cerebral artery flow velocity waveforms in fetal hypoxemia. Br J Obstet Gynaecol 97:797–803

123. Huang SC, Chen CP, Chang FM et al (1993) Serial follow-up of abnormal flow velocity waveforms of dying fetus in case of chronic hypertension. J Clin Ultrasound 21:537–541

124. Rizzo G, Capponi A, Pietropolli LM et al (1994) Fetal cardiac and extracardiac flows preceding intrauterine death. Ultrasound Obstet Gynecol 4:139–142

125. Gramellini D, Folli MC, Raboni S et al (1992) Cerebral umbilical Doppler ratio as a predictor of adverse perinatal outcome. Obstet Gynecol 79:416–420

126. Simon NV, Levisky JS, Shearer DM et al (1988) Predictiveness of sonographic fetal weight estimation as a function of prior probability of intrauterine growth retardation. J Clin Ultrasound 16:285–298

127. Warsof SL, Cooper DJ, Little D et al (1986) Routine ultrasound screening for antenatal detection of intrauterine growth retardation. Obstet Gynecol 76:33–47

128. Mcdearis A (1988) The evaluation and interpretation of ultrasonic assessment of fetal growth. Semin Perinatol 12:31–58

129. Campbell S, Bewley S, Cohen-Overbeek (1987) Investigation of the uteroplacental circulation by Doppler ultrasound. Semin Perinatol 11:362–381

130. Ott WJ (1991) Value of fetal umbilical artery and carotid Doppler flow studies in the evaluation of suspected IUGR. J Matern Fetal Invest 1:185–190

131. Arias F (1994) Accuracy of the middle-cerebral-to-umbilical-artery resistance index ratio in the prediction of neonatal outcome in patients at high risk for fetal and neonatal complications. Am J Obstet Gynecol 171:1541–1545

132. Sterne G, Shields LE, Dubinsky TJ (2001) Abnormal fetal cerebral and umbilical Doppler measurements in fetuses with intrauterine growth restriction predicts the severity of perinatal morbidity. J Clin Ultrasound 29:146–151

133. Akalin-Sel T, Nicolaides K, Peacock J et al (1994) Doppler dynamics and their complex interrelation with fetal oxygen pressure, carbon dioxide pressure, and pH in growth-retarded fetuses. Obstet Gynecol 84:439–444

134. Guzman E, Vintzileos A, Martins M (1995) Relationship between middle cerebral artery velocimetry, computer fetal heart rate assessment and degree of acidemia at birth in intrauterine growth restricted fetuses. Am J Obstet Gynecol 172:337

135. Bada HS, Miller JE, Menke JA, Menten TG, Bashiru M, Binstadt D, Sumner DS, Khanna NN (1982) Intracranial pressure and cerebral arterial pulsatile flow measurement in neonatal intraventricular hemorrhage. J Pediatr 100:291–296

136. Mires GJ, Patel NB, Forsyth JS, Howie PW (1994) Neonatal cerebral Doppler flow velocity waveforms in the pre-term infant with cerebral pathology. Early Hum Dev 36:213–222

137. Ilikkan B, Vural M, Yardimci D, Ozbek S, Perk Y, Ilter O (1998) Intraventricular hemorrhage in premature newborns. Turk J Pediatr 40:195–200

138. Baschat AA, Gembruch U, Viscardi RM, Gortner L, Harman CR (2002) Antenatal prediction of intraventricular hemorrhage in fetal growth restriction: What is the role of Doppler? Ultrasound Obstet Gynecol 19:334–339

139. Chan FY, Pun TC, Lam P, Lam C, Lee CP, Lam YH (1996) Fetal cerebral Doppler studies as a predictor of perinatal outcome and subsequent neurologic handicap. Obstet Gynecol 87:981–988

140. Scherjo SA, Oosting H, Smolders-DeHass H, Zondervan HA, Kok JH (1998) Neurodevelopmental outcome at three years of age after fetal 'brain-sparing'. Early Hum Dev 52:67–79

141. Woo JSK, Liang ST, Lo LS, Chan FY (1987) Middle cerebral artery Doppler flow velocity waveforms. Obstet Gynecol 70:613–616

142. Kurmanavicius J, Florio I, Wisser J, Hebisch G, Zimmermann R, Muller R, Huch R, Huch A (1997) Reference resistance indices of the umbilical, fetal middle cerebral and uterine arteries at 24–42 weeks' gestation. Ultrasound Obstet Gynecol 10:112–120

143. Mullaart RA, Hopman JC, Rotteveel JJ, Daniels O, Stoelinga GB, DeHaan AF (1994) Cerebral blood flow fluctuation in neonatal respiratory distress and periventricular haemorrhage. Early Hum Dev 37:179–185

144. VanBel F, VandeBor M, Stijnen T, Baan J, Ruys JH (1987) Aetiological role of cerebral blood-flow alterations in development and extension of peri-intraventricular haemorrhage. Dev Med Child Neurol 29:601–614

145. Mari G, Abuhamad AZ, Keller M, Verpairojkit B, Ment L, Copel JA (1996) Is the fetal brain-sparing effect a risk factor for the development of intraventricular hemorrhage in the preterm infant? Ultrasound Obstet Gynecol 8:329–332

146. Akalin-Sel T, Nicolaides KH, Peacock J, Campbell S (1994) Doppler dynamics and their complex interrelation with fetal oxygen pressure, carbon dioxide pressure, and pH in growth-retarded fetuses. Obstet Gynecol 84:439–444

147. Rizzo G, Capponi A, Pietropolli LM, Bufalino D, Romanini C (1994) Fetal cardiac and extracardiac flows preceding intrauterine death. Ultrasound Obstet Gynecol 4:139–142

148. Forouzan I, Zhi-Yun T (1996) Fetal middle cerebral artery blood flow velocities in pregnancies complicated by intrauterine growth restriction and extreme abnormality in umbilical artery Doppler velocity. Am J Perinatol 13:139–142

149. Baschat AA, Gembruch U, Harman CR (2001) The sequence of changes in Doppler and biophysical parameters as severe fetal growth restriction worsens. Ultrasound Obstet Gynecol 18:571–577

150. Wladimiroff J, Huisman T, Stewart P (1991) Normal fetal arterial and venous flow-velocity waveforms in early and late gestation. In: Jaffe R, Warsof S (eds) Color Doppler imaging in obstetrics and gynecology. McGraw-Hill, New York, pp 155–173

151. Reed K (1991) Venous flow velocities in the fetus. In: Jaffe R, Warsof S (eds) Color Doppler imaging in obstetrics and gynecology. McGraw-Hill, New York, pp 175–181

152. Appleton C, Hatle L, Popp R (1987) Superior vena cava and hepatic vein doppler echocardiography in healthy adults. J Am Coll Cardiol 10:1032–1039

153. Reuss M, Rudolph A, Dae M (1993) Phasic blood flow patterns in the superior and inferior venae cavae and umbilical vein of fetal sheep. Am J Obstet Gynecol 145:70–78

154. Huisman T, van den Eijnde S, Stewart P et al (1993) Changes in inferior vena cava blood flow velocity and diameter during breathing movements in the human fetus. Ultrasound Obstet Gynecol 3:26–30

155. Reed K, Appleton C, Anderson C et al (1990) Doppler studies of vena cava flows in human fetuses. Circulation 81:498–505

156. Indik J, Chen V, Reed K (1991) Association of umbilical venous with inferior vena cava blood flow velocities. Obstet Gynecol 77:551–557

157. Rizzo G, Capponi A, Talone PE et al (1996) Doppler indices from inferior vena cava and ductus venosus in predicting pH and oxygen tension in umbilical blood at cordocentesis in growth-retarded fetuses. Ultrasound Obstet Gynecol 7:401–410

158. Nakai Y, Miyazaki Y, Masuoka Y (1992) Pulsatile umbilical venous flow and its clinical significance. Br J Obstet Gynaecol 99:977–980

159. Mitra SC (1995) Umbilical venous Doppler waveform without fetal breathing: its significance. Am J Perinatol 12:217–219

160. Reed KL, Chaffin DG, Anderson CF (1996) Umbilical venous Doppler velocity pulsations and inferior vena cava pressure elevations in fetal lambs. Obstet Gynecol 87:617–620

161. Ott WJ (1999) The value of fetal inferior vena cava blood flow analysis for prediction of neonatal outcome. Am J Perinatol 16:429–435

162. Ott WJ, Mora G, Arias F et al (1998) Comparison of the modified biophysical profile to a "new" biophysical profile incorporating the middle cerebral artery to umbilical artery velocity flow systolic/diastolic ratio. Am J Obstet Gynecol 178:1346–1353

163. Rizzo G, Capponi A, Talone PE, Ardunini D, Romanini C (1996) Doppler indices from inferior vena cava and ductus venosus in predicting pH and oxygen tension in umbilical blood at cordocentesis in growth-retarded fetuses. Ultrasound Obstet Gynecol 7:401–410

164. Rizzo G, Capponi A, Talone PE et al (1996) Doppler indices from inferior vena cava and ductus venosus in predicting pH and oxygen tension in umbilical blood at cordocentesis in growth-retarded fetuses. Ultrasound Obstet Gynecol 7:401–410

165. DeVore GR, Horenstein J (1993) Ductus venosus index: a method for evaluating right ventricular preload in the second-trimester fetus. Ultrasound Obstet Gynecol 3:338–342

166. Kiserud T, Eik-Nes SH, Blaas HGK et al (1991) Ultrasonographic velocimetry of the fetal ductus venosus. Lancet 338:1412–1414

167. Reed KL, Chaffin DG, Anderson CF (1996) Umbilical venous Doppler velocity pulsations and inferior vena cava pressure elevations in fetal lambs. Obstet Gynecol 87:617–620

168. Sherer DM, Fromberg RA, Divon MY (1996) Prenatal ultrasonographic assessment of the ductus venosus: a review. Obstet Gynecol 88:626–632

169. Kiserud T, Eik-Nes SH, Blaas HG et al (1994) Ductus venosus blood velocity and the umbilical circulation in the seriously growth-retarded fetus. Ultrasound Obstet Gynecol 4:109–114

170. Harrington KF (2000) Making best and appropriate use of fetal biophysical and Doppler ultrasound data in the management of the growth restricted fetus. Ultrasound Obstet Gynecol 16:399–401

171. Ogundipe EM, Wolfe CDA, Seed P et al (2000) Does the antenatal detection of small-for-gestational age babies influence their two-year outcomes? Am J Perinatol 17:73–81

172. Baschat AA, Gembruch U, Harman CR (2001) The sequence of changes in Doppler and biophysical parameters as severe fetal growth restriction worsens. Ultrasound Obstet Gynecol 18:571–577

173. Hecher K, Bilardo CM, Stigter RH, Ville Y, Hackeloer BJ et al (2002) Monitoring of fetuses with intrauterine growth restriction: a longitudinal study. Ultrasound Obstet Gynecol 19:564–570

174. Ferrazzi E, Bozzo M, Rigano S, Bellotti M, Morabito A, Pardi G et al (2002) Temporal sequence of abnormal Doppler changes in the peripheral and central circulatory systems of the severely growth-restricted fetus. Ultrasound Obstet Gynecol 19:140–146

Chapter 19

Doppler Velocimetry and Hypertension

Hein Odendaal

Introduction

Pre-eclampsia and to a lesser extent hypertension in pregnancy is a vascular disease affecting both maternal and fetal circulations. On the maternal side, one of the very early characteristics of the disease is the deficient infiltration of the spiral arteries by the trophoblast, failing to convert it to uteroplacental arteries [12]. Subsequently, the 10- to 12-fold increase in uterine perfusion, as is seen in normal pregnancy, does not occur. This affects blood flow in the uterine artery [16]. On the fetal side there is poor vascularization of the terminal villi, villous stromal hemorrhage and hemorrhagic endovasculitis [50, 51] or even obliteration of stem villi [26, 27]. As Doppler techniques enable one to study flow velocity waveforms in a non-invasive way, it became one of the most ideal methods to analyze the maternal and fetal circulations and in particular that of the uterine and umbilical arteries. Although Satomura [86] described the feasibility of Doppler ultrasound to determine flow velocity in a peripheral artery, it took almost 20 years until the next important development in this field, when Fitzgerald and Drumm [34] used Doppler ultrasonography to investigate the human fetal circulation. Six years later Campbell et al. [16] reported, for the first time, the importance of uterine artery Doppler in obstetrics. Subsequently, developments have been summarized in very good recent reviews to which the interested reader is referred [13, 24, 26, 27, 36, 50, 51, 64, 65]. Although the research on the umbilical artery preceded that on the uterine artery and the use of its flow velocity waveforms is more established in clinical medicine, the uterine artery is discussed first to follow chronological events in pregnancy.

Uterine Artery

As a result of the trophoblast invasion of the spiral arteries, and increase in uterine perfusion, end-diastolic flow in the uterine artery increases as the pregnancy advances. This gives the flow velocity waveform of the uterine artery a unique shape, character-

ized by high end-diastolic velocities with continuous forward blood flow throughout diastole [27]; however, in abnormal pregnancy there is poor trophoblast invasion of the spiral arteries. Subsequently, the end-diastolic flow does not increase or the diastolic notch does not disappear (Fig. 19.1).

To be able to apply the use of uterine artery flow velocity in clinical practice the following questions need to be answered:
1. How accurate is the screening?
2. When should the screening start?
3. What is the best method of screening?
4. Should any high-risk women be screened?
5. Which risks should be identified?
6. Can intervention in the identified women improve the outcome of pregnancy?

Screening in the First Trimester

Schuchter et al. [87] examined both uterine arteries in 380 singleton pregnancies during the 11–14 weeks of screening for nuchal translucency. They used a pulsatility index at and above the 90th percentile to identify fetal growth restriction, pregnancy-induced hypertension, pre-eclampsia and placental abruption. Their screening was positive in 10% of women. The sensitivity was 25%, and 8.4% of tests were false positive. They also assessed the placental volume at the same examination and found that a combination of the two examinations reduced the sensitivity but increased the number of false-positive tests.

Screening in the Second Trimester

Coleman et al. [21] studied 116 pregnancies in 114 women at high risk of pre-eclampsia. They screened the women between 22 and 24 weeks' gestation using a resistance index (RI) >0.58 as abnormal. Outcome measures were pre-eclampsia, small for gestational age (SGA), placental abruption, intrauterine death and "all" and "severe" outcomes. The sensitivity of any RI >0.58 for pre-eclampsia, SGA, "all" outcomes and "severe" outcomes was 91, 84, 83 and 90%, respectively. Specificity for these outcomes was 42, 39, 47 and 38%, respectively. The positive predictive val-

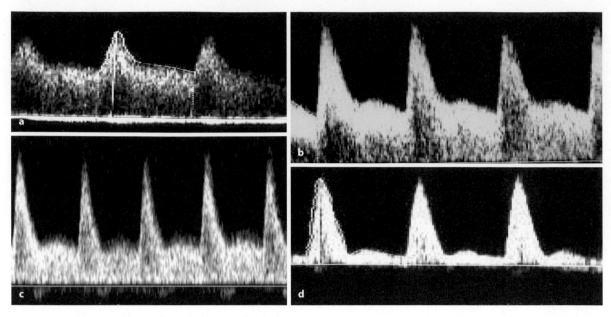

Fig. 19.1. Different flow velocity waveforms of the uterine artery. **a** Good velocity, no notch. **b** Slightly reduced velocity with visible notch. **c** Reduced diastolic velocity with visible notch. **d** Poor diastolic velocity with visible notch

ue for these outcomes was 37, 33, 58 and 24%, respectively. Using both values and a RI of ≥0.7 the positive predictive value improved to 58, 67, 85 and 58%. In the cases of bilateral notches the positive predictive value was 47, 53, 76 and 65%, respectively. They concluded that uterine artery Doppler waveform analysis was better than the clinical risk assessment in the prediction of pre-eclampsia and SGA babies.

Ohkuchi et al. [77] examined 288 normal women attending the antenatal clinic between 16 and 23.9 weeks of gestation, using the notch depth index (NDI) to identify the patient at risk. End points were pre-eclampsia, which developed in 3.1% of women and SGA which occurred in 6.3% of newborns. The sensitivity, specificity and positive predictive values were 67, 92 and 22%, respectively. Using receiver-operating characteristics curves, they found that the NDI was better than the RI or peak systolic to early diastolic velocity ratio in predicting pre-eclampsia or the SGA infant.

Recently, a one-stage screening for pregnancy complications by color Doppler assessment at 23 weeks' gestation was introduced [4]. A mean PI of more than 1.45 was considered increased. Bilateral uterine artery notches were also noted. Increased PI was noted in 5.1% of the 1757 pregnancies. Bilateral notches were noted in 4.4%. Examining how bilateral notches or the mean pulsatility index above 1.45 could predict pre-eclampsia, they found that the sensitivity, specificity and positive predictive value was 45, 94 and 23%, respectively. For pre-eclampsia delivered before 34 weeks these values were 90, 93 and

7%, respectively. They then looked at the PI and bilateral notches individually and in combination and concluded that the screening results were similar for increased PI or bilateral notches. Women with bilateral notches and a high mean PI had a 40% chance of developing pre-eclampsia.

McCowan et al. [66] concentrated on high-risk pregnancies. First of all they selected 224 women with suspected SGA babies (<10th percentile by abdominal circumference on ultrasound) and who were normotensive when the uterine artery Doppler studies were performed. Of the 50 women who developed subsequent hypertension, 42 had gestational hypertension and 8 had eclampsia. When the first uterine artery Doppler examinations were done, both RIs were >0.58 in 7% of pregnancies which remained normotensive, in 17% of pregnancies where gestational hypertension developed and in 50% of pregnancies where pre-eclampsia developed. For bilateral abnormal uterine artery Doppler, in the prediction of gestational hypertension or pre-eclampsia, the sensitivity, specificity and positive predictive value were 22, 93 and 45%, respectively. They also found that more severe uterine artery Doppler abnormalities were associated with more severe fetal disease.

In a different approach, Valensise et al. [100] studied 36 normotensive women with a uterine artery RI >0.58 and bilateral notching at 24 weeks' gestation. Twelve of them developed gestational hypertension and 3 had SGA newborns. When compared with the pregnancies with a normal outcome, these 15 patients (at 24 weeks) had smaller left ventricular outflow tract and left ventricular diastolic diameter. Atrial and ventricular functions were significantly lower in the pathological outcome group. The authors concluded that abnormal placentation has a wide effect on the whole cardiovascular system.

Screening in the Third Trimester

Few studies addressed the significance of abnormal waveforms in the uterine artery in the third trimester. One of these, by Park et al. [81], followed the outcome in 198 pregnant women with an early diastolic notch after 28 weeks' gestation, 9.1% of the pregnant women who were initially screened. Outcome according to the notch index (NI; early diastolic flow/peak diastolic flow) was compared in different categories viz. <0.7, 0.7 to <0.8, 0.8 to <0.9 and ≥0.9. Perinatal outcome improved as the NI increased. For example, there were 9.5% perinatal deaths when the index was <0.7 but no perinatal deaths when the notch index was ≥0.9. Unfortunately, they did not look at the development of hypertension.

Method of Screening (Quantifying Poor Diastolic Flow Velocity)

Aardema et al. [1] compared the PI with NI (peak of notch – nadir of notch/mean flow) at 21–22 weeks' gestation in 531 nulliparous women and 94 multiparous women at risk. Both values were poor predictors for mild gestational hypertension and pre-eclampsia; however, for severe disease the prediction was much better. Logistic regression analysis showed that the NI had no additional value compared with the PI in the prediction of either mild or severe disease.

Using color flow/pulse Doppler, Aquilina et al. [7] examined both uterine arteries at 20 weeks in 614 primiparous women. They then created receiver-operator characteristics curves for systolic/end-diastolic ratio, resistance index and systolic/early diastolic ratio, individually or in the presence or absence of unilateral or bilateral notching. The highest sensitivity (88%) in predicting pre-eclampsia and specificity (83%) was obtained when bilateral notching and mean RI≥0.55 (50th percentile) were used. They concluded that at 20 weeks' gestation, bilateral notches with mean RI cut-offs is the best method if further screening later in pregnancy is proposed.

The Effect of Gestational Age

In studying 88 patients with abnormal uterine Doppler velocimetry at 24 weeks' gestation, it was found that 49% of patients had normalization of uterine artery velocimetry after 28 weeks' gestation, some of which normalized after only 32–34 weeks [91]. No patient developed pre-eclampsia or other severe complications when the uterine artery velocimetry returned to normal. The gestational age when the velocimetry was done therefore has an effect on the predictive value. To study these findings further, Antsaklis et al. [6] examined both uterine arteries in 654 healthy nulliparous women with color Doppler ultrasound at 4-week intervals between 20 and 32 weeks' gestation. Fifteen percent of women had abnormal flow velocity waveforms at their first visit. Preeclampsia developed in 3.2% of women. The sensitivity of the best way declined from 81% at 20 weeks to 71.4% at 32 weeks; however, the specificity and positive value increased significantly. At 24 weeks the sensitivity, specificity and positive predictive power was 76, 95 and 34%, respectively.

Position of the Placenta

Uterine artery impedance is elevated in the contralateral side of the placenta [56]. This finding was also confirmed by Antsaklis et al. [6], who found that the predictive value of the test was lower when the placenta was in a full lateral position on the contralateral side.

Overview

To assess the usefulness of uterine artery Doppler flow velocimetry in the prediction of pre-eclampsia, intrauterine growth restriction and perinatal death, Chien et al. [19] did a semiquantitative review of 27 observational diagnostic studies involving 12,994 women. The measurements studied were the flow velocity waveform ratio ± diastolic notch derived by transabdominal Doppler ultrasound. Likelihood ratios were used to measure diagnostic accuracy. A likelihood ratio of 1 indicated no predictive value for outcome. Likelihood ratios >10 or <0.1 were regarded as conclusive for a positive or negative test result, respectively. Moderate prediction was indicated by likelihood ratios of 5 to 10 or 0.1–0.2. The test was regarded as abnormal when the diastolic notch was present in the velocity waveform of one or both uterine arteries.

In a low-risk population, a positive test result predicted pre-eclampsia with a pooled likelihood ratio of 6.4 (95% CI 5.7–7.1). In a high-risk population a positive test result predicted pre-eclampsia with a pooled likelihood ratio of 2.8 (95% CI 2.3–3.4). A negative test had a likelihood ratio of 0.8 (95% CI 0.7–0.9). They came to the conclusion that uterine artery Doppler flow velocity had limited diagnostic accuracy in predicting pre-eclampsia.

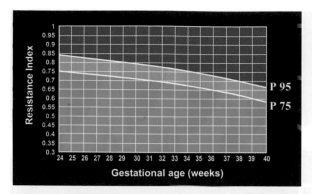

Fig. 19.3. Nomogram for the management of pregnant patients with suspected placental insufficiency according to Doppler flow velocity waveforms of the umbilical artery. The *green area* indicates that the pregnancy could be allowed to continue. No further tests for foetal well-being are indicated unless there is a change in the condition of the mother. The *yellow area* means caution. The test should be repeated and a non-stress test should be done. The *red area* indicates that the patient should be watched very carefully. A resistance index above the 95th percentile mandates an immediate non-stress test and thereafter twice weekly. Patients with absent end-diastolic flow should be admitted for intensive metal monitoring or immediate delivery

pler flow velocity waveforms were therefore of no value in identifying the risk patient for abruption. On the other hand, abnormal fetal heart rate patterns were found in the majority of patients who developed abruptio placentae. The fact that there were only two intra-uterine deaths due to abruptio placentae demonstrates the value of monitoring the fetal heart rate every 6 h in these patients.

Congenital Abnormalities

The risk of euploidy should always be remembered especially in the case of absent end-diastolic velocity without any apparent reason such as hypertension or poor fetal growth [50, 51, 98].

Severe Asphyxia

Several authors [50, 51, 98] also warn against severe IUGR with severe asphyxia; however, this is unlikely when the fetal heart rate is monitored every 6 h [76].

In Utero Treatment in Cases of Poor Umbilical Artery Doppler Velocimetry

It is still uncertain whether treatment of the fetus is possible. In a study of 12 pre-eclamptic women with oligohydramnios and elevated PI in the uterine arteries, Nakatsuka et al. [68] used long-term transdermal nitric oxide donors to reduce the blood pressure.

In addition to lowering the blood pressure, the PI of the umbilical artery was also reduced. It is still uncertain whether this improvement was just symptomatic or whether a real improvement in uteroplacental function was achieved. Further studies are therefore needed to demonstrate the real benefit to the fetus.

When to Deliver for Reverse End-Diastolic Velocity

Several findings have an effect on the maternal and perinatal outcome in patients with severe pre-eclampsia. Unless there is a very clear abnormal finding such as an alarming fetal heart rate pattern or uncontrollable blood pressure, a single abnormality should usually not be an indication for delivery in these patients. One should therefore always take the complete clinical picture into consideration, balancing maternal against perinatal risks but also the risks of further intra-uterine life against that of severe prematurity. Depending on the gestational age and estimated fetal size, reversed end-diastolic flow velocity is usually an indication for delivery; however, if the fetal heart rate pattern is still reassuring, the maternal condition stable and corticosteroids have not yet been administered, one may administer steroids to improve lung maturity and deliver 24–48 h later [29].

When to Deliver for Absent End-Diastolic Velocity

It is still uncertain when to deliver the patient with absent end-diastolic velocity as such. Usually these patients do not reach a gestational age of 34 weeks, when the neonatal outcome is very good. Either fetal or maternal condition often demands earlier delivery.

The GRIT study [94] was done at 67 hospitals in 13 European countries, using Bayesian data monitoring and analysis, to assess the correct timing of delivery between 24 and 36 weeks. In all the cases the umbilical artery Doppler was recorded and there was uncertainty as to when to deliver. The median time-to-delivery intervals were 0.9 days in the immediate group and 4.9 days in the delay group. There was a lack in the overall difference in mortality but the total caesarean sections were 91% in the immediate group and 79% in the delay group (OR 2.7; 95% CI 1.6–4.5). The authors concluded that the timing of delivery was correct as there were not a major delay in delivery (4.9 days) and the morbidity was similar in the two groups; however, in developing countries, later delivery which will enable the baby to start sooner with kangaroo care [52] and the lower caesarean section rate are major advantages. This approach of expectant management of mothers with severe pre-eclampsia helped the group at Tygerberg Hospital to achieve perinatal morbidity rates comparable to those of developed countries [41, 42].

The ACOG [2] recommends that the growth-restricted fetus should be delivered when the risk of fetal death exceeds that of neonatal death; however, if one looks at the reported perinatal morbidity rates in patients with severe pre-eclampsia, even when an expectant regime is followed, there are more neonatal than intrauterine deaths. Concern about the maternal condition could be partly responsible for the early delivery as the safety of the mother should also be considered. On the other hand, a neonatal death may be better explained to the mother than an intrauterine death, and this may sometimes influence the obstetrician towards earlier delivery; however, with intensive fetal monitoring, especially the heart rate, the chances of intrauterine death are very small, even when abruption of the placenta occurs [75]. The timing of delivery should therefore be individualized carefully, balancing the maternal, fetal and neonatal risks.

Method of Delivery

Intrapartum umbilical artery Doppler velocimetry is a poor predictor of adverse perinatal outcome, according to a meta-analysis of 2,700 women in eight studies [32]. There is also no change in the pulsatility index during labor [31]. Patients with an increase in resistance index can be allowed a trial of labor [90]; however, elective delivery is recommended when there is reversed end-diastolic flow or non-reassuming fetal heart rate patterns. Hall et al. [43, 44] examined the route of delivery in 335 women with early onset severe pre-eclampsia. Labor was induced in 103 (31%) of patients of whom 46 (45%) delivered normally. Although non-reassuming fetal heart rate patterns, necessitating delivery for fetal distress, occurred in 38 (37%) of these patients, when compared with elective caesarean section, these babies had lower rates of severe hyaline membrane disease and needed intensive care less often. Fewer developed sepsis; however, they were 1.6 weeks older at birth.

Other Effects on Umbilical Artery Doppler Flow Velocity Waveforms

There is no correlation between the umbilical artery Doppler flow velocity waveforms and coiling index of the umbilical cord [23], and there is a negative correlation between heart rate and the A/B ratio or RI [63, 67, 101, 105]; however, the influence is small when the heart rate varies between 120 and 160 beats per minute. A decrease in the S/D ratio was also found during ritodrine infusion to suppress preterm labor [11]. It is likely that this effect is due to the increase in fetal heart rate caused by ritodrine. Moderately high altitude has no effect on fetal vascular Doppler indices [35].

Neonatal Outcome

As brain sparing in cases of severe IUGR reduces blood supply to the bowel, this ischaemia could facilitate the development of neonatal necrotizing enterocolitis. Kirsten et al. [52] compared the proportion of necrotizing enterocolitis in babies who had absent end-diastolic flow velocity ($n=68$) with those who had a resistance index between the 95th and 99th percentile ($n=43$) or those with normal flow velocity ($n=31$). All these babies were born to mothers with severe pre-eclampsia. No baby who had absent end-diastolic flow velocity developed necrotizing enterocolitis.

Kirsten et al. [52] also followed up these babies for 4 years. There were no differences between the developmental quotients of the infants with normal and absent end-diastolic velocities, either at 24 or 48 months of age; however, looking at fetal aortic blood flow velocity, Ley et al. [59, 60] found an association between abnormal waveforms and intellectual function and minor neurological dysfunction at the age of 7 years.

Conclusion

It has been demonstrated, without doubt, that the clinical use of umbilical artery flow velocity waveforms reduces perinatal deaths and unnecessary admission to hospital or induction of labor for suspected placental insufficiency. It can also be used in primary health care settings to differentiate between a normal fetus with poor growth and placental insufficiency.

Acknowledgements. The author thanks E. Foot for typing the manuscript and L. Geerts for the Doppler flow velocity waveform images.

References

1. Aardema MW, De Wolf BTHM, Saro MCS, Oosterhof H, Fidler V, Aarnoudse JG (2000) Quantification of the diastolic notch in Doppler ultrasound screening of uterine arteries. Ultrasound Obstet Gynecol 16:630–643
2. ACOG practice bulletin (2001) Intrauterine growth restriction. In J Gynecol Obstet 72:85–96
3. Adamson SL (1999) Arterial pressure, vascular input impedance, and resistance as determinants of pulsatile blood flow in the umbilical artery. Eur J Obstet Gynecol Reprod Biol 84:119–125
4. Albaiges G, Missfelder-Lobos H, Lees C, Parra M, Nicolaides KH (2000) One-stage screening for pregnancy

cal artery: a sign of fetal hypoxia and acidosis. Br Med J 297:1026–1027

70. Neilson JP, Alfirevic Z (2003) Doppler ultrasound for fetal assessment in high-risk pregnancies (Cochrane Review). In: The Cochrane Library, issue 3. Update software, Oxford

71. Nienhuis SJ, Vles JSH, Gerver WJM, Hoogland HJ (1997) Doppler ultrasonography in suspected intrauterine growth retardation: a randomized clinical trial. Ultrasound Obstet Gynecol 9:6–13

72. Odendaal HJ, Pattinson RC, Du Toit R (1987) Fetal and neonatal outcome in patients with severe pre-eclampsia before 34 weeks. S Afr Med J 71:555–558

73. Odendaal HJ, Pattinson RC, Du Toit R, Grove D (1988) Frequent fetal heart rate monitoring for early detection of abruptio placentae in severe proteinuric hypertension. S Afr Med J 74:19–21

74. Odendaal HJ, Steyn DW, Norman K, Kirsten GF, Smith J, Theron GB (1995) Improved perinatal mortality rates in 1001 patients with severe pre-eclampsia. S Afr Med J 85:1071–1076

75. Odendaal HJ, Hall DR, Grové D (2000) Risk factors for and perinatal mortality of abruptio placentae in patients hospitalised for early onset severe pre-eclampsia: a case controlled study. J Obstet Gynaecol 20:358–364

76. Oéttle CA, Odendaal HJ (2000) Umbilical artery blood gases in newborns of high-risk mothers delivered within 6 hours of antenatal fetal heart monitoring. S Afr Med J 90:705–706

77. Ohkuchi A, Minakami H, Sato I, Mori H, Nakano T, Tateno (2000) Predicting the risk of pre-eclampsia and a small-for-gestational-age infant by quantitative assessment of the diastolic notch in uterine artery flow velocity waveforms in unselected women. Ultrasound Obstet Gynecol 16:171–178

78. Ott WJ (1997) Sonographic diagnosis of intrauterine growth restriction. Clin Obstet Gynecol 40:787–795

79. Owen P, Harrold AJ, Farrell T (1997) Fetal size and growth velocity in the prediction of intrapartum Caesarean section for fetal distress. Br J Obstet Gynecol 104:445–449

80. Ozeren M, Dinc H, Ekmen U, Senekayli C, Aydemir V (1999) Umbilical and middle cerebral artery Doppler indices in patients with preeclampsia. Eur J Obstet Gynecol Reprod Biol 82:11–16

81. Park YW, Cho JS, Choi HM, Kim TY, Lee SH, Yu JK, Kim JW (2000) Clinical significance of early diastolic notch depth: uterine artery Doppler velocimetry in the third trimester. Am J Obstet Gynecol 182:1204–1209

82. Pattinson RC, Theron GB, Thompson ML, Lai Tung M (1989) Doppler ultrasonography of the fetoplacental circulation: normal references values. S Afr Med J 76:623–625

83. Pattinson RC, Norman K, Odendaal HJ (1993) The use of Doppler velocimetry of the umbilical artery before 24 weeks' gestation to screen for high-risk pregnancies. S Afr Med J 83:734–736

84. Reed KL (1997) Doppler: the fetal circulation. Clin Obstet Gynecol 40:750–754

85. Salafia CM, Pezzullo JC, Minior VK, Divon MY (1997) Placental pathology of absent and reversed end-diastolic flow in growth-restricted fetuses. Obstet Gynecol 90: 830–836

86. Satomura S (1959) Study of the flow patterns in peripheral arteries by ultrasonics. J Acoustical Soc Jap 15:151–158

87. Schuchter K, Metzenbauer M, Hafner E, Philipp K (2001) Uterine artery Doppler and placental volume in the first trimester in the prediction of pregnancy complications. Ultrasound Obstet Gynecol 19:590–592

89. Semchyshyn S, Zuspan FP, Cordero L (1983) Cardiovascular response and complications of glucocorticoid therapy in hypertensive pregnancies. Am J Obstet Gynecol 145:530–533

90. Skinner J, Greene RA, Gardeil F, Stuart B, Turner MJ (1998) Does increased resistance on umbilical artery Doppler preclude a trial of labour? Eur J Obstet Gynecol Reprod Biol 79:35–38

91. Soregaloli M, Valcamonico A, Scalvi L, Danti L, Frusca T (2001) Late normalisation of uterine artery velocimetry in high-risk pregnancy. Eur J Obstet Gynecol Reprod Biol 95:42–45

92. Steyn DW, Odendaal HJ (1997) Randomized controlled trial of ketanserin and aspirin in prevention of pre-eclampsia. Lancet 350:1267–1271

93. Takata M, Nakatsuka M, Kudo T (2002) Differential blood flow in uterine, ophthalmic and brachial arteries of preeclamptic women. Obstet Gynecol 100:931–939

94. The GRIT Study Group (2003) A randomized trial of timed delivery for the compromised preterm fetus: short term outcomes and Bayesian interpretation. Br J Obstet Gynaecol 110:27–32

95. Theron GB, Theron AM, Odendaal HJ (2002) Symphysis-fundus growth measurement followed by umbilical artery Doppler velocimetry to screen for placental insufficiency. Int J Gynecol Obstet 79:263–264

96. Todros T, Ronco G, Fianchino O, Rosso S, Gabrielli S, Valsecchi L, Spagnolo D, Acanfora L, Biolcati M, Segnan N, Pilu G (1996) Accuracy of the umbilical arteries Doppler flow velocity waveforms in detecting adverse perinatal outcomes in a high-risk population. Acta Obstet Gynecol Scand 75:113–119

97. Todros T, Sciarrone A, Piccoli E, Guiot C, Kaufmann P, Kingdom J (1993) Umbilical Doppler waveforms and placental villous angiogenesis in pregnancies complicated by fetal growth restriction. Obstet Gynecol 93: 499–503

98. Trudinger BJ, Cook CM (1985) Umbilical and uterine artery flow velocity waveforms in pregnancy associated with major fetal abnormality. Br J Obstet Gynaecol 92:666–670

99. Vainio M, Kujansuu E, Iso-Mustajärvi M, Mäenpää J (2002) Low dose acetylsalicylic acid in prevention of pregnancy-induced hypertension and intrauterine growth retardation in women with bilateral uterine artery notches. Br J Obstet Gynaecol 109:161–167

100. Valensise H, Vasapollo B, Novelli GP, Larciprete G, Romanini ME, Arduini D, Galante A, Romanini C (2001) Maternal diastolic function in asymptomatic pregnant women with bilateral notching of the uterine artery waveform at 24 weeks' gestation: a pilot study. Ultrasound Obstet Gynecol 18:450–455

101. Van den Wijngaard JAGW, Van Eyck J, Wladimiroff JW (1988) The relationship between fetal heart rate and Doppler blood flow velocity waveforms. Ultrasound Med Biol 14:593–597

102. Venkat-Raman N, Backos M, Teoh TG, Lo WTS, Regan L (2001) Uterine artery Doppler in predicting pregnancy outcome in women with antiphospholipid syndrome. Obstet Gynecol 98:235–242

103. Wallace EM, Baker LS (1999) Effect of antenatal betamethasone administration on placental vascular resistance. Lancet 353:1404–1407

104. Westergaard HB, Langhoff-Roos J, Lingman G, Maršál K, Kreiner S (2001) A critical appraisal of the use of umbilical artery Doppler ultrasound in high-risk pregnancies: use of meta-analyses in evidence-based obstetrics. Ultrasound Obstet Gynecol 17:466–476

105. Yarlagadda P, Willoughby L, Maulik D (1989) Effect of fetal heart rate on umbilical arterial Doppler indices. J Ultrasound Med 8:215–218

Chapter 20

Doppler Velocimetry and Multiple Gestation

Emanuel P. Gaziano, Ursula F. Harkness

The role for fetal Doppler sonography includes detecting fetal growth restriction (FGR), serving as a modality for fetal surveillance, predicting adverse neonatal events, and determining the optimal time for delivery. Multiple-gestation pregnancies afford a unique opportunity for fetal Doppler application, as abnormalities in growth and potential disturbances of the fetal circulation are relatively common. Doppler data add a physiologic parameter not previously available to the clinician. By reflecting downstream resistance to flow in the umbilical artery, it serves as an accurate proxy for placental insufficiency [1]. By including the cerebral circulation, inferences may be made as to the redistribution of fetal blood flow under conditions of chronic asphyxial stress, while multiple vessel interrogation is useful in studying the extremes of circulatory changes seen in some monochorionic twins with twin transfusion syndrome (TTS). In multiple as in singleton pregnancies, application of fetal Doppler velocimetry permits the assessment of the sequence of fetal cardiovascular adjustment to asphyxial stress in the arterial and venous circulations yielding useful insights into the timing of delivery.

Among the risks for multiple gestations listed in Table 20.1, Doppler velocimetry helps define the status of the fetus with restricted growth, TTS, and congenital anomalies. In these instances Doppler information facilitates the appropriate and selective application of perinatal resources. For decisions regarding patient management, Doppler data become a part of

Table 20.1. Major complications: multiple gestation pregnancy

Preterm labor
Fetal malformations
Intrauterine growth restriction
Fetal loss (vanishing twin)
Twin-transfusion syndrome
Amniotic fluid volume changes: polyhydramnios, oligohydramnios
Preeclampsia
Cord prolapse or entanglement
Birth trauma

the clinical mosaic to be used in tandem with other historical, examination, sonographic, laboratory, and biophysical data.

Twin Prevalence

The prevalence of twin gestation varies from 1 to 5% depending on the gestational age at assessment, as a significant number of twins suffer intrauterine fetal demise of one of the pair [2]. The overall incidence of spontaneous twin gestations has declined, but reproductive technologies, including ovulation induction and surgical transfer of gametes or ova, have resulted in an increasing number of high-order multiple gestations [2].

Twin Placentation

Twins are derived from either a single ovum (monozygotic) or two ova (dizygotic). Dizygotic twinning is influenced by maternal central gonadotropin levels [3, 4] and varies among ethnic groups. For example, Nigerian women have a high level and frequency of twinning and Japanese women have a low level and frequency. Occurring at a fixed rate of 1 per 250 births, proportionately more complications occur in twin monozygotic pregnancies probably owing to both placental vascular anastomosis and placental asymmetry [5, 6].

Because dizygotic twin pregnancies arise from two entirely separate placental disks, each gestational sac has one amnion, one chorion, and rare vascular anastomosis [5]. Diamniotic dichorionic gestations account for about 80% of all twin pregnancies, and their placentas may be fused or separate [7]. This type of placentation also may include monozygotic twins if the zygote divides early after fertilization. The type of placentation seen in a given monozygotic twin pregnancy depends on when in development splitting occurs [8]. If division of the ovum occurs before the chorion develops in the first 2 or 3 days, a diamniotic dichorionic gestation will result [8]. If the split occurs between 3 and 8 days post-fertilization, a

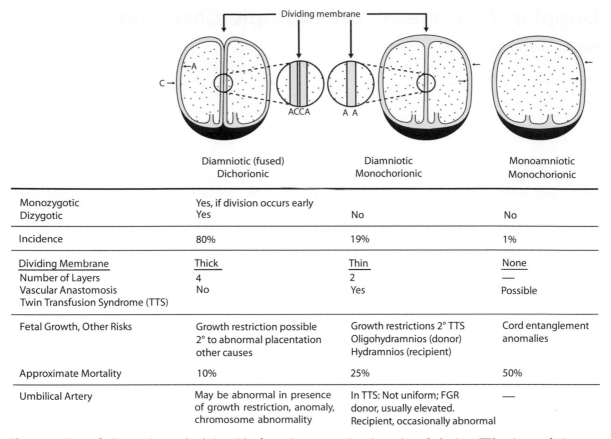

	Diamniotic (fused) Dichorionic	Diamniotic Monochorionic	Monoamniotic Monochorionic
Monozygotic	Yes, if division occurs early		
Dizygotic	Yes	No	No
Incidence	80%	19%	1%
Dividing Membrane	Thick	Thin	None
Number of Layers	4	2	—
Vascular Anastomosis	No	Yes	Possible
Twin Transfusion Syndrome (TTS)			
Fetal Growth, Other Risks	Growth restriction possible 2° to abnormal placentation other causes	Growth restrictions 2° TTS Oligohydramnios (donor) Hydramnios (recipient)	Cord entanglement anomalies
Approximate Mortality	10%	25%	50%
Umbilical Artery	May be abnormal in presence of growth restriction, anomaly, chromosome abnormality	In TTS: Not uniform; FGR donor, usually elevated. Recipient, occasionally abnormal	—

Fig. 20.1. Type of placentation and relative risks for twin pregnancies. *A* amnion, *C* chorion, *TTS* twin-transfusion syndrome, *FGR* fetal growth restriction

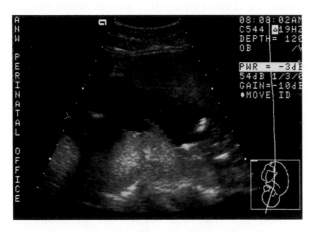

Fig. 20.2. Dividing membrane in dichorionic diamniotic twin pregnancy. Note the anterior and posterior placentas and relative thickness of the dividing membrane

diamniotic monochorionic gestation will result [8]. Monoamniotic monochorionic pregnancies occur when the division occurs between days 8 and 13 after fertilization [8]. Any pregnancy that splits later than this develops into conjoined twins [8]. The type of

placentation is important since this factor defines the relative risks for vascular anastomosis and the complications that result in the greatest fetal morbidity. Growth restriction may have a different mechanism in fetuses from dizygotic pregnancies than in those from a monozygotic pregnancy [9].

Figure 20.1 shows the relation of amnion to chorion and the dividing membrane in diamniotic dichorionic (DADC), diamniotic monochorionic (DAMC), and monoamniotic monochorionic (MAMC) placentation; the latter is rare, accounting for 1% of all twin pregnancies [7]. The number of amnion/chorion layers present in the dividing membrane is also shown in Fig. 20.1. The ultrasonographic appearance of the thicker diamniotic dichorionic dividing membrane is apparent in Fig. 20.2. Monochorionic placentation (20% of all twins) is associated with artery-to-artery (AA), artery-to-vein (AV), and vein-to-vein (VV) superficial anastomosis, although deep capillary villous anastomoses are also possible (Fig. 20.3) [5, 7, 10]. All gradations of anastomoses are possible; hence, the variable clinical presentations and variable Doppler velocimetry findings observed. Most cases of twin transfusion occur with diamniotic monochorio-

Fig. 20.3. Deep arteriovenous anastomosis in monochorionic diamniotic twin placentation. Twin-to-twin transfer. *IUGR* intrauterine growth restriction, *AGA* appropriate-for-gestational age

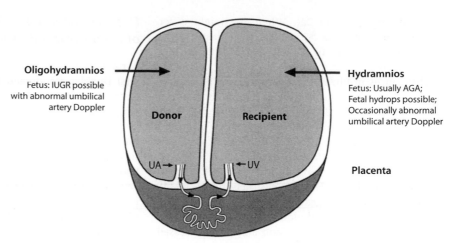

Oligohydramnios
Fetus: IUGR possible with abnormal umbilical artery Doppler

Hydramnios
Fetus: Usually AGA; Fetal hydrops possible; Occasionally abnormal umbilical artery Doppler

Donor   **Recipient**

UA→   ←UV

Placenta

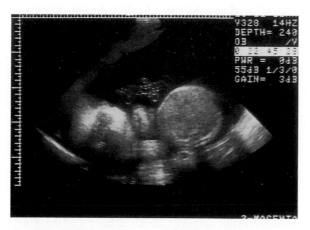

Fig. 20.4. Monochorionic monoamniotic twin placentation with no dividing membrane. Umbilical cords from the twins are entangled

nic placentation, and perinatal mortality (25%–50%) occurs principally with this type of placentation compared with the 10% mortality in the diamniotic dichorionic group [2, 11].

Figure 20.4 demonstrates a monoamniotic monochorionic twin gestation and no dividing membrane. These fetuses are at risk for cord entanglement and death. Recently, 50% mortality was reported for pregnancies with monoamniotic monochorionic placentation [12].

Fetal Doppler and Complications of Multiple Gestation

In the United States, the infant mortality rate among multiple births was more than five times higher than among singleton births in both 1989 and 1999 [13] and the perinatal mortality was similarly increased [14]. Two-thirds of the perinatal losses before 30

weeks occur at gestational ages of 26 weeks or less [15]. Whereas multiple gestations resulted in 3% of live births in 2000, 14% of infant deaths in the same year were multiples [16].

Studies on multiple gestations have focused on using fetal Doppler data in three clinical areas: (a) identification or prediction of growth restriction; (b) the TTS; and (c) prediction of perinatal morbidity and mortality. We address the use of Doppler velocimetry for each of these separately.

Growth Restriction and Discordance

Prior to 30 weeks' gestation, the major causes of neonatal death relate to immaturity while stillbirths due to growth restriction contribute a significant number of perinatal losses after 32 weeks' gestation [15]. Growth restriction occurs in one-fourth of multiple gestations [17]. Representing 1% of pregnancies, twins account for 12% of early neonatal deaths and 17% of all growth-restricted infants [17]. Triplets and other higher-order multiple gestations also lend a disproportionate contribution to the number of growth-restricted fetuses.

Evaluation of Fetal Growth

Two methods are used to evaluate fetal growth in multiple pregnancies: (a) growth discordance (differences in fetal weight frequently expressed as a percent); and (b) longitudinal assessment of the weight or growth for the individual fetus.

Since the introduction of Babson et al.'s correlation between severe growth discordance and neonatal developmental delay [18], the concept of differences in weight (discordance) has gained popularity. No uniform cutoff value is reported for growth discordance, although 15% or more birth-weight difference between twins is considered mild discordance, and more than 25% birth-weight difference is classified as severe discordance [19–22]. When the weight difference between twins is >25%, perinatal death rate is increased by a factor of 2.5 and risk of fetal death is increased by a factor of 6.5 [23].

Differences in ultrasound measurement parameters or Doppler indices in twins are commonly reported as the percent difference and are expressed as delta change or intrapair difference. A number of studies [24–35] rely upon the discordance concept and have reported Doppler results accordingly.

The advent of high-resolution real-time ultrasonography and duplex Doppler systems diminishes the need to view multiple gestations only in terms of discordance because the individual fetus in multiple gestations can be independently and accurately assessed. Expressing either Doppler or estimated fetal weight (EFW) differences between twins is less useful, as neonatal morbidity appears to be best predicted by individual fetal assessment. Using 30% disparity in birth weight, O'Brien et al. [36] were able to determine only one in five growth-restricted twins. Bronsteen and colleagues [37] evaluated 131 consecutive sets of surviving infants and showed that individual evaluation for intrauterine growth was more effective than discordance or other classifications for predicting adverse neonatal outcomes. Regarding neonatal morbidity among twins, neither birth-weight discordance of >20% or >25% was a factor for predicting adverse events compared with individual birth-weight percentiles of <15th and <10th, respectively. The most clinically relevant outcomes, such as neonatal death, congenital anomalies, small for gestational age (SGA) and periventricular leukomalacia, are defined by a birth-weight difference of 30% [38]. In a study of 192 twin pairs who had ultrasound within 16 days of delivery, intertwin estimated fetal weight discordance of 25% or more had a sensitivity of 55%, specificity of 97%, positive predictive value of 82%, and negative predictive value of 91% for predicting actual birth-weight discordance [39]. The antepartum diagnosis of discordance was correct in 4 of 5 cases; however, discordance may be overdiagnosed in almost 20% of cases and almost half of the significantly discordant twin pairs were missed.

Gaziano et al. [33] focus on the individual fetus and classify the Doppler value, EFW, abdominal circumference, or other measurement parameter for each fetus as a percentile for the gestational age at which it is obtained. Deter et al. [40, 41] recommended multiple individual parameter assessment (individualized growth assessment) for the twin fetus suspected of growth restriction. This approach simplifies interpretation of clinical data, allowing the fetus to be followed over time and permitting focused surveillance.

Doppler Sonographic Prediction of Fetal Growth Restriction

A number of difficulties are inherent in assessing the fetal Doppler results and their relationship to growth restriction. Firstly, the heterogeneous cause of FGR in singletons also apply to multiple gestations and can be broadly categorized as follows: (a) malformations, intrauterine infections, or chromosomal abnormalities; (b) maternal vascular and nutritional deficits; and (c) constitutionally small fetuses. In addition, causes specifically related to twins must be considered, such as twin transfusion, primary uterine or placental pathology, and anomalies due to the twinning process. Secondly, although the umbilical arteries are relatively accessible compared with the internal fetal vessels, careful establishment of individual fetal circulations by real-time ultrasonography is necessary to prevent sampling the same umbilical circulation twice. This point is particularly important for suspected TTS, as the smaller "stuck" twin with oligohydramnios may be relatively difficult to image. Thirdly, studies differ in instrumentation, pulsed-wave vs continuous-wave (CW) technology, and the resistance index selected: systolic/diastolic ratio (S/D); pulsatility index (PI); or resistance index (RI). A variety of end points for Doppler-diagnosed abnormalities are reported. Outcomes may be reported as birth-weight differences of >20% or >25% and the cutoff for defining growth restriction is reported at various percentile ranges (<10th, <5th, or <2.5th). Finally, the latter definitions for FGR, as for singletons, are not always satisfactory, as some constitutionally small twins are normal in all other respects, while some "normal"-weight fetuses may be growth restricted.

Pathologic studies suggest an anatomic lesion in some cases of FGR. For example, histologic examination of placentas shows fewer placental tertiary stem villi in twin pregnancies complicated by "placental insufficiency" and abnormal S/D ratios than in fetuses with normal S/D ratios [42]. These findings are similar to those observed in some singleton pregnancies with FGR and suggest a placental vascular pathology rather than a uteroplacental one [1, 42]. Furthermore, in twin pregnancies the PO_2 levels in the individual fetus appear unaffected among a wide range of umbilical RI values [43]. Differences in the RIs for twin fetuses were of little value for detecting PO_2 differences until the differences in the RI between the fetuses was 76% [43].

Doppler prediction for fetal growth restriction has been evaluated by a number of investigators [24–35]. Table 20.2 summarizes the experience of these investigators, indicating the method of assessment, outcome variable measured, and the sensitivity for SGA prediction.

Table 20.2. Fetal growth restriction prediction using umbilical artery in twin-gestation pregnancies. *CW* continuous-wave Doppler, *S/D* systolic/diastolic ratio, *SGA* small-for-gestational age, *GA* gestational age, *PI* pulsatility index, *EFW* estimated fetal weight, *RI* resistance index, *US* ultrasonography

Reference	No. of twin pregnancies	Method of assessment	Outcome variable	Sensitivity (%)
[24]	76	CW; S/D ratio differences of 1.57 or >75th percentile difference	Birth of SGA infant	70
[25]	43	CW; S/D ratio differences between twins of >0.4	Birth of SGA infant	73
[26]	56	Duplex pulsed Doppler; abnormal Doppler value for GA	Weight discordance >25%	82
[27]	30	Duplex pulsed Doppler; percent difference PI umbilical artery	Unfavorable outcome (9 of 11 were SGA)	50
[28]	69	CW after real-time US; S/D difference >0.4	Birth of SGA infant	42 [a]
[29]	58	Real-time US followed by CW; delta S/D or EFW >15%	Birth-weight discordance >15%	78
[30]	89	CW after real-time US	Birth of SGA infant (25th percentile)	29
[31]	31	Duplex pulsed Doppler PI difference >0.5	Birth-weight difference >20%	75
[32]	37	Duplex pulsed Doppler; abnormal Doppler value for GA	Birth of SGA infant (<10th percentile)	58
[33]	94	Duplex pulsed Doppler; abnormal S/D >95th percentile for GA	Birth of SGA infant (<10th percentile)	44
[34]	32	Delta RI	Birth-weight discordance	78
[35]	40	Pulsed Doppler/mechanical sector scanner; PI difference >0.2	Birth of SGA infant	42

[a] Reported as positive predictive value.

Pioneering studies reported by Giles et al. [24] and Farmakides et al. [25] were conducted with CW Doppler, and the S/D ratio (A/B ratio) differences between twins were correlated with the birth of an SGA infant. Index ratio differences of >0.40 or 1.57 demonstrated sensitivities of 73% and 70%, respectively.

In a study of 56 twin pregnancies using real-time and pulsed-wave Doppler ultrasonography, an abnormal Doppler result predicted a weight discordance of >25% with a sensitivity of 82% [26]. Adequate fetal growth was accurately predicted in 44 of 45 normal sets of fetuses and discordant growth in 9 of 11 twin sets. A 50% sensitivity has been demonstrated for unsatisfactory outcomes using abnormal umbilical artery Doppler sonography as an end point. One such adverse outcome was SGA which was found in 9 of 11 fetuses [27]. A 42% positive predictive value for the birth of an SGA infant has been reported when the intrapair difference for the S/D ratio was >0.4 [28]. Some investigators report no difference between ultrasound-derived EFW and the S/D ratio (intrapair differences of >15%) for predicting the birth of discordant-weight twins (>15% birth weight) [29]. Both

methods showed a sensitivity of 78% for these parameters [29]. Yamada et al. [31] demonstrated a sensitivity of 75% for a birth-weight difference of >20% when the umbilical artery PI difference between twins was >0.5, similar to the 78% sensitivity reported by Kurmanvicius et al. for birth weight discordance [34].

In summary, of the studies reviewed, a disparity was observed for FGR prediction among the investigators, and one-third noted sensitivities of <50%.

Ultrasonographic Biometry and Fetal Doppler Studies

Ultrasonographically detected differences in discordant growth pairs can be seen as early as 23–24 weeks, with the smaller twin exhibiting a slow rate of growth between 33 and 37 weeks (Fig. 20.5) [44]. In pathologic twins, differences can be suggested as early as the beginning of the second trimester.

Ultrasound measurements, such as the biparietal diameter (BPD), are insensitive predictors of neonatal growth discordance [23]. In twin gestations the BPD is determined in only 79% of all fetuses, whereas

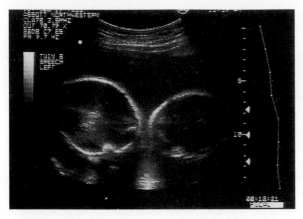

Fig. 20.5. Discordant head size in a monochorionic twin gestation

femur length and abdominal circumference are obtained for 96% and 99% of fetuses, respectively [45]; thus, the ultrasonographically determined EFW is superior to the BPD or femur length for predicting discordance [46]. No apparent advantage is anticipated using abdominal circumference alone for predicting growth discordance or restriction, as it is part of most formulas for estimating fetal weight. In addition, multiple measurements allow potential classification into symmetric and asymmetric patterns of restricted growth.

Sensitivity for SGA prediction is reported as high as 58% in the presence of an abnormal pulsed-wave Doppler result from the umbilical artery, while Doppler abnormality precedes ultrasonographic diagnosis of FGR by an average of 3.7 weeks [32]. Combining sonographic measurements with an abnormal Doppler result may improve the sensitivity to 84% [32]. Both Hastie et al. [30] and Gaziano et al. [33] found relatively low sensitivities (29% and 44%, respectively) for SGA prediction in multiple gestations using abnormal Doppler results in the umbilical artery. Gaziano et al. [33] compared ultrasonographically determined EFW (expressed as a percentile for the gestational age at which it was obtained) with abnormal umbilical artery velocimetry and found biometry to be superior to abnormal Doppler results for SGA prediction. The overall sensitivity for SGA prediction with an ultrasonographic EFW of <10th percentile was 50%, and the best positive predictive value (PPV) was 87.5%, achieved with an ultrasonographic EFW of 35th percentile. Other authors have demonstrated no difference in diagnostic accuracy for twin discordance between Doppler velocimetry and ultrasonography [29].

When Doppler waveform indices and serial measurements of EFW and abdominal circumference were compared in singletons, serial biometric measure-

ments were superior to a number of Doppler indices for FGR prediction [47]. Similar findings are suggested from the limited data on twin pregnancies.

Deter et al. [40, 41] developed a detailed ultrasound biometric assessment technique applicable to the twin fetus. It included measurement of head circumference (HC), abdominal circumference (AC), thigh circumference (ThC), femur diaphysis length (FDL), and EFW. The authors recommended using a multiple-parameter technique rather than standard growth population curves for the detection of FGR in twins. According to their data, single anatomic parameters are inadequate for distinguishing the normal twin from the growth-restricted twin. By assessing the number and magnitude of deviations of the parameter changes, all growth-restricted infants in 34 twin pregnancies were identified; none in the sample were misclassified [41].

Cerebral Vessels

In one study of 17 consecutive twin pregnancies, the sensitivity for FGR prediction was 83% for PI of internal carotid artery (ICA) compared with 33% for the PI of the umbilical artery [48]. Multiple vessel interrogation may increase diagnostic accuracy, and in singletons the ratio between the PI of the umbilical artery and the PI of the internal carotid artery show sensitivities of 84.2% for FGR prediction at a PPV of 97% [49]. The cerebral/umbilical artery ratios may have a greater sensitivity for FGR prediction than does a single-vessel evaluation [50].

Summary

Correlations between ultrasound biometry, Doppler, and FGR identification in multiple gestations are summarized as follows:
1. An abnormal umbilical artery Doppler result is significantly associated with the birth of a growth-restricted infant.
2. A wide range of accuracy for FGR detection is reported, varying according to the population characteristics and the technique employed.
3. Ultrasound biometry is superior to fetal Doppler examination for purposes of diagnosis.
4. Multiple parameter measurements and serial measurements are superior to final individual values for either Doppler studies or biometry.
5. Combinations of biometric with Doppler measurements and cerebral/umbilical artery ratios probably increase the likelihood of FGR detection.

Other than methodologic or technical parameters, a number of factors account for the differences among the studies regarding FGR prediction. Not all

FGR fetuses exhibit abnormal Doppler velocimetry. In singleton fetuses, for example, the birth of an SGA infant was associated with a normal umbilical artery Doppler waveform in 44%–51% of such births [51, 52]. It is unknown what proportion of these infants were constitutionally small instead of growth restricted.

Twin Transfusion Syndrome

Twin transfusion syndrome (TTS) and its manifestations result in a high frequency of fetal loss and significant neonatal morbidity. Becoming clinically evident at the lower limits of fetal viability, intensive maternal and fetal therapy may result in the birth of viable but profoundly ill neonates. The complex vascular arrangements possible within the placental circulations of these monochorionic pregnancies suggest an area of promise for fetal Doppler investigation.

The TTS is characterized by clinical findings which include a recipient fetus who is usually appropriate for gestational age (AGA) or large for gestational age (LGA), and a donor fetus who is small or growth restricted. The recipient's sac demonstrates hydramnios that is sometimes massive. Oligohydramnios is often present in the donor's sac. The marked oligohydramnios results in the "stuck" twin due to compression from the recipient sac [53]. Ultrasonographically, the separating membrane may be difficult to visualize because of its close adherence to the donor and its thin monochorial origin. Signs of fetal hydrops or cardiac failure may develop in either twin, usually the larger.

A scoring system has been proposed for TTS based on sonography, Doppler findings, and cordocentesis [54]. Sonographic and Doppler findings (minor) include an abdominal circumference difference >18 mm, poly- or oligohydramnios, signs of monozygosity, and an intrapair S/D ratio of >0.4. Major criteria include evidence of transplacental shunt, a birth-weight difference of >15%, and a hemoglobin difference of >5 g/dl. Antenatally or postnatally two criteria are needed (two major or one major and one minor). Other authors have suggested variations on these criteria for defining TTS [55, 56].

Although discordant fetal size, amniotic fluid differences, concordant gender, and evidence of monochorial placentation suggest TTS, neonatal criteria for TTS, which include a hemoglobin differential of >5 g/dl, is not uniformly found. In four cases of TTS, cordocentesis was performed and no intrapair hemoglobin differences of >2.7 g/dl were observed [57]. In another study using cordocentesis, others have noted significant hemoglobin differences in only one of nine fetuses with TTS [58]. Ultrasonographic findings in TTS do not always correlate with the classic neonatal

criterion of a hemoglobin difference of >5 g/dl. [59]. Classic TTS was confirmed in only 44% of fetuses by direct injection of transfused blood to the donor while simultaneously assessing evidence for transfused cells in the recipient fetus by direct fetal blood sampling [59].

Ultrasound evaluation of TTS includes a general fetal anatomic survey to rule out gross anomalies and an assessment of the fetuses for signs of fetal hydrops, including scalp edema, ascites, hydrothorax, and pericardial effusion. The sex of the fetuses should be determined and membrane thickness assessed for evidence of zygosity. To infer zygosity, placental localization in multiple pregnancies is best assessed during the early part of the second trimester (12–14 weeks) when fused or separate placentas can be distinguished.

The amniotic fluid volume in each sac should be assessed, and detection of hydramnios or oligohydramnios by a modified four-quadrant technique may be helpful. A cutoff of 8 cm vertical depth for amniotic volume is suggested [60]. In addition, the degree of hydramnios is correlated with the probability of fetal abnormality [60]. For twin pregnancies, abnormal monochorionic placentation (TTS) is the most frequently cited association with hydramnios [60].

The fetal weight should be estimated ultrasonographically for each fetus using the formulas of Hadlock et al. [61], Shepard et al. [62], or others and then the EFW classified into a percentile ranking for the gestational age at which it was determined. The individual fetal growth can then be classified as appropriate for gestational age (AGA), SGA, or LGA. On the basis of Rossavik growth models and using detailed measurements in normal twins, individual assessment for the growth of the twins can be performed with the same methods used for singletons and the results are similar [63]. A multiple parameter individualized growth assessment technique as described by Deter et al. [40, 41] may be the most precise biometric method, but its clinical application remains to be evaluated.

Standards of birth weight in twin gestation stratified by placental chorionicity are a recent contribution. Singleton charts tend to underestimate twin growth at earlier gestational ages and overestimate twin growth at later gestational ages [64].

Irrespective of the neonatal findings regarding hemoglobin differences, the ultrasonographic findings described previously portend a poor prognosis. Based on ultrasound findings, Pretorius et al. [12] noted possible TTS in nine twin pairs. Patients in their series with TTS had a relatively high death rate. The overall mortality rate for TTS depends on birth weight and gestational age at delivery and is reported to be as high as 70% [6]. Among pregnancies delivering at <28 weeks, a survival rate of only 21% was reported for TTS and neither decompression amniocentesis nor tocolysis altered this outcome [65].

Pathology of Monochorionic Placentation

When placentas from monochorionic twins are compared with the presence or absence of TTS, placentas from pregnancies with TTS had fewer anastomoses overall, and fewer anastomoses for each specific type, such as arterioarterial (AA), venovenous (VV) and arteriovenous (AV) [66, 67]. In addition, anastomoses in the TTS group tended to be indirect or AV, rather than direct AA or VV when compared to monochorionic twins without TTS. Hemodynamic models of TTS in monochorionic twins support the pathologic findings that fewer anastomoses effect greater discordance between monochorionic twins and that the discordance increases beyond fetal compensatory capacity [68]. Color Doppler insonation of placental vasculature in monochorionic twins also demonstrates an absence of functional AA anastomoses in monochorionic twins with TTS [69]. In assessment of clinical outcomes, AV anastomoses in the absence of AA and VV, especially if present with placental asymmetry, carry the worse prognosis [67]. Unidirectional AV flow in the absence of compensatory bidirectional anastomoses results in adverse fetal effects and poor outcomes for some monochorionic gestations.

The placenta of the donor twin may have a small, inconspicuous vascular supply and may demonstrate a large number of villi per unit volume of placenta, whereas the recipient twin demonstrates an increase in the volume of fetal capillaries [70]. Donor twins may have a deficiency of maternally transferred immunoglobulin G (IgG), indicating impaired intervillous maternal-fetal transfer [71].

Placental Symmetry and TTS

Abnormalities of monochorionic placental symmetry have received less attention than the anastomoses but are of importance. Monochorionic twin placental asymmetry has been variously described as unequal sharing of venous return zones, unequal allocation of parenchyma, and discordant vascular perfusion zones, but a precise quantitative definition is lacking [6].

The morphogenesis of MC placental asymmetry is also unknown, but the monochorionic monozygotic (monochorionic MZ) twin blastocyst has an intrinsic polarity defect at implantation [6]. The portions of the monochorionic twin placenta in TTS are often asymmetrical with the donor twin's placenta typically the smaller [5, 67, 72]. The threshold for significant asymmetry (e.g., 60:40, 70:30, 80:20, 90:10, etc.) and clinical placental insufficiency in one twin may vary in each case and depend on gestational age and

type and number of anastomotic vessels. In the absence of anastomoses, unequal sharing is an important cause of growth discordance in monochorionic twins [73]. The vascular anastomoses place an monochorionic twin with an adequate placental share at risk for pathophysiologic processes of the twin with placental insufficiency. Conversely, the anastomoses may sustain a twin with a small share by supplementing nutrients, which would otherwise be deficient. In addition to quantitative differences, the asymmetric monochorionic portions may differ qualitatively in placental circulation relative to umbilical cord insertions, chorion surface vessel pattern, and villous capillaries. In monochorionic twin gestations, the relative roles of reduced placental mass, abnormal cord insertions, and intertwin vascular anastomoses are difficult to ascertain and often occur together.

Umbilical Artery Doppler Velocimetry – TTS

A summary of fetal Doppler evaluation of TTS is presented in Table 20.3, including the method of assessment, principal findings, and conclusions.

Umbilical artery velocimetry was first reported in 5 of 76 twin pregnancies with TTS [24]. Using CW Doppler technology and a cutoff for A/B (S/D) ratio difference of 1.57 (greater than the 75th percentile), TTS pregnancies showed normal A/B ratios that were concordant. Growth restriction was present in 12 of 18 monochorionic pairs, but an elevated A/B ratio was present only in 7 pairs. The authors concluded that the A/B ratios in TTS are normal and concordant, and that differences in size on ultrasonography in the presence of no S/D difference suggest TTS.

Another report described TTS in two twin pregnancies – one at 20 weeks and one during labor [25]. The amniotic fluid volume assay indicated hydramnios/oligohydramnios in the first case and a normal state in the second case. Using CW Doppler technology, the S/D ratio of the umbilical artery was abnormal in the SGA donor twin and normal in the recipient, and the S/D ratio difference was 1.9 (an S/D ratio of >0.4 was the cutoff for twin abnormality).

Serial Doppler and ultrasound examinations were reported in a twin pregnancy with TTS [74]. The donor twin showed abnormal velocimetry with cyclic variations thought to be due to an arterial anastomosis. This donor fetus demonstrated abnormal flow (zero and reversal) and died in utero. The recipient survived, demonstrating normal velocimetry.

Pretorius et al. [75] reported fetal Doppler ultrasound findings in eight cases of TTS. Pulsed-wave duplex Doppler sonography was employed with high-resolution ultrasound, and A/B ratios were determined for the umbilical artery. Significant A/B ratio differences were noted in seven of the eight cases,

Table 20.3. Fetal Doppler evaluation of the umbilical artery in TTS. *CW* continuous-wave Doppler, *S/D* systolic/diastolic ratio, *US* ultrasonography, *PI* pulsatility index, *IUGR* intrauterine growth retardation, *UA* umbilical artery, *MCA* middle cerebral artery

Reference	Technique	No. of pregnancies	Method of assessment	Doppler findings	Conclusions
[24]	CW	5	CW; S/D ratio differences	No S/D ratio differences; 2 of 10 perinatal deaths	No S/D ratio difference in presence of size (US) difference suggests TTS
[25]	CW	2	CW; S/D ratio differences >0.4 abnormal	S/D ratio difference	TTS: high/low resistance values
				Case 1: 1.9, SGA twin: abnormal value	
				Case 2: one twin with abnormal value	
[74]	Pulsed Doppler	1	CW/real-time US; serial PI values in donor and recipient	PI in small donor cyclical but showed 0 to reversal during diastole; PI recipient normal	Artery-to-artery anastomosis suspected; morbidity not confined to volume exchange alone in TTS
[75]	Pulsed Doppler duplex	8	Pulsed Doppler; individual S/D ratios	All S/D differences between twins >0.4	Variable findings unable to differentiate donor and recipient; poor outcome with abnormal Doppler
				Five fetuses had absent/ reversal of diastolic flow One recipient and 6 donors with abnormal Doppler	
[31]	Pulsed Doppler	6	Pulsed Doppler; PI differences	Of 31 sets of twins, PI difference >0.5 in 7 cases; 6 of the 7 were associated with TTS	Of 12 infants with abnormal ratios, 5 suffered perinatal death
[76]	Pulsed Doppler; individual Doppler values	11	Pulsed Doppler; high-resolution US	Of 11 donor twins, 7 showed severe IUGR and elevated S/D ratios; 2 of recipient fetuses also showed abnormal values	Variable Doppler findings, but donor SGA fetuses more commonly had high S/D ratios than did recipient fetuses
				Oligohydramnios in donor sac; hydramnios in recipient sac	
[78]	Pulsed Doppler	4	Pulsed Doppler; PI in MCA, UA	UA increased resistance in 3, absent end-diastolic flow in 1 (recipient)	Doppler velocimetry helps explain changes in fetal hemodynamics in TTS
				MCA decreased resistance in 3 that could be measured (recipient) UA and MCA PI in donors were normal	

and in all cases the A/B ratio differences were >0.4. Pretorius et al. [75] concluded that Doppler findings are commonly abnormal in the presence of TTS, differing with Giles et al. [24], and that the Doppler findings were variable, suggesting "an extremely complex dynamic physiologic state."

Later, in 31 twin pregnancies, Doppler ultrasound findings were described for six pregnancies with TTS [31]. The PI was determined using pulsed-wave Doppler interrogation of the umbilical artery. Of the 31 twin pregnancies, 7 had intrapair differences for PI of >0.5; 6 of the 7 were associated with TTS.

Gaziano et al. [76] described 11 pregnancies with TTS from 101 multiple-gestation pregnancies using high-resolution real-time ultrasonography and a comprehensive assessment of the fetus that included detailed biometry and a fetal anatomic survey with amniotic fluid and placental assessment. Donor twins tended to be severely growth restricted, with 7 of the 11 showing elevated S/D ratios. Amniotic fluid tended to be decreased in the donor's sac and normal or increased in the recipient's sac. Normal S/D ratios were seen most frequently in the recipient fetus, although abnormal velocimetry was seen in two fetuses.

Other authors studying suspected TTS patients noted normal blood flow measurements in the umbilical artery of some fetuses [77]. They confirmed the observations that pathologic velocimetry patterns usually affect the smaller (donor) fetus.

In another study, four pairs of twins with TTS were described [78]. The three recipients for whom blood flow in the middle cerebral artery (MCA) could be measured had a decreased PI and each of the four recipients had abnormal umbilical artery waveforms (increased PI or absent end-diastolic flow). The middle cerebral and umbilical artery PIs were normal in the donors.

The heterogeneity of placental and clinical findings for, and the lack of strict criteria for, the diagnosis of TTS may explain some of the variability of findings reported for Doppler in TTS.

Venous Waveforms

Umbilical venous blood flow sampling in twin pregnancies using fetal Doppler ultrasonography was described by Gerson et al. [26]. The sampling was normal in cases of discordant growth due to abnormal placentation but was abnormal in one fetus with TTS. Pretorius et al. [75] described a biphasic venous waveform in the umbilical vein at 29 weeks' gestation in a fetus with TTS who also had Doppler echocardiographic findings suggestive of tricuspid insufficiency. Abnormal umbilical venous flow has been seen in other cases of fetal hydrops and most likely reflects right-sided cardiac failure. Figures 20.6 and 20.7 illustrate a case of fetal hydrops in TTS with an abnormal venous waveform pattern and fetal abdominal ascites.

Findings of reversed flow in the inferior vena cava and reversed flow in the ductus venosus is suggestive of right heart failure in a larger recipient twin [78]. In addition, echocardiography may demonstrate mitral and tricuspid regurgitation in twins with ultrasound evidence of hydrops [78].

Doppler velocimetry may differentiate between twin pregnancies complicated by FGR and TTS. This distinction is important since the death of one fetus

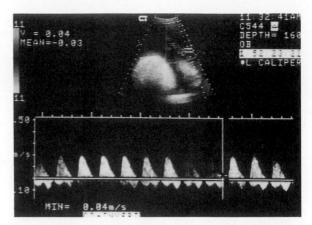

Fig. 20.6. Zero diastolic flow and abnormal venous waveform in the recipient fetus with TTS

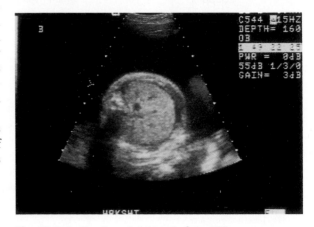

Fig. 20.7. Ascites in recipient twin from TTS

in TTS can be deleterious to the other, whereas death of an FGR fetus in a diamniotic dichorionic twin gestation poses less risk to the co-twin. Abnormal uterine artery Doppler values and brain sparing can be seen with both FGR and TTS [79]. Venous flow of the larger twin in TTS can be abnormal [79]. If FGR is due to poor placental function or chromosomal abnormality, venous flow in the larger twin is expected to be normal [79].

Outcome in TTS Pregnancies

Absent or reversed flow in five of the eight fetuses with TTS was associated with perinatal death in each instance [75]. Doppler abnormality in the setting of TTS portends a poor outcome [75]. Gaziano et al. [76] also noted increased morbidity and mortality in TTS fetuses with abnormal velocimetry. The PI difference in twins was greater in those destined to develop fetal hydrops [31]. In another study of 23 sets of twins with TTS, the following factors independently predicted poor survival: absent or reversed end-diastolic flow in the donor umbilical artery; abnormal pulsatility in the venous system of the recipient; and absence of an arterioarterial anastomosis [80].

Unbalanced arteriovenous shunting is probably the major pathophysiologic event in TTS, while the variety of potential vascular arrangements does not allow for uniformity of the fetal Doppler findings. In most cases the donor twin becomes progressively hypovolemic and sometimes, but not always, relatively anemic [57, 58]. The donor twin is not infrequently oliguric following delivery [76]. In the donor these events most likely result in increased umbilical vascular resistance, as reflected in an abnormal umbilical artery waveform. Because of the hypovolemia, urine output diminishes in the donor fetus, resulting in significant oligohydramnios. Mari et al. [81] found that the PI of the renal artery in the twin with oligohydramnios was higher than that in the renal artery of the twin with hydramnios. The hypervolemia in the larger twin results in right-sided cardiac failure, abnormal venous waveforms, and fetal hydrops. With increased urine output and possibly decreased fetal swallowing, hydramnios usually occurs in the recipient's sac [82]. Occasionally, the shunt reverses with high resistance, which is then reflected in the umbilical circulation of the larger (recipient) twin, with the smaller (donor) twin consequently developing hydrops. We have observed spontaneous reversal of these events, indicating the likely development of a compensatory anastomosis. Other authors have reported resolution of hydrops following the death of one of the twins [83].

The rigid neonatal standards (e.g., hemoglobin and birth-weight differences) for the diagnosis of TTS seem no longer tenable. Any number of weight and hemoglobin differences are possible (reflecting varied hemodynamic arrangements) in monochorionic twin pregnancies [84, 85].

Quintero et al. [86] proposed a staging system for TTS which considers a sequence of events in progressive TTS. A negative correlation was noted between survival of at least one fetus and stage and TTS was defined as polyhydramnios (maximum vertical pocket >8 cm) in the recipient and oligohydramnios (maximum vertical pocket of <2 cm) in the donor. All cases also had a single placenta, absent twin-peaks sign, and same-sex fetuses. The individual stages are as follows:

1. Stage I: polyhydramnios in the recipient, severe oligohydramnios in donor but visible bladder in the donor (BDT)
2. Stage II: polyhydramnios in the recipient, a stuck donor, BDT not visible, diastolic flow present in the umbilical artery and forward flow in the ductus venosus
3. Stage III: polyhydramnios and oligohydramnios, BDT not visible, critically abnormal Doppler (at least one of absent or reverse end-diastolic flow in the umbilical artery, reverse flow in the ductus venosus, or pulsatile umbilical venous flow)
4. Stage IV: presence of ascites or frank hydrops (fluid collection in two or more cavities) in either donor or recipient
5. Stage V: demise of either fetus

In Quintero et al.'s report [86] on staging, a number of patients were treated with laser or umbilical cord ligation. Taylor et al. [87] applied this staging methodology on a population treated with serial amnioreduction, septostomy, and selective reduction alone or in combination. They found no significant influence of staging at presentation with survival in their conservatively treated group. Survival was significantly poorer where stage increased rather than decreased. These authors concluded that the Quintero et al. [86] staging system should be used with caution for determining prognosis at the time of diagnosis, but may be better suited for monitoring disease progression.

Treatment

Options to improve prognosis in TTS include serial amnioreduction for hydramnios (Fig. 20.8), laser ablation of anastomoses between twins, septostomy, and selective feticide.

In a study of eight pregnancies with severe polyhydramnios secondary to TTS, uterine artery mean blood velocity, and volume of flow was significantly increased after amnioreduction [88]. The RI and PI in the same vessel were decreased after amnioreduction compared with Doppler values prior to the procedure, although the difference was not significant. Four of the eight RI measurements were >97.5th percentile of published reference for twins before the

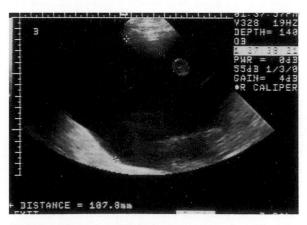

Fig. 20.8. Massive hydramnios in recipient sac of a fetus with TTS

procedure compared with only one such measurement after amnioreduction.

Improvement in TTS has been reported after therapeutic amniocentesis [89]. At 22 weeks after several amniocenteses, the smaller twin developed signs of congestive heart failure and absent diastolic flow. Another amniocentesis was performed after which the hydrops resolved and the diastolic flow in the umbilical artery improved.

Doppler values in the MCA have been monitored in women undergoing therapeutic amnioreduction [90]. Pulsatility index of the MCA fell after amniocentesis in all fetuses, although there was no consistent trend in response of the umbilical artery PI. Fetal stress is expected to cause a reduction in PI of the MCA as a brain-sparing response. An acute fall in amniotic fluid pressure likely creates an effective hypovolemia to which the fetus responds with dilation of resistance vessels in the brain reflected as a decrease in cerebral artery PI. Close fetal monitoring is recommended to avoid acute changes in pressure during amnioreduction [90].

Long-term outcomes were reported in 33 women with TTS who underwent amnioreduction [91]. None of the infants (16 sets of twins) developed major neurological handicap if both twins met the following conditions: were delivered after 27 weeks; were without congenital malformations; and both twins survived the neonatal period. Eight sets of twins had at least one twin with absent end-diastolic flow in the umbilical artery before the first amnioreduction; all except one of these twins either died in utero or after birth.

Survival was reported [92] for 13 of 14 co-twins (93%) after selective reduction using bipolar diathermy of either the donor or recipient twin in pregnancies complicated by stage III/VI TTS as defined by the staging system of Quintero et al. [86]. Three donors and four recipients had absent or reversed end-diastolic flow in the umbilical artery prior to the procedure. In all those with absent end-diastolic flow before the procedure, positive end-diastolic flow was restored, in the majority of cases, within 24 h following selective reduction. None of the co-twins later developed absent end-diastolic flow.

Laser ablation of the connecting vessels in TTS is an appealing option in the management of the worse forms of TTS since it is the sole treatment modality which corrects one of the underlying pathophysiologic defects and has been demonstrated to be effective [6]. Randomized clinical trials are now underway to assess laser ablation. All treatment options are subject to failure since many cases of TTS are in pregnancies in which there is significant asymmetrical distribution of the placental mass (see placental symmetry) as well as the presence of abnormal cord insertions in the affected twins.

Summary

Given the limited data from multiple relatively small studies and the causes of the fetal Doppler findings in TTS, the following list attempts to summarize current observations:

1. Twin transfusion syndrome is a complex pathophysiologic event for which there is no predictable pattern of vascular anastomosis and no uniform pattern of Doppler abnormality.
2. Differences in umbilical artery Doppler parameters are relatively common in twin pairs with TTS.
3. Abnormal umbilical artery velocimetry may be seen in either the donor or the recipient fetus, but it is more common in the growth-restricted donor fetus with oligohydramnios.
4. Abnormal umbilical venous flow may be seen in the circulation of the hydropic recipient fetus.
5. Abnormal velocimetry in TTS, particularly low diastolic velocities in the umbilical artery, is associated with a poor outcome and justifies the use of intensive surveillance.
6. Clinical criteria for TTS are difficult to define because of the individual and varying complexity of the vascular arrangements.
7. There may be a role for Doppler velocimetry in TTS staging, to determine the most appropriate treatment options, and to monitor disease progression.

Doppler Velocimetry and Outcome in Twin Pregnancies

Third-Trimester Doppler Studies

Velocimetry of the umbilical artery appears superior to that in the fetal ascending aorta, pulmonary artery, or internal carotid artery [93]. Singleton SGA infants with abnormal umbilical artery velocimetry have increased admission rates and prolonged courses in the neonatal intensive care unit (NICU) [51]. Fetuses with growth restriction and normal Doppler values have less morbidity than growth-restricted fetuses with abnormal values [94]. A variety of adverse events, including fetal distress, premature delivery, the presence of SGA, and low birth weight, are more common in Doppler-abnormal than in Doppler-normal fetuses [95].

The outcome of fetal growth restriction can be classified according to umbilical artery Doppler values [96], and the increased neonatal morbidity in SGA infants with abnormal antenatal umbilical artery Doppler findings has been repeatedly supported [97]. Abnormal resistance in the descending fetal aorta is associated with increased perinatal risk for death, necrotizing enterocolitis, and hemorrhage, whereas 75% of SGA infants with normal values had uncomplicated courses [52]. Gaziano et al. [98] demonstrated that preterm growth-restricted infants with abnormal umbilical artery Doppler studies were admitted to the NICU more frequently and remained twice as long as preterm growth-restricted infants with normal values. Finally, studies suggest that the perinatal mortality rate in pregnancies complicated by growth restriction and/or hypertension is higher in fetuses with reversed end-diastolic flow (33%–73%) or absent end-diastolic flow in the umbilical artery (9%–41%) [99–101]. These data in singletons support a role for fetal Doppler velocimetry as a predictor for adverse neonatal events. Although present outcome data are modest for multiple gestations and abnormal velocimetry, the initial information parallels that reported for singleton pregnancies.

Table 20.4 shows studies in twins that correlate abnormal Doppler studies with adverse outcome. In four fetuses from twin pregnancies with persistently absent end-diastolic velocities, three were born SGA, and one died in utero [30]. In seven fetuses the RI was normal early but later showed absent end-diastolic velocities; six of seven of these infants were subsequently born SGA.

Abnormal Doppler velocimetry in the fetal descending aorta and the umbilical artery are correlated with unsatisfactory outcomes including preterm delivery before 32 weeks, > 500 g birth weight discrepancy, < 10th percentile birth weight, and admission to an NICU [27]. Measures of the PI of the umbilical artery had a 50% sensitivity for adverse outcome prediction, while PI abnormality in the descending aorta showed a 44% sensitivity for unsatisfactory outcome.

Gaziano et al. [76] described outcomes relative to umbilical artery velocimetry in 207 fetuses from multiple-gestation pregnancies and noted 17 with an abnormal Doppler result; 15 of the 17 had adverse perinatal outcomes. Infants with abnormal waveforms delivered 3–4 weeks earlier and were more likely to have structural malformations (12% vs 1%), to be < 1500 g at birth, to suffer intrauterine death, and to have lower 5-min Apgar scores than twins with normal antenatal waveforms. Most of the morbidity and mortality occurred in the Doppler-abnormal group, which accounted for 8% of this twin population.

Joern et al. [102] studied 130 women with multiple gestations and compared cardiotocography, sonography, and Doppler for prediction of intrauterine growth restriction and "pathological fetal outcome"; included in the latter were umbilical artery pH < 7.20, 5-min Apgar < 8, or NICU admission for primarily asphyxia and only secondarily prematurity. These authors correctly identified 63 of 81 neonates with birth weights below the 10th percentile (sensitivity 76%) and 47 of 76 children who would have a "pathological fetal outcome" using Doppler data (sensitivity

Table 20.4 Fetal Doppler and adverse outcome among twin studies. *PI* pulsatility index

Reference	Vessel interrogated	Comment
[30]	Umbilical artery	Persistently absent end-diastolic velocities associated with poor outcome
[27]	Umbilical artery; descending fetal aorta	For unsatisfactory outcomes: PI of umbilical artery = 50% sensitivity; abnormal PI of descending aorta = 44% sensitivity
[76]	Umbilical artery	Abnormal waveforms in 8% of fetuses; 15 of 17 infants with abnormal waveforms showed significant morbidity; abnormal waveforms associated with earlier delivery (by 3 weeks), < 1500 g birth weight, increased structural malformations and stillbirths
[102]	Umbilical artery, middle cerebral artery, descending aorta	Doppler better than biometry or cardiotocography at predicting growth restriction (76%) and "pathologic fetal outcome" (sensitivity 60%)
[103]	Umbilical artery	Increased risk of adverse outcome if abnormal PI

60%). Fetuses were said to have a pathological "total Doppler result" if any of the following were abnormal: fetal descending aorta; umbilical artery; or middle cerebral artery. Doppler sonography appeared superior to cardiotocography and ultrasound biometry in detection of acute and chronic placental insufficiency, although better for prediction of chronic placental insufficiency as manifested by growth restriction.

In another study of outcomes in 206 twin pregnancies [103], 32 of which had at least one twin with an abnormal umbilical artery PI, the group with abnormal Doppler values had an increased risk of FGR or preeclampsia, cesarean section for fetal distress, premature birth, small-for-gestational-age infant, umbilical artery pH ≤ 7.15, neonatal intensive care unit admission and birth weight < 500, 1000, and 1500 g.

Giles et al. [104] studied fetal Doppler velocimetry and twin pregnancy outcomes in 272 pregnancies. They reported a decrease in uncorrected perinatal mortality from 42.1/1000 to 8.9/1000, after the Doppler result was made available to the referring obstetrician. The Doppler data was made available to the clinician at 28 weeks' gestation, allowing focused, and intensive surveillance for the pregnancies at risk.

Abnormal velocimetry in the umbilical artery reflects increased resistance to flow in the uteroplacental circulation. These changes most likely reflect long-standing compromise of the maternal-fetal gaseous and nutrient exchange, which corresponds to an alteration in fetal growth and a marked reduction in fetal reserves.

Questions remain relative to the morbidity issue. What is the frequency of normal velocimetry in the FGR fetus from a twin pregnancy, and is this finding prognostic? Are all growth-restricted neonates with normal umbilical artery Doppler findings constitutionally small, or are they growth-restricted but at low risk for adverse events? Can fetal vascular interrogation change the need for, or the frequency of, fetal surveillance?

Brain-Sparing Effect

There is a relative increase in blood flow to the brain in the growth-restricted fetus which has been called the "brain-sparing effect." This event is more likely to be seen in the fetus with placental insufficiency and chronic asphyxial stress, manifested by increased resistance in the umbilical artery. Blood flow redistribution occurs when resistance in the cerebral circulation is less than the resistance in umbilical circulation. The cerebroplacental ratio (CPR) was first defined by Arbeille et al. in 1997 [105]. The CPR is equal to the cerebral resistance index (CRI) divided by the umbilical resistance index (URI). The CPR has been shown to be a more sensitive predictor for poor perinatal outcome in growth-restricted fetuses than either cerebral RI or placental RI alone [105].

The work of Gaziano et al. [106] suggests that CPR is also superior to the umbilical artery RI and middle cerebral RI in predicting adverse neonatal events in twins. Birth weight, total length of stay, and total length of stay in special care nursery correlated more closely with CPR than with umbilical artery resistance index or MCA resistance index. The CPR was also significantly lower in diamniotic monochorionic vs diamniotic dichorionic twins. Finally, among the Doppler variables, CPR showed the highest sensitivity for growth restriction (67%).

The predictive benefits of comparing velocity recordings in the cerebral and umbilical arterial systems has been substantiated in studies showing improved risk prediction using ratios of cerebral to umbilical PI. These studies were done on singletons at risk for intrauterine growth restriction or growth-restricted fetuses [107–109]. Akiyama et al. [110] evaluated alterations in various fetal regional arterial PIs with increasing gestational age in appropriates for gestational-age singletons, twins, and triplets, and found no significant differences based on number of fetuses.

Gaziano et al. [111] used the ratio of the MCA and umbilical artery RIs to measure blood flow redistribution in 83 twin pairs. Brain sparing was seen significantly more frequently in growth-restricted (≤10th percentile) babies. Brain sparing was seen in 67% of growth-restricted babies and only 7% of non-growth-restricted babies. Diamniotic monochorionic twins from the lower birth weight group more often demonstrated blood flow redistribution compared with dizygotic twins of similar low birth weights. Placental vascular connections in diamniotic monochorionic pregnancies and the associated hemodynamic changes are likely responsible for the difference.

Second-Trimester Doppler Studies

Can fetal Doppler measurements taken in the second trimester predict uteroplacental complications which might occur later in pregnancy? For multiples, many complications, such as growth restriction, are likely to occur at higher rates than in singletons.

Transvaginal uterine artery Doppler measurements were taken at 22–24 weeks' gestation in 351 twin pregnancies [112]. Using mean PI above the 95th percentile and bilateral notches, screening with Doppler data identified women destined to develop complications related to uteroplacental insufficiency. Pregnancies with a high mean PI and bilateral notches were particularly worrisome. Women with a high mean PI had a 10-fold increased risk of becoming preeclamptic, a 14-fold increased risk of having an abruptio placenta, and a 7-fold increased risk of having an intrauterine fetal demise.

The frequency of complications in women with normal uterine artery RIs is higher in twin compared with singleton pregnancies [113]. Twin compared with singleton nomograms yield a higher sensitivity for the occurrence of complications such as preeclampsia, growth restriction, and growth discordance of ≥20%. Still, the sensitivities for developing preeclampsia, fetal growth restriction, birth-weight discordance, and any adverse outcome using the twin nomograms were relatively low at 36%, 27%, 29%, and 27%, respectively.

Uterine artery Doppler nomograms are different in dichorionic twins compared with singletons [114]. Twins showed lower RIs at all gestational ages (18–40 weeks). For both twins and singletons, uterine artery RI decreased linearly with increasing gestational age. Abnormal Doppler values at 20–24 weeks demonstrated low predictive value for gestational hypertension and/or preeclampsia.

Future Research

The value of Doppler velocimetry in twin and other pregnancy applications is questioned since this modality has yet to demonstrate an improvement in pregnancy outcome by prospective studies [115]. While this remains a challenge, those who apply Doppler studies to their at-risk patients appreciate its utility in improving diagnostic precision by allowing a greater understanding of pathophysiology, and permitting an insight into therapeutic interventions. As evidence supports the association of abnormal Doppler values with poor perinatal outcome, studies will focus on using Doppler velocimetry to alter treatment patterns in an effort to decrease perinatal morbidity and mortality.

Reverse end-diastolic umbilical artery flow can be seen as early as 11 weeks [116], while differences in fetal size and amniotic fluid volume may be appreciated at as early as 9 weeks of gestation [117]; thus, early ultrasound and continued improvements in amniotic fluid estimation in twin pregnancies will facilitate early diagnosis of twin disorders [118, 119].

Continued advances are expected detailing the pathophysiology of twin pregnancies. Doppler observations in the fetal circulation of discordant twins allow differentiation between growth discordance due to placental insufficiency and twin-to-twin transfusion [120]; for the latter, continued Doppler investigations into the venous side of the fetal circulation will clarify right-sided failure and cardiac function in affected fetuses [121, 122]. In addition, cordocentesis studies in monochorionic twins can assess the diagnostic value of serum erythropoietin, pancuronium bromide, and hematological and other biochemical studies in TTS [123–125].

Finally, Doppler sonography may play a role in the early identification of pregnancies at risk for TTS by color Doppler identification of communicating vessels. Less clear is color Doppler's role in supporting surgical approaches to this disorder by defining the location of these vessels. Furthermore, the inclusion of Doppler parameters into the evaluation of patients with TTS will prove useful in counseling patients, monitoring disease progression, and determining appropriate interventions. There is a need for randomized trials to determine the most effective treatments for TTS.

Conclusion

Doppler velocimetry supplements ultrasound biometry in multiple pregnancies for detection of the growth-restricted fetus. Fetal Doppler abnormality may precede alterations in growth and allow early identification of the at-risk fetus [32]. Similarly, abnormal velocimetry may precede other adverse events, such as the development of fetal hydrops [31] or the development of hypertensive disorders of pregnancy. Initial reports also suggest a role in predicting neonatal outcome. This technology adds to our understanding and knowledge of the complex hemodynamic changes in the TTS. Finally, Doppler velocimetry in multiple gestations serves as an important and accurate indicator of fetal vulnerability, allowing for appropriate surveillance and intervention for these at-risk pregnancies.

References

1. Trudinger BJ, Giles WB, Cook CM, Bombarieri J, Collins L (1985) Fetal umbilical artery flow velocity waveforms and placental resistance: clinical significance. Am J Obstet Gynecol 92:23–30
2. Hollenbach HA (1990) Epidemiology and diagnosis of twin gestation. Clin Obstet Gynecol 33:3–9
3. Nylander PPS (1978) Causes of high twinning frequencies in Nigeria. In: Navce WE, Allen G, Parisi P (eds) Twin research: biology and epidemiology. Liss, New York, pp 35–43
4. Nylander PPS (1981) The factors that influence twinning ratios. Acta Genet Med Gemellol 30:189–202
5. Benirschke K (1990) The placenta in twin gestation. Clin Obstet Gynecol 33:18–31
6. Gaziano EP, Lia JE de, Kuhlmann RS (2000) Diamniotic monochorionic twin gestations: an overview. J Matern Fetal Med 9:89–96
7. Cameron AH (1968) The Birmingham twin survey. Proc R Soc Med 61:229–234
8. Gersell DJ, Kraus FT (1994) Disease of the placenta. In: Kurman RJ (ed) Blaustein's pathology of the female genital tract. Springer, Berlin Heidelberg New York, pp 975–1048
9. Bleker PO, Oosting J, Hemrika DJ (1988) On causes of the retardation of fetal growth in multiple gestations. Acta Genet Med Gemellol 37:41–46
10. Bryan EM (1992) The biology of twinning. In: Twins and higher multiple births. Edward Arnold, London, pp 9–30
11. Pretorius DH, Mahony BS (1990) Twin gestation. In: Nyberg DA, Mahoney BS, Pretorius DH (eds) Diagnostic ultrasound of fetal anomalies. Mosby Year Book, St. Louis, pp 592–622
12. Pretorius DH, Budorick NE, Scioscia AI (1993) Twin pregnancies in the second trimester in women in an alpha-fetoprotein screening program: sonographic evaluation and outcome. AJR 161:1007–1013
13. Russell RB, Petrini JR, Damus K et al. (2003) The changing epidemiology of multiple births in the United States. Obstet Gynecol 101:129–135
14. Jones JM, Sbarra AJ, Cetrulo CL (1990) Antepartum management of twin gestation. Clin Obstet Gynecol 33:32–41
15. Fliegner JR (1989) When do perinatal deaths in multiple pregnancies occur? Aust NZ J Obstet Gynaecol 29:371–374
16. Mathews TJ, Menacker F, MacDorman MF (2002) Infant mortality statistics from the 2000 period linked birth/infant death data set. Nat Vital Stat Reports 50:12–13

17. Manlan G, Scott KE (1978) Contribution of twin pregnancy to perinatal mortality and fetal growth retardation after birth. Can Med Assoc J 118:365–367

18. Babson SG, Phillips DS (1973) Growth and development of twins dissimilar at birth. N Engl J Med 289:937–940

19. Babson S, Kangas J, Young N et al. (1964) Growth and development of twins dissimilar at birth. Pediatrics 33:327–333

20. Socol M, Tamura R, Sabbagha R et al. (1984) Diminished biparietal diameter and abdominal circumference growth in twins. Obstet Gynecol 64:235–238

21. Blickstein I, Lancet M (1988) The growth discordant twin. Obstet Gynecol Surv 43:509–515

22. Blickstein I (1991) The definition, diagnosis, and management of growth-discordant twins: an international census survey. Acta Genet Med Gemellol 40:345–351

23. Erkkola R, Ala-Mello S, Piiroinen O et al. (1985) Growth discordancy in twin pregnancies: a risk factor not detected by measurements of biparietal diameter. Obstet Gynecol 66:203–206

24. Giles WB, Trudinger BJ, Cook CM (1985) Fetal umbilical artery flow velocity-time waveforms in twin pregnancies. Br J Obstet Gynaecol 92:490–497

25. Farmakides G, Schulman H, Saldana LR et al. (1985) Surveillance of twin pregnancy with umbilical arterial velocimetry. Am J Obstet Gynecol 153:789–792

26. Gerson AG, Wallace DM, Bridgens NK et al. (1987) Duplex Doppler ultrasound in the evaluation of growth in twin pregnancies. Am J Obstet Gynecol 70:419–423

27. Nimrod C, Davies D, Harder J et al. (1987) Doppler ultrasound prediction of fetal outcome in twin pregnancies. Am J Obstet Gynecol 156:402–406

28. Saldana LR, Eads MC, Schaefer TR (1987) Umbilical blood waveform in fetal surveillance of twins. Am J Obstet Gynecol 157:712–715

29. Divon MY, Girz BA, Sklar A et al. (1989) Discordant twins: a prospective study of the diagnostic value of real-time ultrasonography combined with umbilical artery velocimetry. Am J Obstet Gynecol 161:757–760

30. Hastie SJ, Danskin F, Neilson JP et al. (1989) Prediction of the small for gestational age twin fetus by Doppler umbilical artery waveform analysis. Obstet Gynecol 74:730–733

31. Yamada A, Kasugai M, Ohno Y et al. (1991) Antenatal diagnosis of twin–twin transfusion syndrome by Doppler ultrasound. Obstet Gynecol 78:1058–1061

32. Degani S, Gonen R, Shapiro I et al. (1992) Doppler flow velocity waveforms in fetal surveillance of twins: a prospective longitudinal study. J Ultrasound Med 11:537–541

33. Gaziano EP, Calvin S, Bendel RP et al. (1992) Pulsed Doppler umbilical artery waveforms in multiple gestation: comparison with ultrasound estimated fetal weight for the diagnosis of the small-for-gestational-age (SGA) infant. J Matern Fetal Invest 1:277–280

34. Kurmanavicius J, Hesbisch G, Huch R et al. (1992) Umbilical artery blood flow velocity waveform in twin pregnancies. J Perinat Med 20:307–312

35. Ferrazzi E, Pardi G (1993) Doppler assessment of multiple pregnancy. In: Chervenak FA, Isaacson GC, Campbell S (eds) Ultrasound in obstetrics and gynecology. Little Brown, Boston, pp 625–634

36. O'Brien WF, Knuppel RA, Scerbo JC et al. (1986) Birth weight in twins: an analysis of discordancy and growth retardation. Obstet Gynecol 67:483–486

37. Bronsteen R, Goyert G, Bottoms SF (1989) Classification of twins and neonatal morbidity. Obstet Gynecol 74:98–101

38. Cheung VYT, Bocking AD, Dasilva OP (1995) Preterm discordant twins: What birth weight difference is significant? Am J Obstet Gynecol 172:955–959

39. Gernt PR, Mauldin JG, Newman RB et al. (2001) Sonographic prediction of twin birth weight discordance. Obstet Gynecol 97:53–56

40. Deter RL, Stefos T, Harrist RB et al. (1992) Detection of intrauterine growth retardation in twins using individualized growth assessment. I. Evaluation of growth outcome at birth. J Clin Ultrasound 20:573–577

41. Deter RL, Stefos T, Harrist RB et al. (1992) Detection of intrauterine growth retardation in twins using individualized growth assessment. II. Evaluation of third-trimester growth and prediction of growth outcome at birth. J Clin Ultrasound 20:579–585

42. Giles W, Trudinger B, Cook CM et al. (1993) Placental microvascular changes in twin pregnancies with abnormal umbilical artery waveforms. Obstet Gynecol 81:556–559

43. Jensen OH (1993) Doppler velocimetry and umbilical cord blood gas assessment of twins. Eur J Obstet Gynecol Reprod Biol 49:155–159

44. Rodis JF, Vintzileos AM, Campbell WA et al. (1990) Intrauterine fetal growth in discordant twin gestations. J Ultrasound Med 8:443–448

45. Rodis JF, Vintzileos AM, Campbell WA et al. (1990) Intrauterine fetal growth in concordant twin gestations. Am J Obstet Gynecol 162:1025–1029

46. Storlazzi E (1987) Ultrasound diagnosis of discordant fetal growth in twin gestations. Obstet Gynecol 69:363–367

47. Chang TC, Robson SC, Spencer JAD et al. (1993) Identification of fetal growth retardation: comparison of Doppler waveform indices and serial ultrasound measurements of abdominal circumference and fetal weight. Obstet Gynecol 82:230–236

48. Degani S, Paltiely J, Lewinsky R et al. (1990) Fetal blood flow velocity waveforms in pregnancies complicated by intrauterine growth retardation. Isr J Med Sci 26:250–254

49. Degani S, Paltiely J, Lewinsky R et al. (1988) Fetal internal carotid artery flow velocity time waveforms in twin pregnancies. J Perinat Med 16:405–409

50. Arduini D, Rizzo G (1993) Doppler studies of deteriorating growth-retarded fetuses. Curr Opin Obstet Gynecol 5:195–203

51. Berkowitz GS, Mehalek KE, Chitkara U et al. (1988) Doppler velocimetry in the prediction of adverse outcome in pregnancies at risk for intrauterine growth retardation. Obstet Gynecol 71:742–746

52. Hackett GA, Campbell S, Gamsu H et al. (1987) Doppler studies in the growth retarded fetus and prediction of neonatal necrotising enterocolitis, hemorrhage, and neonatal morbidity. Br Med J 294:13–17

53. Mahoney G, Filly R, Callen P (1985) Amnionicity and chorionicity in twin pregnancies: prediction using ultrasound. Radiology 155:205–209

54. Blickstein I (1990) The twin–twin transfusion syndrome. Obstet Gynecol 76:714–722

55. Shah DM, Chaffin D (1989) Perinatal outcome in very preterm births with twin–twin transfusion syndrome. Am J Obstet Gynecol 161:1111–1113

56. Brown DL, Benson CB, Driscoll SG et al. (1989) Twin–twin transfusion syndrome: sonographic findings. Radiology 170:61–63

57. Saunders NJ, Snijders RJM, Nicolaides KH (1991) Twin–twin transfusion syndrome during the 2nd trimester is associated with small intertwin hemoglobin differences. Fetal Diagn Ther 6:34–36

58. Fisk NM, Borrell A, Hubinont C et al. (1990) Fetofetal transfusion syndrome: Do the neonatal criteria apply in utero? Arch Dis Child 65:651–661

59. Bruner JP, Rosemond RL (1991) Twin-to-twin transfusion syndrome: a subset of the twin oligohydraminos–polyhydraminos oligohydraminos sequence. Am J Obstet Gynecol 169:925–930

60. Damato N, Filly RA, Goldstein RB et al. (1993) Frequency of fetal anomalies in sonographically detected polyhydraminos. J Ultrasound Med 12:11–15

61. Hadlock FP, Harrist RB, Carpenter RJ et al. (1984) Sonographic estimation of fetal weight. Radiology 150: 535–540

62. Shepard MJ, Richards VA, Berkowitz RL et al. (1982) An evaluation of two equations for predicting fetal weight by ultrasound. Am J Obstet Gynecol 142:47–54

63. Stefos T, Deter RL, Hill RM et al. (1989) Individual growth curve standards in twins: prediction of third-trimester and birth characteristics. Am J Obstet Gynecol 161:179–183

64. Anath CV, Vintzileos AM, Shen-Schwarz S et al. (1998) Standards of birth weight in twin gestations stratified by placental chorionicity. Obstet Gynecol 91:917–924

65. Gonsoulin W, Moise KJ, Kirshon B et al. (1990) Outcome of twin–twin transfusion diagnosed before 28 weeks of gestation. Obstet Gynecol 75:214–216

66. Bajora R, Wigglesworth J, Fisk NM (1995) Angioarchitecture of monochorionic placentas in relation to the twin–twin transfusion syndrome. Am J Obstet Gynecol 172:856–863

67. Machin G, Still K, Lalani T (1996) Correlations of placental vascular anatomy and clinical outcomes in 69 monochorionic twin pregnancies. Am J Med Genet 61: 229–236

68. Van Gemert MJ, Sterenborg HJ (1998) Haemodynamic model of twin–twin transfusion syndrome in monochorionic twin pregnancies. Placenta 19:195–208

69. Denbow ML, Coz P, Talbert D et al. (1998) Colour Doppler energy insonation of placental vasculature in monochorionic twins: absent arterio-arterial anastomoses in association with twin-to-twin transfusion syndrome. Br J Obstet Gynaecol 105:760–765

70. Sala MA, Matheus M (1989) Placental characteristics in twin transfusion syndrome. Arch Gynecol 246:51–56

71. Bryan EM (1977) IgG deficiency in association with placental edema. Early Hum Dev 1:133–143

72. Bendon RW (1995) Twin transfusion: pathologic studies of the monochorionic placenta in liveborn twins and the perinatal autopsy in monochorionic twin pairs. Pediatr Pathol Lab Med 15:363–376

73. Fries MH, Goldstein RB, Kilpatrick SJ et al. (1993) The role of velamentous cord insertion in the etiology of twin–twin transfusion syndrome. Obstet Gynecol 81: 569–574

74. Erskine RLA, Ritchie JWK, Murnaghan GA (1986) Antenatal diagnosis of placental anastomosis in a twin pregnancy using Doppler ultrasound. Br J Obstet Gynaecol 93:955–959

75. Pretorius DH, Manchester D, Barkin S et al. (1988) Doppler ultrasound of twin transfusion syndrome. J Ultrasound Med 7:117–124

76. Gaziano EP, Knox GE, Bendel RP et al. (1991) Is pulsed Doppler velocimetry useful in the management of multiple-gestation pregnancies? Am J Obstet Gynecol 164: 1426–1433

77. Kainer F, Rodriquez J, Maier R et al. (1993) Diastolic zero-flow in the umbilical artery in twin pregnancies. J Perinat Med 21:273–277

78. Ropacka M, Markwitz W, Ginda W et al. (1998) Ultrasound in the diagnosis of twin-to-twin transfusion syndrome: a preliminary report. Acta Genet Med Gemellol 47:227–237

79. Soikkeli P, Dubiel M, Gudmundsson S (2002) Doppler velocimetry for predicting fetal death in a twin pregnancy. Acta Obstet Gynecol Scand 81:783–785

80. Taylor MJO, Denbow ML, Duncan KR et al. (2000) Antenatal factors at diagnosis that predict outcome in twin–twin transfusion syndrome. Am J Obstet Gynecol 183:1023–1028

81. Mari G, Kirshon B, Abuhamad A (1993) Fetal renal artery flow velocity waveforms in normal pregnancies and pregnancies complicated by polyhydramnios and oligohydramnios. Obstet Gynecol 81:560–564

82. Kirshon B (1989) Fetal urine output in hydramnios. Obstet Gynecol 73:240–242

83. Kirshon B, Moise KJ, Mari G et al. (1990) In utero resolution of hydrops fetalis following the death of one twin in twin–twin transfusion. Am J Perinatol 2:107–109

84. Danskin FH, Neilson JP (1989) Twin-to-twin transfusion syndrome: What are appropriate diagnostic criteria? Am J Obstet Gynecol 161:365–369

85. Wenstrom KD, Tessen JA, Zlatnik FJ et al. (1992) Mechanisms of hematologic and weight discordance in monochorionic twins. Obstet Gynecol 80:257–261

86. Quintero RA, Morales WJ, Allen MH et al. (1999) Staging of twin–twin transfusion syndrome. J Perinatol 19:550–555

87. Taylor MJO, Govender L, Jolly M et al. (2002) Validation of the Quintero staging system for twin–twin transfusion syndrome. Obstet Gynecol 100:1257–1265

88. Bower SJ, Flack NJ, Sepulveda W et al. (1995) Uterine artery blood flow response to correction of amniotic fluid volume. Am J Obstet Gynecol 173:502–507

89. Smith JF, Pesterfield W, Day LD et al. (1997) Doppler evidence of improved fetoplacental hemodynamics following amnioreduction in the stuck twin phenomenon. Obstet Gynecol 90:681–682

90. Mari G, Wasserstrum N, Kirshon B (1992) Reduction in the middle cerebral artery pulsatility index after decompression of polyhydramnios in twin gestation. Am J Perinatol 9:381–384

91. Mari G, Detti L, Oz U et al. (2000) Long-tern outcome in twin–twin transfusion syndrome treated with serial aggressive amnioreduction. Am J Obstet Gynecol 183: 211–217

92. Taylor MJO, Shalev E, Tanawattanacharoen S et al. (2002) Ultrasound-guided umbilical cord occlusion using bipolar diathermy for stage III/IV twin–twin transfusion syndrome. Prenat Diagn 22:70–76
93. Gorenenberg IA, Bearts W, Hop WC et al. (1991) Relationship between fetal cardiac and extra-cardiac Doppler flow velocity waveforms and neonatal outcome in intrauterine growth retardation. Early Hum Dev 26: 185–192
94. Reuwer PJHM, Rietman GW, Sijmons EA et al. (1987) Intrauterine growth retardation: prediction of perinatal distress by Doppler ultrasound. Lancet 2:415–418
95. Mulders LGM, Jongsma HY, Hein PR (1989) Uterine and umbilical artery blood flow velocity waveforms and their validity in the prediction of fetal compromise. Eur J Obstet Gynecol Reprod Biol 31:143–154
96. Burke G, Stuart B, Crowley P et al. (1990) Is intrauterine growth retardation with normal umbilical artery blood flow a benign condition? Br Med J 300:1044–1045
97. McCowan LM, Erskine LA, Ritchie K (1987) Umbilical artery Doppler blood flow studies in the preterm small for gestational age fetus. Am J Obstet Gynecol 156:655–659
98. Gaziano EP, Knox H, Ferrera B et al. (1994) Is it time to reassess the risk for the growth retarded fetus with normal velocimetry of the umbilical artery? Am J Obstet Gynecol 170:1734–1741
99. Brar H, Platt LD (1988) Reverse end-diastolic flow velocity on umbilical artery velocimetry in high-risk pregnancies: an ominous finding with adverse pregnancy outcome. Am J Obstet Gynecol 159:559–561
100. Karsdorp VHM, van Vugt JMG, van Geijn HP et al. (1994) Clinical significance of absent or reversed end diastolic velocity waveforms in umbilical artery. Lancet 344:1665–1668
101. Zelop CM, Richardson DK, Heffner LJ (1996) Outcomes of severely abnormal umbilical artery Doppler velocimetry in structurally normal singleton fetuses. Obstet Gynecol 87:434–438
102. Joern H, Schroeder W, Sassen R et al. (1997) Predictive value of a single CTG, ultrasound and Doppler examination to diagnose acute and chronic placental insufficiency in multiple pregnancies. J Perinat Med 25:325–332
103. Joern H, Rath W (2000) Correlation of Doppler velocimetry findings in twin pregnancies including course of pregnancy and fetal outcome. Fetal Diagn Ther 15: 160–164
104. Giles WB, Trudinger BJ, Cook CM et al. (1988) Umbilical artery flow velocity waveforms and twin pregnancy outcome. Obstet Gynecol 72:894–897
105. Arbeille P (1997) Fetal arterial Doppler: IUGR and hypoxia. Eur J Obstet Gynecol Reprod Biol 75:51–53
106. Gaziano EP, Gaziano C, Terrell CA et al. (2001) The cerebroplacental Doppler ratio and neonatal outcome in diamniotic monochorionic and dichorionic twins. J Matern Fetal Med 10:371–375
107. Gramellini D, Folli MC, Raboni S et al. (1992) Cerebral-umbilical Doppler ratio as a predictor of adverse perinatal outcome. Obstet Gynecol 79:416–420
108. Bahado-Singh RO, Kovanci E, Jeffres A et al. (1999) The Doppler cerebroplacental ratio and perinatal outcome in intrauterine growth restriction. Am J Obstet Gynecol 180:750–756
109. Wladimiroff JW, Wijngaard JAGW, Degani S et al. (1987) Cerebral and umbilical arterial blood flow velocity waveforms in normal and growth-retarded pregnancies. Obstet Gynecol 69:705–709
110. Akiyama M, Kuno A, Tanaka Y et al. (1999) Comparison of alterations in fetal regional arterial vascular resistance in appropriate-for-gestational-age singleton, twin and triplet pregnancies. Hum Reprod 14:2635–2643
111. Gaziano E, Gaziano C, Brandt D (1998) Doppler velocimetry determined redistribution of fetal blood flow: correlation with growth restriction in diamniotic monochorionic and dizygotic twins. Am J Obstet Gynecol 178:1359–1367
112. Yu CKH, Papageorghiou AT, Boli A et al. (2002) Screening for pre-eclampsia and fetal growth restriction in twin pregnancies at 23 weeks of gestation by transvaginal uterine artery Doppler. Ultrasound Obstet Gynecol 20:535–540
113. Geipel A, Berg C, Germer U et al. (2002) Doppler assessment of the uterine circulation in the second trimester in twin pregnancies: prediction of pre-eclampsia, fetal growth restriction and birth weight discordance. Ultrasound Obstet Gynecol 20:541–545
114. Rizzo G, Arduini D, Romanini C (1993) Uterine artery Doppler velocimetry waveforms in twin pregnancies. Obstet Gynecol 82:978–983
115. Kochenour NK (1993) Doppler velocimetry in pregnancy. Sem Ultrasound CT MRI 14:249
116. Montenegro N, Beires J, Leite LP (1995) Reverse end-diastolic umbilical artery blood flow at 11 weeks' gestation. Ultrasound Obstet Gynecol 5:141–142
117. Tadmor O, Nitzan M, Rabinowitz R et al. (1995) Prediction of second trimester intrauterine growth retardation and fetal death in a discordant twin by first trimester measurements. Fet Diagn Ther 10:17–21
118. Watson WJ, Harlass FE, Menard MK et al. (1995) Sonographic assessment of amniotic fluid in normal twin pregnancy. Am J Perinatol 12:122–124
119. Magann EF, Whitworth NS, Bass JD et al. (1995) Amniotic fluid volume of third-trimester diamniotic twin pregnancies. Obstet Gynecol 85:957–960
120. Rizzo G, Arduini D, Romanini C (1994) Cardiac and extracardiac flows in discordant twins. Am J Obstet Gynecol 170:1321–1327
121. Hecher K, Ville Y, Snijders R et al. (1995) Doppler studies of the fetal circulation in twin–twin transfusion syndrome. Ultrasound Obstet Gynecol 5:318–324
122. Mitra SC (1995) Umbilical venous Doppler waveform without fetal breathing; its significance. Am J Perinatol 12:217–219
123. Lemery DR, Santolaya-Forgas J, Serre AF et al. (1995) Fetal serum erythropoietin in twin pregnancies with discordant growth. A clue for the prenatal diagnosis of monochorionic twins with vascular communications. Fet Diagn Ther 10:86–91
124. Tanaka M, Natori M, Ishimoto H et al. (1992) Intravascular pancuronium bromide infusion for prenatal diagnosis of twin–twin transfusion syndrome. Fet Diagn Ther 7:36–40
125. Berry SM, Puder KS, Uckele JE et al. (1995) Comparison of intrauterine hematologic and biochemical values between twin pairs with and without stuck twin syndrome. Am J Obstet Gynecol 172:1403–1410

Doppler Sonography in Pregnancies Complicated with Pregestational Diabetes Mellitus

Dev Maulik, Genevieve Sicuranza, Andrzej Lysikiewicz, Reinaldo Figueroa

Introduction

During the past few decades, tremendous advances have been made in the medical and obstetrical management of pregnancies complicated with pregestational diabetes resulting in considerable improvements in maternal and perinatal outcomes [1]. Stringent periconceptional glycemic control and advances in fetal surveillance have significantly contributed to this improvement. The successful management of a pregestational diabetic mother requires timely and appropriate antepartum fetal surveillance which permits the pregnancy to progress while identifying the fetus who may be compromised and may benefit from delivery. Doppler velocimetry enables the investigation of fetal circulatory decompensation, and thus provides a noninvasive monitoring tool for assessing fetal well-being. There is considerable evidence affirming the efficacy of umbilical arterial Doppler sonography in predicting and improving adverse perinatal outcome in pregnancies with fetal growth restriction (FGR) and preeclampsia; however, the utility of Doppler fetal surveillance in managing uncomplicated pregnancies with pregestational diabetes remains controversial.

This chapter presents a review of the role of Doppler sonography in assessing the fetus of a pregestational diabetic mother and recommends a management plan based on the current evidence.

Maternal Glycemic State and Fetal Hemodynamics

Fetal circulatory response to altered maternal glycemic state appears to be complex. This section briefly addresses this issue pertaining to both hyper- and hypoglycemia.

In an experimental model involving late gestation ewes, induction of acute maternal hyperglycemia produced a 27%–29% reduction in the placental share of the cardiac output which was redistributed to fetal carcass, heart, renal, adrenal, and splanchnic circulations [2]. Concordant with the changes in perfusion, the fetuses also developed systemic hypoxemia and mixed acidemia during induced maternal hyperglycemia without any alterations in fetal cardiac, brain, and renal oxygenation. The response to hyperglycemic challenge, however, was different in the fetuses of ewes rendered diabetic by streptozocin administration [3]. The umbilical–placental blood flow did not change significantly in these fetuses but significantly declined in the controls, whereas fetal brain and renal perfusion was significantly higher in the former at all times than in the controls. The fetuses of the diabetic mothers were also more hypoxemic than the controls. Fetal hypoxemia induced by maternal hyperglycemia could be explained by the earlier observation that chronic fetal hyperglycemia is associated with accelerated fetal oxidative metabolism. In the latter study, chronic fetal hyperglycemia produced by fetal glucose infusion via chronic in utero catheterization led to an increase in calculated fetal O_2 consumption by approximately 30% ($p < 0.01$) [4]. The intensity of fetal hyperglycemia, and not the degree of fetal hyperinsulinemia, was the prime determinant of the magnitude of fetal O_2 consumption which was associated with a significant increase in fetal O_2 extraction with no alterations in either fetal O_2 delivery or fetal blood O_2 affinity.

The relationship between fetal hypoxemia and acidemia, and fetal and uterine hemodynamics, was investigated in a cross-sectional study involving women with well-controlled diabetes mellitus [5]. Of the 65 patients who had Doppler investigations performed, 41 had cordocentesis performed. The changes in the umbilical arterial Doppler indices correlated well with the changes in fetal pH (correlation coefficient –0.402; $p < 0.01$) and in pO_2 (correlation coefficient –0.544; $p < 0.001$); however, this correlation was limited to the cases with FGR or preeclampsia as the Doppler findings were abnormal only in the presence of these complications. This finding is consistent with the known association between umbilical arterial abnormality and fetal growth restriction and preeclampsia. As the mothers' glycemic state was well controlled, this study did not address the issue of human fetal hemodynamic response to in utero hyperglycemia.

The effect of maternal hypoglycemia on fetal cardiovascular system has been investigated in an animal model and also in humans. Maternal hypoglycemia induced by infusion of insulin in a ewe model led to increased fetal plasma catecholamine and free fatty acid levels ($p < 0.01$) [6]; however, no significant effects were noted on the fetal heart rate, blood pressure, or arterial blood gases. Moreover, fetal insulin and glucagon levels were also unaffected. The studies in pregnant diabetic mothers were experimental in design and involved the use of the insulin clamp method for inducing hypoglycemia. Moderate maternal hypoglycemia induced by the insulin clamp technique in ten insulin-dependent diabetic women in the third trimester was associated with no consistent changes in the umbilical arterial Doppler waveform. No significant alterations were observed in fetal breathing movements or the heart rate, although maternal epinephrine and growth hormone levels were significantly ($p < 0.001$) increased [7]. In a similar study, the effect of hypoglycemia induced by hyperinsulinemic hypoglycemic clamp on the fetal heart rate and the umbilical artery flow velocity waveforms was investigated in a prospective experimental study in ten women with insulin-dependent diabetes mellitus in the third trimester of pregnancy. Maternal hypoglycemia led to increases in the frequency and amplitude of fetal heart rate accelerations and maternal catecholamine levels but only a slight decline in the pulsatility index of the umbilical artery [8].

In summary, the above experimental and clinical studies enhance our understanding of maternal diabetes-induced modifications in fetal circulatory homeostasis. Fetal response to hyperglycemic challenge is modulated by the chronic glycemic state and the intensity of the glycemic challenge. In the presence of maternal diabetes, the fetus increases its oxidative metabolism becoming more hypoxemic. Perfusion of the brain and kidneys increases without any significant changes in the fetoplacental perfusion and the Doppler velocimetry of the umbilical arteries remains unchanged unless FGR is also present. Cordocentesis data confirm that significant hypoxemia and acidemia in maternal diabetes mellitus may not be associated with Doppler-recognizable changes in fetal flow impedance unless the pregnancy is complicated with FGR or preeclampsia. Human and animal studies indicate that the fetal response to moderate maternal hypoglycemia is unremarkable and inconsistent.

Umbilical Artery Doppler Sonography in Diabetic Pregnancies

This section reviews the role of Doppler ultrasound investigation of the umbilical artery in relation to adverse perinatal outcome and also in relation to maternal glycemic state.

Umbilical Artery Doppler and Perinatal Outcome

The efficacy of umbilical arterial Doppler indices for predicting adverse perinatal outcomes in high-risk pregnancies has been affirmed by numerous studies. Abnormally elevated umbilical arterial Doppler indices have been associated with low Apgar score, fetal distress (late and severe variable decelerations), absent variability, low fetal scalp and umbilical cord arterial pH, presence of thick meconium, and admission to the neonatal intensive care unit [9]. As presented in Chap. 25, an absent or reversed end-diastolic velocity in the umbilical arterial Doppler waveform is particularly ominous and is associated with markedly adverse perinatal outcome including a high perinatal mortality rate.

It remains somewhat controversial whether such diagnostic efficacy of Doppler sonography also encompasses pregnancies with diabetes. The studies in this area differ in several respects including the sample size, the Doppler parameter used and its threshold value, the measures of perinatal outcome, and prevalence of complications such as vasculopathy. Although there is no complete unanimity in the conclusions regarding efficacy, critical appraisal of these studies reveal that the controversy is mostly apparent. The relevant studies regarding adverse perinatal outcome are summarized in Table 21.1 and are selectively discussed below.

Bracero and associates [10] observed a significant correlation between elevated umbilical arterial S/D and adverse perinatal outcome including increased stillbirths and neonatal morbidity such as hypoglycemia and hyperbilirubinemia in a mixed population of class A and insulin-dependent diabetic mothers. In a more recent report, the same investigator noted that umbilical arterial SD ratio was superior to biophysical profile or nonstress test in predicting preterm labor (< 37 weeks), FGR, hypoglycemia, hyperbilirubinemia, respiratory distress and cesarean for fetal distress (relative risk 2.6, 1.7, and 1.7, respectively; $p < 0.001$).

Landon and colleagues [11] performed multiple umbilical arterial S/D measurements in 35 insulin-dependent diabetic women and observed significantly elevated mean second- and third-trimester S/D values in women with vasculopathy compared with women without the complication (4.34±0.7 and 3.2±0.65 vs 3.72±0.42 and 2.55±0.32, respectively; $p < 0.03$). The elevated ratio preceded development of preeclampsia and fetal growth restriction.

Johnstone and associates [12] prospectively investigated the efficacy of the umbilical arterial resistance

Table 21.1. Diagnostic efficacy of umbilical arterial Doppler in diabetic pregnancy. *PPV* positive predictive value, *NPV* negative predictive value, *LR+* positive likelihood ratio, *LR–* negative likelihood ratio, *FGR* fetal growth restriction, *FD* fetal distress, *C/S* cesarean section. (From [36])

Reference	Outcome	Prevalence	Sensitivity	Specificity	PPV	NPV	LR+	LR–	Accuracy
[10]	Stillbirth	0.04	1	0.83	0.22	1	7.6	0	0.85
[11]	FGR, FD	0.09	1	0.89	0.51	1	9.7	0	0.90
[12]	FD	0.05	0.42	0.95	0.33	0.96	8.6	0.6	0.92
[15]	C/S for FD	0.30	0.93	0.93	0.75	0.75	6.0	0.7	0.75
[16]	Composite	0.23	0.32	0.92	0.57	0.81	4.2	0.7	0.78
[17]	C/S for FD	0.27	0.61	0.75	0.48	0.84	2.5	0.5	0.71

Table 21.2. Umbilical arterial Doppler and maternal glycemic control. *S/D* systolic to diastolic ratio, *RI* resistance index, *Δ* the change, *r* correlation coefficient, *NS* not statistically significant. (From [36])

Reference	Doppler index	HbA1c	Δ HbA1c	Mean blood glucose
[10]	S/D			$r = 0.52$, $p < 0.001$
[11]	S/D	$r = 0.25$, NS		$r = 0.15$, NS
[12]	RI		$r = 0.02$–0.17, NS	
[14]	S/D	$r = 0.28$, NS		0.19
[13]	S/D	NS		NS
[15]	PI	NS		
[5]	Δ PI		0.011, NS	

index in 128 pregnancies with uncomplicated diabetes mellitus. Abnormally elevated umbilical arterial RI significantly predicted nonassuring antepartum fetal heart rate tracing and/or a low biophysical profile score requiring immediate caesarean delivery; however, the RI was not predictive in four of seven pregnancies with fetal compromise which led the authors to caution against undue dependence on umbilical arterial RI in uncomplicated diabetic pregnancies.

In a patient population of 56 diabetic mothers including 14 with vasculopathy, Reece and associates [13] observed higher mean umbilical arterial indices in those with vasculopathy than those without vasculopathy or diabetes. Elevated Doppler indices were significantly associated with FGR and neonatal metabolic complications. This relationship between abnormal umbilical arterial Doppler indices, and the presence of maternal vasculopathic complication and various adverse perinatal outcomes has been corroborated by other investigators [14–17].

Umbilical Arterial Doppler Sonography and Maternal Glycemic Control

In contrast to adverse outcome, the relationship between abnormal umbilical arterial Doppler indices

and the quality of glycemic control remains highly controversial. Bracero and associates [10] first noted a significant positive correlation between umbilical arterial S/D and mean serum glucose values ($r = 0.52$, $p < 0.001$). This finding however was refuted by Landon and associates [11] who found no significant correlation between mean third-trimester umbilical arterial S/D, and glycosylated hemoglobin ($r = 0.25$) or mean blood glucose levels ($r = 0.15$). This lack of correlation was corroborated by other investigators. These studies are summarized in Table 21.2.

In summary, most studies suggest significant diagnostic efficacy in diabetic pregnancies complicated by the presence of FGR or hypertension. It is noteworthy that these studies were heterogeneous regarding the outcome measures and the population size, and that the Doppler method demonstrated varying degrees of diagnostic efficacy. Moreover, the presence of normal Doppler may not always rule out fetal compromise. The ability of the umbilical artery Doppler indices to reflect maternal glycemic control remains controversial.

Doppler Sonography of Other Fetal and the Uterine Circulations in Pregestational Diabetic Pregnancies

Fetal Middle Cerebral Artery Doppler

There is insufficient information regarding the clinical value of Doppler investigation of the fetal cerebral circulation. In the neonate, Van Bel and associates found unaffected cerebral hemodynamics in the macrosomic infants of insulin-dependent diabetic mothers during the first 4 days of life even in the presence of ventricular septal hypertrophy with reduced cardiac output and stroke volume [18]. Salvesen and co-workers found no significant changes in the fetal circulation in a longitudinal Doppler study of 48 relatively well-controlled diabetic pregnancies except when complicated by preeclampsia or FGR [5]. The study included Doppler velocimetry of the middle cerebral artery. In a separate report, the authors found normal Doppler results in the uterine and fetal circulations including the middle cerebral artery of most patients (five of six) with diabetic nephropathy despite the cordocentesis evidence of fetal acidemia within 24 h before delivery [19]. Ishimatsu and colleagues observed that the Doppler waveforms of the middle cerebral artery in 43 pregnant women with diabetes mellitus between 24 and 38 weeks of gestation were unaffected by maternal glycemic control [20].

Fetal Cardiac Doppler

Rizzo and colleagues studied fetal cardiac function in 37 mothers with type-I diabetes [21, 22]. The ratio between the peak velocities during early passive ventricular filling and active atrial filling (E/A ratio) were measured at the level of mitral and tricuspid valves. The investigators demonstrated that the E/A ratios were significantly lower in fetuses of diabetic mothers than in control fetuses, and were significantly and independently affected by the interventricular wall thickness, heart rate, and hematocrit values. No significant alterations were observed in aortic and pulmonary peak velocities or in time-to-peak velocity values. The investigators also noted interventricular septal hypertrophy despite adequate glycemic control. This was corroborated by Miyake who observed significantly smaller E/A ratios of the left and right ventricles in later gestation in the fetuses of diabetic mothers than those in the controls [23].

Rizzo and associates also investigated the venous blood flow patterns in insulin-dependent diabetic mothers in early gestation, and observed higher values of percent reverse flow in inferior vena cava and a significantly higher frequency of umbilical venous pulsations at 12 weeks which lasted until 16 weeks [24]. These abnormalities were more pronounced in pregnancies with poorer glycemic control. In fetuses of well-controlled insulin-dependent diabetic mothers, Gandhi and co-workers demonstrated that the ratio of the right ventricular shortening fraction/left ventricular shortening fraction was significantly higher from that in the control group indicating increased right ventricular hypercontractility in late diabetic pregnancy [25].

The cardiac dysfunction apparently continues in the neonatal period as shown by Kozak-Barany and colleagues who investigated the left ventricular systolic and diastolic functions in term neonates of mothers with well-controlled pregestational and gestational diabetes between 2 and 5 days after birth [26]. Prolonged deceleration time of early left ventricular diastolic filling was observed. The authors speculated that this probably reflected an impaired left ventricular relaxation related to maternal hyperglycemia leading to subsequent fetal hyperinsulinemia and cardiac hypertrophy.

Uterine Artery Doppler

The efficacy of uterine artery Doppler for managing pregnancies with pregestational diabetes remains unproven despite initial enthusiasm.

Bracero and associates noted abnormal uterine artery velocity waveforms in 15.4% of 52 diabetic pregnancies compared with 2% in a nondiabetic population ($p < 0.001$) [27]. Those with abnormal uterine Doppler had a higher occurrence of suboptimal glycemic control, chronic hypertension, polyhydramnios, vasculopathy, preeclampsia, cesarean delivery for fetal distress, and neonates with respiratory distress syndrome. In 37 pregnant patients with pregestational and gestational diabetes, uterine Doppler demonstrated a sensitivity of 44.5%, specificity of 100%, positive predictive value of 100%, and negative predictive value of 84.3% in predicting the later development of vascular complications [28].

Bracero and associates studied the association between uterine artery Doppler velocimetry discordance and perinatal outcome in 265 women with singleton pregnancies complicated by diabetes who underwent Doppler examinations within 1 week before delivery [29]. Adverse outcome was defined as stillbirth, intrauterine growth restriction, delivery before 37 weeks' gestation, or cesarean delivery for fetal risk. Considerable overlap in discordance was present between the good and adverse outcome groups. The discordance between right and left uterine artery systolic–diastolic ratios was significantly higher in pregnancies with adverse outcome ($p = 0.018$). The uterine artery S/D ratio differences of 0.60 or greater was predictive of cesarean delivery for fetal risk. In diabetic women with chronic hypertension the discordance was not predictive of adverse outcome.

Grunewald and associates noted the absence of the normal third trimester decline in uteroplacental pulsatility indices in 24 well-controlled insulin-dependent pregestational diabetics [30]. The pulsatility index was not influenced by glycemic control. Barth and co-workers investigated the uterine arcuate artery Doppler and decidual microvascular pathology in 47 gravidas with type-I diabetes mellitus [31]. Significant correlation was noted between the abnormal Doppler indices from the uterine arcuate arteries and decidual microvascular pathology including fibrinoid necrosis, atherosis, and thrombosis ($p < 0.05$).

In contrast to the above findings, other studies failed to confirm any predictive utility of the uterine Doppler velocimetry in pregnancies complicated with diabetes. Kofinas and associates observed that in gravidas with gestational ($n = 31$) and insulin-dependent ($n = 34$) diabetes mellitus, the umbilical and uterine artery flow velocity waveforms could not differentiate between good and poor glycemic control, although it discriminated the patients with preeclampsia from those without preeclampsia [32]. The investigators concluded that the clinical utility of Doppler waveform analysis in diabetic pregnancies might be limited to only those with preeclampsia.

In a cross-sectional study of 65 well-controlled diabetic pregnancies, Salvesen and co-investigators found that the Doppler indices of the placental and fetal circulations were essentially normal, except when complicated by preeclampsia or FGR [5]. In a study involving 43 pregnancies with insulin-dependent diabetes mellitus, Zimmermann and colleagues reported that long- and short-term glycemic control were unrelated to vascular resistance in the uterine artery, although the latter was higher in the presence of vasculopathy; however, more than half of the diabetics without vasculopathic complications showed a persistent notch in the uterine artery Doppler waveforms. Furthermore, uterine artery Doppler velocimetry did not demonstrate efficacy in predicting diabetes-related adverse fetal outcome [33].

In summary, the Doppler sonographic investigations of fetal central and cerebral circulations, and the maternal uterine circulation have yielded information of varying degrees of importance on maternal and fetal hemodynamic changes in pregnancies complicated with pregestational diabetes; however, there is no evidence that they are clinically useful in managing these pregnancies.

Clinical Effectiveness and Guidelines

As discussed in Chap. 30, the clinical effectiveness of umbilical Doppler velocimetry has been demonstrated in high-risk pregnancies by randomized clinical trials. But no such level of evidence exists for other biophysical tests of fetal well-being, which still constitute a critical component of the antepartum management of these pregnancies, and most often include the nonstress test (NST) and the biophysical profile (BPP). These tests are usually initiated at 32 weeks and performed twice a week. Daily fetal movement count is also used as an adjunct screening test. There are no randomized trials dealing exclusively with the clinical effectiveness of Doppler fetal surveillance in pregnancies complicated with pregestational diabetes mellitus; however, in a randomized trial recently reported by Williams and colleagues, umbilical artery Doppler was compared with NST as a test for fetal well-being in a population of 1,360 high-risk gravidas 11% of whom had diabetes mellitus [34]. The Doppler group had a significantly lower

cesarean delivery rate for fetal distress than the NST group (4.6% vs 8.7%, respectively; $p < 0.006$). The greatest effect was observed in pregnancies with hypertension and suspected FGR suggesting diabetic pregnancies with these complications may benefit from the use of Doppler velocimetry of the umbilical artery.

In utilizing the Doppler results, the clinical practice guidelines derived from the available evidence are also applicable to managing selected pregnant patients with pregestational diabetes. These guidelines are summarized here. It is emphasized that the overall obstetrical management in pregestational diabetes in pregnancy depends on multiple factors which include the severity of diabetes, adequacy of glycemic control, presence of vasculopathic complications, gestational age, assurance of fetal well-being, and past obstetrical history.

In diabetic pregnancies with FGR or preeclampsia, umbilical artery Doppler sonography should be added to the current standards of practice for fetal surveillance involving the NST and the BPP. If the Doppler index remains within the normal limits or is not progressively rising, weekly Doppler tests should continue. A high or increasing S/D ratio warrants more intense fetal surveillance consisting of umbilical Doppler ultrasound twice a week or more along with NST and BPP. If absent end-diastolic flow velocity (AEDV) develops, the likelihood of poor perinatal outcome is high and urgent clinical response is indicated. At or near term, the development of AEDV should prompt immediate consideration for delivery. Cesarean delivery may be preferable in the presence of reversed end-diastolic velocity or other ominous fetal monitoring findings (nonreactive NST, poor FHR baseline variability, persistent late decelerations, oligohydramnios, and BPP score < 4). In preterm pregnancies, further assurance of fetal well-being is sought by daily surveillance with umbilical Doppler, NST, and BPP. Determination of fetal lung maturity may also assist in timing the delivery in this circumstance. In preterm pregnancies, considerations should also be given to steroid administration along with the modification of glycemic management as needed. Delivery is indicated when a single or a combination of the fetal tests indicate imminent fetal danger irrespective of lung maturity or when fetal risk from a hostile intrauterine environment is judged to be greater than that from pulmonary immaturity in a given neonatal service.

Current concepts and controversies on the general management of diabetic pregnancies and also on fetal surveillance may also be found elsewhere [35–37].

Conclusion

Antepartum fetal surveillance constitutes an essential component of the standards of care in managing pregnancies complicated with pregestational diabetes mellitus. Fetal hyperglycemia is associated with increased oxidative metabolism, hypoxemia, and increased brain and renal perfusion without any significant changes in fetoplacental perfusion. Moreover, the relationship between abnormal umbilical arterial Doppler indices and the quality of glycemic control remains unproven; however, observational studies suggest significant diagnostic efficacy of the umbilical arterial Doppler method in diabetic pregnancies complicated with FGR or hypertension. Although there are no randomized trials specifically addressing this issue, existing evidence suggests that Doppler velocimetry of the umbilical artery may be beneficial for antepartum fetal surveillance in diabetic pregnancies in the presence of these complications. Such utilization should be integrated with the existing standards of practice.

References

1. Garner P (1995) Type I diabetes mellitus and pregnancy. Lancet 346:157–161
2. Crandell SS, Fisher DJ, Morriss FH Jr (1985) Effects of ovine maternal hyperglycemia on fetal regional blood flows and metabolism. Am J Physiol 249:E454–E460
3. Dickinson JE, Meyer BA, Palmer SM (1998) Fetal vascular responses to maternal glucose administration in streptozocin-induced ovine diabetes mellitus. J Obstet Gynaecol Res 24:325–333
4. Philipps AF, Porte PJ, Stabinsky S, Rosenkrantz TS, Raye JR (1984) Effects of chronic fetal hyperglycemia upon oxygen consumption in the ovineuterus and conceptus. J Clin Invest 74:279–286
5. Salvesen DR, Higueras MT, Mansur CA, Freeman J, Brudenell JM, Nicolaides KH (1993) Placental and fetal Doppler velocimetry in pregnancies complicated by maternal diabetes mellitus. Am J Obstet Gynecol 168:645–652
6. Harwell CM, Padbury JF, Anand RS, Martinez AM, Ipp E, Thio SL, Burnell EE (1990) Fetal catecholamine responses to maternal hypoglycemia. Am J Physiol. 259:R1126–R1130
7. Reece EA, Hagay Z, Roberts AB, DeGennaro N, Homko CJ, Connolly-Diamond M, Sherwin R, Tamborlane WV, Diamond MP (1995) Fetal Doppler and behavioral responses during hypoglycemia induced with the insulin clamp technique in pregnant diabetic women. Am J Obstet Gynecol 172:151–155
8. Bjorklund AO, Adamson UK, Almstrom NH, Enocksson EA, Gennser GM, Lins PE, Westgren LM (1996) Effects of hypoglycaemia on fetal heart activity and umbilical artery Doppler velocity waveforms in pregnant women with insulin-dependent diabetes mellitus. Br J Obstet Gynaecol 103:413–420
9. Maulik D, Yarlagadda P, Youngblood JP et al. (1990) The diagnostic efficacy of the umbilical arterial systolic/diastolic ratio as a screening tool: a prospective blinded study: Am J Obstet Gynecol 162:1518–1523
10. Bracero L, Schulman H, Fleischer A, Farmakides G, Rochelson B (1986) Umbilical artery velocimetry in diabetes and pregnancy. Obstet Gynecol 68:654–658
11. Landon MB, Gabbe SG, Bruner JP, Ludmir J (1989) Doppler umbilical artery velocimetry in pregnancy complicated by insulin-dependent diabetes mellitus. Obstet Gynecol 73:961–965
12. Johnstone FD, Steel JM, Haddad NG, Hoskins PR, Greer IA, Chambers S (1992) Doppler umbilical artery flow velocity waveforms in diabetic pregnancy. Br J Obstet Gynaecol 99:135–140
13. Reece EA, Hagay Z, Assimakopoulos E, Moroder W, Gabrielli S, DeGennaro N, Homko C, O'Connor T, Wiznitzer A (1994) Diabetes mellitus in pregnancy and the assessment of umbilical artery waveforms using pulsed Doppler ultrasonography. J Ultrasound Med 13:73–80
14. Dicker D, Goldman JA, Yeshaya A, Peleg D (1990) Umbilical artery velocimetry in insulin dependent diabetes mellitus (IDDM) pregnancies. J Perinat Med 18:391–395
15. Grunewald C, Divon M, Lunell NO (1996) Doppler velocimetry in last trimester pregnancy complicated by insulin-dependent diabetes mellitus. Acta Obstet Gynecol Scand 75:804–808
16. Bracero LA, Figueroa R, Byrne DW, Han HJ (1996) Comparison of umbilical Doppler velocimetry, nonstress testing, and biophysical profile in pregnancies complicated by diabetes. J Ultrasound Med 15:301–308
17. Fadda GM, D'Antona D, Ambrosini G, Cherchi PL, Nardelli GB, Capobianco G, Dessole S (2001) Placental and fetal pulsatility indices in gestational diabetes mellitus. J Reprod Med 46:365–370
18. Van Bel F, Van de Bor M, Walther FJ (1991) Cerebral blood flow velocity and cardiac output in infants of insulin-dependent diabetic mothers. Acta Paediatr Scand 80:905–910
19. Salvesen DR, Higueras MT, Brudenell JM, Drury PL, Nicolaides KH (1992) Doppler velocimetry and fetal heart rate studies in nephropathic diabetics. Am J Obstet Gynecol 167:1297–1303
20. Ishimatsu J, Matsuzaki T, Yakushiji M, Hamada T (1995) Blood flow velocity waveforms of the fetal middle cerebral artery in pregnancies complicated by diabetes mellitus. Kurume Med J 42:161–166
21. Rizzo G, Arduini D, Romanini C (1991) Cardiac function in fetuses of type I diabetic mothers. Am J Obstet Gynecol 164:837–843
22. Rizzo G, Pietropolli A, Capponi A, Cacciatore C, Arduini D, Romanini C (1994) Analysis of factors influencing ventricular filling patterns in fetuses of type I diabetic mothers. J Perinat Med 22:149–157
23. Miyake T (2001) Doppler echocardiographic studies of diastolic cardiac function in the human fetal heart. Kurume Med J 48:59–64
24. Rizzo G, Arduini D, Capponi A, Romanini C (1995) Cardiac and venous blood flow in fetuses of insulin-dependent diabetic mothers: evidence of abnormal hemodynamics in early gestation. Am J Obstet Gynecol 173:1775–1781

25. Gandhi JA, Zhang XY, Maidman JE (1995) Fetal cardiac hypertrophy and cardiac function in diabetic pregnancies. Am J Obstet Gynecol 173:1132–1136

26. Kozak-Barany A, Jokinen E, Kero P, Tuominen J, Ronnemaa T, Valimaki I (2004) Impaired left ventricular diastolic function in newborn infants of mothers with pregestational or gestational diabetes with good glycemic control. Early Hum Dev 77:13–22

27. Bracero LA, Schulman H (1991) Doppler studies of the uteroplacental circulation in pregnancies complicated by diabetes. Ultrasound Obstet Gynecol 1:391–394

28. Haddad B, Uzan M, Tchobroutsky C, Uzan S, Papiernik-Berkhauer E (1993) Predictive value of uterine Doppler waveform during pregnancies complicated by diabetes. Fetal Diagn Ther 8:119–125

29. Bracero LA, Evanco J, Byrne DW (1997) Doppler velocimetry discordancy of the uterine arteries in pregnancies complicated by diabetes. J Ultrasound Med 16: 387–393

30. Grunewald C, Divon M, Lunell NO (1996) Doppler velocimetry in last trimester pregnancy complicated by insulin-dependent diabetes mellitus. Acta Obstet Gynecol Scand 75:804–808

31. Barth WH Jr, Genest DR, Riley LE, Frigoletto FD Jr, Benacerraf BR, Greene MF (1996) Uterine arcuate artery Doppler and decidual microvascular pathology in pregnancies complicated by type I diabetes mellitus. Ultrasound Obstet Gynecol 8:98–103

32. Kofinas AD, Penry M, Swain M (1991) Uteroplacental Doppler flow velocity waveform analysis correlates poorly with glycemic control in diabetic pregnant women. Am J Perinatol 8:273–277

33. Zimmermann P, Kujansuu E, Tuimala R (1994) Doppler flow velocimetry of the uterine and uteroplacental circulation in pregnancies complicated by insulin-dependent diabetes mellitus. J Perinat Med 22:137–147

34. Williams KP, Farquharson DF, Bebbington M, Dansereau J, Galerneau F, Wilson RD, Shaw D, Kent N (2003) Screening for fetal well-being in a high-risk pregnant population comparing the nonstress test with umbilical artery Doppler velocimetry: a randomized controlled clinical trial. Am J Obstet Gynecol 188:1366–1371

35. Gabbe SG, Graves CR (2003) Management of diabetes mellitus complicating pregnancy. Obstet Gynecol 102: 857–868

36. Maulik D, Lysikiewicz A, Sicuranza G (2002) Umbilical arterial Doppler sonography for fetal surveillance in pregnancies complicated by pregestational diabetes mellitus. J Matern Fetal Neonatal Med 12:417–422

37. Landon MB, Vickers S (2002) Fetal surveillance in pregnancy complicated by diabetes mellitus: Is it necessary? J Matern Fetal Neonatal Med 12:413–416

Chapter 22

Doppler Velocimetry in Maternal Alloimmunization

Andrzej Lysikiewicz

Obstetrical management of isoimmunized pregnancy is determined by the severity of fetal anemia. Early and accurate diagnosis of anemia makes safe and effective clinical management. In fetal Rh disease, fetal anemia leads to cardiovascular changes in blood flow through the major fetal vessels, detectable by Doppler velocimetry. Diagnosis by Doppler velocimetry is particularly attractive since examination can be quick, safe, and cost-effective.

Doppler Velocimetry as the Preferred Diagnostic Tool

The most accurate assessment of fetal anemia is by direct fetal blood examination obtained by cordocentesis; however, it is also the most invasive diagnostic method with substantial maternal morbidity and fetal mortality reported at 1%–2.7% [1, 2]. Even when no immediate fetal mortality results, lesser complications of the procedure have the potential for delayed fetal adverse effect; therefore, this diagnostic method is used if no safer alternative exists and only when fetal health and survival are in question. Those limitations, however, make clinical diagnosis of fetal anemia less available to the clinician.

Another common diagnostic procedure, amniocentesis, which has become the standard for diagnosis [3] is also not without risks and is less accurate than cordocentesis [4]. These risks have long been recognized and various management schemes have been suggested [5] to minimize maternal/fetal exposure in diagnosis. No management proposals, however, eliminate procedure-related risks completely unless invasive procedures can be avoided. Doppler velocimetry measurements are noninvasive and could be superior in terms of safety, patient comfort, and cost.

The natural disease process in alloimmunization leads to increased dynamics of fetal circulation, well suited for Doppler studies. The need for cordocentesis for presumed fetal anemia initially provided an opportunity to compare fetal Doppler velocimetry before and after the procedure with actual fetal blood hemoglobin values. Such studies have, however, the disadvantage of cross-sectional data that may not be representative to the extent of prospective longitudinal observations [6]. Prospective longitudinal studies avoid this limitation [7, 8].

Maternal Alloimmunization and Fetal Disease

Most maternal alloimmunizations occur due to the presence of D antigen Rh blood group system incompatibility, but other fetal antigens will also result in alloimmunization if they are absent in the mother [9]. The clinical picture varies in those cases when fetal anemia is inconsistent with the antibody concentrations as correlated in Rh disease. There is no evidence, however, that fetal blood velocities are related to any other factors than fetal anemia, and no specific findings of Doppler velocimetry have been reported in alloimmunizations of different antigens.

Fetal Pathophysiology in Alloimmunization

Fetal Anemia

Destruction of fetal red cells by maternal antibodies in the reticulo-endothelial system is the mechanism of fetal Rh disease [9]. Erythrocyte destruction is initially well compensated by fetal intramedullary hematopoesis. This process increases with increased maternal antibody production leading to increased fetal red cell turnover. As more immature cells are released into the fetal circulation, their maturation decreases. Eventually, medullary fetal red cell production is complemented by erythropoiesis in the liver and the spleen [10]. Initially this process compensates for red cell destruction with little or no fetal anemia; however, in time, this fetal reserve becomes exhausted and fetal anemia results.

Increased red cell production in the fetal liver is associated with increased hematopoietic cellular mass that affects liver portal circulation, producing portal hypertension, and compromising fetal liver function

[11]. Hypoproteinemia that develops from impaired protein synthesis in the liver contributes to development of fetal hypervolemia and hydrops. Fetal hydrops can present as a spectrum of ultrasonographic findings, from a mild form with little fetal circulatory overload to an end-stage disease, involving all major systems that, with no intervention, will progress to fetal death. Development of fetal hydrops is associated with significantly increased fetal loss even if intervention with fetal intravascular transfusion is attempted [12].

The fetus appears to be resistant to decreased oxygen-carrying capacity in fetal anemia as there is little of fetal hypoxemia in anemic fetuses [13]. Increased dynamic of fetal circulation compensates well initially for the decreased fetal erythrocyte mass, maintaining adequate oxygenation. Fetal hypoxia develops relatively late in the process as fetal hemoglobin oxygen-carrying capacity is efficient even at low concentrations.

Fetal Cardiovascular Changes in Alloimmunization

A substantial amount of information has been collected about fetal circulation during the course of alloimmunization. Fetal anemia consists of reduced red cell mass/cc and "thinning" of the fetal blood. Significant fetal anemia has been reported as 5 g/dl below the mean hemoglobin concentration for gestational age, since at this level risk for development of fetal hydrops increases [14]. Lower fetal hemoglobin levels reduce oxygen-carrying capacity that could eventually lead to fetal hypoxia. Hypoxia is, however, not observed until late in the process, presumably due to increased 2,3-diphosphoglycerate concentration and increased cardiac output that maintain adequate tissue oxygen delivery [15]. At this level, anemia leads to reduction of fetal blood viscosity that is further multiplied by decreased fetal plasma protein production in the fetal liver. The compensatory increase of cardiac output and faster blood circulation, a combination described as the fetal hyperdynamic state [16], prevents development of hypoxia and acidosis early in the process.

Increase of the fetal blood flow velocities is not equally consistent in all vessels. Selective redistribution of the blood flow, similar to those of chronic hypoxic growth restriction, has not been confirmed [16]. With terminal hydrops, however, hypoxia is likely and some redistribution of the fetal blood flow may be expected. In early fetal anemia, however, the selection of the most representative vessels reflecting the fetal condition is important to obtain pertinent measurements [17].

Cardiac Blood Flow

In early fetal Rh disease, in the absence of fetal hydrops, there are no indications that fetal anemia of less than 5 g/dl of hemoglobin deficit from the mean hemoglobin concentration expected for gestational age value affects fetal cardiac functions.

At the end stage of alloimmunization generalized fetal hydrops develops. Decreased serum oncotic pressure owing to reduced liver albumin production, umbilical venous and portal hypertension, hypoxic endothelial damage, and congestive heart failure are postulated as mechanisms of hydrops, with congestive heart failure being infrequent. Hecher et al. [15] examined fetal flow-velocity waveforms from the atrioventricular valves, ductus venosus, right hepatic vein, inferior vena cava, middle cerebral artery (MCA), and descending thoracic aorta with concurrent cordocentesis in 38 fetuses with red blood cell isoimmunized pregnancies. Increased blood flow velocities in the thoracic aorta, MCA, and the ductus venosus were consistent with hyperdynamic state. In this study, increased velocity in the thoracic aorta was associated with fetal anemia as in other previous reports [18, 19]. The authors did not notice major changes in the venous blood flow. They concluded that congestive heart failure is not a major factor in development of fetal hydrops and that it happens late in the process, if at all.

Fetal Heart Rate

Fetal hypoxia is often a concern in anemic fetuses in alloimmunization because of presumed reduced oxygen-carrying capacity. Hypoxic fetal response can be expected to involve compensatory tachycardia and redistribution of the fetal blood flow similar to chronic hypoxia in intrauterine growth restriction; however, several studies have shown that the correlation between fetal anemia and fetal acid base is inconsistent [13, 20]. Fetal hypoxia does not appear until late in the process and fetal hemoglobin, even if diluted, can carry a sufficient amount of oxygen. Fetal tachycardia that may be observed is more likely to result from the fetal hyperdynamic state [16]; therefore, only in the very late stage of fetal disease in alloimmunization, reduced oxygen-carrying capacity will lead to hypoxia and fetal tachycardia. With fetal tachycardia a higher end-diastolic flow can be recorded with shortened diastole period. This represents a nonspecific finding related to tachycardia itself.

Sinusoidal Fetal Heart Rate

Abnormal cardiac rhythm characteristic for fetal anemia is a sinusoidal rhythm (Fig. 22.1). It has been observed in severely anemic fetuses, regardless of the

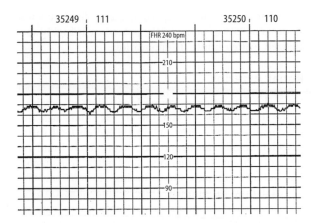

Fig. 22.1. Sinusoidal fetal heart rate pattern

cause of fetal anemia. Intermittent, low-frequency 3- to 5-Hz sinusoidal variations of the fetal heart rate are more likely a result of stressed cardiac neuroregulation than actual changes in fetal blood flow [21, 22].

The inability of the medullary centers to control the fetal heart rate results in a sinusoidal heart rate pattern. Observations of fetal heart rate in severe anemia, fetal brain maldevelopment, cytomegalovirus infection and during alfaprodine or pancuronium bromide administration as reported by various authors appear to confirm this mechanism [23, 24].

In the absence of significant hypoxia a mechanism of sinusoidal heart rate pattern is not well understood. It is likely that more than one compensatory mechanism is involved in such a severely affected fetus. Decreased fetal blood viscosity, increased blood volume, increased preload, baroreceptor, and volume receptor stimulation all affect fetal heart rate. Hecher et al. [15] reported increased fetal blood viscosity after fetal intravascular transfusion that occurred only in whole blood but not in serum, suggesting that it is increased erythrocyte mass that leads to increased blood viscosity. In anemic fetuses the cumulative effects of increased blood volume and decreased blood viscosity may lead to increased venous blood return and increased preload as reflected by the preload index in inferior vena cava velocimetry.

No systematic studies of Doppler velocimetry during sinusoidal rhythm have been reported. In our one case fetal Doppler velocimetry in umbilical artery, descending aorta, MCA, and inferior vena cava were recorded. The elevation of "a" wave in the inferior vena cava was noted, and fetal anemia was confirmed by cordocentesis. Subsequently, sinusoidal rhythm was relieved by fetal intravascular transfusion with the return of the inferior vena cava Doppler waveform to normal values shortly after transfusion. Association of abnormal Doppler velocimetry with a sinu-

soidal heart rate pattern has not been definite and needs more observations; however, the presence of fetal sinusoidal rhythm has been reported consistently as an ominous sign and an emergency requiring prompt diagnosis and treatment [21].

Changes in Fetal Systemic Arterial Blood Flow

Doppler Flow Velocity Measurements

Fetal blood flow velocity is the parameter that can be adequately measured, provided that the angle of insonation is known and laminar blood flow is taken into consideration [25]. Accuracy of these measurements depends on the angle of insonation, $< 60°$ being acceptable [26]. Volumetric flow measurements are also possible but require accurate data on the size of the vessel that are not easy to obtain. With current technology, they are not of practical use in fetal Rh disease.

According to the law of physics, low viscosity "thinned" fetal blood in anemia flows faster in fetal blood vessels [16]. With unchanged peripheral resistance that translates into increased systolic and diastolic velocities. A similar increase in both systolic and diastolic blood flow velocities may be an explanation for generally unchanged S/D ratios and other indices in fetal arterial circulation. An increase in blood flow velocity does occur and to measure this change in flow the maximum velocity (or "peak velocity") may be a more appropriate measurement [17]. This single measurement of absolute velocity at its maximum peak is angle dependent and as such requires consistency in the technique of measurements. In extreme conditions, in a terminally ill fetus, additional factors (hypoxia, neural regulation) may be affecting blood flow distribution and blood flow velocity in specific vessels, but it is not observed in mild to moderate anemia.

Fetal Aortic Arch

Increased fetal blood flow velocity in the aortic arch can be expected in anemic fetuses consistent with increased blood flow velocity in the fetal descending aorta but specific studies are lacking. The standard measurements have not been established for this complex blood flow velocity pattern that varies according to changing physiologic conditions [26].

Fetal Descending Aorta

An example of blood flow velocity measured in the fetal aorta in an anemic fetus is presented in Fig. 22.2.

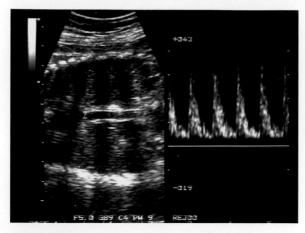

Fig. 22.2. Fetal descending aorta Doppler velocity in the anemic fetus

Blood flow mean velocity measured in the fetal descending aorta was inversely correlated with fetal hematocrit [27, 28]. Rightmire et al. [27] compared the fetal umbilical artery Pourcelot index with fetal hematocrit and a numerical correlation allowed for retrospective development of a formula predicting fetal hematocrit. Prospective clinical confirmation of the accuracy of this method has not been published. A similar study by Copel et al. [29] led to development of formulas that had limited accuracy for predicting fetal hematocrit when based on fetal descending aorta Doppler velocities alone.

Descending aorta Doppler velocities were again studied by Nicolaides et al. [17] and the conclusion of this group did not support use of fetal descending aorta Doppler velocities for prediction of fetal hematocrit. A correlation with fetal hematocrit was shown only when descending aorta velocimetry data was analyzed in relation to gestational age [30]. The authors concluded that the correlation, although statistically significant, has no sufficient predictive value for clinical application.

Splenic Artery

The splenic artery, a branch of the celiac axis, can be identified with color Doppler and, within its straight segment, a Doppler velocity measurement can be carried out. If done at an insonation angle of close to 0°, a high accuracy of such a measurement can be expected [30, 31].

According to this study, the deceleration angle of Doppler waveform correlates well (r = 0.68) with fetal hemoglobin deficit (mean expected for gestational age minus actual hemoglobin). Also splenic artery mean velocity is a good predictor of fetal anemia, with sensitivity approaching 100%. Although the authors re-

ported success in obtaining satisfactory blood flow waveforms in 95% of patients, the procedure is highly specialized, which limits its application.

Renal Arteries

Limited information exists on blood flow in renal arteries in Rh disease. Mari et al. [32] indicates improvement in the pulsatility index before fetal intravascular blood transfusion in anemic fetuses and return of absent end-diastolic flow after transfusion. The authors attribute these findings to fetal increase in renal flow to eliminate excess fluid after transfusion. Diagnostic applications of renal artery velocity measurements in fetal anemia have not been established.

Umbilical Arteries

No significant correlation has been found between umbilical artery S/D ratio, pulsatility index, or resistance index and fetal anemia [33, 34]. Perhaps steady placental resistance and consistent umbilical vessel diameter does not alter systolic/diastolic flow ratio even with increased flow of both.

Doppler velocimetry of the fetal umbilical artery reflects fetal placental resistance. There is no evidence that placental vascular resistance is affected by maternal alloimmunization; hence, no changes in umbilical artery indices should be expected.

Internal Carotid Artery

A significant association between the degree of fetal anemia and the increase in mean velocity in the fetal common carotid artery has been reported by Bilardo et al. [34]. In their series of 12 fetuses with primary anemia (previously untransfused) measurements were made immediately before cordocentesis. They suggested that increased fetal cardiac output associated with fetal anemia is an underlying mechanism and not the redistribution in blood flow that occurs in chronic hypoxia in growth-restricted fetuses.

Middle Cerebral Artery

Middle cerebral artery peak blood flow velocity can be visualized on an axial view of the cranium (Fig. 22.3).

Significant and consistent increase of peak flow velocity in the MCA was seen in anemic fetuses when measured at the bifurcation from the circle of Willis and at an angle of insonation of < 30° [35]. This finding was reported in several other studies [16, 36, 37], including a multicenter clinical trial [7], and was linearly correlated with the degree of fetal anemia (Fig. 22.4) [16].

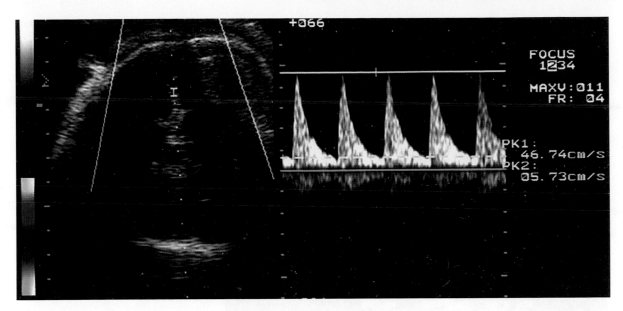

Fig. 22.3. Middle cerebral artery peak velocity

Fig. 22.4. Fetal middle cerebral artery peak velocity in anemic and nonanemic fetuses. *Open circles* indicate fetuses with either no anemia or mild anemia [0.65 multiples of the median (MoM) hemoglobin concentration]. *Triangles* indicate fetuses with moderate or severe anemia (<0.65 MoM hemoglobin concentration). The *solid circles* indicate the fetuses with hydrops. The *solid curve* indicates the median peak systolic velocity in the middle cerebral artery and the *dotted curve* indicates 1.5 MoM. (From [16])

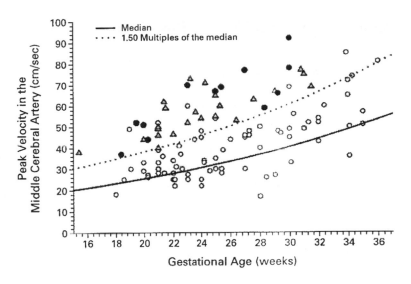

The accuracy of Doppler diagnosis of fetal anemia varies depending on previous history of fetal blood transfusions. In anemic, previously untransfused, nonhydropic fetuses, MCA peak velocity correlates well with fetal hemoglobin level obtained at cordocentesis [36]. When there is a history of a previous transfusion given to the fetus, the correlation is not as strong [37]. These cross-sectional studies have also been confirmed recently by observational data of fetal MCA peak velocity in a longitudinal study of fetal blood flow in alloimmunization reported by Zimmerman [7].

In this multicenter study, 125 fetuses at risk of anemia were longitudinally monitored in 7- to 14-day intervals for abnormal velocimetry or signs of hy-drops. Cordocentesis or delivery was performed if signs of fetal anemia were detected. Sensitivity of 88%, specificity of 87%, positive predictive value of 53%, and negative predictive value of 98% was achieved. The method was not effective after 35 weeks. The authors' recommendation of this method as primary fetal surveillance in alloimmunization appears well founded and may reduce the need for invasive diagnosis.

Middle cerebral artery peak velocity was compared with other sonographic methods for diagnosis of fetal anemia. In 16 fetuses with isoimmunization, Doppler evaluation of MCA peak systolic velocity was a better predictor than intrahepatic umbilical maximum velocity, liver length, or spleen perimeter [39].

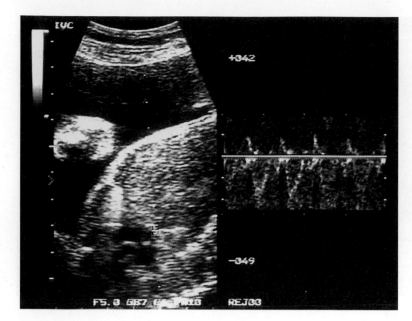

Fig. 22.5. Fetal preload index and fetal hematocrit at cordocentesis

Changes in Fetal Venous Blood Flow

High arterial fetal blood flow velocity and increased tissue perfusion in the fetal hyperdynamic cardiovascular state is followed by a blood volume shift from arterial to venous circulation resulting from decreased blood viscosity [40]. The resulting high venous return may lead to right heart overload and right heart failure that can be detectable by Doppler velocimetry [41]; therefore, fetal venous flow has been extensively studied as an indicator of fetal condition in alloimmunization.

Umbilical Vein

An early study by Jouppila reported an inverse correlation between umbilical venous flow and fetal hemoglobin at birth within 4 days from delivery [42]. It was later confirmed by Warren et al. [40] and Iskaros et al. [6] who noted increased venous blood flow in the umbilical vein associated with development of fetal hydrops. Dukkler et al. [39] attempted to correlate intrahepatic umbilical venous maximum velocity and MCA peak velocity with fetal anemia in six fetuses with alloimmunization. They found that in prediction of fetal anemia, the MCA was 100% specific, while intrahepatic umbilical venous blood flow had specificity of 83%.

Inferior Vena Cava Blood Flow

Inferior vena cava blood flow has been described as the A/S index or the atrial flow velocity to atrial regurgitation velocity ratio (Fig. 22.5) [41]. This index

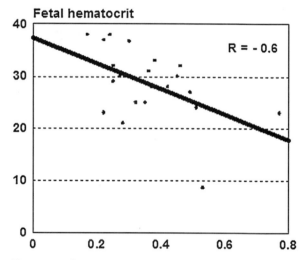

Fig. 22.6. Inferior vena cava A/S ratio

is a sensitive indicator of the right cardiac function, especially fetal right heart failure.

In fetal hyperdynamic circulation in anemic fetuses with isoimmunization, an increased venous return could lead to right heart failure. Studies of inferior vena cava blood flow do not, however, support this assumption. In an early study by Rightmire et al. [27] inferior vena cava average velocity was elevated prior to the first blood transfusion in anemic fetuses, but the correlation with fetal hematocrit was not significant. In our own series, 20 fetal preload index measurements were followed by fetal hematocrit evaluations by immediate cordocentesis in 13 fetuses in alloimmunized pregnancies (Fig. 22.6) [43]. An association with low fetal hematocrit was weak with 66% sensitivity, 75% specificity, 50% positive predictive value, and 86% negative predictive value.

Diagnostic use of the preload index is further limited by the difficulty in obtaining consistent measurements from a specific site [44].

Ductus Venosus

The ductus venosus in anemic fetuses demonstrates higher flow, reflecting increased venous return, and cardiac preload. Oepkes found the ductus venosus elevated in anemic fetuses with marked improvement following fetal transfusion [37]. A study by Hecher did not, however, show any significant association with fetal anemia sufficient for use as a diagnostic tool [15].

Maternal Uterine Artery

The pulsatility index of the uterine arteries and thoracic aorta peak velocity were used in a multiple regression model to predict fetal hematocrit following fetal transfusion on the assumption that resolving placental edema after transfusion improves uteroplacental circulation. The uterine artery pulsatility index alone has not been found to change in fetal anemia.

Fetal Morphologic Changes and Doppler Velocimetry in Alloimmunization

Fetal cardiovascular changes reflected in Doppler velocimetry precede development of fetal hydrops. During development of anemia in alloimmunization fetal hydrops develops gradually and relatively late in the process. Fetal signs of hydrops appear infrequently if the fetal hemoglobin level is within 5 g of the median value for gestational age. With more severe anemia fetal hydrops appears, often gradually, over a period of days. The following conditions are observed:
1. Increased amniotic fluid volume
2. Increase in placental thickness
3. Fetal liver enlargement
4. Fetal pericardial effusions
5. Ascites
6. Free loops of bowel in ascites
7. Double-walled bladder
8. Scalp edema ("halo")
9. Facial swellings
10. Pleural effusions
11. Extremities edema
12. Umbilical cord pulsation

Moderate increase in amniotic fluid volume enhances the resolution of ultrasound imaging and often facilitates detection of even small amounts of fluid in fetal body cavities. Findings of fluid in any fetal compartment in isoimmunized pregnancy should prompt a complete fetal morphology review for signs of fetal hydrops. Polyhydramnios in alloimmunization may reach a significant degree that is detrimental to the clarity of the imaging. Preterm labor, that often follows, can make fetal examination even more difficult. Polyhydramnios will frequently regress with correction of fetal anemia.

Placental thickness also increases as part of the process of isoimmunization; however, it is not a reliable indicator of fetal anemia [45].

Liver enlargement is often seen during fetal anemia in alloimmunization as a result of increased fetal extramedullary erythropoiesis [46]. This increased liver size is associated with increased venous Doppler blood flow velocity in fetal intrahepatic venous flow as reported by Oepkes et al. [37]. Although it was postulated by Vintzileos to be a good indicator of fetal compromise [47], it was not as accurate as evaluation with MCA peak velocity measurements [39].

A certain amount of fluid is not unusual in the pericardium. When measured at the valvular level, 2 mm of fluid is often found and is not abnormal. This small fluid collection is not associated with abnormal Doppler velocimetry; however, large pericardial effusions are one of the signs of fetal hydrops and indicates fetal anemia.

Ascites are defined as sonolucent areas in the fetal abdomen with loops of bowel visible, floating in the ascites and the fetal bladder visible with fluid inside and outside the bladder wall (Fig. 22.7). The presence of ascites is commonly associated with fetal anemia and abnormal Doppler velocimetry of the MCA and other vessels. Pleural effusions when present in hydrops fetalis suggest advanced disease.

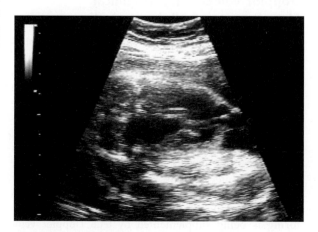

Fig. 22.7. Fetal ascites

Scalp edema and generalized edema are nonspecific changes that may not be related to fetal anemia and changes of Doppler velocimetry.

In summary, it appears that fetal hydropic changes occur as a result of severe fetal anemia. They should not be used as predictors of fetal disease because of their poor predictive value [11, 45]. Abnormal Doppler velocimetry detects changes in fetal circulation that precede fetal hydrops and therefore can detect fetal anemia early. According to data by Mari et al. [35] early detection of fetal anemia is feasible using fetal cardiovascular monitoring with Doppler velocimetry.

A finding of severe fetal hydrops in isoimmunization should be considered as evidence of advanced fetal disease but may be avoidable with intensive fetal diagnosis and active clinical management.

Fetal Blood Redistribution and Fetal Hypoxia in Alloimmunization

Fetal blood redistribution in chronic fetal hypoxia has been reported in growth-restricted fetuses. With decreased oxygen-carrying capacity in fetal anemia, similar findings could be expected due to presumed fetal hypoxia. Initial response to fetal hypoxia is an increase in fetal heart rate [21]. In alloimmunization, however, this heart rate increase may more likely be related to the blood volume increase and blood viscosity decrease resulting in increased fetal circulation [16]. Contrary to expectations, fetal hypoxia is not common in isoimmunized fetuses. Fetal hemoglobin, even if diluted, is able to transport oxygen without developing significant fetal hypoxia [48]. There is no evidence that fetal blood redistribution plays a significant role in fetal cardiovascular changes in isoimmunization [16].

Doppler Velocimetry in Clinical Management of Alloimmunization

Fetal anemia determines the management of alloimmunization.

Use of specific Doppler velocimetry measurements requires a selective, evidence-based approach in choice of measurements. Multiple Doppler-detectable changes of the fetal circulation do not have equal diagnostic value. Methods not adequately studied should only be used with caution, if at all, for diagnostic purposes as those findings often prompt major therapeutic interventions.

The standard of care in alloimmunization has been changing rapidly. The traditional biochemical monitoring is being supplemented by fetal Doppler velocimetry supported by clinical studies.

History of Previous Pregnancy

A history positive for a previous pregnancy with complications should increase the index of suspicion as it is predictive of the general severity of fetal involvement. Maternal history of alloimmunization, previous affected pregnancy or previous neonatal disease are risk factors for development of fetal anemia. Although the correlation is strong, history alone is not sufficient to guide obstetrical management.

Maternal Antibody Titer

Maternal antibody titer has been a landmark in management of alloimmunization for several decades. Maternal antibody, if present, should prompt paternal blood type zygosity evaluation to determine the likelihood of the presence of an antigen in the fetal blood. If such a risk is not 100%, as in paternal homozygosity, then fetal blood typing should be carried out. Absence of an antigen in the fetal blood rules out fetal involvement and makes further testing unnecessary (Fig. 22.8).

Maternal antibody concentration has been correlated with the presence and severity of fetal disease but is not accurate in prediction of specific cases. High initial titer or rising titer indicates the possibility of fetal anemia, but specific critical titers requiring intervention are difficult to define. Depending on laboratory methods, commonly, values 1:16 or higher are being investigated because of the probability of fetal hemolytic anemia. In this range fetal anemia and hemodynamic changes may be better detected by Doppler velocimetry than by antibody titer alone [7].

Amniotic Fluid Densitometry

A change in optical density at 450 nm wavelength detects the presence of bilirubin, an end product of fetal hemolysis. It has been used for four decades in combination with standards developed by Liley [3] to predict severely anemic fetuses that could benefit from intervention. A recent review of values by Queenan et al. improved accuracy of the curve, especially for early pregnancy [5]. According to their report, specificity of detecting severe anemia was 79%. In 21% of fetuses, however, severe anemia would not be detected by this method. This low accuracy of the Liley curves has been a concern in management of fetal anemia [5]. Doppler velocimetry is expected to improve accuracy of this diagnosis.

Detecting Fetal Anemia

For management of alloimmunization an accurate diagnosis of fetal anemia is essential. High specificity is mandatory for this testing to avoid development of

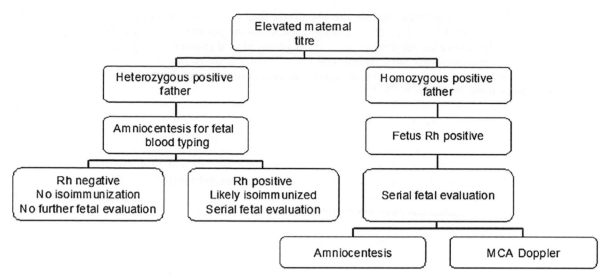

Fig. 22.8. Management of alloimmunization – maternal antibodies

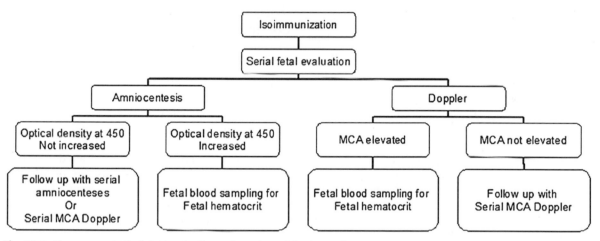

Fig. 22.9. Management of alloimmunization – detection of fetal anemia

severe fetal disease and fetal losses. Figure 22.9 presents diagnostic options for detecting fetal anemia in alloimmunization.

Physical signs, such as fetal tachycardia, polyhydramnios, fetal movements, and fetal heart changes have historically guided physicians; those, however, were not accurate enough to assure fetal survival.

Detecting fetal anemia by sonography is not accurate. Morphologic markers do not predict the severity of fetal anemia [11] sufficiently enough to guide clinical management. Detection of fetal anemia using umbilical vein diameter (intrahepatic portion) [49], liver size [46], spleen size [30, 31], placental thickness, abdominal circumference, abdominal diameter, and other parameters have been developed. Although some were reported as accurate predictors, those methods did not gain widespread use. Methodology,

experience and reproducibility were likely limiting factors as much as the fact that fetal hemodynamic changes are first to occur in fetal anemia, preceding other changes. Abnormal fetal morphology occurs as a result of this process and absence of those signs does not prove fetal normality. Monitoring fetal morphology should not be used alone in management of alloimmunization.

Detection of fetal hyperdynamic state indicates fetal anemia. According to a longitudinal study of 125 pregnancies monitored by MCA peak velocity in pregnancies with red cell isoimmunization, 88% sensitivity can be achieved [7].

Methodologic considerations are important. Appropriate training and experience is required to correctly measure the peak velocity in the fetal MCA. Insonation angle is a potential source of error, as is selection of the level of measurement outside the bifurcation of the MCA from the circle of Willis. An insonation angle of $< 30°$ allows for minimal error.

Other blood flow measurements await clinical validation before they can be adopted as clinical tools; some already have been shown to be ineffective. For example, the umbilical artery blood flow indices are not informative in alloimmunization and normal values do not represent useful clinical information. A study reported by Bilardo et al. [34] found no correlation between umbilical artery pulsatility index and fetal anemia. A highly specialized measurement of flow velocities within the splenic artery requires specific techniques and experience that may not be universally available. This method of interrogation has not been widely used in clinical management. A study by Dukkler et al. [39] did not show intrahepatic vein velocity to be more predictive than the MCA peak velocity.

Without reliable estimation of fetal blood vessel size, attempts to quantitatively measure fetal blood flow do not yield any new information. In addition, with no changes in vessel size in the process of fetal anemia, blood flow measurements will provide no more information than peak velocities.

Middle cerebral artery peak velocity appears to contain the most accurate information on fetal circulation to allow for noninvasive diagnosis of fetal hyperdynamic circulation in fetal anemia and to select patients for invasive procedures.

A review by Divakaran included eight primary studies with 362 pregnancies affected by red cell alloimmunization evaluated by noninvasive methods. The cumulative metaanalysis of studies with the highest methodologic quality reported a positive likelihood ratio of 8.45 (95% CI 4.69–15.56) and negative likelihood ratio of 0.02 (95% CI 0.001–0.025) [8]. Although those results are encouraging, more clinical data may be needed before Doppler velocimetry will be recommended as a primary standard evaluation of fetal anemia.

Diagnostic Invasive Procedures to Detect Fetal Anemia and Doppler Velocimetry

Diagnostic procedures have to be weighted between risk of procedure and quality of information obtained for fetal anemia in alloimmunization.

Amniocentesis is considered a safe procedure with a complication rate of less than 1%. A major risk in using this method lies in the low accuracy of predictions. According to Queenan et al. [5], if used for detection of fetal anemia in combination with the OD curve, it is only 89% specific, whereas 21% of anemic fetuses remain undetected. Frigoletto et al. [50] conservatively managed 11 zone-III fetuses with no adverse fetal outcomes. Fetal Doppler velocimetry of the MCA has the potential to replace amniocentesis in diagnosis of fetal anemia (Fig. 22.8).

Cordocentesis is the most accurate procedure for detection of fetal anemia. It is also the most risky of all procedures with associated fetal loss of 1% [1] and as high as 4%. If cordocentesis is used as a primary diagnosis, a large number of fetuses will be exposed to this risk unnecessarily since only 25% of all fetuses develop severe anemia requiring fetal blood transfusion, but all will have multiple cordocenteses to confirm normal hemoglobin concentration.

With five diagnostic cordocenteses during pregnancy the cumulative fetal mortality risk may reach 10%–20%, too high for a diagnostic procedure. Clearly, fetal Doppler velocimetry may not be as accurate but is safer and should be considered as an alternative to cordocentesis.

Doppler Monitoring During Cordocentesis

Fetal Intravascular Transfusions

Accurate estimation of fetal anemia by cordocentesis, before and after intravascular blood transfusion, can be compared with Doppler velocimetry and numerous cross-sectional data sets were obtained in this fashion.

Fetal MCA Doppler velocimetry can detect fetal anemia and provide timing for initiation of intravascular transfusion prior to the development of fetal hydrops. The role of Doppler velocimetry is to guide timing of transfusions frequently enough to maintain sufficient fetal hemoglobin levels, but not too often, in order to avoid unnecessary risks from the procedure.

Clinical guidance for fetal intravascular transfusions currently rely on clinical findings and the observation that fetal hematocrit decreases at the rate of 0.3%–1.0% per day. Using mathematical formulas and known hematocrit at the time of cordocentesis, an estimate can be made regarding appropriate amount of time for repeated intrauterine intravascular fetal transfusion. Longitudinal Doppler velocimetry assessment of fetal anemia is the other alternative in guiding frequency and timing of fetal intravascular transfusions.

Several management schemes have been developed to guide frequency of transfusions. Less frequent, larger volume transfusions can be safer by reducing the total number of fetal intravascular blood transfusions [51], thereby reducing the risk of fetal blood volume overload [52]. Use of Doppler velocimetry during transfusion to assess fetal condition has not been widely used except for detecting acute fetal bradycardia.

Posttransfusion hemodynamic changes can be detected by Doppler velocimetry. Rizzo et al. reported changes consistent with transient right and left heart overload following transfusion that lasted up to 2 h after transfusion [53] and overall reduction of the hyperdynamic state.

In our own series [43], in 18 cases that required blood transfusion due to hematocrit level, a less significant decrease in the fetal preload index was noted following fetal intravascular transfusion $p < 0.05$. There is a fall in the fetal preload index following fetal intravascular transfusion. The fetal preload index predicts fetal anemia with a sensitivity of 66% and a negative predictive value of 86% (Fig. 22.5).

Increased blood viscosity, congestive heart failure, and cardiac humoral regulation are likely all involved in the posttransfusion changes. It is still unclear if such changes can be used to guide the physician regarding the amount of blood necessary to be transfused and the timing for consecutive transfusion.

Posttransfusion changes occurred immediately but delayed effects are also observed:

- Immediate posttransfusion changes:
  - Increase of fetal red cell mass
  - Increase of blood viscosity and peripheral resistance
  - Vascular overload
  - Decreased cardiac output
  - Fetal humoral response
- Delayed changes:
  - Fetal fluid resorption and loss within hours after transfusion
  - Decrease of fetal venous return
  - Relief of the acute fluid overload and hyperdynamic state.

Rizzo et al. [53] found a temporary decrease in cardiac output after intravascular transfusions due to an increase in fetal vascular resistance that returned to normal 2 h later. Similarly, Mari et al. [54] found decreased middle cerebral peak velocity following fetal intravascular transfusion. Copel et al. [29] studied blood flow velocities in the descending aorta and found no significant changes following the transfusion. In a series by Weiner et al., a decrease in resistance after blood transfusion was attributed to vasodilatory humoral fetal response [52].

Clearly more than one fetal physiologic response is observed after blood transfusion. Severity of fetal anemia, amount of blood transfused, dynamic of transfusion, and fetal humoral response all have an effect on fetal Doppler velocimetry and represent limitations in fetal evaluation.

Early Delivery

Historically early delivery has been advised for severe alloimmunization; however, prematurity, fetal anemia, and hydrops are associated with high mortality and morbidity. Early delivery is therefore advised after fetal lung maturity can be confirmed or if additional fetal indices are non-reassuring and fetal conditions worsen despite adequate intrauterine treatment. Fetal biophysical profile is often used for fetal surveillance. Decreased fetal activity unresponsive to fetal transfusions may result from additional pathology other than alloimmunization, requiring delivery. Biophysical fetal assessment has been used in those circumstances as a primary method of fetal surveillance. Fetal umbilical artery blood flow can occasionally reveal absent end-diastolic flow that is more likely to be a reflection of placental vascular pathology. Abnormal umbilical Doppler indices are often difficult to interpret in severe fetal anemia. If fetal lung maturity can be confirmed, an early delivery is preferable.

Noninvasive Therapies, Gamma Globulin, Plasmapheresis, Nonintervention

None of these treatments have gained wide use, and since advances in fetal diagnosis and intravascular transfusion therapy have been developed, these methods have been largely abandoned.

Conclusion

Fetal anemia with low fetal blood viscosity and hyperdynamic fetal circulation is a mechanism of fetal disease in isoimmunization. Doppler-detectable changes occur in arterial and venous circulation. Doppler velocimetry in specific vessels and specific measurements can be used in clinical management.

Fetal MCA peak velocity is the best studied, specific Doppler marker for fetal anemia, and is preferable to other Doppler-based diagnostic methods.

Intravascular fetal blood transfusions are associated with temporary cardiovascular overload that can be detected by Doppler velocimetry.

The role of Doppler velocimetry in technical aspects of fetal intravascular transfusions remains to be determined.

References

1. Daffos F, Capella-Pavlovsky M, Forestier F (1983) Fetal blood sampling via the umbilical cord using needle guided by ultrasound. Report of 66 cases. Prenatal Diagn 3:271–277

2. Ghidini A, Sepulveda W, Lockwood CJ et al. (1993) Complications of fetal blood sampling. Am J Obstet Gynecol 168:1339–1344

3. Liley AW (1961) Liquor amnii analysis in management of pregnancy complicated by rhesus immunization. Am J Obstet Gynecol 82:1359–1365

4. Nicolaides KH, Rodeck CH, Mibashan RS, Kemp JR (1986) Have Liley charts outlived their usefulness? Am J Obstet Gynecol 155:90–94

5. Queenan JT, Tomai TP, Ural SH et al. (1993) Deviation in amniotic fluid optical density at a wavelength of 450 nm in Rh isoimmunized pregnancies from 14–40 weeks gestation: a proposal for clinical management. Am J Obstet Gynecol 168:1370–1376

6. Iskaros I, Kingdom J, Morrison J, Rodeck C (1998) Prospective non-invasive monitoring of pregnancies complicated by red cell alloimmunization. Ultrasound Obstet Gynecol 11:432–437

7. Zimmerman R, Durig P, Carpenter R, Mari G (2002) Longitudinal measurement of peak systolic velocity in the fetal middle cerebral artery for monitoring pregnancies complicated by red cell alloimmunisation: a prospective multicentre trial with intention-to-treat. BJOG 109:746–752

8. Divakaran TG, Waugh J, Clark TJ, Khan KS, Whittle MJ, Kilby MD (2001) Noninvasive techniques to detect fetal anemia due to red blood cell alloimmunization: a systematic review. Obstet Gynecol 98:509–517

9. Bowman JM (1999) Hemolytic disease (Erythroblastosis fetalis). In: Creasy RK, Resnik R (eds) Maternal–fetal medicine. Saunders, Philadelphia, pp 736–767

10. Nicolaides KH, Warenski JC, Rodeck CH (1985) The relationship of fetal protein concentration and hemoglobin level to the development of hydrops in Rhesus isoimmunization. Am J Obstet Gynecol 152:341–344

11. Nicolaides KH, Fontanarosa M, Gabbe SG, Rodeck CH (1988) Failure of ultrasonographic parameters to predict the severity of fetal anemia in rhesus isoimmunization. Am J Obstet Gynecol 158:920–926

12. Schumacher B, Moise KJ (1966) Fetal transfusion for red blood cell alloimmunization in pregnancy. Obstet Gynecol 88:137–150

13. Soothill PW, Nicolaides KH, Rodeck CH (1987) Effects of anaemia on fetal acid-base status. Br J Obstet Gynaecol 94:880–883

14. Nicolaides KH, Soothill PW, Clewell WH, Rodeck CH, Mibashan R, Campbell S (1988) Fetal haemoglobin measurement in the assessment of red cell isoimmunization. Lancet i:1073–1076

15. Hecher K, Snijders R, Campbell S, Nicolaides K (1995) Fetal venous, arterial and intracardiac blood flows in red blood-cell isoimmunization. Obstet Gynecol 85:122–128

16. Mari G, Deter RL, Carpenter RL, Rahman F, Zimmerman R, Moise KJ et al. for the Collaborative Group for Doppler Assessment of the Blood Velocity in Anaemic Fetuses (2000) Non-invasive diagnosis by Doppler ultrasonography of fetal anemia due to maternal red-cell alloimmunization. N Engl J Med 342:9–14

17. Nicolaides KH, Bilardo CM, Campbell S (1990) Prediction of fetal anemia by measurement of the mean blood flow in the fetal aorta. Am J Obstet Gynecol 162:209–212

18. Nagy D (2000) Noninvasive diagnosis of fetal anemia by Doppler ultrasonography. N Engl J Med 343:66–68

19. Copel JA, Grannum PA, Green JJ, Belanger K, Hobbins JC (1989) Pulsed Doppler flow-velocity waveforms in the prediction of fetal hematocrit of the severely isoimmunized pregnancy. Am J Obstet Gynecol 161:341–344

20. Legarth J, Lingman G, Stangenberg M, Rahman F (1992) Lack of relationship between fetal blood gases and fetal blood flow velocity waveform indices found in rhesus isoimmunized pregnancies. Br J Obstet Gynaecol 99:813–836

21. Modanlou H, Freeman R (1982) Sinusoidal fetal heart rate pattern: its definition and clinical significance. Am J Obstet Gynecol 142:1033–1038

22. Verma U, Tejani N, Weiss R, Chatterjee S, Halitsky V (1980) Sinusoidal fetal heart rate patterns in severe RH disease. Obstet Gynecol 55:666–669

23. Young B, Katz M, Wilson S (1980) Sinusoidal fetal heart rate: clinical significance. Am J Obstet Gynecol 138:587

24. Street P, Dawes GS, Moulden M, Redman CW (1991) Short-term variation in abnormal antenatal fetal heart rate records. Am J Obstet Gynecol 165:515–523

25. Burns P (1993) The physics of Doppler. In: Chervenak FA, Isaacson G, Campbell S (eds) Ultrasound in obstetrics and gynecology. Little Brown, Boston, p 33

26. Tortoli P, Bambi G, Guidi F, Muchada R (2002) Toward a better quantitative measurement of aortic flow. Ultrasound Med Biol 28:249–257

27. Rightmire DA, Nicolaides KH, Rodeck CH, Campbell S (1986) Fetal blood velocity in Rh isoimmunization relationship to gestational age and fetal hematocrit. Obstet Gynecol 68:233–236

28. Steiner H, Schaffer H, Spitzer D, Batka M, Graf AH, Staudach A (1995) The relationship between peak velocity in the fetal descending aorta and hematocrit in rhesus isoimmunization. Obstet Gynecol 85:659–662

29. Copel JA, Grannum PA, Belanger K, Green J, Hobbins JC (1988) Pulsed Doppler flow velocity waveforms before and after intrauterine intravascular transfusion for severe erythroblastosis fetalis. Am J Obstet Gynecol 158:768–774

30. Bahado-Singh R, Oz U, Deren O, Pirhonen J, Kovanci E, Copel J et al. (1999) A new splenic artery Doppler velocimetric index for prediction of severe fetal anemia associated with Rh alloimmunization. Am J Obstet Gynecol 180:49–54

31. Bahado-Singh R, Oz U, Mari G, Jones D, Paidas M, Onderoglu L (1998) Fetal splenic size in anemia due to Rh-alloimmunization. Obstet Gynecol 92:828–832

32. Mari G, Moise KJ Jr, Deter RL, Carpenter RJ Jr (1991) Doppler assessment of renal blood flow velocity waveform in the anaemic fetus before and after intravascular transfusion for severe red cell alloimmunization. J Clin Ultrasound 19:9–15

33. Warren PS, Gill WR, Fisher CC (1987) Doppler flow studies in rhesus isoimmunization. Semin Perinatol 11:375–378

34. Bilardo CM, Nicolaides KH, Campbell S (1989) Doppler studies in red cell isoimmunization. Clin Obstet Gynecol 32:719–727

35. Mari G, Andringolo A, Abuhamad AZ et al. (1995) Diagnosis of fetal anemia with Doppler ultrasound in the pregnancy complicated by maternal blood group isoimmunization. Ultrasound Obstet Gynecol 5:400–405

36. Vyas S, Nicolaides KH, Campbell S (1990) Doppler examination of the middle cerebral artery in anaemic fetuses. Am J Obstet Gynecol 162:1066–1068

37. Oepkes D, Band R, Vandenbussche FP, Meermen RH, Khanhai HH (1994) The use of ultrasonography and Doppler in the prediction of fetal haemolytic anaemia: a multivariate analysis. Br J Obstet Gynaecol 100:680–684

38. Nicolaides KH, Kaminopetros P (1992) Red-cell isoimmunization. In: Pearce M (ed) Doppler ultrasound in perinatal medicine. Oxford University Press, Oxford, pp 244–257

39. Dukkler D, Oepkes D, Seaward G, Windrim R, Ryan G (2003) Noninvasive tests to predict fetal anemia: a study comparing Doppler and ultrasound parameters. Am J Obstet Gynecol 188:1310–1314

40. Warren PS, Gill RW, Fisher CC (1987) Doppler blood flow studies in rhesus isoimmunization. Semin Perinatol 11:375–378

41. Kanzaki T, Chiba Y (1990) Evaluation of the preload condition of the fetus by inferior vena caval blood flow pattern. Fetal Diagn Ther 5:168–174

42. Jouppila P, Kirkinen P (1984) Umbilical vein blood flow in the human fetus in cases of maternal and fetal anemia and uterine bleeding. Ultrasound Med Biol 10:365–370

43. Lysikiewicz A, Jaffe R, Bracero LA, Evans R (2001) Fetal Preload index predicts fetal anemia. J Med Ultrasound 9:123–126

44. Huisman TWA, van den Eijnde SM, Stewart PA, Wladimiroff JW (1996) Changes in inferior vena cava blood flow velocity and diameter during fetal breathing. Ultrasound Obstet Gynecol 3:26–30

45. Chitkara U, Wilkins I, Lynch L, Mehalek K, Berkowitz RL (1988) The role of sonography in assessing severity of fetal anemia in Rh- and Kell-isoimmunized pregnancies. Obstet Gynecol 71:393–398

46. Nicolaides KH, Thilaganathan B, Rodeck CH, Mibashan RS (1988) Erythroblastosis and reticulocytosis in anemic fetuses. Am J Obstet Gynecol 159:1063–1065

47. Vintzileos AM, Campbell WA, Storlazzi E, Mirochnick MH, Escoto DT, Nochimson DJ (1986) Fetal liver ultrasound measurement in isoimmunized pregnancies. Obstet Gynecol 68:162–167

48. Soothill PW, Lestas AN, Nicolaides KH, Rodeck CH, Bellingham AJ (1988) 2,3-Diphosphoglycerate in normal, anaemic and transfused human fetuses. Clin Sci 74:527–530

49. DeVore GR, Mayden K, Tortora M, Berkowitz RL, Hobbins JC (1981) Dilation of the fetal umbilical vein in rhesus hemolytic anemia: a predictor of severe disease. Am J Obstet Gynecol 141:464–466

50. Frigoletto FD, Greene MF, Benacerraf BR, Barss VA, Saltzman DH (1986) Ultrasonographic fetal surveillance in the management of isoimmunized pregnancy. N Engl J Med 315:430–432

51. Inglis SR, Lysikiewicz A, Sonnenblick AL, Streltzoff JL, Bussel JB, Chervenak FA (1996) Advantages of larger volume, less frequent intrauterine red blood cell transfusions for maternal red cell isoimmunization. Am J Perinatol 13:27–33

52. Weiner C, Wenstrom KD, Sipes SL, Williamson RA (1991) Risk factors for cordocentesis and fetal intravascular transfusion. Am J Obstet Gynecol 165:1020–1025

53. Rizzo G, Nicolaides KH, Arduini D, Campbell S (1990) Effects of intravascular fetal blood transfusion on fetal intracardiac Doppler velocity waveforms. Am J Obstet Gynecol 163:569–571

54. Mari G, Rahman F, Olofsson P, Ozcan T, Copel JA (1997) Increase of fetal hematocrit decreases the middle cerebral artery peak systolic velocity in pregnancies complicated by rhesus alloimmunization. J Matern Fetal Med 6:206–208

Chapter 23

Doppler Velocimetry in Prolonged Pregnancy

Ray O. Bahado-Singh, Maria Segata, Chin-Chien Cheng, Giancarlo Mari

Introduction

Registry data [1] indicate that the increased risk of stillbirth in post-term pregnancies is partly due to an increased risk of small-for-gestational-age (SGA) fetuses; the latter is in turn partly due to an increased risk of congenital anomalies. When malformations were excluded, the post-term SGA had a higher stillbirth rate than term SGA and post-term appropriate-for-gestational-age fetuses. Similarly, the risk of 5-min Apgar score <5 was higher among the post-term SGA than the other two groups. Naeye [2] estimated that 50% of the excess perinatal mortality in post-term pregnancy was due to problems related to uteroplacental perfusion inadequacy (25%) or congenital malformations (25%).

As a result of data indicating an elevated risk of adverse perinatal outcomes, antenatal testing is now a standard feature of the clinical management of prolonged gestations [3]. There is convincing scientific evidence that Doppler velocimetry of the umbilical vessels identifies uteroplacental insufficiency in high-risk pregnancies. Furthermore, it has been shown that when umbilical Doppler information is made available to clinicians it improves decision making and ultimately the outcomes in such pregnancies [4]. Not surprisingly, therefore, there was initial interest and optimism in deploying Doppler for the management of prolonged gestation.

Whether or not umbilical Doppler velocimetry proves to be beneficial depends on a single overriding consideration, namely, the pathological basis of poor perinatal outcome in prolonged gestations. The answer to this question remains unresolved. If uteroplacental vascular insufficiency is the principal cause of poor outcome, then it is reasonable to expect that umbilical artery Doppler will identify the prolonged pregnancies destined for poor outcome; if not, then Doppler is likely to be of little value in clinical management.

Umbilical Artery Doppler

In one of the earliest studies, Rightmire and Campbell [5] prospectively evaluated the umbilical artery Pourcelot index (PI) in 35 singleton pregnancies between 42 and 44 2/7 weeks' gestation. A "labor-compromised" fetus was defined as one with either Apgar score <7, asphyxia or meconium aspiration requiring neonatal intensive care unit (NICU) admission, or operative delivery for fetal distress. The eight pregnancies with adverse outcome had a mean ± standard deviation (SD) PI of 0.56±0.027 compared with cases with acceptable outcome (0.49±0.017). The difference was statistically significant. This study suggested that compromise in postdates pregnancy is due to fetoplacental rather than uteroplacental insufficiency.

Guidetti et al. [6] evaluated the umbilical artery S/D ratio in 46 pregnancies at ≥41 weeks' gestation using continuous-wave Doppler. An abnormal outcome included an abnormal non-stress test (NST), oligohydramnios in which the largest fluid pocket was <2 cm, moderate or thick meconium, intrapartum distress, or low 5-min Apgar. Postmaturity syndrome was diagnosed based on neonatal physical exam. The mean gestational age of the study population was 42.4±0.4 weeks at delivery. There was no statistically significant difference in the umbilical S/D ratios of the 21 infants with normal intrapartum and postnatal outcome compared with the 25 cases experiencing complications. The authors reported that the study was sufficiently powered to detect a statistically significant difference. They concluded that postmaturity may be due to placental changes that compromise nutrient transfer to the fetus rather than clinical uteroplacental vascular insufficiency.

In a larger study of 82 patients at ≥41 weeks' gestation at the time of Doppler, Battaglia et al. [7] did not find a significant difference in the umbilical artery Doppler resistance index (RI) between 58 cases with normal-descending thoracic aorta mean Doppler velocity compared with the 24 cases with decreased mean aortic velocity (umbilical artery RI 0.52±0.06 vs 0.53±0.07, p=NS). The authors did demonstrate a statistically significantly higher frequency of oligohydramnios and meconium staining of the amniotic fluid and abnormal non-stress test in the group with decreased time-averaged mean velocities in the thoracic aorta. There was no direct comparison of umbilical Doppler values in the adverse outcome compared to normal groups; however, this study as designed did not appear to find umbilical artery velocimetry to be a useful tool for the prediction of intrapartum compromise in prolonged gestation.

Fischer et al. [8] did a detailed analysis of 75 postdates pregnancies, ≥41 weeks at the time of evaluation. Cases suspected of having intrauterine growth restriction (IUGR) based on prenatal ultrasound or those having chronic vascular disorders, such as hypertension, diabetes, and renal disease, and other conditions predisposing to IUGR, were excluded. Abnormal perinatal outcome was defined as non-reassuring fetal heart rate patterns, low cord arterial and venous pH, and meconium below the vocal cords, NICU admission, and birth weight below the 10th percentile. Continuous-wave Doppler ultrasound was used to measure the umbilical artery S/D ratio. Fairly detailed statistical analyses were performed. The mean (SD) umbilical S/D ratio was significantly higher in the 21 cases with abnormal outcome compared with the normal group (2.43 ± 0.43 vs 2.19 ± 0.25; $p = 0.03$). When a threshold S/D ratio value of ≥2.40 was used to define abnormal umbilical Doppler, a sensitivity of 57.1%, specificity of 77.8%, positive predictive value of 50.0%, and negative predictive value of 82.4% was obtained for the prediction of complications. Multiple logistic regression confirmed that S/D ≥2.40 was a statistically significant predictor of abnormal perinatal outcome with adjusted odds ratio 2.40 (1.50–13.56). This was a fairly well-designed study and had stringent criteria for adverse outcome. Their adverse outcome groups are therefore more likely to be truly clinically compromised and therefore likely to manifest Doppler abnormalities. Consistent with this view is the finding that 16.7% of the newborns in the abnormal Doppler group, i.e., S/D ≥2.40, had birth weights less than the 10th percentile vs 0% in the others ($p = 0.009$).

Malcus et al. [9] found no difference in umbilical artery PI when 102 pregnancies ≥42 completed weeks were compared with previously derived normative data. Subgroup analysis of postdates pregnancies with normal testing and spontaneous labor, a subgroup with induced labor, a group with abnormal NST, and finally a subgroup with asphyxia, defined as umbilical artery pH ≤7.10, low Apgar score, or operative delivery for fetal distress, did not yield umbilical Doppler values outside of the normative range. Overall, the prolonged-pregnancy group did not have a significantly different rate of acute fetal asphyxia during labor compared with the contemporaneous group of 2,630 cases <294 days

delivered at the same institution. Along with the small number of study and subgroup patients and the low rate of compromise it is possible that this study was not sufficiently powered to detect Doppler differences in the prolonged-pregnancy group.

Pearce and McParland [10] studied 534 pregnancies exceeding 42 weeks with twice weekly umbilical Doppler velocimetry using a continuous-wave Doppler machine. Abnormal umbilical waveforms were defined as those with S/D ratio greater than the 95% confidence limits or absent end-diastolic velocity. Absent umbilical artery end-diastolic velocity, which occurred in 11 fetuses (2.1%), was highly sensitive (91%) and specific (100%) for detecting fetal distress in the first stage of labor. Fetal distress was defined as operative delivery for fetal distress, confirmed by scalp pH <7.25, low Apgar scores, or low umbilical venous pH at birth. Doppler was not, however, effective in predicting fetal distress in the second stage of labor. The latter finding may reflect the fact that distress in the second stage is largely the result of acute factors, e.g., cord compression due to the descent of the fetal presenting part or nuchal cord. Such problems have no relationship to chronic placental insufficiency and are unable to be detected by antepartum testing. A reasonable overall conclusion from this study is that milder impairment of placental function in prolonged pregnancies does not have an identifiable effect on umbilical Doppler measurements. Severe grades of dysfunction can, however, result in umbilical artery Doppler abnormalities that strongly correlate with perinatal outcome.

Stokes and coworkers [11] could find no difference in the umbilical S/D ratios in a study of 70 singleton pregnancies at ≥41 weeks. Abnormal outcome categories included abnormal fetal heart tracing, reduced amniotic fluid volume, intrapartum fetal distress, or moderate to thick meconium. There was no significant difference in the mean S/D ratio between paired subgroups with and without particular categories of abnormal outcomes. There were 48 neonates with no abnormal tests or outcomes and 22 with one or more abnormal outcomes. No significant differences in umbilical S/D ratios were noted between these two groups. The authors posited that failing placental transport of nutrients and byproducts likely occur in the ageing placenta without affecting vascular resistance. This then would explain the lack of sensitivity of umbilical Doppler velocimetry.

In a prospectively designed study of 142 sonographically dated pregnancies >41 weeks, Weiner et al. [12] evaluated umbilical Doppler RI greater than the 95th percentile as a predictor of adverse outcome; the latter was defined as either 5-min Apgar <7, NICU admission, cesarean for fetal distress, and birth weight less than the 5th percentile. There were 12 cases with one or more abnormal outcome of which 6 had IUGR. A total of 5 (3.8%) compared with 2 (16.7%) of abnormal vs normal groups had abnormal umbilical artery Doppler measurements. This difference was not statistically significant. The mean umbilical artery RI was not significantly different between the two groups. Doppler had a low sensitivity for predicting an adverse outcome, as did other antepartum tests such as NST and amniotic fluid volume.

Anteby et al. [13] studied 79 well-dated pregnancies ≥41 weeks. Patients at known risk for adverse outcome based on medical conditions or with abnormal antepartum testing based on NST or fluid volume were excluded. In addition, patients scheduled for cesarean section or planned induction were also excluded. The authors therefore considered only low-risk patients with prolonged pregnancy. The outcome measures used were moderate to thick meconium and moderate to severe persistent intrapartum heart rate abnormality and finally heart rate abnormalities requiring operative delivery. The umbilical artery S/D ratio was statistically elevated in cases with FHR abnormalities requiring operative delivery. No such difference was observed when the PIs of the two groups were compared. An umbilical S/D > 2.5 had 60% sensitivity and 71% specificity for fetal distress requiring intervention. The authors suggested that a normal umbilical Doppler identifies post-term pregnancies at low risk for intrapartum fetal distress.

Zimmerman et al. [14] studied umbilical artery Doppler RI in 153 well-dated pregnancies ≥41 weeks. Cases with maternal diseases, prolonged rupture of membranes, malpresentation, and growth-restricted fetuses were excluded. Outcomes included asphyxia defined by Apgar scores, low arterial pH or encephalopathy, thick meconium, neonatal signs of postmaturity, abnormal FHR patterns in labor, and non-asphyxial causes of operative delivery such as arrest of labor. Pregnancies with normal and abnormal outcomes had umbilical RI values within the 95% confidence interval used to define normal. Thirty-eight pregnancies had asphyxial-related complications, whereas 30 had non-asphyxial complications. The umbilical RI for the prediction of asphyxia had a sensitivity of 37% with a specificity of 75%. For non-asphyxial complications these values are 7% and 75%, respectively. Overall, the umbilical Doppler was not a significant predictor of asphyxial or non-asphyxial outcome based on inspection of the respective receiver-operating characteristics curves.

Olofsson et al. [15] performed longitudinal comparison of umbilical Doppler in 34 women who delivered after 43 weeks. Doppler values were also compared with those of 32 controls delivered at <41 weeks. All pregnancies were well dated with the assistance of mid-trimester ultrasound. The mean Doppler velocity and estimated blood volume flow in the umbilical vein was noted to increase significantly on longitudinal evaluation of the 34 study cases from 42 weeks to delivery. There was no significant change in the umbilical artery RI over time. Compared with the control group, the umbilical artery RI was significantly reduced, consistent with reduced vascular resistance and increased blood flow in prolonged gestation. Of the entire study group, 41.2% experienced one or more complications, namely oligohydramnios, meconium staining, fetal distress in labor, or birth asphyxia. The study findings were novel in that the authors demonstrated reduced placental resistance and enhanced blood flow in post-term pregnancies. Presumably enhanced flow would facilitate further fetal growth in such patients. These findings are at odds with the generally accepted view of compromised placental function with aging. An explanation might be that in the "normal" prolonged gestations, even though placental senescence limits nutrient transfer, this bottleneck is overridden by enhanced placental flow. Indeed, it would explain the observation that macrosomia is a common feature of prolonged pregnancies. The study by Olofsson et al. [15] had findings that deviated significantly from the published literature cited above. Forty-four study cases were booked from the first trimester and had dating confirmed based on 16–19 weeks ultrasound. There were no cases of perinatal death, thick meconium of the amniotic fluid, meconium aspiration, or low 5-min Apgar. There were 16 cases with light meconium, fetal distress requiring operative delivery or birth asphyxia based on cord pH values. The umbilical artery pH was significantly less in this compromised group than in the 28 patients without complications (0.73 ± 0.14 vs 0.82 ± 0.14; p = 0.03). Dichotomized analysis of cases with and without fetal distress showed significantly lower umbilical artery RI in the group with distress. The same was found when comparing groups with and without light meconium staining. The authors explained these unlikely results by hypothesizing that vasodilatation developed in response to mild hypoxia possibly through the release of vasoactive agents. Contradistinction was drawn to the situation where severe or prolonged hypoxia results in increased vascular resistance. A transient increase in placental perfusion reflecting reduced vascular resistance reportedly has been demonstrated with acute hypoxia in healthy lambs [16].

Every effective screening test has varying sensitivity values depending on the false-positive (1-specificity) threshold that is chosen. As the false-positive threshold increases, e.g., 10% compared with 5%, the sensitivity value will generally also increase. It is therefore misleading and erroneous to compare the sensitivities of two screening tests without regard to

Table 23.1. Umbilical artery Doppler: diagnostic performance for adverse outcome in prolonged pregnancies. *AEDF* absent end-diastolic flow, *PPV* positive predictive value, *NPV* negative predictive value, *LR* likelihood ratio (sensitivity/false-positive rate)

Reference	Test	Sensitivity (%)	Specificity (%)	PPV	NPV	LR[a]
[8]	S/D≥2.4	57.1	77.8	50.0	82.4	2.6
[10]	AEDF	91	100	91	180	_[a]
[12]	RI	16.7	96.2	28.6	92.6	4.4
[13]	S/D	80	55	30	97	1.8
[4]	RI>0.62	37	75	40	73	1.5

[a] LR=infinity.

their respective false-positive rates (or their specificities). The various Doppler studies quoted different specificity values for their reported sensitivities. This makes it very difficult to compare the diagnostic accuracy of umbilical Doppler between different studies. One way of surmounting this limitation is to calculate the so-called likelihood ratio (LR). The likelihood ratio is calculated by dividing the sensitivity value by the false-positive rate. The false-positive rate in turn is equal to 1–specificity expressed as a decimal or alternatively 100%–specificity expressed as a percentage. The higher the LR of a test, the stronger is the correlation between the test measurement and outcome; thus, a test with a higher LR is generally a better test than one with a lower value. Table 23.1 lists the diagnostic indices of umbilical artery Doppler velocimetry in prolonged pregnancies from studies reporting more complete data.

The issue of whether umbilical artery Doppler consistently predicts adverse outcome in prolonged pregnancy remains unresolved. Of the 10 studies reviewed, only three reported increased vascular resistance identifiable on Doppler in prolonged pregnancy with adverse outcome. Indeed, one study paradoxically found a reduction in placental resistance in prolonged pregnancies as determined by umbilical Doppler. There is currently insufficient evidence to propose that Doppler velocimetry of the umbilical artery should be used in routine management of prolonged gestation. The significant variability in the design of these various studies quite predictably makes it impossible to draw any strong conclusions regarding the value of umbilical Doppler in prolonged gestations. The many areas of differences in study designs included differences in defining prolonged pregnancies, varying umbilical Doppler thresholds used to define abnormal variation in ultrasound equipment, and Doppler modality used, i.e., continuous- vs pulsed-wave Doppler and, most importantly, significant variation in outcome end points used to define perinatal complications. Very few of the studies with negative association performed power analysis. There is a significant possibility that many of the negative trials were underpowered.

Umbilical Artery Doppler Versus Other Antepartum Tests

Currently, the most commonly employed protocols for the antepartum monitoring of prolonged pregnancies incorporate the NST and amniotic fluid volume assessment. A few studies compared umbilical Doppler velocimetry to these more commonly used tests. In a study that found a correlation between Doppler and perinatal complications, Fischer et al. [8] compared umbilical Doppler S/D to NST and amniotic fluid measurements (Table 23.2). The umbilical artery Doppler was a better test than NST and amniotic fluid volume assessment combined.

In another study that found the umbilical artery to be a useful predictor of outcome in prolonged pregnancy Pearce and McParland [10] compared absent end-diastolic flow velocity (AEDF) umbilical Doppler to NST and largest fluid pocket < 3 cm for prediction of fetal distress. The Cohen kappa statistic was used. Kappa values vary from 0 to 1.0. Values of 0–0.2 denote test results that may be chance findings, 0.2–0.8 indicates increasing agreement, and values > 0.8 show strong correlation between the test results and the outcome of interest. Based on the kappa statistic, umbilical Doppler AEDF appeared to be a superior predictor of fetal distress in the first stage of labor compared with either the NST or amniotic fluid pocket. Kappa statistic for AEDF, NST, and fluid pocket fetal distress in the first stage of labor was 0.91, 0.41, and 0.68, respectively. Fluid pocket and Doppler AEDF were modest predictors of second-stage distress with NST showing no meaningful correlation with this particular outcome (kappa values 0.39, 0.29, and 0.05). All except fluid volume had poor correlation with 5-min Apgar < 5 (kappa statistic 0.03, 0.07, and 0.37 for NST, AEDF, and fluid pocket, respectively).

Weiner et al. [12] compared NST, oligohydramnios (< 5 cm), and umbilical RI >0.68 for the detection of perinatal compromise; the latter consisted of 5-min Apgar < 7, NICU admission, cesarean for fetal distress, and birth weight less than the 5th percentile. The umbilical artery Doppler performance based on

Table 23.2. Comparison of umbilical artery Doppler velocimetry to other biophysical tests in prolonged pregnancies. *NST* non-stress test, *AF* amniotic fluid, *CST* contraction stress test, *Doppler* umbilical artery Doppler, *MCA/UA* ratio of the Doppler S/D ratio of the middle cerebral artery to the umbilical artery, *LR* likelihood ratio (sensitivity/false-positive rate)

Reference	Test	Sensitivity	Specificity	PPV	NPV	LR
[8]	NST+AF	19.1	84.9	33.3	72.6	1.3
	Doppler	57.1	77.8	50.0	82.4	2.6
	NST	8.3	95.4	14.3	91.6	1.8
[12]	AF	25.0	93.8	27.3	93.1	4.0
	Doppler	16.7	96.2	28.6	92.6	4.4
	NST/CST	8	96	63	71	2.0
[4]	AF	16	95	60	72	3.2
	Doppler	37	75	40	73	1.5
	NST	40	89.7	50.0	85.4	3.9
[17]	AF	20	97.4	66.7	82.6	7.7
	BPP	30	92.3	50	83.7	3.9
	MCA/UA	80	94.9	80.0	94.9	15.7

All values except LR are expressed as percentages.

LR values appear superior to NST, with slightly higher diagnostic accuracy compared with the amniotic fluid volume measurement (Table 23.2). When an abnormal test was defined as either NST, Doppler, or fluid-volume abnormal, the test performance appeared to be substantially improved.

In the study by Zimmerman et al. [14], abnormal umbilical Doppler velocimetry, defined as RI ≥0.62, was a poor predictor of perinatal asphyxia. Doppler appeared to be inferior to fluid volume assessment, while fetal heart rate monitoring using the NST or CST appeared slightly better than Doppler.

Finally, Devine et al. [17] compared middle cerebral artery to umbilical artery S/D ratio to a biophysical profile (≤6), amniotic fluid index ≤5 cm, and NST for the prediction of adverse outcome. This was defined as meconium aspiration syndrome, cesarean delivery for fetal distress, or fetal acidosis in a total group of 49 pregnant women ≥41 weeks' gestation. Of this group, 10 (20.4%) experienced adverse outcome. Middle cerebral to umbilical artery ratio (<1.05) was the only significant predictor of adverse perinatal outcome.

Three of the four studies reviewed in Table 23.2 suggested that Doppler involving umbilical artery by itself or as a component of a Doppler index was superior to NST and amniotic fluid assessment in prolonged gestations. Only one study, that by Devine et al. [17], confirmed statistical significance of this apparent superiority of Doppler. In the other two studies, those by Fischer et al. [8] and Weiner et al. [12], tests of significance were not performed to evaluate apparent differences in diagnostic accuracy between Doppler and other biophysical markers. The study by Pearce and McParland [10] also indicated the superiority of umbilical Doppler for fetal distress in the first stage of labor over fluid volume and NST and superiority to NST for second-stage fetal distress.

The apparent trend in observed superiority is interesting, not the least because both NST and fluid volume assessment are the de facto clinical standards for monitoring prolonged pregnancies. A large-scale study of this observation would have not only scientific interest but also possible clinical value.

Middle Cerebral Artery Doppler Velocimetry

Redistribution of fetal cardiac output with an enhanced flow to the brain is an important finding in IUGR due to placental insufficiency. This phenomenon, called the "brain-sparing effect," is recognizable on Doppler interrogation [18]. A few investigators have studied whether a similar phenomenon occurs in prolonged pregnancy. Battaglia et al. [7] used reduction in the time-averaged mean Doppler velocity changes in the fetal descending thoracic aorta to identify those at increased risk for complications including oligohydramnios and cesarean section for fetal distress. There was no significant difference observed in the middle artery RI between groups with normal and decreased aortic mean velocity. This suggested no significant alteration of cerebral flow velocity even in compromised post-term fetuses. Anteby et al. [13], in contrast, found decreased middle cerebral artery PI in fetuses >41 weeks who developed moderate to severe variable decelerations in labor. Decreased middle cerebral artery vascular resistance was demonstrated in the study by Weiner et al. [19], of post-term pregnancies manifesting compromise. The middle cerebral artery PI was significantly lower in 16 post-term fetuses with oligohydramnios defined as AFI ≤5 cm compared with 104 with normal fluid. The findings are consistent with preferential perfusion of the brain at the expense of the kidney resulting in oligohydramnios. Bar-Hava et al. [20] found no such difference in the middle cerebral artery RI when a group of 15 post-term fetuses with oligohydramnios was compared with 42 with normal fluid volume defined as amniotic fluid indexes >5 cm. As mentioned previously, the study by Devine et al. [17] found cerebral redistribution defined as middle cerebral artery umbilical artery Doppler ratio <1.05 to be reduced in compromised post-term pregnancies. This ratio was found to be a significant predictor, with 80.0% sensitivity and 94.9% specificity for the detection of adverse outcomes in such fetuses. Zimmerman et al. [14] did not find significant differences in the middle cerebral Doppler RI values when subgroups of post-term patients with complications such as low Apgar scores, low cord pH, postmaturity syndrome, or thick meconium, among others, were compared with a normal group. No power analysis was performed to determine adequacy of the sample size. It is likely based on numbers presented that the study was underpowered for these analyses. Selam et al. [21] studied the middle cerebral artery PI in 10 post-term cases with amniotic fluid index >5 cm compared with 25 cases with normal fluid. The middle cerebral artery PI was significantly lower in the post-term group with oligohydramnios (median value 0.89 vs 1.33, respectively; $p = 0.004$). The placental–cerebral ratio derived as umbilical to middle cerebral PI value was significantly higher in the oligohydramnios vs normal fluid group (median value 0.88 vs 0.67, respectively; $p = 0.027$). This supports the notion that cardiovascular redistribution occurs in pregnancies complicated by oligohydramnios.

The study by Brar et al. [22] also found reduced cerebral placental (umbilical) S/D ratios in 19 post-term patients with abnormal antepartum test defined as either an abnormal NST or amniotic fluid index <5 cm compared with a group of 26 with normal test results. Cerebral to placental resistance in the compromised group was 1.1 ± 0.3 vs 1.8 ± 0.3 in normal ($p < 0.05$).

Aortic Blood Flow Doppler

Rightmire and Campbell [5] measured the time-averaged mean velocity in the thoracic aorta in 35 pregnancies ≥ 42 weeks. Mean Doppler velocities, corresponding to blood flow, diminished with prolongation of gestation beyond term. Although the 8 fetuses with compromised outcome had lower mean velocities than other postdates pregnancies, the difference did not achieve significance. The authors speculated that the decreasing velocities resulted from hypovolemia and hemoconcentration (hyperviscosity) in the compromised fetuses.

Battaglia et al. [7] found a "generally high predictive value" of decreased mean descending thoracic aorta Doppler velocity for various outcomes such as oligohydramnios, meconium staining, and abnormal NST. Aortic Doppler had an 80% sensitivity, 78% specificity, 33% PPV, and 78% NPV for cesarean done for fetal distress. Reduced mean aortic velocity correlated with shorter interval to delivery and preceded an abnormal NST by greater than 36 h on average.

In the study by Malcus et al. [9], there was no significant reduction in mean fetal descending aortic Doppler velocity with advanced gestation in prolonged pregnancies. This is in contrast to that reported by Rightmire and Campbell [5]. There were no significant differences found in aortic Doppler PI in 23 cases experiencing asphyxia defined by low Apgar or arterial cord pH <7.10 compared with 23 with normal outcome in the study by Malcus et al. [9]. Power analysis was not used to help to explain the lack of significance observed. Anteby et al. [13] found a negative correlation between the mean time-averaged aortic blood flow Doppler velocity and adverse perinatal outcome in their study of 71 women >41 weeks. Time-averaged velocity of the descending thoracic aorta was significantly decreased in cases with meconium, moderate to severe variable decelerations and operative delivery for fetal distress compared with their unaffected peers. Olofsson et al. [23] compared mean thoracic aortic Doppler velocities and estimated aortic blood flow using vessel diameter measurements in 34 women delivered after 43 weeks compared with 32 controls delivered <40 weeks. Mean aortic velocity and relative volume flow was significantly lower in the post-term group vs controls. When study cases experiencing complications, such as oligohydramnios, meconium, fetal distress, and birth asphyxia, were excluded, there was no significant difference in aortic flow values between normal prolonged gestation cases and controls. This finding suggests that the differences initially observed between prolonged gestation and controls was due to compromised cases with altered aortic Doppler flow indices.

Weiner et al. [19] found no significant difference between the abdominal aorta PI values when term patients were compared with post-term cases >41 weeks who had either normal or reduced amniotic fluid volume. The 16 post-term cases with low AFI (<5 cm) had significantly worse perinatal outcome including cesarean section for fetal distress, NICU admission, and 5-min Apgar score <7 when compared with the post-term group with normal fluid volume.

The cumbersome and time-consuming nature of fetal aortic Doppler measurements combined with equivocal reports reviewed above would militate against its use in clinical care. Furthermore, variability in technique and defined outcomes once again limits our ability to arrive at definitive conclusions. There does, however, appear to be some observable changes in aortic Doppler indices in compromised prolonged gestations with reduced velocity, possibly indicating a degree of compromise.

Aorta and Pulmonary Artery Doppler

Hemodynamic changes in cardiac function have been described in growth-restricted fetuses. Weiner et al. [24] suggested that abnormal cardiac Doppler precedes the occurrence of abnormal fetal heart rate (FHR) pattern in these fetuses. These authors [19] also investigated the aorta and pulmonary outflow tracts by Doppler ultrasound in uncomplicated prolonged pregnancies to determine if changes of cardiac function can cause the development of oligohydramnios and the occurrence of an abnormal FHR pattern. They found that both the aortic peak velocity and the estimated aortic blood flow calculated using vessel diameter measurements correlated significantly with both the amniotic fluid index and the FHR pattern. On the other hand, the pulmonary peak velocity and estimated outflow volume correlated with the FHR pattern only; thus, left cardiac output was reduced in post-term pregnancies with oligohydramnios and both left and right output were reduced in the presence of abnormal fetal heart rate. It is well known that the left cardiac output is directed mainly to the brain. It is possible that reduced renal perfusion occurred in association with the lower left cardiac output directed mainly to the brain, leading to oliguria and oligohydramnios.

Renal Artery Doppler

Doppler velocimetry of the renal artery, while of limited practical value in the day-to-day management of prolonged pregnancies, has the potential to shed light on the mechanism of fetal deterioration. A limited number of studies have been published in this area. Arduini et al. [25] compared the Doppler changes in the fetal renal artery in IUGR and post-term fetuses to determine whether the mechanisms of fetal compromise were the same. Changes in the renal PI in 114 IUGR and 97 post-term fetuses >42 weeks were compared. In each population the relationship between renal PI and fluid volume categorized as adequate reduced or oligohydramnios was evaluated. The renal PI in IUGR fetuses was significantly increased above normal. This increase was most marked in the oligohydramnios group. This contrasted with findings

in the post-term fetuses where there were no significant differences in renal artery PI compared with normative data. Furthermore, there was no correlation between renal Doppler and amniotic fluid volume. The authors concluded that while IUGR results have classic utero-placental insufficiency with redistribution of fetal cardiac output, a different mechanism occurred in prolonged gestation. Specifically, it was noted that animal studies demonstrated increased sensitivity of the fetal kidney to vasopressin with advancing gestation. Vasopressin promotes reabsorption of water by the kidney resulting in reduced urine volume [26]. Arduini et al. [25] suggested that this might be the mechanism of oligohydramnios in prolonged human pregnancies. Veille et al. [27] compared the renal artery S/D in 33 patients with normal amniotic fluid volume vs 17 with oligohydramnios defined as AFI ≤5 cm. The mean gestational age in the normal group and the group with low amniotic fluid volume was 41.3 weeks; however, the number of cases that were post-term was not given. Despite the fact that there was no difference in the umbilical artery S/D (normal fluid group 2.36 ± 0.05 vs oligohydramnios group 2.24 ± 0.05; $p = NS$), the renal S/D was significantly higher in the oligohydramnios group (renal S/D: 6.5 ± 0.3 vs 7.8 ± 0.4; $p < 0.009$). Overall, there was a significant negative correlation between AFI and fetal renal S/D ($Y = -0.435$, $p = 0.01$). This study suggested that the reduction in amniotic fluid volume was indeed secondary to reduced renal perfusion and conflicts with the findings of Arduini et al. [25]. The number of cases with IUGR in the Veille et al. study [27] was not given, whereas IUGR cases were excluded from consideration among the post-term fetuses in the study of Arduini et al. [25]. Along with the differences in the gestational age of inclusion the prolonged pregnancy groups of the two studies may not be comparable.

Bar-Hava et al. [20] compared renal and umbilical artery RI in 57 post-term pregnancies >41 weeks. Fifteen patients had oligohydramnios (AFI<5), while the other 42 had normal fluid volume and served as controls. There were no differences in either the umbilical (0.51 ± 0.1 vs 0.052 ± 0.06) or renal (0.71 ± 0.08 vs 0.73 ± 0.05) artery RI values between oligohydramnios and control groups, respectively. Power analysis done by the authors reportedly confirmed the adequacy of the patient numbers. They therefore did not find evidence or renal blood flow redistribution in post-term pregnancies with oligohydramnios.

Studies in laboratory animals [28] indicate that angle-independent Doppler indices, such as S/D, PI, and RI, correlate poorly with actual blood flow measured by more direct methods. Direct velocity measurements, such as peak systolic (PSV) and end-diastolic velocities (EDV), were found to correlate more closely with actual volume flow. Oz et al. [29] studied renal artery RI, PSV, and EDV in 147 patients > 41 weeks; of these, 21 (14.3%) had oligohydramnios. Adverse outcome was defined as cesarean for fetal distress, 5-min Apgar < 7, prolonged NICU stay, or perinatal death. The renal artery RI was significantly higher in the oligohydramnios group (0.884 vs 0.860; $p < 0.05$).

Interestingly, renal artery Doppler EDV below the mean for gestation significantly increased the risk of oligohydramnios: RR (95% CI) 1.5 (1.1, 2.0). This finding suggested that the changes in EDV accounted for the different RI values. Reduced renal EDV would reflect increased renal vascular resistance. This study provided the most specific evidence as to the mechanism of oligohydramnios in prolonged pregnancies.

A smaller study of 38 patients > 41 weeks was performed by Selam et al. [21]. They compared the renal artery RI in 10 oligohydramnios cases (AFI < 5 cm) with 28 cases with normal fluid. An increase in the renal artery PI was observed. Differences in study design, inclusion, and exclusion criteria and different outcomes of interest account for some of the variability in the studies conclusions. It is possible that more than one mechanism accounts for oligohydramnios in prolonged pregnancies. At this point we are unable to explain why a different mechanism might predominate in different patients.

Uterine and Uteroplacental Artery Doppler

As reported for placental insufficiency in IUGR fetuses, it is possible that a decrease in uteroplacental flow could also occur as a consequence of prolonged pregnancy. Several studies, therefore, have been undertaken to investigate whether Doppler waveform analysis of uteroplacental circulations could have a role in the identification of at-risk fetuses in post-date pregnancies. Uterine arteries, uterine–arcuate arteries, and radial spiral arteries have been assessed with Doppler ultrasonography by investigators in different studies.

A study on 82 pregnancies of at least 287 days gestation found normal Doppler findings in uterine arteries but a significant reduction of time-averaged mean velocity in the descending aorta was associated with oligohydramnios, meconium-stained fluid, abnormal NST, and cesarean delivery for fetal distress [7].

The prospective study of Malcus et al. [9] involving 102 women with more than 294 completed gestational days found similar Doppler PIs in the uterine artery compared with values at term. The study found that abnormal flow velocity waveforms in the uterine artery had no significant relationship to fetal asphyx-

ia defined as the presence of umbilical artery pH ≤7.10 and/or an Apgar score < 7 at 1 or 5 min and/or operative delivery for fetal distress.

Uterine–arcuate arteries were assessed by continuous-wave Doppler ultrasound in 75 pregnancies of at least 41 weeks' gestation and systolic–diastolic ratio (S/D) and RI were calculated by Fischer et al. [8]. There was no significant difference in the mean uterine–arcuate artery S/D or resistance index between pregnancies with normal and abnormal perinatal outcome.

In the study by Weiner et al. [12] uterine artery blood flow velocity waveforms were measured transvaginally in 142 post-term pregnancies combined with umbilical artery Doppler and antepartum tests, namely, NST and estimation of amniotic fluid volume. The authors concluded that in post-term pregnancies Doppler velocimetry alone (either the uterine or the umbilical artery) did not by itself improve the ability to predict abnormal outcome but may increase the ability to predict the compromised fetus when combined with additional antepartum tests.

Zimmerman et al. [14] measured Doppler waveforms in the uteroplacental arteries in the region of placental implantation in a total of 153 prolonged pregnancies. The uteroplacental arteries were localized within the myometrium close to the placental bed. These corresponded anatomically to the radial-spiral arteries and RI values were calculated. The investigators showed that Doppler resistance indices in the uteroplacental arteries in the region of placental implantation did not change significantly with increasing gestation from 41 to 43 weeks' gestation and sonographic grading of placenta maturity was also not related to vascular resistance in the uteroplacental arteries nor to fetal outcome. Finally, they did not find any correlation between uteroplacental RIs and perinatal outcome in post-term pregnancy.

Some data are available for very prolonged pregnancies beyond 43 weeks' gestation. In a study population of 44 women proceeding to 43 completed weeks' gestation, perinatal complications were not associated with an increased uteroplacental vascular resistance [15].

Taken together, the results of these studies indicate that there is no major alteration to maternal uteroplacental flow in those prolonged pregnancies that are destined to be complicated by fetal compromise. The underlying mechanism of fetal complication in post-date pregnancies therefore appears different from the uteroplacental insufficiency responsible for IUGR occurring at earlier gestational ages. Even if placental histological modifications are present in post-date pregnancies, they do not appear to result in major changes in Doppler flow velocity in the uteroplacental circulation. Indeed, whether or not such changes consistent with placental senescence even exist has been called into question [30]. We can therefore conclude that uterine artery and uteroplacental Doppler, when used for the routine assessment of prolonged pregnancies, do not predict fetuses that will subsequently develop perinatal complications.

Conclusion

A comprehensive review of Doppler velocimetry revealed significant variability in the design and conduct of these studies. Areas of variability include differences in ultrasound machines used, Doppler modality (continuous value vs pulsed Doppler), Doppler indices used, and definition of prolonged pregnancy and precision of pregnancy dating. The Doppler technique requires experience and precision that are difficult to ensure and maintain across different trials. The extreme variability observed is likely to overwhelm any small or moderate correlation between Doppler measurements and outcomes, should they exist. The generally small size of the study samples and the near universal lack of power analysis for studies with negative results represent significant additional hurdles. Properly designed and sufficiently powered trials would therefore still be of benefit. An interesting empirical observation was that umbilical Doppler velocimetry appeared to better predict outcome in prolonged pregnancy when compared with the standard antenatal tests such as NST and fluid volume assessment. This is certainly an observation that merits further investigation.

References

1. Clausson B, Cnattingius S, Axelsson (1999) Outcomes of post-term births: the role of fetal growth restriction. Obstetric Gynecol 94:758–762
2. Naeye R (1978) Causes of perinatal mortality excess in prolonged gestations. Am J Epidemiol 108:429–433
3. ACOG Practice Patterns (1997) Management of post-term pregnancy. #6, October
4. Alfirevic Z, Nielson JP (1995) Doppler ultrasonography in high-risk pregnancies: systematic review with meta-analysis. Am J Obstet Gynecol 172:1379
5. Rightmire DA, Campbell S (1987) Fetal and maternal Doppler blood flow parameters in post-term pregnancies. Obstet Gynecol 69:891–894
6. Guidetti DA, Divon MY, Cavalieri RL, Langer O, Merkatz IR (1987) Fetal umbilical artery flow velocimetry in postdate pregnancies. Am J Obstet Gynecol 57:1521–1523
7. Battaglia C, Larocca E, Lanzani A, Coukos G, Genazzani AR (1991) Doppler velocimetry in prolong2ed pregnancy. Obstet Gynecol 77:213–216
8. Fischer RL, Kuhlman KA, Depp R, Wapner RJ (1991) Doppler evaluation of umbilical and uterine arcuate arteries in postdates pregnancy. Obstet Gynecol 78:363–368
9. Malcus P, Maršál K, Persson PH (1991) Fetal and uteroplacental blood flow in prolonged pregnancies. A clinical study. Ultrasound Obstet Gynecol 1:40–45
10. Pearce JM, McParland PI (1991) A comparison of Doppler flow velocity waveforms, amniotic fluid columns, and non-stress test as a means of monitoring postdates pregnancies. Obstet Gynecol 77:204–208
11. Stokes HJ, Roberts RV, Newnham JP (1991) Doppler flow velocity waveform analysis in postdate pregnancies. Aust NZ J Obstet Gynecol 31:27–30
12. Weiner Z, Reichler A, Zlozover M, Mendelson A, Thaler I (1993) The value of Doppler ultrasonography in prolonged pregnancies. Eur J Obstet Gynecol Reprod Biol 48:93–97
13. Anteby EY, Tadmor O, Revel A, Yagel S (1994) Post-term pregnancies with normal cardiotocographs and amniotic fluid columns: the role of Doppler evaluation in predicting perinatal outcome. Eur J Obstet Gynecol Reprod Biol 54:93–98
14. Zimmerman P, Alback T, Kiskinen J, Vaalamo R, Tuimala R, Ranta T (1995) Doppler flow velocimetry of the umbilical artery, uteroplacental arteries and fetal middle cerebral artery in prolonged pregnancy. Ultrasound Obstet Gynecol 5:189–197
15. Olofsson P, Saldeen P, Maršál K (1996) Fetal and uterolplacental circulatory changes in pregnancies proceeding beyond 43 weeks. Early Hum Dev 46:1–13
16. Block BSB, Llanas AJ, Creasy RK (1984) Responses of growth retarded fetus to acute hypokemia. Am J Obstet Gynecol 148:878–883
17. Devine PA, Bracero LA, Lysikiewicz A, Evans R, Womack S, Byrne DW (1994) Middle cerebral to umbilical artery Doppler ratio in postdate pregnancies. Obstet Gynecol 84:856–860
18. Bahado-Singh RO, Kovanchi E, Jeffres A, Oz U, Deren O, Copel J, Mari G (1999) The Doppler cerebroplacental ratio and perinatal outcome in intrauterine growth restriction. Am J Obstet Gynecol 180:750–756
19. Weiner Z, Farmakides G, Schulman H, Casale A, Itskovitz-Eldor J (1996) Central and peripheral haemodynamic changes in post-term fetuses: correlation with oligohydramnios and abnormal fetal heart rate pattern. Br J Obstet Gynecol 103:541–546
20. Bar-Hava I, Divon MY, Sardo M, Barnhard Y (1995) Is olighydramnios in post-term pregnancy associated with redistribution of fetal blood flow? Am J Obstet Gynecol 173:1523–1527
21. Selam B, Koksal R, Ozcan T (2000) Fetal arterial and venous Doppler parameters in the interpretation of oligohydramnios in post-term pregnancies. Ultrasound Obstet Gynecol 15:403–406
22. Brar HS, Horenstein J, Medearis AL, Platt LD, Phelan JP, Paul RH (1989) Cerebral, umbilical, and uterine resistance using Doppler velocimetry in post-term pregnancy. J Ultrasound Med 8:187–191
23. Olofsson P, Saldeen P, Maršál K (1997) Association between a low umbilical artery pulsatility index and fetal distress in very prolonged pregnancies. Eur J Obstet Gynecol Reprod Biol 73:23–29

24. Weiner Z, Farmakides G, Barnhard Y, Bar-Hava I, Divon MY (1996) Doppler study of fetal cardiac function in prolonged pregnancies. Obstet Gynecol 88:200–202

25. Arduini D, Rizzo G (1991) Fetal renal artery velocity wavelength and amniotic fluid volume in growth-retarded and post-term fetuses. Obstet Gynecol 77:370–373

26. Robillard JE, Weitzman RE, Burmeister L, Smith FG Jr (1981) Developmental aspects of renal response to hypoxemia in the fetal lamb in utero. Circ Res 48:128–130

27. Veille JC, Penry M, Mueller-Heubach E (1993) Fetal renal pulsed Doppler waveform in prolonged pregnancies. Am J Obstet Gynecol 169:882–884

28. Batten DG, Hellman J, Hernandez MJ, Maisels MJ (1983) Regional cerebral blood flow, cerebral blood velocity and pulsatility index in newborn dogs. Pediatr Res 17:908–912

29. Oz AV, Holub B, Mendilcioglu I, Mari G, Bahado-Singh RO (2002) Renal artery Doppler investigation of the etiology of oligohydramnios in post-term pregnancy. Obstet Gynecol 100:715–718

30. Fox H (1997) Aging of the placental. Arch Dis Child 77:165–170

Doppler Velocimetry for Fetal Surveillance: Adverse Perinatal Outcome and Fetal Hypoxia

Dev Maulik, Reinaldo Figueroa

The primary objective of fetal surveillance is to detect fetal compromise arising from nutritive and respiratory deficiencies. A variety of obstetric complications, including fetal growth restriction and hypertension, may expose the fetus to such risks. There is emerging evidence that the growth-restricted human fetus suffers from chronic hypoxia and acidosis. Although an immense amount of information is available on acute and subacute fetal respiratory deficit, the mechanism of chronic nutritional and respiratory deficiency in the fetus has remained relatively ill-understood.

Encountering unfavorable circumstances, the fetus appears to mobilize a spectrum of compensatory responses, including preferential preservation of fetal growth over placental growth, changes in fetal movement pattern, and eventual deceleration of the fetal growth rate (Fig. 24.1). In the face of deepening deprivation, compensation gives way to decompensa-tion. It has also been shown that a central component of the fetal homeostatic response involves flow redistribution, which favors the vital organs (i.e., brain, heart, adrenals), whereas flow to muscle, viscera, skin, and other less critical tissues and organs declines [1]. Underlying this phenomenon are the diverse changes in impedance in these vascular systems.

The introduction of Doppler velocimetry has not only enabled us to investigate this phenomenon in the human fetus but it has opened up the potential of its use for detecting fetal compromise. A significant amount of information exists on the diagnostic efficacy of the Doppler method for identifying the fetus with adverse outcome as defined by various clinical parameters. What constitutes adverse perinatal outcome, however, is a highly controversial and problematic issue. It is well recognized that many of these

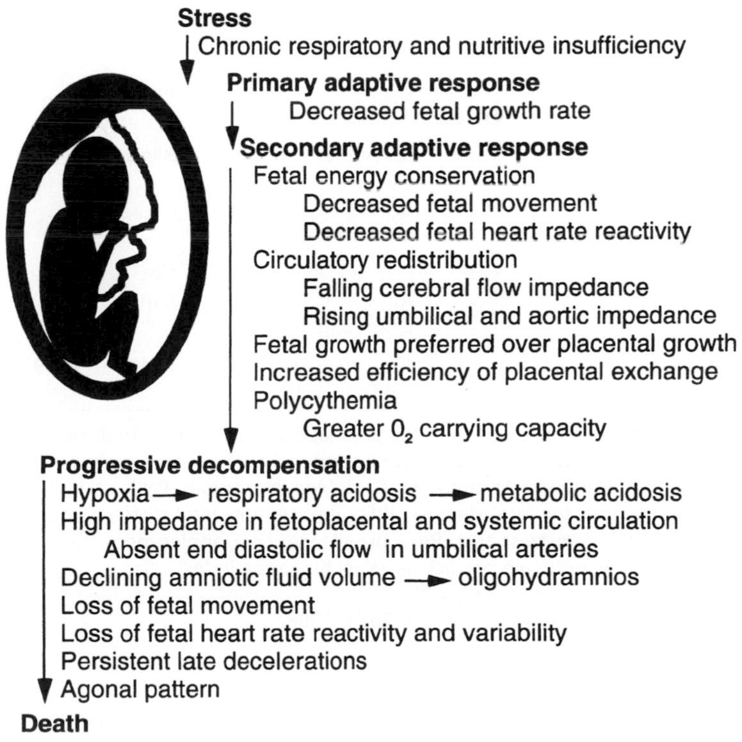

Stress
Chronic respiratory and nutritive insufficiency
Primary adaptive response
Decreased fetal growth rate
Secondary adaptive response
Fetal energy conservation
Decreased fetal movement
Decreased fetal heart rate reactivity
Circulatory redistribution
Falling cerebral flow impedance
Rising umbilical and aortic impedance
Fetal growth preferred over placental growth
Increased efficiency of placental exchange
Polycythemia
Greater O_2 carrying capacity
Progressive decompensation
Hypoxia → respiratory acidosis → metabolic acidosis
High impedance in fetoplacental and systemic circulation
Absent end diastolic flow in umbilical arteries
Declining amniotic fluid volume → oligohydramnios
Loss of fetal movement
Loss of fetal heart rate reactivity and variability
Persistent late decelerations
Agonal pattern
Death

Fig. 24.1. Summary of fetal sequential response to progressive stress. Note that the depicted sequence is an approximation; the actual course may vary depending on the characteristics of the chronic deprivation and the individual fetal ability to cope

clinical indicators do not necessarily reflect chronic respiratory or nutritive deficit of the fetus. It is important therefore to consider the efficacy of fetal Doppler velocimetry also with regard to detecting fetal hypoxia or asphyxia, although it may not prognosticate the long-term neurologic outcome of the infant.

This chapter provides a general review of the efficacy of fetal Doppler velocimetry for predicting adverse perinatal outcome and identifying fetal hypoxia and acidosis in high-risk and unselected pregnancies. The efficacy of the method in relation to specific pregnancy disorders is considered in other dedicated chapters in this book.

Doppler Velocimetry and Adverse Perinatal Outcome

This section presents a critical appraisal of the effectiveness of fetal Doppler velocimetry for identifying the fetus at risk. During this inquiry it is important to ascertain whether the technique is used in complicated pregnancies or in an unselected obstetric population. Although such risk categorization is merely a relative distinction of high or low prevalence of adverse outcome in population, it significantly influences the efficacy measures of a test. Thus for a given diagnostic test, the efficacy is greater among patients with a high prevalence of the disorder than among those with a low prevalence. The efficacy of the Doppler technique should therefore be appraised according to the risk category of the study population.

Table 24.1. Diagnostic efficacy of umbilical Doppler velocimetry for high-risk pregnancies

Study, first author	No. of patients	Risk	Outcome	Prev (%)	Design	DI	Sens (%)	Spec (%)	PPV (%)	NPV (%)	KI
Trudinger [2]	170	GHR	SGA <10th C, AS$_5$<7	31	?	S/D≥3	60	85	64	83	
Laurin[a]	159	SGA	IUGR<2SD	47	Blind	BFC II–III	50	97	93	69	0.48
			ODFD	19			83	90	66	96	0.66
Dempster[b]	205	GHR	Late deceleration	16	Blind	S/D≥97th C	70	89	54	94	
Berkowitz[c]	172	Risk of IUGR	ODFD, AF, Mec, AS, PND, RDS, SGA	21	Blind	S/D≥3	47	84	57	86	
	43	SGA	Complications	43			67	63	57	71	
Chambers[d]	145	SGA, HTN	CSFD	17	Blind	RI≥2SD	100[f]	77	46	100	
Maulik [7]	350	GHR	SGA<10th C, IPFD, AS$_5$<7, UApH<7.2, NICU admission	28	Blind	S/D≥3	79	93	83	91	0.73
Devoe [3]	1,000	GHR	PND, IPFD, AS$_5$<7, UApH<7.2	19	Not blind	S/D≥90th C, AEDV	21	95	49	85	
Pattinson[e]	369	GHR	Abnormal NST	8	Blind	RI≥95th C	93	78	8	100	
			CSFD	3			92	89	22	100	

Risk, risk characteristics of the study population; GHR, general high risk; SGA, small for gestational age; HTN, hypertension; IUGR, intrauterine growth restriction; C, percentile; AS$_5$, Apgar score at 5 min; SD, standard deviation; ODFD, operative delivery for fetal distress; AF, amniotic fluid; Mec, meconium; PND, perinatal death; RDS, respiratory distress syndrome; CSFD, cesarean section for fetal distress; IPFD, intrapartum fetal distress; UApH, umbilical arterial pH; NICU, neonatal intensive care unit; NST, nonstress test; Prev, prevalence; DI, Doppler index; Sens, sensitivity; Spec, specificity; PPV, positive predictive value; NPV, negative predictive value; KI, kappa index.
[a] Br J Obstet Gynecol 69:895, 1987.
[b] Eur J Obstet Gynecol Reprod Biol 29:21, 1988.
[c] Obstet Gynecol 71:742, 1988.
[d] Br J Obstet Gynaecol 96:803, 1989.
[e] Obstet Gynecol 78:353, 1991.
[f] Analysis done with the sensitivity kept fixed at 100% (i.e., no cases of adverse outcome would be missed).

Diagnostic Efficacy of Doppler Velocimetry Among High-Risk Pregnancies

The efficacy of fetal Doppler investigations for predicting adverse perinatal outcome in complicated pregnancies has been widely investigated. A selection of these studies is summarized in Table 24.1, some of which are also discussed later.

Most studies indicated that the Doppler results were efficacious for identifying the fetus at risk in complicated pregnancies. There are, however, wide variations in the performance of the technique, with the sensitivity ranging from 21% to more than 90% and the specificity from 63% to 97%. This range may not be surprising, as the studies were heterogeneous in several ways, including the population selection criteria, the method of using Doppler surveillance (e.g., the frequency of examination), the diagnostic threshold value of the test result, and the outcome parameters. As is evident, the investigators were not uniform in their selection criteria of an adverse perinatal outcome, which included fetal smallness for gestational age (SGA), operative delivery for fetal distress, Apgar score, the need for admission to the neonatal intensive care unit (NICU), and various other

conditions. These variations are not surprising as the criteria for morbid perinatal outcome remain controversial. Many of the traditional measures of morbidity are now known to be of little significance for long-term prognosis of the infant. Despite these limitations, traditional measures of perinatal morbidity have not yet been replaced by any more insightful alternatives.

In addition, some of these studies were deficient in their experimental approach. For example, many investigators did not employ a blind technique, which might have compromised the studies' validity as the clinicians' preconceived notion about the efficacy of the test would inevitably introduce bias. If the physician was already favorably disposed toward the test, the results could be erroneously affirmative; on the other hand, the chances of obtaining false-negative results would increase if the physician had no confidence in the test. Thus blind evaluations significantly enhance the validity of the study results. In one of the first studies reported on the diagnostic efficacy of Doppler velocimetry, the investigators [2] did not state whether the clinicians were blind to the Doppler results. Moreover, in one of the largest studies on Doppler efficacy, which also included a nonstress test (NST) and biophysical

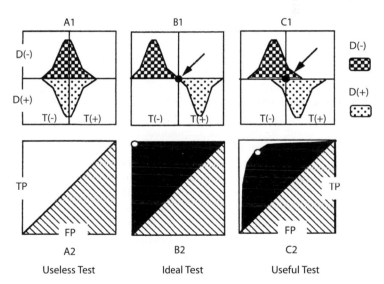

Fig. 24.2. Principle of receiver operating characteristic (ROC) curve analysis for assessing the efficacy of a diagnostic test. *D(–)* disease-free, *D(+)* diseased, *T(–)* test negative, *T(+)* test positive, *TP* true positive, *FP* true negative. *Top:* Distribution pattern of the diseased and disease-free populations along the test value represented by the *horizontal line* in the middle of each panel. *Bottom:* ROC curves. Note that with a useless test there is an equal chance of being diseased or disease-free at any given value of the test (*A1*); the corresponding curve (*A2*) is the *diagonal* from the *lower* left to the *upper right corner*. In contrast, a perfect test completely discriminates between the two populations (*B1*). The *arrow* points to the most discriminatory value of

the test. The corresponding ROC curve (*B2*) is represented by the *left* and *upper margins* of the graph with no false positives. The *upper left corner* corresponds to only true-positive and no false-positive results and therefore represents the absolute discriminatory value of the test. A useful, but less than perfect, test predominantly separates the two populations with some degree of overlap that contributes to the false-positive and false-negative results (*C1*). The *arrow*, as in the previous case, points to the most discriminatory value of the test. The ROC curve covers an area (*black shaded*) that is a measure of the test's overall efficacy (*C2*). The test value nearest to the *upper left corner* is the most efficacious

profile [3], the clinicians had ready access to the Doppler and other fetal monitoring results, which obviously compromised the reliability of the conclusions drawn from this investigation.

Despite such limitations, most investigators have confirmed that fetal Doppler velocimetry is an effective method for identifying fetal jeopardy in high-risk pregnancies with the significant exception of postdatism, for which it may not be a reliable discriminator of fetal status (see Chap. 23 for an in-depth discussion).

This affirmative conclusion remains valid irrespective of whether the study utilized the Bayesian or signal analytic approach or both. The Bayesian approach determines the probabilistic measures of efficacy, such as the sensitivity, specificity, or predictive values, at a given test value. The signal analysis method measures the overall discriminatory performance of a test from its true- and false-positive rates for all available values and assists in determining its optimal threshold for a particular application. This technique is also known as the receiver operating characteristic (ROC) method [4] and is explained in Fig. 24.2. In addition to these two techniques, the kappa index [5] has been used. The kappa index measures the degree of concordance between the test result and the diagnosis beyond chance; the value of this index has been utilized to assess the magnitude of the test's efficacy [6]. A kappa index more than 0.8 is regarded as near perfect, at 0.6–0.8 as "substantial", at 0.4–0.6 as moderate, and less than 0.4 as fair to poor.

These analytic techniques were utilized by Maulik et al. [7] to evaluate the diagnostic efficacy of the umbilical arterial systolic/diastolic (S/D) ratio for predicting adverse perinatal outcome. As indicated, the study was blind, so that those responsible for clinical management of the patient did not have access to the Doppler results. A free-standing continuous-wave Doppler device with a 4-MHz transducer and a fast Fourier analyzer was used. The criteria for abnormal perinatal outcome included (1) SGA at birth (<10th percentile); (2) 5-min Apgar score <7; (3) umbilical cord arterial pH below 7.2; (4) fetal distress during labor (late and severe variable deceleration, subnormal short-term variability, and fetal scalp pH <7.20); (5) presence of thick meconium; and (6) NICU admission. The ROC curve assisted in determining the optimal cutoff value of the S/D ratio (demonstrated in Fig. 24.3). The ROC analysis indicated that this test had an impressive but less than perfect capability of discriminating between an adverse and a normal outcome. Ratios of 2.9 and 3.0 exhibited the maximum inherent discriminatory power: The former of the two values exhibited greater sensitivity, and the latter, which is the more prevalent standard, showed greater specificity and a higher kappa index (Table 24.2). Furthermore, when fetal SGA status was excluded

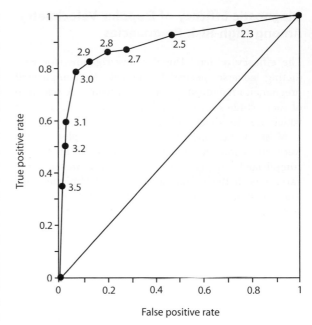

Fig. 24.3. Receiver operating characteristic curve of the umbilical arterial systolic/diastolic (S/D) ratio. Note that the S/D ratio cutoff point (2.9) closest to the *upper left corner* of the graph has the best ability to discriminate between the normal and abnormal outcome groups. (Reprinted from [7] with permission)

Table 24.2. Test performance values for various systolic/diastolic ratio cutoff points (from [7] with permission)

Cutoff point	Sensitivity	Specificity	PPV	NPV	KI
2.5	0.93	0.53	0.47	0.94	0.36
2.9	0.83	0.87	0.74	0.92	0.68
3.0	0.79	0.93	0.83	0.91	0.73
3.5	0.35	0.99	0.93	0.77	0.41

PPV, positive predictive value; NPV, negative predictive value; KI, kappa index.

from the outcome, the S/D ratio had the best diagnostic efficacy; in contrast, when small fetal size was the only outcome criterion, the test demonstrated the worst efficacy. This result further confirms that the umbilical arterial Doppler indices are more capable of identifying fetal compromise than small fetal size.

Fetal Doppler Velocimetry, Nonstress Test, and Biophysical Profile: Comparative Efficacy for Predicting Adverse Perinatal Outcome

When appraising the diagnostic efficacy of fetal Doppler, an important consideration is to compare it with that of the currently utilized fetal surveillance procedures. This section presents the comparative effectiveness of these modalities in relation to the prediction of adverse perinatal outcome. Other relevant aspects of this issue (i.e., the prediction of fetal asphyxia and the sequence of occurrence of abnormal tests) are discussed later in the chapter.

The effectiveness of the umbilical arterial A/B (S/D) ratio for predicting adverse outcome was investigated by Trudinger et al. [2] in 170 high-risk patients. The parameters of fetal compromise included birth weight below the 10th percentile or an Apgar score of less than 7 at 5 min. The fetal heart rate was assessed in terms of reactivity and a modified Fischer score. In this study, the umbilical arterial S/D ratio appeared to be more sensitive, but less specific, than electronic fetal heart rate monitoring. Farmakides et al. [8] investigated the diagnostic efficacy of the NST and the umbilical arterial S/D ratio in 140 pregnancies. The measures of outcome included intrauterine growth restriction (IUGR), fetal distress, cesarean section for fetal distress, and admission to the NICU. Fetuses with a normal NST but abnormal S/D ratio had an outcome worse than those with an abnormal NST and a normal S/D ratio; those for whom both tests were abnormal experienced the worst outcome.

Further corroboration came from Arduini et al. [9], who noted in a cross-sectional study involving 1,000 unselected pregnancies at 36–40 weeks' gestation that umbilical velocimetry was more effective than NST for identifying fetuses at risk of adverse outcome (cesarean section for fetal distress, lower birth weight, 5-min Apgar score <7, admission to the NICU). The relative strengths of the individual and combined use of the various tests were investigated by Hastie et al. [10] in 50 pregnant patients. These investigators observed that the repeat nonreactive NST was highly sensitive (92%) and the S/D ratio highly specific (83%); they therefore suggested the effectiveness of combining the two tests for predicting adverse perinatal outcome. The suggestion of a combined approach also came from Nordstrom et al. [11], who determined the umbilical arterial S/D ratio and biophysical profile in 69 high-risk pregnancies within 10 days preceding the delivery. Intrapartum fetal distress and SGA occurred in 43% of the infants. The S/D ratio demonstrated a higher sensitivity (37%), specificity (92%), positive predictive value (PPV) (79%), and negative predictive value (NPV) (66%) than the biophysical profile (27%, 82%, 53%, and 59%, respectively).

These observational studies, though highly informative, do not provide evidence for a greater effectiveness of any of the tests in regard to altering outcome. Such conclusions can be achieved only by randomized trials. This issue is discussed in Chap. 26.

Fetal Doppler Sonography and Neurodevelopmental Outcome

As indicated above, the currently utilized immediate measures of outcome may not effectively prognosticate the long-term effects of in utero fetal compromise on subsequent neurologic development. This point is particularly relevant when assessing the efficacy of antepartum surveillance, which is a relatively difficult area of investigation. Not surprisingly, there are few studies in this area, and those published so far are contradictory. Maršál and Ley [12] in their long-term investigation found a significant correlation between the abnormalities of fetal aortic Doppler waveforms and deficient neurologic development of the infant assessed at 7 years of age. Similarly, Fouron et al. [13] measured the ratio of antegrade to retrograde velocity integrals in the aortic isthmus of 44 fetuses with abnormal umbilical artery Doppler velocimetry and studied the neurodevelopmental condition of the children between the ages of 2 and 4 years. The investigators found a significant correlation between the flow patterns in the fetal aortic isthmus and neurodevelopmental deficit, with a relative risk of 2.05 (95% CI 1.49–2.83) when predominantly retrograde flow was observed in the fetal aortic isthmus. These findings are significant and require corroboration. In a group of fetuses from high-risk pregnancies delivered before 34 weeks Todd et al. [14] found that when compared with umbilical Doppler velocimetry, antepartum fetal heart rate monitoring was more strongly associated with poor cognitive function of the infant at 2 years of age. Obviously, additional investigations are required before any definitive conclusions can be reached on this issue.

Efficacy of Doppler Sonography for Screening Low-Risk and Unselected Pregnancies

Although the diagnostic efficacy of the Doppler technique in a high-risk population is encouraging, its performance in a low-risk population is disappointing, as indicated by several studies summarized below.

In a prospective study involving 2,097 singleton pregnancies, Beattie and Dornan [15] evaluated the capability of umbilical arterial Doppler indices [pulsatility index (PI), S/D ratio, resistance index (RI)] to detect fetal growth restriction and perinatal compromise. It was noted that the indices did not adequately predict any of the parameters of adverse perinatal outcome. It is noteworthy, however, that elevated Doppler indices were the only abnormal findings in three cases of unexplained fetal death in this population. Moreover, although the investigators did not find the indices to be useful for timing the death, there were no indications that these fetuses underwent adequate surveillance after the abnormal Doppler findings, as up to 6 weeks transpired between the abnormal findings and the fetal death. There is an important methodologic issue related to the Doppler examination technique. The high-pass filter, which screens out low frequency components of the Doppler signal, was set at 200 Hz, thereby increasing the odds of a false-positive diagnosis of an absent end-diastolic velocity. Regrettably, such an inappropriately high setting of the high-pass filter has been used by many other investigators, which may have compromised the validity of their results. Despite these limitations, the main finding that Doppler insonation of the umbilical arteries may not be efficacious in a low-risk population has been corroborated by others [16–18].

Hanretty and coworkers [16] investigated the association between the uteroplacental and umbilical arteries and the obstetric outcome in unselected pregnant mothers. Only the results of the umbilical Doppler studies are discussed here. Their study utilized a prospective blind design and the populations of 326 women at 26–30 weeks' gestation and 356 women at 34–36 weeks' gestation. There was a significant ($p < 0.05$–0.002) decrease in the birth weight of fetuses with an abnormal umbilical artery S/D ratio at either gestation. There were no statistically significant differences between the groups in relation to other obstetric outcomes, including antepartum admission, preeclampsia, preterm delivery, antepartum and intrapartum cesarean section, Apgar score, and NICU admission.

Newnham and associates [17] evaluated the umbilical arterial S/D ratio as a screening tool in a prospective double-blind study of 535 pregnancies at medium risk for fetal compromise. Ultrasound biometry and Doppler measurements were performed at 18, 24, 28, and 34 weeks' gestation. Umbilical artery S/D ratios at 24, 28, and 34 weeks' gestation were found to be predictive of IUGR. This predictive capability was enhanced in the growth-restricted fetuses in whom hypoxia developed but was weak when umbilical artery S/D ratios were evaluated as primary screening tests for fetal hypoxia. The results confirm a role for Doppler-determined S/D ratios in the evaluation of high-risk pregnancies but do not support a role as primary screening tests in low-risk obstetric populations.

Sijmons and colleagues [18] conducted a prospective blind assessment of the efficacy of umbilical arterial PI screening for predicting infants with SGA (birth weight < 2.3rd and 10th percentile) and a low ponderal index (< 3rd and 10th percentile). The population consisted of 400 women at 28 and 34 weeks' gestation attending a university tertiary medical center. The prevalence of the outcome varied between 3.3% and 22.1%. For the different outcome parameters, the test sensitivity ranged from 6.9% to 41.7%, specificity from 91.5% to 99.7%, the PPV from 10.0% to 52.9%, and the NPV from 79.1% to 97.8%.

Doppler Velocimetry and Fetal Hypoxia-Asphyxia

In this section we examine the efficacy of Doppler velocimetry of the various fetal circulations to detect fetal hypoxia and acidosis.

Fetal Asphyxia and Umbilical and Aortic Doppler Indices

A number of clinical studies have been reported on the efficacy of umbilical arterial and aortic Doppler measurements for detecting fetal hypoxia and asphyxia (Table 24.3). The studies employed two distinct approaches for assessing fetal asphyxia. In four studies, umbilical cord blood sampling was performed at the time of elective cesarean section. Blood gases measured in this manner, however, may not reflect the antepartum acid-base status of the fetus. In the remaining five studies, blood gases in fetal blood samples were determined by cordocentesis. Most studies used Doppler assessment of the umbilical artery, although one used the aortic mean velocity and another added aortic and carotid Doppler assessments. In three studies the efficacy of umbilical arterial Doppler and biophysical profile was compared, and one included a comparison with fetal heart rate monitoring. All studies measured pH, most determined the PO_2, and some also measured PCO_2 and lactate. There was also a considerable variability in the patient populations, ranging from those with sonographic diagnosis of fetal growth compromise to those without recognized risks. Most investigators found a significant association between fetal acid-base compromise and Doppler indices from the umbilical and aortic circulations. As expected, the higher the risk category of the pregnancy, the greater the association of the Doppler results with fetal asphyxia. The association between fetal hypoxia and the umbilical artery Doppler index was less impressive. These studies are discussed below according to whether the investigations were restricted to the Doppler method or included other methods of fetal surveillance.

Efficacy of Doppler Method

Soothill et al. [19] were the first to use cordocentesis to assess the efficacy of fetal Doppler velocimetry for reflecting fetal oxygenation and acidosis. Umbilical ve-

Table 24.3. Association between fetal Doppler results and fetal blood gases

Study, first author	No. of patients	Patient risk category	Cord blood sampling	Doppler assessment	Acid-base parameters	Association correlation
Soothill [19]	29	SGA	Cordocentesis	Aortic MV	pH, PO_2, PCO_2	Present
Nicolaides [20]	59	SGA	Cordocentesis	UA AEDV	pH, PO_2	Present
Ferrazzi [31]	14	High risk	C/S	UA PI	pH, PCO_2, lactate	Present
Tyrrell [22]	112	Unselected	C/S	UA AEDV	pH, PO_2	Present
Bilardo [27]	51	SGA AGA	Cordocentesis	UA, aortic, carotid PI, RI, MV	pH, PO_2	Present
Vintzileos [24][a]	62	High risk	C/S	UA S/D	pH	Absent
Yoon [25][a]	105	Unselected	C/S	UA PI	pH, PO_2, PCO_2	Present
Pardi [22][b]	21	SGA	Cordocentesis	UA PI	pH, PO_2, PCO_2, lactate	Present
Yoon [25][a]	24	High risk	Cordocentesis	UA PI	pH, PO_2, PCO_2	Present

SGA, small for gestational age; AGA, appropriate for gestational age; C/S, cesarean section; UA, umbilical artery; AEDV, absent end-diastolic velocity; MV, mean velocity; PI, pulsatility index; RI, resistance index; S/D, systolic/diastolic ratio.
[a] Studies compared the Doppler method with the biophysical profile.
[b] Study compared fetal heart rate monitoring with the Doppler method.

nous blood PO_2, PCO_2, pH, and plasma lactate were measured in 29 fetuses with growth restriction (abdominal circumference < 5th percentile for gestational age). A duplex Doppler device was used to determine the mean velocity of aortic blood flow, which demonstrated significant negative correlations with the severity of fetal hypoxia ($r = -0.73$, $p < 0.0001$), hypercapnia ($r = -0.48$, $p < 0.02$), and hyperlactemia ($r = -0.54$, $p < 0.005$) and a positive correlation with fetal venous acidemia ($r = 0.58$, $p < 0.001$). These investigators subsequently demonstrated the efficacy of the continuous-wave Doppler interrogation, a simpler, more cost-effective technique for indirectly reflecting fetal blood gas status [20]. Umbilical venous blood gases were determined by cordocentesis in 59 fetuses with abdominal circumferences below the 5th percentile for gestational age who also suffered from the absence of umbilical artery end-diastolic flow. In 88% of the cases the blood gases were abnormal; 42% were hypoxic, 37% were asphyxiated, and 9% were acidotic. Furthermore, there was poor correlation between the degree of fetal smallness and the acidosis or severity of hypoxia.

Additional support for the efficacy of umbilical artery Doppler indices for detecting fetal hypoxia and acidosis has come from other investigators. Ferrazzi et al. [21] used cord blood sampling at cesarean section on 14 high-risk pregnant patients, 10 of whom also underwent cordocentesis. A significant relation was found between the umbilical artery PI and the fetal blood pH, PCO_2, and lactate concentrations. Um-

bilical venous oxygen content failed to show this association. A noteworthy observation was the sharp rise in umbilical venous lactate concentration when the umbilical arterial PI exceeded 1.5. Tyrrell et al. [22] observed a significant association between the absence of end-diastolic flow in the umbilical artery and hypoxia and acidosis. The absent end-diastolic velocity detected hypoxia with a sensitivity of 78%, specificity 98%, PPV 88%, and NPV 98%. Similarly, acidosis was detected with a sensitivity of 90%, specificity 92%, PPV 53%, and NPV 100%. When umbilical artery Doppler sonography revealed the presence of the end-diastolic velocity, an S/D ratio elevated beyond 4.5 was diagnostic of hypoxia (sensitivity 89%, specificity 97%, PPV 40%, NPV 98%) and acidosis (sensitivity 100%, specificity 88%, PPV 20%, NPV 100%). Although the authors were confident about the method's diagnostic efficacy for both fetal hypoxia and acidosis, it should be noted that the umbilical arterial response was greater with acidosis than with hypoxia.

Comparative Efficacy of Doppler Velocimetry and Other Methods of Fetal Surveillance

The diagnostic efficacy of umbilical arterial Doppler velocimetry has been compared with that of other modalities of antepartum fetal surveillance. Pardi and colleagues [23] studied SGA fetuses (abdominal circumference < 5th percentile) regarding the umbilical artery PI and by cardiotocography to detect cordocentesis-derived fetal blood gas abnormalities. Fetuses with normal cardiotocography and a normal PI did not demonstrate hypoxia or acidemia. In contrast, when both tests were abnormal, two-thirds of the fetuses had lactic acidosis, low blood oxygen content, and low pH values. These observations indicate that the combination of Doppler indices and cardiotocography is a powerful tool for identifying asphyxia in the SGA fetus. Use of this approach should improve management of this condition by identifying the infants who are not only small but also compromised, which in turn should promote more timely intervention and at the same time minimize unnecessary procedures.

More extensive investigations exist regarding the comparative efficacy of Doppler velocimetry and the biophysical profile in recognizing fetal asphyxia. Among these studies the report by Vintzileos and co-investigators [24] is the only one that contradicts the rest of the investigations discussed in this chapter. They found no association between the Doppler results and cord arterial and venous pH. Fetal biophysical assessment was made and the umbilical artery S/D ratio determined in 62 patients with pregnancy complications (mostly preeclampsia or SGA) within 3 h of delivery by cesarean section, which was performed before the onset of labor. Cord blood gases were measured on samples collected immediately after delivery of the baby. The relation between the cord arterial and venous pH and the biophysical profile score and NST were statistically significant ($p < 0.05$–< 0.0005), whereas that between the S/D ratio and cord arterial or venous pH was not significant. Furthermore, the NST had the best sensitivity (100%) and NPV (100%). The fetal biophysical profile had the best specificity (91%), PPV (62%), and overall efficiency (90%). The S/D ratio had the lowest sensitivity (66%), specificity (42%), PPV (16%), NPV (88%), and overall efficiency (45%). The authors concluded that the umbilical arterial S/D ratio, as determined by continuous-wave Doppler velocimetry, is inferior to the biophysical profile and the NST, and it has no value for antepartum surveillance for fetal acidosis.

These findings, however, were contradicted by Yoon et al., who used both approaches of cord blood sampling: collection from the cord vessels at cesarean section or from the umbilical vein by antepartum cordocentesis. In the first study [25] the comparative efficacy of Doppler umbilical velocimetry and the biophysical profile for identifying fetal acidosis was investigated in 105 singleton pregnancies in which umbilical blood gases were determined at cesarean section performed before the onset of labor. The biophysical profile and Doppler velocimetry showed comparable effectiveness for detecting fetal acidosis.

Patients with abnormal Doppler results showed a significantly higher prevalence of fetal acidosis, and all the fetuses with abnormal Doppler results were either acidotic or growth-restricted. Upon recognizing the limited validity of cord blood gases sampled at cesarean section for reflecting antepartum fetal acid-base status, the investigators conducted a second study [26], which used cordocentesis to assess fetal acidemia, hypoxemia, and hypercarbia in 24 patients (at 26–40 weeks' gestation). Umbilical arterial PI was determined using pulsed Doppler equipment. The prevalence of fetal acidemia (pH at 2 SD below the mean for gestational age) was 41.7%. A statistically significant relation was noted between the change in umbilical artery PI and fetal acidemia ($p < 0.001$) and hypercarbia ($p < 0.001$) but not hypoxemia ($p > 0.1$). Similarly, a significant relation was noted between the biophysical profile score and fetal acidemia ($p < 0.001$) and hypercarbia ($p < 0.005$) but not hypoxemia ($p > 0.1$). Stepwise multiple logistic regression and ROC analyses demonstrated that umbilical artery Doppler velocimetry was a better predictor for acidemia and hypercarbia than the biophysical profile score.

Fetal Asphyxia and Cerebral Doppler Sonography

In contrast to the umbilical artery Doppler indices, the cerebral artery Doppler indices demonstrate a consistent relation with fetal hypoxia. The human fetal cerebral circulation is uniquely sensitive to a decline in PO_2 and a rise in PCO_2. As hypoxia develops, vasodilation and a concomitant fall in the middle cerebral arterial Doppler index occur. When hypoxia becomes severe, the Doppler index tends to rise, suggesting increasing cerebral vascular impedance, which is probably caused by cerebral edema. It is also apparent that the umbilical artery Doppler indices are sensitive to acidosis but not to the partly compensated respiratory acidosis.

Bilardo et al. [27] performed multiple ultrasound biometric and pulsed Doppler measurements in 41 SGA and 10 appropriate-for-gestational-age (AGA) fetuses at 19–37 weeks' gestation. Fetal asphyxia was assessed from umbilical venous blood sampled by cordocentesis. In addition to the PO_2, PCO_2, and pH measurements, an asphyxia index was formulated from the three blood gas parameters by principal component analysis. Of the various ultrasonographic biometric and Doppler parameters, those encompassing the hemodynamic changes in the vascular supply to the fetal brain (internal carotid) and abdominal viscera (aorta) were the best predictors of fetal asphyxia. A more specific study on the middle cerebral artery PI and fetal oxygenation [28], which utilized cordocentesis for fetal blood sampling, showed a significant quadratic relation between fetal hypoxemia and the degree of reduction in the PI. The maximum fall in PI occurred when the fetal PO_2 was 2–4 SD below the normal mean for gestation. When the oxygen deficit increased, the PI tended to rise. The authors speculated that this increase reflected the development of fetal brain edema.

The fetal cerebral and umbilical circulatory responses to hypoxia, hypercapnia, and acidosis were investigated by Chiba and Murakami [29] in 17 SGA fetuses. Cordocentesis was performed to determine umbilical venous blood gases and pH. The fetal circulatory response was evaluated by gestation-adjusted RI values from the middle cerebral and umbilical arteries. The middle cerebral artery demonstrated decreased impedance in the presence of hypoxia and acidosis. In contrast, the umbilical artery impedance increased with acidosis but was insensitive to hypoxia and hypercapnia. These observations were corroborated by Akalin-Sel et al. [30], who found a low PO_2 and pH and a high PCO_2 in the umbilical venous blood sampled by cordocentesis from the SGA fetuses compared to the gestation-related normal values. The cerebral circulation was responsive to hypoxia and hypercapnia, whereas the aortic and umbilical circulations were responsive to hypercapnia and acidosis but not to hypoxia. Decreased impedance in the cerebral arterial system was associated with increased impedance in the aortic, umbilical, and uteroplacental arteries.

These findings have significant clinical implications for managing high-risk pregnancies. Although some animal studies suggest that fetal Doppler velocimetry may not be efficacious for identifying fetal asphyxia, it may not be applicable to the human situation, as indicated by the results of clinical research summarized above. Obviously, the fetal cardiovascular response to chronic and progressive hypoxia and acidosis is complex. Doppler investigation helps us to elucidate this phenomenon and may contribute to improving the perinatal outcome. The differential response of the umbilical and cerebral hemodynamics to hypoxia and acidosis may be utilized to sequence the progression of fetal compromise, which may significantly enhance the diagnostic efficacy of the Doppler technique. Moreover, integration of the current modes of fetal surveillance, such as antepartum cardiotocography or biophysical profile scoring with the Doppler mode, offers exciting possibilities for improving the clinical value of this diagnostic approach.

Sequence of Changes in Fetal Surveillance Parameters with Progressive Antepartum Fetal Compromise

Although comparisons have been made between Doppler velocimetry and other prevalent modes of fetal surveillance, no single testing modality should be regarded as the exclusive choice for fetal surveillance, as these tests reveal different aspects of fetal pathophysiology, often in a complementary manner. Obviously, more work is needed to determine the optimal integration of the various surveillance methods for improving the perinatal outcome in a cost-effective manner: It is important to establish the sequence in which the various signs of fetal compromise manifest during surveillance of the fetus at risk. It is known that not all of these signs appear simultaneously. We have witnessed a variable chronology of falling cerebral Doppler indices, rising umbilical arterial Doppler indices, eventual disappearance of the end-diastolic flow, and the occurrence of ominous cardiotocographic patterns. It is also critical to examine the prognostic significance of the pattern of these occurrences. A few studies have systematically addressed this issue.

Arduini et al. [31] followed 36 SGA fetuses with an abnormal elevation of the umbilical and middle cerebral artery PI ratios (>95th percentile) until the onset of antepartum late deceleration of the fetal heart rate. Comprehensive Doppler evaluation of the fetal circulation was performed along with fetal cardiotocographic examination. Statistically significant changes in PI occurred in all the vessels (umbilical artery, descending aorta, renal artery, internal carotid artery, middle cerebral artery). The most significant fall in the middle cerebral PI occurred 2 weeks before the onset of late deceleration, indicating the maximum compensatory vasodilatory response of the cerebral circulation. In contrast, significant increases in the peripheral and umbilical PI occurred close to the onset of abnormal fetal heart rate patterns. James et al. [32] evaluated the chronology of abnormalities of: (1) umbilical artery Doppler results; (2) fetal growth as indicated by ultrasound measurement of the fetal abdominal circumference; and (3) biophysical profile score. The retrospective study of 103 fetuses at risk of chronic fetal asphyxia revealed that the umbilical artery Doppler result deteriorated first, followed by the abdominal circumference, and then the biophysical profile score. Whereas an abnormality of one of these parameters in isolation did not result in any adverse consequences, abnormality of all three ultrasonographic features led to the worst outcome.

A prospective longitudinal investigation was conducted by Ribbert et al. [33] that included the following indicators of fetal well-being: fetal heart rate variability, body movements, breathing movements, and Doppler hemodynamic evaluation of the umbilical and internal carotid arteries. The study population consisted of 19 SGA fetuses who eventually required delivery by cesarean section because of fetal distress. In 14 of 19 fetuses, abnormal velocity waveforms were present from the beginning of the study. The heart rate variability was initially marginal but declined further during the last 2 days preceding delivery. Decreased body and breathing movements occurred subsequently and less frequently. The worst outcome was in fetuses with reversed end-diastolic velocities and a rapid fall in the variability. The authors concluded that with the progressive decline of the fetal condition fetal test abnormalities occur in the following sequence: Abnormal velocity waveform patterns occur first followed by a progressive decrease in the heart rate variability; fetal general body and breathing movements are the last to decline.

Weiner et al. [34], studying hemodynamic changes in the middle cerebral artery and the aortic and pulmonic outflow tracts, correlated these changes with the computerized fetal heart rate pattern in fetuses with absent end-diastolic velocity in the umbilical artery. They observed that with progressive deterioration of the fetal status the cerebral circulation loses its autonomic reactivity first, followed within a few days by a similar response in the heart, as shown by the decreased fetal heart rate variability. This study is discussed in greater detail in Chap. 25.

A prospective longitudinal study was conducted by Hecher et al. [35] that included short-term variation of the fetal heart rate, PIs of fetal arterial and venous waveforms, and the amniotic fluid index. The study population included 110 singleton pregnancies with growth-restricted fetuses after 24 weeks of gestation and was divided into two groups: pregnancies delivered at 32 weeks or less and pregnancies delivered after 32 weeks. The first variables to become abnormal were the amniotic fluid index and the umbilical artery PI. Abnormalities of the middle cerebral artery, aorta, fetal heart rate short-term variation, ductus venosus, and inferior vena cava then followed. The decrease in PI of the middle cerebral artery followed the abnormalities in the umbilical PI, and became progressively abnormal until delivery in the pregnancies delivered before 32 weeks. In pregnancies delivered after 32 weeks the authors found a normalization of the middle cerebral artery PI before abnormalities in the fetal heart rate. In the pregnancies delivered before 32 weeks of gestation, the increase in the ductus venosus PI and the decrease in short-term variation were more pronounced than the changes in the other variables and became abnormal a few days before delivery. In addition, perinatal mortality was

significantly higher if the short-term variation and ductus venosus PI were abnormal compared to only one or neither being abnormal.

Baschat et al. [36] examined longitudinally 44 growth-restricted fetuses with elevated umbilical artery PI (>2 standard deviations above mean) and birth weight below the 10th percentile who required delivery for abnormal scores in the biophysical profile. Fetal well-being was assessed serially using all five components of the biophysical profile and concurrent Doppler evaluations of the umbilical artery, middle cerebral artery, ductus venosus, inferior vena cava, and free umbilical vein. The majority of the fetuses did not have reactivity of the fetal heart rate. The investigators observed significant deterioration of the biophysical profile and Doppler studies between the first examination and time of delivery. First, there was a change in the Doppler variables. In 42 (95.5%) fetuses one or more of the Doppler variables were abnormal. The umbilical artery and ductus venosus PI abnormalities progressed rapidly a median of 4 days before the biophysical profile worsened. Fetal breathing movement began to decline 2–3 days before delivery, followed by a decrease in the amniotic fluid volume. Loss of fetal movement and tone were observed on the day of delivery. Additionally, in 31 fetuses deterioration in the Doppler parameters was complete 23 h before a worsening of the biophysical profile, while in 11 fetuses deterioration of the Doppler parameters and the biophysical profile occurred simultaneously.

The above studies indicate that Doppler velocimetry and existing fetal monitoring techniques can be integrated to provide greater pathophysiologic insight into the mechanism of progressive fetal decompensation. Such integration may provide a rational, effective alternative to the current standards of fetal surveillance.

Summary

There is ample evidence that Doppler indices from the fetal circulation can reliably predict adverse perinatal outcome in an obstetric patient population with a high prevalence of complications, such as fetal growth restriction and hypertension. This efficacy is not evident, however, in populations with a low prevalence of pregnancy complications. It is also apparent that fetal Doppler indices are capable of reflecting fetal respiratory deficiency with varying degrees of efficiency. The umbilical arterial Doppler indices are more sensitive to asphyxia than to hypoxia, whereas cerebral Doppler indices demonstrate significant sensitivity to hypoxia. Compared to fetal heart rate monitoring and the biophysical profile, umbilical artery

Doppler velocimetry shows mostly similar and often superior efficacy. Furthermore, progressive fetal deterioration manifests in sequential abnormalities of the various fetal assessment parameters, starting with middle cerebral artery vasodilation and eventual progression to disappearance of the fetal heart rate variability, late deceleration, and the absence or reversal of the end-diastolic velocity in the umbilical artery. Evidently, no single testing modality should be regarded as the exclusive choice for fetal surveillance, as these tests reveal different aspects of fetal pathophysiology, often in a complementary manner. Clearly, more work is needed to determine the optimal integration of the various surveillance methods for improving perinatal outcome in a cost-effective manner.

References

1. Cohn H, Sachs E, Heymann M, Rudolph A (1974) Cardiovascular responses to hypoxemia and acidemia in fetal lambs. Am J Obstet Gynecol 120:817–823
2. Trudinger BJ, Cook CM, Jones L, Giles WB (1986) A comparison of fetal heart rate monitoring and umbilical artery waveforms in the recognition of fetal compromise. Br J Obstet Gynaecol 93:171–175
3. Devoe LD, Gardner P, Dear C, Castillo RA (1990) The diagnostic values of concurrent nonstress testing, amniotic fluid measurement, and Doppler velocimetry in screening a general high-risk population. Am J Obstet Gynecol 163:1040–1047
4. Swets JA, Pickett RM (1982) Evaluation of diagnostic systems: methods from signal detection theory. Academic Press, Orlando, FL
5. Cohen J (1960) A coefficient of agreement for nominal scales. Educ Psychol Meas 20:37–44
6. Landis JR, Koch GG (1977) The measurement of observer agreement for categorical data. Biometrics 33:159–160
7. Maulik D, Yarlagadda P, Youngblood JP, Ciston P (1990) The diagnostic efficacy of the umbilical arterial systolic/diastolic ratio as a screening tool: a prospective blinded study. Am J Obstet Gynecol 162:1518–1523
8. Farmakides G, Schulman H, Winter D et al (1988) Prenatal surveillance using non-stress testing and Doppler velocimetry. Obstet Gynecol 71:184–189
9. Arduini D, Rizzo G, Soliani A, Romanini C (1991) Doppler velocimetry versus nonstress test in the antepartum monitoring of low-risk pregnancies. J Ultrasound Med 10:331–335
10. Hastie SJ, Brown MF, Whittle MJ (1990) Predictive values of umbilical artery waveforms and repeat cardiotocography in pregnancies complicated by nonreactive cardiotocography. Eur J Obstet Gynecol Reprod Biol 34:67–72
11. Nordstrom UL, Patel NB, Taylor DJ (1989) Umbilical artery waveform analysis and biophysical profile: a comparison of two methods to identify compromised fetuses. Eur J Obstet Gynecol Reprod Biol 30:245–251
12. Maršál K, Ley D (1992) Intrauterine blood flow and postnatal neurological development in growth-retarded fetuses. Biol Neonate 62:258–264
13. Fouron JC, Gosselin J, Amiel-Tison C et al (2001) Correlation between prenatal velocity waveforms in the aortic isthmus and neurodevelopmental outcome between the ages of 2 and 4 years. Am J Obstet Gynecol 184:630–636
14. Todd AL, Trudinger BJ, Cole MJ, Cooney GH (1992) Antenatal tests of fetal welfare and development at age 2 years. Am J Obstet Gynecol 167:66–71
15. Beattie RB, Dornan JC (1989) Antenatal screening for intrauterine growth retardation with umbilical artery Doppler ultrasonography. BMJ 298:631–635
16. Hanretty KP, Primrose MH, Neilson JP, Whittle MJ (1989) Pregnancy screening by Doppler uteroplacental and umbilical waveforms. Br J Obstet Gynaecol 96:1163–1167
17. Newnham JP, Patterson LL, James IR, Diepeveen DA, Reid SE (1990) An evaluation of the efficacy of Doppler flow velocity waveform analysis as a screening test in pregnancy. Am J Obstet Gynecol 162:403–410
18. Sijmons EA, Reuwer PJ, van Beek E, Bruinse HW (1989) The validity of screening for small-for-gestational-age and low-weight-for-length infants by Doppler ultrasound. Br J Obstet Gynaecol 96:557–561
19. Soothill PW, Nicolaides KH, Bilardo K, Campbell S (1986) Relation of fetal hypoxia in growth retardation to mean blood velocity in the fetal aorta. Lancet 2:1118–1120
20. Nicolaides KH, Bilardo CM, Soothill PW, Campbell S (1988) Absence of end diastolic frequencies in umbilical artery: a sign of fetal hypoxia and acidosis. BMJ 297:1026–1127
21. Ferrazzi E, Pardi G, Bauscaglia M (1988) The correlation of biochemical monitoring versus umbilical flow velocity measurements of the human fetus. Am J Obstet Gynecol 159:1081–1087
22. Tyrrell S, Obaid AH, Lilford RJ (1989) Umbilical artery Doppler velocimetry as a predictor of fetal hypoxia and acidosis at birth. Obstet Gynecol 74:332
23. Pardi G, Cetin I, Marconi AM et al (1993) Diagnostic value of blood sampling in fetuses with growth retardation. N Engl J Med 328:692–696
24. Vintzileos AM, Campbell W, Rodis J et al (1991) The relationship between fetal biophysical assessment, umbilical artery velocimetry, and fetal acidosis. Obstet Gynecol 77:622–627
25. Yoon BH, Syn HC, Kim SW (1992) The efficacy of Doppler umbilical velocimetry in identifying fetal acidosis: a comparison with fetal biophysical profile. J Ultrasound Med 11:1–6
26. Yoon BH, Romero R, Roh CR et al (1993) Relationship between the fetal biophysical profile score, umbilical artery Doppler velocimetry, and fetal blood acid-base status determined by cordocentesis. Am J Obstet Gynecol 169:1586–1594
27. Bilardo CM, Nicolaides KH, Campbell S (1990) Doppler measurements of fetal and uteroplacental circulations: relationship with umbilical venous blood gases measured at cordocentesis. Am J Obstet Gynecol 162:115–120
28. Vyas S, Nicolaides KH, Bower S, Campbell S (1990) Middle cerebral artery flow velocity waveforms in fetal hypoxaemia. Br J Obstet Gynaecol 97:797–803

29. Chiba Y, Murakami M (1992) Cerebral blood flow dynamics in fetus. No To Hattatsu 24:136–142
30. Akalin-Sel T, Nicolaides KH, Peacock J, Campbell S (1994) Doppler dynamics and their complex interrelation with fetal oxygen pressure, carbon dioxide pressure, and pH in growth-retarded fetuses. Obstet Gynecol 84:439–446
31. Arduini D, Rizzo G, Romanini C (1992) Changes of pulsatility index from fetal vessels preceding the onset of late decelerations in growth-retarded fetuses. Obstet Gynecol 79:605–611
32. James DK, Parker MJ, Smoleniec JS (1992) Comprehensive fetal assessment with three ultrasonographic characteristics. Am J Obstet Gynecol 166:1486–1491
33. Ribbert LS, Visser GH, Mulder EJ, Zonneveld MF, Morssink LP (1993) Changes with time in fetal heart rate variation, movement incidences and haemodynamics in intrauterine growth retarded fetuses: a longitudinal approach to the assessment of fetal well being. Early Hum Dev 31:195–208
34. Weiner Z, Farmakides G, Schulman H, Penny B (1994) Central and peripheral hemodynamic changes in fetuses with absent end-diastolic velocity in umbilical artery: correlation with computerized fetal heart rate pattern. Am J Obstet Gynecol 170:509–515
35. Hecher K, Bilardo CM, Stigter RH et al (2001) Monitoring of fetuses with intrauterine growth restriction: a longitudinal study. Ultrasound Obstet Gynecol 18:564–570
36. Baschat AA, Gembruch U, Harman CR (2001) The sequence of changes in Doppler and biophysical parameters as severe fetal growth restriction worsens. Ultrasound Obstet Gynecol 18:571–577

Absent End-Diastolic Velocity in the Umbilical Artery and Its Clinical Significance

Dev Maulik, Reinaldo Figueroa

Among the characteristics of the umbilical arterial Doppler waveform, the end-diastolic velocity is of primary hemodynamic and clinical significance. As discussed in Chap. 10, the end-diastolic velocity demonstrates an impressive continuous increase throughout the gestation which is attributable to an ever-increasing decline of the fetoplacental flow impedance. It results in a concomitant decrease in the pulsatility of the waveform and is reflected in the Doppler indices such as the systolic/diastolic (S/D) ratio and the resistance index (RI), both of which progressively decline with the advancing gestation. These changes are prognostically reassuring. In contrast, any decline in the end-diastolic velocity with the consequently rising Doppler indices indicates rising impedance in the fetoplacental vascular bed and signifies a worsening prognosis. With the further increase of impedance, the end-diastolic velocity eventually becomes absent. Such a development, though rare, is ominous and results in a profoundly adverse perinatal outcome. An example of absent end-diastolic velocity (AEDV) is shown in Fig. 25.1. Occasionally, further hemodynamic deterioration occurs, resulting in reversal of the end-diastolic velocity (Fig. 25.2). The impressive amount of information [1–26] now available on the clinical significance of the absent and reversed end-diastolic velocity in the umbilical artery is appraised in this chapter.

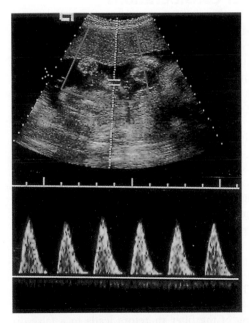

Fig. 25.1. Example of absent end-diastolic velocity in the umbilical artery. *Top*: Color Doppler-directed pulsed Doppler interrogation of the umbilical vessels. *Bottom*: umbilical arterial Doppler waveforms. Note that there is no noticeable loss of low frequency shift information, as the high-pass filter was set at 50 Hz

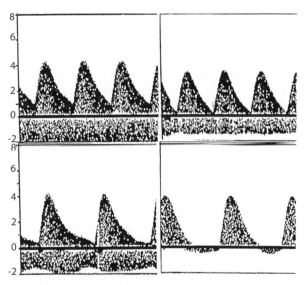

Fig. 25.2. Progressive disappearance of the end-diastolic frequency shift in the umbilical arterial Doppler waveforms from a pregnancy complicated with severe fetal growth restriction at 33 weeks' gestation. *Top left*: Presence of the end-diastolic frequency shift, although the Doppler indices were high for the gestational age (systolic/diastolic ratio 5; resistance index 0.8). *Top right*: Absence of the end-diastolic frequency shift. *Bottom left*: Spontaneous deceleration with prolongation of the diastolic phase and the appearance of umbilical venous pulsation. *Bottom right*: Progression to the reversal of the end-diastolic frequency shift

Table 25.1. Incidence of absent and reversed end-diastolic velocity in high- and low-risk populations

Study, first author	No. of patients	Risk category	Doppler type	High-pass filter (Hz)	AEDV No.	AEDV %
Johnstone [7]	380	High	PW, CW	150	24	6.30
Beattie [27]	2,097	Low	CW	200	6	0.29
Huneke [14]	226	High	CW	200	18	8.00
Malcolm [15]	1,000	High	PW	100	25	2.50
Wenstrom [17]	450	High	PW	100	22	4.90
Weiss [19]	2,400	Unselected	PW	50	51	2.10
Battaglia [23][a]	46	Very high	PW	100	26	56.20
Pattinson [22]	342	Very high	PW, CW	150 200	120	34.50
Rizzo [25]	6,134	High	PW	100	192	3.10
Karsdorp [24][a]	459	Very high	?PW	Lowest	245	53.40

CW, continuous wave; PW, pulsed wave; AEDV, absent end-diastolic velocity.
[a] Fetuses with congenital anomalies and dyskaryosis were clearly excluded. The other studies either included these fetuses or are unclear about it.

Incidence

The frequency with which absent or reversed end-diastolic velocity (AREDV) is encountered in the umbilical artery varies according to the risk category of the obstetric population, the time of gestation at which the observation is made, and the Doppler examination technique. For high-risk pregnancies the incidence varies from 2.1% to 56.0% (Table 25.1). Such a wide range may be explained by the differing definitions of high-risk pregnancy used by the investigators and by the level of the high-pass filter used. For example, the basis for high-risk categorization of a pregnancy may range from clearly defined clinical criteria, such as hypertension, to ill-defined groupings of various clinical conditions. In contrast to that in the high-risk population, the incidence of AREDV may be as low as 0.29% in an obstetric population with a low prevalence of pregnancy complications. The following two examples illustrate this point. In probably the largest reported series on AREDV, Karsdorp et al. [24] used well-defined criteria for selecting the population for a multicenter study. Only patients with hypertension or fetal growth restriction (or both) were included. Hypertension was defined as a diastolic pressure of 110 mmHg by a single measurement or 90 mmHg by two or more measurements. Also included were patients with hypertension plus proteinuria; the latter was defined as urinary protein loss of more than 300 mg in 24 h. Intrauterine growth restriction (IUGR) was defined as the abdominal circumference measuring less than the 5th percentile for gestational age based on local population-specific nomograms. The lowest possible high-pass filter threshold was used. Of the 459 patients selected in this manner, 245 developed AREDV, for an incidence of 53.4%. In comparison, Beattie and Dornan [27] found that only 6 of 2,097 singleton pregnancies developed AREDV for an incidence of 0.29%. The actual rate might even be lower if we consider that the high-pass filter setting was 200 Hz, which is relatively high for umbilical arterial Doppler insonation.

Technical Considerations

As alluded to above and discussed elsewhere in this book, the procedure used for Doppler measurement may affect the measured magnitude of the end-diastolic frequency shift. It is apparent from the basic principles of the Doppler shift that shifted frequencies can only be underestimated, not overestimated. There are two technical sources of this problem: (1) the threshold setting of the high-pass filter; and (2) the angle of insonation between the Doppler beam and the flow axis. The high-pass filter (see Chap. 3) eliminates from the Doppler signal the low-frequency/high-amplitude frequency component and is used to remove signals generated by movement of the vascular wall or other adjacent tissues. This filter, however, also removes low-frequency components generated from the slow-moving blood flow as encountered during the end-diastolic phase of the cardiac cycle. Thus end-diastolic frequencies are removed from the umbilical Doppler waveform. A relatively high setting of the filter therefore leads to a false diagnosis of AEDV. It is strongly recommended that the high-pass filter should be at the lowest possible setting, which may not exceed 100 Hz. The second consideration is related to the angle of insonation, which is inversely related to the magnitude of the estimated Doppler shift because of the cosine function of the angle in the Doppler equation (see Chap. 2). A larger angle therefore leads to a lower frequency measurement, which leads to disappearance of the end-diastolic frequency even in the presence of end-diastolic flow.

Absent End-Diastolic Velocity and Adverse Perinatal Outcome

There is an ominous association between the AREDV in the umbilical artery and adverse perinatal outcome (Table 25.2). The latter includes not only morbid states, such as fetal growth restriction, developmental anomalies, and abnormal chromosomes, but also a substantial increase in perinatal deaths. In addition, there is a significant association with pregnancy complications, such as hypertensive disease of pregnancy and oligohydramnios.

Perinatal Mortality

One of the most remarkable features of umbilical arterial absent and reverse flow is the catastrophic increase of deaths of fetuses in utero and of neonates. From a total of 1,126 cases of AREDV reviewed in this chapter, 193 were stillborn and 312 died during the neonatal period. These data translate into a 170/1,000 stillbirth rate and 280/1,000 neonatal mortality rate, respectively – hence a 450/1,000 perinatal mortality rate. Most deaths are attributable to obstetric complications, such as growth restriction and hypertension with the underlying pathology of chronic in utero respiratory and nutritional deprivation, but they also may be attributed to the higher frequency of anomalies and aneuploidy encountered in these infants, as well as prematurity. It is difficult to correct the mortality figures for congenital malformations and chromosomal abnormalities, as most studies do not explicitly report this information. However, it appears that the corrected perinatal mortality is approximately 340/1,000 births. When the end-diastolic flow in the umbilical artery is reversed, the outcome is abysmal. The European Multicenter Study observed that 98% of such infants required NICU admission, and the odds ratio for perinatal mortality was 10.6 when compared to those with positive end-diastolic velocity. The reverse flow therefore indicates severe fetal decompensation and, if unattended, eventually leads to an agonal pattern and fetal death. An example is presented in Fig. 25.3.

Table 25.2. Absent and reverse end-diastolic velocity in the umbilical artery and adverse perinatal outcome

Perinatal outcome	Mean	Range
Death (%)	45	17–100
Gestational age (weeks)	31.6	29–33
Birth weight (g)	1,056	910–1,481
Small-for-gestational age (%)	68	53–100
Cesarean section for fetal distress (%)	73	24–100
Apgar score <7 at 5 min (%)	26	7–69
Admission to neonatal intensive care unit (%)	84	77–97
Congenital anomalies (%)	10	0–24
Aneuploidy (%)	6.4	0–18

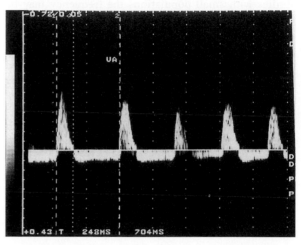

Fig. 25.3. Umbilical arterial Doppler velocimetry showing an agonal pattern. Note that reverse end-diastolic velocity was present for most of the cardiac cycle (60%–70%). This pattern signifies that fetoplacental perfusion, which is normally present for the duration of the cardiac cycle, was seen in this case for only a fraction of that time

Perinatal Morbidity

Not only is there a high rate of perinatal loss, the surviving fetuses and infants demonstrate signs of profound compromise, with a marked increase in the incidence of various measures of morbidity (Table 25.2). One of the main complications of AREDV is a high frequency of fetal anatomic malformations and aneuploidy. In addition, there is a great preponderance of preterm births and low birth weight infants, which are mostly attributable to fetal or maternal complications mandating early intervention. Thus there is a three- to fourfold increase in the number of cesarean deliveries because of fetal distress. These infants are of low birth weight because they are not only preterm but also suffer from growth deficit.

There is a much higher frequency of fetal acidosis, ominous cardiotocographic findings, low Apgar score, and the need for NICU admission. Furthermore, the combination of fetal asphyxia and prematurity exposes the fetus to the additional danger of end-organ damage, such as necrotizing enterocolitis and cerebral hemorrhage.

Congenital Malformation and Chromosomal Abnormalities

There is a preponderance of congenital malformations and abnormal chromosomes in fetuses afflicted with umbilical arterial AREDV. Cumulative data, as summarized in Table 25.2, demonstrate that one in ten fetuses with AREDV have anatomic maldevelopment. There is heterogeneity, however, in the reported incidence. In studies with small populations the frequency may be in excess of one in five. On the other hand, not all studies encountered fetal anomalies associated with AREDV that frequently. Pattinson and associates [22], in a reported series of 120 AREDV infants, observed no anomalies independent of aneuploidy. The largest series of malformations in relation to umbilical arterial AREDV was reported by Rizzo and colleagues [25], who found 25 fetuses with anomalies among 192 with AREDV; of these anomalies, 14 were associated with aneuploidy.

The AREDV-associated anomalies involve most organ systems (Table 25.3), although anomalies of the cardiovascular system are encountered most frequently. Isolated and multiple malformations are encountered with equal frequency, and most cases of multiple anomalies are seen with aneuploidy. Hence most cases with normal chromosomes have isolated malformations, whereas most cases of aneuploidy are associated with multiple malformations.

The frequency of chromosomal abnormalities is 1 in 16. Autosomal trisomy dominates, with trisomy 18 being the most frequently encountered aneuploidy. The relative distribution of various chromosomal anomalies in AREDV fetuses is shown in Fig. 25.4. The risk factors for chromosomal aberrations include (1) an absence of obstetric complications, such as gestational hypertension or preeclampsia; (2) the presence of fetal malformations; and (3) the appearance of absent end-diastolic velocity (AEDV) at an early gestational age. Although these fetuses are severely growth-restricted, there is no difference in the pattern of growth compromise between those with abnormal chromosomes and those without. Snijders and associates [28] studied a population of 458 growth-restricted fetuses and observed that the fetuses with chromosomal abnormalities had a higher mean head-circumference/abdominal circumference ratio than fetuses with a normal karyotype. More specifically, Rizzo and associates [25], in their investigation of fetuses with AEDV, found no signifcant difference in head/abdomen circumference between those with abnormal karyotype and those with a normal karyotype. This finding is contrary to the conventional wisdom, which holds that fetuses with chromosomal aberrations suffer from symmetric growth compromise.

Many of these infants also tend to develop abnormal fetal heart rate patterns during labor, which may lead to cesarean delivery unless the fetal karyotype is known. The mechanism of increased fetoplacental impedance is not fully understood. The work of Rochelson and colleagues [29], however, shed considerable light on this phenomenon. A quantitative morphometric analysis of placentas revealed a significant reduction in the small muscular artery count and the small muscular artery/villus ratio. Abnormal Doppler

Table 25.3. Absent end-diastolic velocity and congenital malformations

Cardiovascular system
  Ventricular septal defect
  Hypoplastic left heart syndrome
  Double-outlet right ventricle
  Ebstein anomaly
  Arrhythmia: congenital heart block

Central nervous system
  Hydrocephaly
  Holoprosencephaly
  Agenesis of corpus callosum

Urogenital system
  Renal agenesis
  Hydronephrosis

Gastrointestinal system/abdominal wall
  Esophageal atresia
  Omphalocele
  Gastroschisis

Skeletal system
  Polydactyly
  Dysplasia

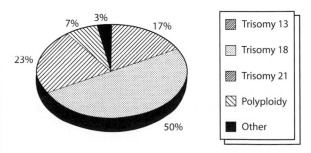

Fig. 25.4. Relative frequency of the various chromosomal abnormalities associated with umbilical arterial absent end-diastolic velocity

waveforms correlated closely with reduced small muscular artery counts. It is apparent that aneuploidy adversely affects fetoplacental vascularization, which results in increased fetoplacental circulatory impedance and may contribute to fetal growth restriction.

Recently, Doppler flow studies in the umbilical artery were performed in first trimester fetuses. Borrell and colleagues [30] screened 2,970 pregnancies at 10–14 weeks' gestation and observed 11 cases of reversed end-diastolic flow for an incidence of 0.4%. Seven of the 11 fetuses had an autosomal trisomy and two other fetuses had a congenital heart defect.

Earlier, Martinez and associates [31] had prospectively recorded the umbilical artery pulsatility index (PI) in 1,785 pregnancies before undergoing chorionic villus sampling or genetic amniocentesis. They had shown that fetuses with trisomy 18 had an elevated PI. The PI was measured transvaginally for pregnancies from 10 to 13 weeks and transabdominally for pregnancies from 14 to 18 weeks. Seven of the ten fetuses with trisomy 18 had an elevated PI above the 95th percentile; nine fetuses had an elevated PI above the 90th percentile. PI as a marker for trisomy 18 had good sensitivity (70%–90%), specificity (>90%), and negative predictive value (99%) but a poor positive predictive value (5%–7%). Reversed end-diastolic flow was detected in two cases, both of which had trisomy 18.

Intrauterine Growth Restriction

The strength of the relation between AREDV and fetal growth compromise depends on the stringency of the definition of growth restriction. A small-for-gestational-age (SGA) fetus is not necessarily growth-restricted, as fetal "smallness" may also be constitutional in nature. It is also probable that a fetus who fails to realize its full growth potential may not necessarily be SGA. Indeed, the terms IUGR and SGA demonstrate diagnostic uncertainty and lack prognostic reliability. Being SGA does not necessarily indicate a compromised outcome. Despite these ambiguities, fetuses experiencing a substantial defined growth failure often suffer from in utero asphyxia and its adverse consequences. These fetuses also have Doppler evidence of increasing fetoplacental arterial impedance. Thus 50% or more of the fetuses with AREDV demonstrate a growth disturbance (Table 25.2). A similar proportion of fetuses with sonographic evidence of growth restriction develop AREDV. Thus Battaglia and associates [23] noted that 57% of the fetuses identified as being growth restricted by serial ultrasound measurements developed AEDV. Similarly, Pattinson and colleagues [22] observed that 48% of the fetuses suspected of severe growth restriction in their series developed umbilical

arterial AREDV. It is noteworthy that pregnancies complicated by both growth restriction and hypertension demonstrate a greater propensity for developing AREDV than those with either growth restriction or hypertension [24].

Fetal Asphyxia and Hypoxia

Fetal asphyxia and hypoxia can largely be attributed to fetal exposure to chronic hypoxic and asphyxial insult. The significant association between abnormal umbilical arterial Doppler indices and fetal hypoxia and acidosis is discussed in Chap. 24. It is apparent that the umbilical hemodynamics are affected more by asphyxia or acidosis and less by hypoxia. One of the most impressive pieces of evidence has been provided by Nicolaides and associates [32], who measured umbilical venous blood gases by cordocentesis in 59 fetuses suspected of growth restriction (abdominal circumference below the 5th percentile for gestational age). These fetuses also demonstrated absent umbilical arterial end-diastolic flow. In 88% of the cases the blood gases were abnormal; 42% of the fetuses were hypoxic, 37% asphyxiated, and 9% acidotic. Futhermore, there was a poor correlation between the degree of fetal smallness and acidosis or severity of hypoxia. Other investigators [33] have also observed this efficacy of absent end-diastolic flow and fetal acidosis. The AEDV identified acidosis with a sensitivity of 90%, specificity 92%, positive predictive value (PPV) 53%, and negative predictive value (NPV) 100%.

It is important to note that not all fetuses with AREDV are hypoxic or acidotic. Normal fetal blood gas values, however, do not ensure fetal well-being. Several investigators have noted progressive fetal deterioration and adverse perinatal outcome in fetuses with AREDV despite normal fetal acid-base status as determined by cordocentesis [34, 35]. It appears that progressive fetal hemodynamic decline, as manifested by umbilical arterial AREDV, is not necessarily related to fetal asphyxia and presents a serious threat to the fetus independent of fetal hypoxia or acidosis.

Cerebral Hemorrhage

One of the major concerns regarding chronic intrauterine asphyxia is its effect on the fetal brain. Although the risk of fetal brain damage due to prematurity and birth asphyxia has been well investigated, the role of antepartum asphyxia in fetal neurologic damage due to hypoxemic ischemic injury requires elucidation. One of the gross lesions from such injury is cerebral hemorrhage, which has been reported in association with AREDV. The main question is whether this association is independent of the preterm birth of these infants.

Table 25.4. Umbilical arterial absence of end-diastolic velocity and cerebral hemorrhage

Study, first author	Cerebral hemorrhage		p
	Control group	AREDV group	
Weiss [19][a]	3/47 (6%)	7/47 (15%)	>0.05
Pattinson [21][a]	3/16 (19%)	4/16 (25%)	>0.05
Karsdorp [24][b]	1/124 (1%)	27/168 (16%)	<0.02

[a] Case-control study, matched for gestational age.
[b] Corrected for gestational age by multiple logistic regression.

Weiss and associates [19] conducted a case-control study, comparing 47 fetuses with AREDV of the umbilical artery to 47 control fetuses matched for gestational age and with normal umbilical artery flow velocity waveforms. Fetuses with AREDV showed an increased incidence of cerebral hemorrhage (Table 25.4), but it was not statistically significant. Pattinson and associates [21] also performed a case-control study that showed no difference in cerebral hemorrhage between the 16 matched pairs of fetuses with the presence or absence of umbilical artery end-diastolic velocity. Both of the above findings were refuted by the much larger European Community Multicenter Study [24], which found a significantly increased incidence of severe cerebral hemorrhage in the fetuses with AREDV (Table 25.4). Although it was not a case-control study, the contribution of prematurity was corrected by multiple logistic regression. The odds for cerebral hemorrhage increased by 2.6 when the end-diastolic velocity was absent and by 4.8 when the velocity was reversed. It appears that in a pregnancy complicated with fetal growth restriction or hypotension (or both) AREDV may be associated with an increased risk of fetal cerebral hemorrhage. Such hemorrhagic complication may be related to hypoxemic ischemic injury induced by antepartum asphyxial insult and may be causally related to reperfusion. This consideration is important when critically examining the role of Doppler velocimetry of the fetal circulation as an indicator for antepartum asphyxia-related gross brain injury. Obviously, more work is needed in this area to clarify these issues.

Necrotizing Enterocolitis

Several investigators have reported on the increased risk of necrotizing enterocolitis in neonates who had suffered in utero from AREDV of the umbilical artery or the aorta. This serious complication is typically seen in premature neonates who experienced perinatal asphyxia, often secondary to the respiratory distress syndrome caused by pulmonic immaturity. Most infants with AREDV are delivered before 32 weeks

(Table 25.2) and are therefore more apt to develop these complications independent of the existence of AREDV.

The issue is again whether AREDV contributes to this complication independent of prematurity. Hackett and colleagues [4] investigated 82 consecutive cases of fetal growth restriction and identified 29 fetuses with an absence of end-diastolic frequencies in the fetal aorta. These fetuses were significantly more growth-restricted ($p<0.001$), delivered earlier ($p<0.001$), and were more apt to suffer perinatal death ($p<0.05$), necrotizing enterocolitis ($p<0.01$), or hemorrhage ($p<0.05$). Malcolm and coinvestigators [15] studied 25 high-risk pregnancies with AREDV in the umbilical artery and observed a highly significant increased risk of necrotizing enterocolitis in the morphologically normal fetuses (53%) compared with the controls (6%), who demonstrated umbilical artery end-diastolic flow in utero. This increased risk appeared to be independent of the degree of growth restriction, prematurity, or perinatal asphyxia. These findings were supported by those of McDonnell and colleagues [36], who noted that the infants who had AREDV were started on enteral feeds later, were more likely ro receive parenteral nutrition, and developed necrotizing enterocolitis more frequently than a gestationally matched control group.

The conclusion that AREDV may increase the risk of developing necrotizing enterocolitis independent of prematurity, however, was not supported by Karsdorp and associates [24] in their European multicenter research project. Although proportionately more infants with AREDV developed necrotizing enterocolitis, the difference was not statistically significant ($p=0.20$). Moreover, when corrected for gestational age, the absence or reversal of umbilical arterial end-diastolic flow did not influence the risk of respiratory distress syndrome or necrotizing enterocolitis of the neonate.

Other investigators have not confirmed the findings of Hackett [4] and Malcolm [15]. Kirsten and colleagues [37] evaluated 242 infants born to women with severe early preeclampsia (before 34 weeks' gestation). Sixty-eight (28%) of these infants had AEDV while 131 (54%) had normal umbilical artery Doppler flow velocities. Twenty infants developed definite (grade 2) and advanced (grade 3) necrotizing enterocolitis and 21 infants had suspected (grade 1) necrotizing enterocolitis. None of the infants with definite necrotizing enterocolitis had AEDV. In addition, the prevalence of suspected necrotizing enterocolitis between the infants with AEDV and the infants with normal umbilical artery Doppler flow studies was similar (48% versus 43%). Kirsten and associates postulated that the suspected necrotizing enterocolitis could have been a disturbance of the motility of the gastrointestinal tract as a result of the preeclampsia or the administration of magnesium sulfate to the mother and not necessarily necrotizing enterocolitis. Suspected necrotizing enterocolitis is a clinical diagnosis and, in the majority of cases, the condition improves with conservative management.

Hematologic Changes

Neonates with AREDV during fetal life are apt to develop thrombocytopenia and anemia. They may have a low platelet count at birth and are more likely to become significantly thrombocytopenic during the first week of life [36]. They are also at increased risk of being anemic. It has also been reported [24] that the infants with absent or reversed end-diastolic velocity had odds ratios of 3.0 and 6.1, respectively, for developing anemia compared to a control group of infants. The latter were growth-restricted and their mothers had hypertension, but they had umbilical arterial end-diastolic forward flow. The reason for developing anemia independent of prematurity and other known complications remains to be determined [24].

Baschat and colleagues [38] have also shown that AREDV in growth-restricted fetuses is associated with an increased risk of neonatal thrombocytopenia. In a study comparing 67 fetuses with elevated PI (more than two standard deviations above the mean) to 48 fetuses with AREDV, 22 of the 48 fetuses with AREDV had thrombocytopenia ($<100,000$ mm^3) compared to 3 of the 67 fetuses in the control group. Neonates with AREDV had a relative risk of 10.3 or a tenfold increase in the incidence of thrombocytopenia when compared to the control group. In addition, neonates with AREDV had a higher nucleated red blood cell count than the control group. High numbers of nucleated red blood cells in the umbilical cord have been associated with hypoxemia during intrauterine life and subsequent neurologic impairment.

Similarly, Axt-Fliedner and coinvestigators [39] reported an increased number of nucleated red blood cells in the umbilical artery at birth in growth–restricted neonates with AREDV during fetal life when compared to neonates with elevated Doppler studies. Moreover, the nucleated red blood cells persisted in the neonatal circulation for a longer period of time in the neonates with AREDV. Nucleated red blood cells are immature erythrocytes. They are seen in variable numbers in the newborn circulation. Although an increased number of nucleated red blood cells has been attributed to increased erythropoiesis in the fetal liver as a result of chronic hypoxemia, these studies [38, 39] have shown that the neonates with a higher number of nucleated red blood cells have lower hematocrits, hemoglobin levels, and platelet counts that the other neonates studied.

Hypoglycemia

Infants with AREDV become hypoglycemic more frequently, and it cannot be fully attributable to preterm gestational age or IUGR. The odds for developing hypoglycemia is 5.0 compared to growth-compromised fetuses without AREDV [24]. The reason for this metabolic problem remains unclear.

Neurodevelopmental Sequelae

Any examination of the efficacy of umbilical arterial AREDV for fetal prognostication must go beyond looking for gross cerebral lesions (e.g., hemorrhage) and encompass immediate and long-term neurologic performance. Furthermore, its imperative that neurologic outcome measures should be extended to include not only moderate to severe neurologic deficits but also more subtle compromises in cognitive and motor performance. Although there it is a paucity of information in this area, a few preliminary reports are available concerning the neurodevelopmental significance of AREDV. Weiss and associates [19] observed in their case-control study (see above) an increase in abnormal neurologic signs in the AREDV group. The pediatric neurologic assessment was blinded to the fetal Doppler results. The adverse signs included persistent hyperreflexia, hypo- or hypertonia, seizures, and cerebral palsy. Fourteen fetuses in the index group (30%) and three fetuses in the control group (6%) demonstrated abnormal neurologic signs at the time of discharge. The results were statistically significant ($p < 0.006$).

In a more comprehensive and long-term investigation, Valcamonico and associates [40] conducted a cohort study in a group of 31 fetuses with IUGR and AREDV in the umbilical artery and 40 growth-restricted fetuses with detectable diastolic flow in the umbilical artery divided into two control groups. The survivors of the perinatal period were followed for a mean of 18 months (range 12–24 months). Twenty surviving neonates with AREDV demonstrated a greater risk of permanent neurologic sequelae (35% versus 0% and 12%) than the two control groups. Although the results suggest that growth-compromised fetuses with AREDV are at a significant risk of sustaining long-term permanent neurologic damage, it may be premature to draw a definitive conclusion on the neurodevelopmental significance of AREDV. This hesitation is based on such observations as those of Pillai and James [41], who performed serial behavioral observations in four severely growth-restricted singleton fetuses who had persistent AREDV for 2–9 weeks. Comparison with 45 low-risk singleton fetuses at comparable gestations revealed no significant differences in the development of behavioral cycles, the proportion of time spent in quiet cycles, or the amount of fetal breathing. The heart rate pattern remained normal in all the fetuses. Kirsten and associates [42a] evaluated the neurodevelopmental outcome of a group of infants of 242 women with severe early preeclampsia (<34 weeks). Sixty-eight of these women had neonates with AEDV in fetal life. In total, 193 infants, 51 with AEDV, survived to hospital discharge and were evaluated every 6 months until 48 months of age. In all, 126 infants were assessed at 24 months of age. The infants with AEDV scored significantly lower in the performance subscale compared to the infants who had normal or elevated umbilical artery flow studies. In total, 157 infants were assessed at 48 months of age. No differences were noted in developmental quotients, verbal and nonverbal quotients, or in any of the nonverbal intelligence subscales based on umbilical artery flow velocities. Multiple regression analysis showed that socioeconomic status was significantly associated with lower developmental quotients. Cerebral palsy was identified in four of the infants evaluated; AEDV was not associated with cerebral palsy. The mean developmental quotient at 24 and at 48 months of age was not associated with AEDV. It appears that prenatal neurobehavioral development is not necessarily compromised even by long-term AREDV. Although the above investigations did not utilize similar or even comparable methods of neurologic assessment, it is obvious that additional in-depth and long-term investigations are necessary to reconcile these apparently contradictory findings and to elucidate their implications for clinical management.

See Chap. 12 for further discussions on Doppler ultrasound and neurological outcomes.

Maternal Hypertension and Absent End-Diastolic Velocity

The most frequent maternal complications seen in conjunction with AREDV are the various types of hypertensive disorders encountered during pregnancy, with a preponderance of primary preeclampsia and preeclampsia superimposed on chronic hypertensive disease. The frequency with which hypertension is associated with AREDV varies from 40% to 70%. On the other hand, the proportion of hypertensive mothers who develop umbilical artery AREDV may be as high as 36% [22]. It is noteworthy that when pregnancy is complicated with hypertension alone the risk of developing AREDV is significantly lower than when fetal growth restriction complicates hypertension. This risk was quantified by Karsdorp and his colleagues [24], who noted that in comparison with hypertension the odds ratio for developing AREDV was 3.1 with growth restriction alone and 7.4 when hypertension was complicated by growth restriction.

Other maternal disorders associated with the development of AREDV in the umbilical artery include systemic lupus erythematosus and diabetes mellitus of long duration with vasculopathy. Most such cases are also complicated by fetal growth restriction or hypertension.

Reappearance of End-Diastolic Velocity

Once AREDV develops in the umbilical artery, it is usually regarded as a nonreversible phenomenon during the course of progressive fetal decompensation. Several investigators, however, have reported apparent improvement of the hemodynamic situation, as indicated by reappearance of forward flow during the umbilical artery end-diastolic phase. Hanretty and colleagues [42b] were among the first to report the reappearance in a case report where the mother was treated for hypertension. Subsequently, Brar and Platt [10] reported improvement of the end-diastolic velocity in 5 of 31 cases of AREDV followed closely during hospitalization. The improved fetuses had better perinatal outcome than those with continuing AREDV. This observation received support from others. Sengupta and associates [16] used prospective conservative management (bed rest and fetal surveillance) in pregnancies complicated by AREDV and found those who improved had a better outcome. Bell and associates [20] used retrospective data analysis and also found improved outcome. The above three studies noted the reappearance of end-diastolic velocity in 19.0%–51.5% cases of AREDV and a consequent increase in the diagnosis-delivery interval by 11–37 days, gestational age by 2–4 weeks, and birth weight by 400–1,400 g. These results, particularly the frequency of reappearance and the impressive improvements in the perinatal outcome noted in one of the studies [20], are remarkable, are not encountered in common experience, and require corroboration.

The study design of Karsdorp and associates [43] differed from those described above. Theirs was a controlled intervention study with seven patients in each arm. The study group received daily volume expansion in addition to management by bed rest and antihypertensive medications, which were also used in the control group. The Doppler waveform improved in the volume-expansion group, which demonstrated statistically significant improved survival (five of seven in the study and one of seven in the control group, $p < 0.05$). There were no significant differences between the groups with regard to birth weight or gestational age. Although the results are encouraging, this investigation should be regarded as preliminary because of the lack of randomization and

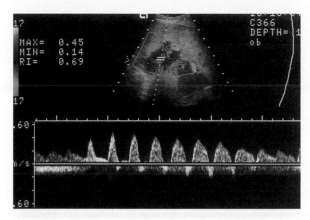

Fig. 25.5. Doppler sonogram of the umbilical artery showing transient absence and reversal of end-diastolic velocity followed by prompt recovery of a discordant twin

AREDV and Other Emergent Signs of Fetal Compromise

The homeostatic significance of absent end-diastolic velocity in relation to alterations in other components of the fetal circulation and other parameters of fetal well-being needs clarification. Some of these issues, particularly those related to the diagnostic efficacy of fetal Doppler indices, are discussed in Chap. 24. Although some degree of overlap is inevitable, the focus of this chapter is specifically on the umbilical arterial AREDV. Reports provide considerable insight in this area. Teyssier et al. [45] observed in an animal model a hierarchic sequence in the decline of the end-diastolic flow when fetoplacental vascular resistance increased; flow in the aortic isthmus was affected first, followed by flow in the descending aorta and the umbilical artery. Preliminary clinical observations tend to confirm this sequence [46].

Bekedam and associates [13] performed longitudinal measurements of the umbilical arterial PI in 29 growth-restricted fetuses with antepartum late heart rate decelerations. In 17 of these fetuses (59%), AEDV preceded the occurrence of decelerations, with a median interval of 12 days. Arduini and colleagues [47] evaluated 37 fetuses without structural and chromosomal abnormalities regarding the various maternal and fetal factors that affect the time interval between the occurrence of AEDV in the umbilical artery and either the development of abnormal fetal heart rate patterns or delivery. The interval between the first occurrence of umbilical arterial AEDV and delivery ranged from 1 to 26 days. Multivariate analysis revealed that gestational age, the presence of hypertension, and the appearance of umbilical venous pulsation are the principal determinants of this time interval. Finally, Weiner and associates [48] studied hemodynamic changes in the middle cerebral artery and the aortic and pulmonic outflow tracts, correlating these changes with the computerized fetal heart rate pattern in fetuses with AREDV in the umbilical artery. They observed that when the middle cerebral artery began to lose its compensatory vasodilatation other ominous fetal cardiovascular signs emerged, including decreases in the left cardiac output ($p < 0.05$) and the fetal heart rate long-term variability (< 30 ms) and the occurrence of repetitive fetal heart rate decelerations. These observations contribute to elucidation of the evolving cardiovascular responses to progressive fetal decompensation and should lead to the development of more effective fetal surveillance and clinical intervention.

the small sample size. As the authors suggested, randomized trials should be conducted to confirm their observations.

It should be recognized that the appearance of AREDV does not necessarily lead to immediate fetal demise. Days to weeks may pass before the emergence of other ominous signs of fetal jeopardy necessitating delivery. In some cases the end-diastolic velocity returns, and the fetal risk is diminished, although it is highly unlikely that this occurrence is as frequent as some investigators have reported. On rare occasions, apparently normal waveforms may change to the ominous pattern of disappearance and reversal of the end-diastolic flow, returning quickly to the previous pattern; we observed this pattern in a discordant twin (Fig. 25.5). Although the hemodynamic mechanism of this phenomenon remains to be elucidated, the fetus eventually developed persistent AREDV.

Variable end-diastolic velocity in the umbilical artery of a donor fetus with twin-twin transfusion syndrome has been documented [44]. The umbilical artery end-diastolic velocity in the donor fluctuated between positive, absent, and reversed. Eventually the fetus was delivered at 28 weeks because of fetal distress of the donor. A velamentous cord insertion, suspected during the ultrasound evaluation, was confirmed. The significance of finding variable end-diastolic velocity is unknown at this time.

Finally, it should be emphasized that for reliable assessment of the end-diastolic velocity an appropriate Doppler procedure must be used, ensuring a low filter setting and a consistent sampling site in the cord if a pulsed-wave duplex system is used. The use of a high, inconsistent filter setting or different sampling sites can lead to erroneous diagnosis of disappearance and reappearance of the end-diastolic frequency.

Recently, Williams and associates [49] conducted a prospective randomized study where women who had been referred to their antepartum fetal testing unit because of perceived increased fetal risk were randomized to either umbilical artery Doppler studies or nonstress testing as a screening test of fetal well-being. In this investigation, normal studies were repeated with the same technique as initially assigned. Women with umbilical artery S/D ratios over the 90th percentile or equivocal nonstress testing were subjected to an additional test, the amniotic fluid index. When the amniotic fluid index was below the 5th percentile, the S/D ratio had AREDV, or when the nonstress test was abnormal, induction and delivery were recommended. More women in the Doppler group than in the nonstress group underwent induction of labor (4.8% versus 1.9%, $p < 0.005$). The main outcome variable studied was the presence of peripartum morbidity and was measured by the cesarean delivery rate for fetal distress in labor. The incidence of cesarean delivery for fetal distress was lower in the Doppler group compared with the nonstress group (4.6% versus 8.7%, $p < 0.006$). The women with hypertension and intrauterine growth restriction sustained the greatest reduction in cesarean delivery for fetal distress. The neonatal morbidity between the two groups was similar.

Some investigators have obtained more information from the umbilical artery waveforms in cases of reverse end-diastolic flow. This has been done to try to improve the timing of the delivery and to predict the outcome of the pregnancy. Brodszki and associates [50] measured the highest amplitude and the area below the maximum velocity curve of forward and reverse flow; and they also measured the duration of forward and reverse flow in 44 fetuses with reverse end-diastolic flow. They calculated three ratios: (1) the ratio of the highest amplitude of the forward and reverse flow, (2) the ratio of the area of the forward and reverse flow, and (3) the ratio of the duration of the forward and reverse flow. Then, they established cut-off values for each ratio for the prediction of perinatal death. The ratio of the highest amplitude of the forward and reverse flow and the ratio of the area of forward and reverse flow had the best capacity to predict perinatal death. They found that survivors had higher ratios than the nonsurvivors did. In addition, more fetuses with ratios below the established cut-off values had pulsations in the venous system. The calculation of these ratios may provide additional information when these fetuses are evaluated.

Summary

It is apparent from cumulative experience that the end-diagnostic component of the umbilical arterial Doppler waveform is of crucial importance for fetal prognostication. AREDV is known to be associated with an unusually adverse perinatal outcome. Most remarkably, these infants suffer from high perinatal mortality and morbidity rates and demonstrate an increased frequency of malformations and chromosomal abnormalities, with a predominance of trisomies 13, 18, and 21. Most infants with AREDV require intensive care. Furthermore, the risk of cerebral hemorrhage, anemia, and hypoglycemia is increased. It has been observed, however, that absent end-diastolic flow may improve, although often only transiently, and that weeks or more may elapse before the fetus shows additional evidence of compromise. Obviously, the presence of absent end-diastolic flow should warn the physician of significantly increased fetal risk. Appropriate surveillance measures should be immediately undertaken. If the pregnancy is significantly preterm, consideration for delivery should include additional signs of fetal compromise. A more aggressive approach should be taken to ensure fetal maturity. If fetal anomalies are present or AEDV cannot be explained by pregnancy complications such as preeclampsia, then fetal karyotype should also be determined to rule out lethal aneuploidies. Although the benefits of emergency delivery for this phenomenon remain controversial, randomized clinical trials have shown improved outcome from intervention in pregnancies with absent end-diastolic velocity. This subject is discussed comprehensively in Chap. 26.

References

1. Rochelson B, Schulman H, Framakides G et al (1987) The significance of absent end-diastolic velocity in umbilical artery velocity waveforms. Am J Obstet Gynecol 156:1213–1218

2. Woo JS, Liang ST, Lo RL (1987) Significance of an absent or reversed end diastolic flow in Doppler umbilical artery waveforms. J Ultrasound Med 6:291–297

3. Reuwer PJ, Sijmons EA, Rietman GW, van Tiel MW, Bruines HW (1987) Intrauterine growth retardation: prediction of perinatal distress by Doppler ultrasound. Lancet 2:415–418

4. Hackett GA, Campbell S, Gamsu H, Cohen-Overbeek T, Pearce JM (1987) Doppler studies in the growth retarded fetus and prediction of neonatal necrotising enterocolitis, haemorrhage, and neonatal morbidity. BMJ 294:13–16

5. Arabin B, Siebert M, Jimenez E, Saling E (1988) Obstetical characteristics of a loss of end-diastolic velocities in the fetal aorta and/or umbilical artery using Doppler ultrasound. Gynecol Obstet Invest 25:173–180

6. Hsieh FJ, Chang FM, Ko TM, Chen HY, Chen YP (1988) Umbilical artery flow velocity waveforms in fetuses dying with congenital anomalies. Br J Obstet Gynaecol 95:478–482

7. Johnstone FD, Haddad NG, Hoskins P et al (1988) Umbilical artery Doppler flow velocity waveform: the outcome of pregnancies with absent end diastolic flow. Eur J Obstet Gynecol Reprod Biol 28:171–178

8. Brar HS, Platt LD (1988) Reverse end-diastolic flow velocity on umbilical artery velocimetry in high-risk pregnancies: an ominous finding with adverse pregnancy outcome. Am J Obstet Gynecol 159:559–561

9. Tyrrell S, Obaid AH, Lilford RJ (1989) Umbilical artery Doppler velocimetry as a predictor of fetal hypoxia and acidosis at birth. Obstet Gynecol 74:332–337

10. Brar HS, Platt LD (1989) Antepartum improvement of abnormal umbilical artery velocimetry: does it occur? Am J Obstet Gynecol 160:36–39

11. Divon MY, Girz BA, Lieblich R, Langer O (1989) Clinical management of the fetus with markedly diminished umbilical artery end-diastolic flow. Am J Obstet Gynecol 161:1523–1527

12. McParland P, Steel S, Pearce JM (1990) The clinical implications of absent or reversed end-diastolic frequencies in umbilical artery flow velocity waveforms. Eur J Obstet Gynecol Reprod Biol 37:15–23

13. Bekedam DJ, Visser GH, van der Zee AG, Snijders RJ, Poelmann-Weesjes G (1990) Abnormal velocity waveforms of the umbilical artery in growth retarded fetuses: relationship to antepartum late heart rate decelerations and outcome. Early Hum Dev 24:79–89

14. Huneke B, Carstensen MH, Schroder HJ, Gunther M (1991) Perinatal outcome in fetuses with loss of end-diastolic blood flow velocities in the descending aorta and/or umbilical arteries. Gynecol Obstet Invest 32: 167–172

15. Malcolm G, Ellwood D, Devonald K, Beilby R, Henderson-Smart D (1991) Absent or reversed end diastolic flow velocity in the umbilical artery and necrotising enterocolitis. Arch Dis Child 66:805–807

16. Sengupta S, Harrigan JT, Rosenberg JC, Davis SE, Knuppel RA (1991) Perinatal outcome following improvement of abnormal umbilical artery velocimetry. Obstet Gynecol 78:1062–1066

17. Wenstrom KD, Weiner CP, Williamson RA (1991) Diverse maternal and fetal pathology associated with absent diastolic flow in the umbilical artery of high-risk fetuses. Obstet Gynecol 77:374–378

18. Schmidt W, Ruhle W, Ertan AK, Boos R, Gnirs J (1991) Doppler ultrasonography – perinatal data in cases with end-diastolic block and reverse flow. Geburtshilfe Frauenheilk 51:288–292

19. Weiss E, Ulrich S, Berle P (1992) Condition at birth of infants with previously absent or reverse umbilical artery end-diastolic flow velocities. Arch Gynecol Obstet 252:37–43

20. Bell JG, Ludomirsky A, Bottalico J, Weiner S (1992) The effect of improvement of umbilical artery absent end-diastolic velocity on perinatal outcome. Am J Obstet Gynecol 167:1015–1020

21. Pattinson RC, Hope P, Imhoff R et al (1993) Obstetric and neonatal outcome in fetuses with absent end-diastolic velocities of the umbilical artery: a case-controlled study. Am J Perinatol 10:135–138

22. Pattinson RC, Odendaal HJ, Kirsten G (1993) The relationship between absent end-diastolic velocities of the umbilical artery and perinatal mortality and morbidity. Early Hum Dev 33:61–69

23. Battaglia C, Artini PG, Galli PA et al (1993) Absent or reversed end-diastolic flow in umbilical artery and severe intrauterine growth retardation: an ominous association. Acta Obstet Gynecol Scand 72:167–171

24. Karsdorp VH, van Vugt JM, van Geijn HP et al (1994) Clinical significance of absent or reversed end diastolic velocity waveforms in umbilical artery. Lancet 344: 1664–1668

25. Rizzo G, Pietropolli A, Capponi A, Arduini D, Romanini CC (1994) Chromosomal abnormalities in fetuses with absent end-diastolic velocity in umbilical artery: analysis of risk factors for an abnormal karyotype. Am J Obstet Gynecol 171:827–831

26. Poulain P, Palaric JC, Milon J et al (1994) Absent end diastolic flow of umbilical artery Doppler: pregnancy outcome in 62 cases. Eur J Obstet Gynecol Reprod Biol 53:115–119

27. Beattie RB, Dornan JC (1989) Antenatal screening for intrauterine growth retardation with umbilical artery Doppler ultrasonography. BMJ 298:631–635

28. Snijders RJ, Sherrod C, Gosden CM, Nicolaides KH (1993) Fetal growth retardation: associated malformations and chromosomal abnormalities. Am J Obstet Gynecol 168:547–555

29. Rochelson B, Kaplan C, Guzman E et al (1990) A quantitative analysis of placental vasculature in the third-trimester fetus with autosomal trisomy. Obstet Gynecol 75:59–63

30. Borrell A, Martinez JM, Farre MT, Azulay M, Cararach V, Fortuny A (2001) Reversed end-diastolic flow in first-trimester umbilical artery: an ominous new sign for fetal outcome. Am J Obstet Gynecol 185:204–207

31. Martinez JM, Antolin E, Borrell A, Puerto B, Casals E, Ojuel J, Fortuny A (1997) Umbilical Doppler velocimetry in fetuses with trisomy 18 at 10–18 weeks' gestation. Prenatal Diagnosis 17:319–322

32. Nicolaides KH, Bilardo CM, Soothill PW, Campbell S (1988) Absence of end-diastolic frequencies in umbilical artery: a sign of fetal hypoxia and acidosis. BMJ 297:1026–1027

33. Tyrrell S, Obaid AH, Lilford RJ (1989) Umbilical artery Doppler velocimetry as a predictor of fetal hypoxia and acidosis at birth. Obstet Gynecol 74:332–337

34. Ashmead GG, Lazebnik N, Ashmead JW, Stepanchak W, Mann LI (1993) Normal blood gases in fetuses with absence of end-distolic umbilical artery velocity. Am J Perinatol 10:67–70

35. Warren W, Ronkin S, Chayen B, Needleman L, Wapne RJ (1989) Absence of end-diastolic umbilical artery blood flow predicts poor fetal outcome despite normal blood gases. Am J Obstet Gynecol 160:197

36. McDonnell M, Serra-Serra V, Gaffney G, Redman CW, Hope PL (1994) Neonatal outcome after pregnancy complicated by abnormal velocity waveforms in the umbilical artery. Arch Dis Child 70:F84–89

37. Kirsten GF, van Zyl N, Smith M, Odendaal H (1999) Necrotizing enterocolitis in infants born to women with severe early preeclampsia and absent end-diastolic umbilical artery Doppler flow velocity waveforms. Am J Perinat 16:309–314

38. Baschat AA, Gembruch U, Reiss I, Gornter L, Weiner CP, Harman CR (2000) Absent umbilical artery end-diastolic velocity in growth-restricted fetuses: a risk factor for neonatal thrombocytopenia. Obstet Gynecol 96:162–166

39. Axt-Fliedner R, Hendrik HJ, Schmidt W (2002) Nucleated red blood cell counts in growth-restricted neonates with absent or reversed-end-diastolic umbilical artery velocity. Clin Exp Obst Gyn 29:242–246

40. Valcamonico A, Danti L, Frusca T et al (1994) Absent end-diastolic velocity in umbilical artery: risk of neonatal morbidity and brain damage. Am J Obstet Gynecol 170:796–891

41. Pillai M, James D (1991) Continuation of normal neurobehavioural development in fetuses with absent umbilical arterial end diastolic velocities. Br J Obstet Gynaecol 98:277–281

42a. Hanretty KP, Whittle MJ, Rubin PC (1988) Reappearance of end-diastolic velocity in a pregnancy complicated by severe pregnancy-induced hypertension. Am J Obstet Gynecol 158:1123–1124

42b. Kirsten GF, van Zyl JI, van Zijl F, Maritz JS, Odendaal HJ (2000) Infants of women with severe early preeclampsia: the effect of absent end-diastolic umbilical artery Doppler flow velocities on neurodevelopmental outcome. Acta Paediatr 89:566–570

43. Karsdorp VH, van Vugt JM, Dekker GA, van Geijn HP (1992) Reappearance of end-diastolic velocities in the umbilical artery following maternal volume expansion: a preliminary study. Obstet Gynecol 80:679–683

44. Kush ML, Jenkins CB, Baschat AA (2003) Variable umbilical artery end-diastolic velocity: a possible sign of velamentous cord insertion in monochorionic gestation. Ultrasound Obstet Gynecol 21:95–96

45. Teyssier G, Fouron JC, Maroto D, Sonesson SE, Bonnin P (1993) Blood flow velocity in the fetal aortic isthmus: a sensitive indicator of changes in systemic peripheral resistance. I. Experimental studies. J Matern Fetal Invest 3:213–218

46. Fouron JC, Teyssier G, Bonnin P et al (1993) Blood flow velocity in the fetal aortic isthmus: a sensitive indicator of changes in systemic peripheral resistances. II. Preliminary observations. J Matern Fetal Invest 3:219–224

47. Arduini D, Rizzo G, Romanini C (1993) The development of abnormal heart rate patterns after absent end-diastolic velocity in umbilical artery: analysis of risk factors. Am J Obstet Gynecol 168:43–50

48. Weiner Z, Farmakides G, Schulman H, Penny B (1994) Central and peripheral hemodynamic changes in fetuses with absent end-diastolic velocity in umbilical artery; correlation with computerized fetal heart rate pattern. Am J Obstet Gynecol 170:509–515

49. Williams KP, Farquharson DF, Bebbington M, Dansereau J, Galerneau F, Wilson RD, Shaw D, Kent N (2003) Screening for fetal well-being in a high-risk pregnant population comparing the nonstress test with umbilical artery Doppler velocimetry: a randomized controlled clinical trial. Am J Obstet Gynecol 188:1366–1371

50. Brodszki J, Hernandez-Andrade E, Gudmundsson S, Dubiel M, Mandruzzato GP, Laurini R, Maršál K (2002) Can the degree of retrograde diastolic flow in abnormal umbilical artery flow velocity waveforms predict pregnancy outcome? Ultrasound Obstet Gynecol 19:229–234

Doppler Velocimetry for Fetal Surveillance: Randomized Clinical Trials and Implications for Practice

Dev Maulik, Reinaldo Figueroa

The cumulative clinical evidence indicates that Doppler velocimetry of the fetal circulation is an effective tool for recognizing fetal compromise in high-risk pregnancies. It has prompted many to propose its introduction as a standard for fetal surveillance. However, such enthusiasm must be tempered by a critical appraisal of the efficacy and benefits of the technique. Introduction of a new diagnostic test involves the sequential and often parallel research process of generating evidence that transforms the promises of a new technique into an effective diagnostic tool that delivers measurable benefits (Fig. 26.1).

The process begins with recognition of the potential of a new technology to measure a clinically relevant variable, followed by demonstration of the feasibility of using the technology. This phase is followed by the collection and analysis of normative data on the test, which includes determining the physiologic variations in the test value and establishing its range under normal circumstances. Any possible association between the test and the disease process is then investigated. The next step involves studying the diagnostic efficacy of the test for discriminating between the diseased and nondiseased states. Often a test is introduced into clinical practice at this stage based on the affirmative demonstration of its diagnostic efficacy. However, the diagnostic efficacy may not translate into any tangible benefit for the patient. Indeed, a new test may not be more beneficial than the existing tests; its introduction may unnecessarily increase the cost of care, and it may even be detrimental. It is imperative therefore to demonstrate without bias that utilization of the test improves clinical outcome, which can be accomplished by randomized clinical trials. It is regrettable that most modalities of fetal surveillance in current practice are not based on such evidence.

It is encouraging to note that with regard to Doppler velocimetry for fetal surveillance, 21 clinical trials [1–21] have been fully reported from 1987 until 2003 in the peer-reviewed literature. In addition, during that period limited information was available on five published or presented randomized trials comprising two review articles [2, 22] and three abstracts [23–25]. All the studies evaluated umbilical arterial velocimetry; a few also used uterine arterial velocimetry. There have been ongoing meta-analyses of these studies as they became available first in the Oxford Perinatal Database and subsequently in the Cochrane Center electronic publications. The initial comprehensive meta-analysis by Alfirevic and Neilson [26] was published in 1995. Since that initial meta-analysis the data have been reanalyzed various times evaluating high- and low-risk pregnancies separately, or evaluating high-risk pregnancies with well-defined candidates (IUGR, hypertension) [27–31]. The original studies are comprehensively reviewed here, and the implications of their findings on the clinical practice of high-risk obstetrics are discussed. The review process included both the traditional and meta-analytic approaches.

Doppler Randomized Trials: A Summary

The essential features of the 21 published randomized trials are listed in Table 26.1 and are summarized below both individually and as a group. The sequence is according to the chronology of their publication.

Trudinger and associates [1] were the first to report a randomized trial on umbilical arterial Doppler velocimetry. The aim was to assess the impact of

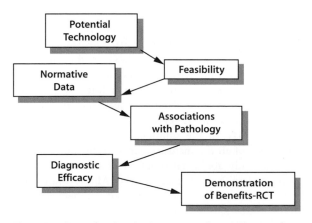

Fig. 26.1. Steps for developing a new diagnostic test, from the feasibility study to the introduction to clinical practice

Table 26.1. Randomized trials of Doppler ultrasonography for fetal surveillance

First Author, Year (Reference)	Population	Doppler Index*	Doppler in Controls	Treatment Protocol	Clinical Benefits**
Trudinger, 1987 (1)	300 High risk	UA S/D	Concealed	No	Yes
Tyrrell, 1990 (3)	500 High risk	UA S/D Ut S/D	Selective	No	Yes
Hofmeyr, 1991 (4)	897 High risk	UA S/D	Selective	No	No
Newnham, 1991 (5)	505 High risk	UA S/D Ut S/D	Concealed	No	No
Almstrom, 1992 (6)	426 High risk	UA BFC	No Doppler	Yes	Yes
Davies, 1992 (7)	2475 Unselected	UA S/D Ut S/D	No Doppler	No	No
Mason, 1993 (8)	2025 Unselected	UA S/D	No Doppler	No	No
Johnstone, 1993 (9)	2289 High risk	UA RI	No Doppler	No	No
Newnham, 1993 (10)	2834 Unselected	UA S/D Ut S/D	Selective	No	No
Omtzigt, 1994 (11)	1598 Unselected	UA S/D	No Doppler	Yes	Yes
Pattinson, 1994 (12)	212 High risk	UA S/D	Concealed	Yes	Yes
Whittle, 1994 (13)	2986 Unselected	UA S/D	Concealed	No	Yes
Nienhuis, 1997 (14)	150 High risk	UA PI	Concealed	Limited	No
Doppler French Study Group, 1997 (15)	4187 Low risk	UA RI	No Doppler	No	No
Haley, 1997 (16)	150 High risk	UA S/D	No Doppler	Yes	No
Ott, 1998 (17)	665 High risk	Ratio of UA S/D & MCA S/D	UA S/D only in 11%	No	Yes
McCowan, 2000 (18)	167 High risk	UA RI	MCA RI Ut A RI	No	No
Williams, 2003 (19)	1340 High risk	UA S/D	No	Yes	Yes
GRIT Group, 2003 (20)	547 High risk	UA EDV	Post-test randomization	Yes	No
Giles, 2003 (21)	526 Twins	UA S/D	No Doppler	Yes	No

* BFC = blood flow classes; EDV = end diastolic flow velocity; MCA = middle cerebral artery; PI = pulsatility index; RI = resistance index; S/D = systolic/diastolic ratio; UA = umbilical artery; Ut = uterine artery.
** Clinical benefits refer to clinical outcomes only.

using this approach for identifying potential fetal compromise on the timing of delivery and obstetric intervention. Despite the randomization, more patients were assigned to the control group ($n = 167$) than to the study group ($n = 133$). The Doppler results were revealed for the study group, and no specific management protocol was assigned to the providers. Information on the incidence of absent end-diastolic velocity (AEDV) is not given in this paper. A significant reduction was noted in the incidence of intrapartum fetal distress after spontaneous onset of labor (study group 0.8%, control group 4.9%, $p < 0.05$) and of emergency cesarean section (study group 13%, control group 23%, $p < 0.05$).

MacParland and Pierce [2] reported briefly a randomized trial in a review article involving 509 patients. The complete study was not published. The preliminary report showed improved outcomes. However, serious allegations on the credibility of one of the authors led to the exclusion of the study from any further considerations.

Tyrrell et al. [3] described a randomized comparison of the effect of routine versus highly selected use of umbilical and uterine arterial Doppler ultrasonography and the biophysical profile on gestational age at delivery, the rate of obstetric intervention, and short-term neonatal morbidity in 500 pregnant women (study group 250, control group 250) at risk for fetal growth restriction and fetal death. The investigators used a modified version of the biophysical profile and devised a scoring system for the Doppler result incorporating the umbilical arterial systolic/diastolic (S/D) ratio and the uterine arterial resistance index (RI). The test results were available to the physician apparently with no defined intervention protocol. The study group mothers underwent a total of 902 biophysical profiles and Doppler measurements, which were performed in 12 patients in the control group (4.8%). AEDV in the umbilical artery was found in only 2.7% of all the measurements in the study group. A persistently abnormal biophysical score was always associated with umbilical arterial AEDV. Main outcome measures were gestational age at delivery, obstetric intervention rates, and short-term neonatal morbidity. The mean gestational age at induction of labor and the intervention rates were similar in the two groups. However, in the study group a significant decrease was noted in low 5-min Apgar scores [odds ratio (OR) 0.24; 95% confidence interval (CI) 0.06–0.86] and serious neonatal morbidity (OR 0.12, CI 0.02–0.98). The authors concluded that access to Doppler velocimetry improves the efficacy of fetal surveillance.

Hofmeyr and associates [4] conducted a randomized trial of umbilical arterial Doppler velocimetry in 897 women (Doppler group 438, control group 459). The objective was to determine the impact of Doppler assessment on reducing the need for fetal heart rate (FHR) monitoring and on the time required for fetal testing. In the study group initial assessment was by umbilical arterial resistance index (RI) determination, and in the fetal heart rate (FHR) group it was done by computerized FHR analysis. In the Doppler group 66% underwent FHR monitoring, whereas 39% of the control (FHR) group underwent Doppler velocimetry. The study design permitted such additional evaluation using the nonallocated method based on broad criteria of fetal risk. The study group and the control group were found to be comparable. It was observed that the primary Doppler screening did not reduce the time needed for fetal assessment. There were no significant differences in perinatal outcome between the groups, except that emergency cesarean sections were less frequent in the Doppler group than in the control group (14% versus 20%, $p < 0.05$; OR 0.69, CI 0.49–0.98).

Newnham and associates [5] investigated whether the introduction of umbilical and uterine Doppler assessment into an ultrasonography department of a tertiary level hospital reduces neonatal morbidity and improves obstetric management. The population consisted of 505 women (study group 254, control group 251) with pregnancy complications referred for fetal ultrasonographic investigation during the third trimester. Results were revealed to patients and clinicians. The main outcome measure was the duration of neonatal stay in the hospital; other measures of the perinatal outcome included the number of examinations, the type of FHR monitoring, obstetric interventions, frequency of fetal distress, birth weight, Apgar score, and the need for neonatal intensive care. Umbilical arterial Doppler revealed a 2.9% incidence of AEDV; noteworthy is the high-pass filter setting of 280 Hz, which is considered too high and might have generated false-positive results. The introduction of Doppler waveform studies did not reduce neonatal morbidity and therefore did not change the duration of neonatal hospitalization. Compared to the control group, the Doppler group showed an increase in the 1-min Apgar score (32% versus 22%, respectively) and 5-min Apgar score (3.3% versus 2.6%, respectively), but these differences were not significant. The

study group patients had fewer contraction stress tests and less likelihood of antepartum fetal distress; they were, however, more prone to fetal distress after induction of labor leading to emergency cesarean section. Again, none of these differences was significant.

Davies et al. [7] reported a randomized trial in a general obstetric population to assess the effect on primary management and outcome of routine Doppler velocimetry. The study group of 1,246 patients were allocated to routine umbilical and uterine artery Doppler ultrasound examinations, which were done first at 19–22 weeks' gestation and monthly thereafter if the pregnancy was considered high risk ($n = 192$) or once at 32 weeks if considered low risk ($n = 1,054$). The control group consisted of 1,229 women who received standard, antenatal care without Doppler testing. Doppler sonography was performed in 1.2% of the control group. The frequency of AEDV was low (0.1%). The study and control groups were comparable in terms of the frequency of antenatal admissions, cardiotocographs, gestational age at delivery, mode of delivery, frequency of deliveries with fetal distress, the need for resuscitation, and admission to the neonatal intensive care unit (NICU). The authors failed to demonstrate any improvement in neonatal outcome after routine Doppler ultrasound screening of a general obstetric population. However, the Doppler group experienced significantly more perinatal deaths. Abnormal umbilical arterial Doppler results occurred in 1 of 11 normally formed stillborn infants and in none of the four normally formed neonates who died after 24 weeks' gestation. Although the incidence of stillbirths was increased in the Doppler group, the difference from controls was not significant [16 versus 9; relative risk (RR) 1.75, 95% CI 0.78–3.95]. When corrected for malformations, the perinatal death rate was significantly higher in the Doppler group (16 versus 4; RR 3.95, 95% CI 1.32–11.77). This factor obviously remains a matter of concern and requires clarification. Interestingly, this trial is the only randomized one where such an adverse effect was observed.

In a Swedish multicenter trial, Almstrom and associates [6, 23] compared umbilical arterial Doppler velocimetry with antepartum cardiotocography (CTG) in 426 pregnant women (Doppler group 214, CTG group 212) with fetuses found to be small for gestational age (SGA) (<2 SD) on ultrasound examination at 31 weeks' gestation or later. The objective was to investigate whether the Doppler technique was superior to CTG reducing fetal mortality in these pregnancies. This study had a predefined protocol that was described in the report. In the control group, 16 (7.5%) had abnormal CTG. In the study group, 4 (1.8%) had blood flow class III (AEDV). Interestingly, 14% of the Doppler group also underwent CTG. Compared to the CTG group, the Doppler group experienced significant decreases in antepartum hospitalization (31% versus 46%, $p < 0.01$), induction of labor (10% versus 22%, $p < 0.01$), and emergency cesarean section for fetal distress (5.1% versus 14.2%, $p < 0.01$). There were no perinatal deaths in the Doppler group, but there were two stillbirths and one neonatal death in the CTG group. One stillbirth was due to placental abruption. The second intrauterine death occurred at 35 weeks' gestation following a normal CTG; there was no apparent cause, and the fetal weight was 27% below the norm. The authors concluded that umbilical arterial Doppler velocimetry is a more effective fetal surveillance tool for SGA fetuses than antepartum FHR monitoring.

Mason and associates [8] performed a randomized trial on 2,016 low-risk primigravid women (Doppler group 1,015, control group 1,001) to determine the effect of routine pregnancy screening with umbilical arterial Doppler testing on obstetric intervention rates and shortterm neonatal morbidity. The incidence of abnormal Doppler results was low (1.7%); that of AEDV was only 0.3%. In the control group, 42 women (3.9%) underwent Doppler examination. The investigators observed no significant differences between the control and study groups for any of the outcomes measured. There was only one perinatal death in the study, which occurred in the Doppler group; the pregnancy was complicated by spontaneous rupture of membranes at 34 weeks, fetal bradycardia for which cesarean section was performed, tight nuchal cord, and grade 3 intraventricular hemorrhage. This study demonstrated no beneficial or detrimental effect of routine Doppler ultrasound screening of low-risk women.

Johnstone and coinvestigators [9] performed a randomized controlled trial on 2,289 pregnant mothers (Doppler group 1,114, control group 1,175). The objective was to assess the effect of clinicians' access to umbilical Doppler results in obstetric practice. Continuous-wave Doppler studies of the umbilical artery were performed and the results made immediately available to clinicians. The outcome measures included perinatal mortality, Apgar score, and admission to the NICU. Fetal surveillance included cardiography, biophysical profile, and ultrasound biometry. Doppler was performed in three patients (0.26%) in the control group. Obstetric interventions measured were admission to hospital, induction of labor, and cesarean section. The treatment and control groups were well matched and showed no appreciable differences in perinatal outcome, obstetric intervention, or use of fetal monitoring. However, use of Doppler in the high-risk subgroup led to greater use of FHR monitoring ($p = 0.007$). There were no significant differences in the perinatal mortality between the

groups. The results indicated that obstetricians do not use the test to modify their risk assessment or therefore the need for fetal surveillance.

Newnham and colleagues [10] used a randomized trial to investigate the effects of frequent ultrasound imaging and Doppler velocimetry during pregnancy. The principal outcome parameters were the duration of neonatal hospital stay and the rate of preterm births. The population comprised 2,834 women with single pregnancies at 16–20 weeks' gestation attending the ultrasonography department. The study group consisted of 1,415 who underwent ultrasound imaging and continuous-wave Doppler studies at 18, 24, 28, 34, and 38 weeks' gestation. The control group of 1,419 women underwent single ultrasound imaging at 18 weeks. The only difference between the two groups was a significantly higher incidence of SGA fetuses in the intensively studied group, when expressed as birth weight in the 10th percentile (RR 1.35; CI 1.09–16.7) and birth weight in the 3rd percentile (RR 1.65; CI 1.09–2.49). Although it is possible that this finding was a chance effect, it is also plausible that frequent exposure to ultrasound may have influenced fetal growth. In terms of the efficacy of the Doppler examination, because the study group had frequent sonographic biometry in addition to the Doppler testing it is difficult to distinguish the influence of biometric assessments from those of the Doppler examination.

Whittle and associates [13] performed a randomized trial of Doppler sonography in a nonselected population of 2,986 women (Doppler group 1,642, control group 1,344) to investigate the impact of umbilical arterial Doppler velocimetry screening on obstetric outcome in a nonselected population of mixed low-risk and high-risk pregnancies. The main outcome measure was perinatal mortality corrected for malformations. The eligibility for entry into the study was physicians' concerns regarding "fetal well-being." Subgroup analysis was performed on those with hypertension and suspected growth restriction. The Doppler results were made available only for the study group. There were no significant differences between groups regarding antenatal admissions to hospital, preterm deliveries, rate of cesarean section, admission to the neonatal unit, or need for assisted ventilation. The results of the subgroup analysis were similar. Fewer stillbirths occurred in the Doppler group but the difference did not reach significance (8 versus 3; OR 0.34, CI 0.10–1.07).

Omtzigt et al. [11, 32] conducted a randomized trial of umbilical Doppler velocimetry in a nonselected hospital population of 1,598 (control group 789, study group 809). More than 40% were at high risk. The objective was to investigate the effect of Doppler velocimetry on the rate and duration of maternal hospital admission, obstetric management, and perinatal outcome. In the study group, umbilical arterial Doppler investigation was conducted only when indicated (46%). Abnormal pulsatility index (PI) values prompted intensified fetal monitoring. AEDV was observed in 3.5% of the patients. This study not only had a predefined protocol, it was described in the report and is discussed in detail later in this chapter. The study group demonstrated a significant reduction in perinatal mortality of normally formed fetuses and infants weighing 500 g or more (RR 0.33, CI 0.13–0.82) compared to the control group. As the neonatal mortality rate did not differ between the groups, the reduction in perinatal mortality was attributable to the use of umbilical arterial Doppler surveillance and not to any delay in the timing of fetal death. Neonatal seizure activity was noted in two infants in the control group and none in the Doppler group, but the difference was not statistically significant.

Pattinson et al. [12] investigated the effect of Doppler fetal surveillance in a randomized trial of pregnant women of more than 27 weeks' gestation with hypertensive disease or suspected SGA fetuses. The outcome measures were perinatal mortality and morbidity, antenatal hospitalization, maternal intervention, admission to the NICU, and hospitalization until discharge from the neonatal wards. Doppler velocimetry was performed in all patients, but the results were revealed only for the study group. The groups were clinically comparable. Physicians received management guidelines for patients with AEDV. Twenty patients (9.4%) developed AEDV in the umbilical artery; all were SGA fetuses. Among the SGA patients (study group 61, control group 63), there was one perinatal death in the study group (neonatal death related to respiratory distress syndrome) and six perinatal deaths in the control group (five stillbirths and one neonatal death). None of the infants who had end-diastolic velocity in the umbilical artery died. The reduction of stillbirths in the Doppler group was significant ($p = 0.029$; OR 0.13, CI 0.02–0.78). For those with SGA fetuses with end-diastolic velocity, the women in the Doppler group spent significantly fewer days in the hospital before delivery (median stay 0 versus 2 days, $p = 0.05$) and tended to have fewer maternal interventions (27% versus 43%; OR 0.49, CI 0.20–1.25), cesarean sections (13% versus 27%; OR 0.43, CI 0.14 and 1.32), and NICU stay (median stay 1.5 versus 4.0 days, $p < 0.05$). There were no differences in outcome when the end-diastolic velocity was present in conjunction with hypertension. There was one neonatal death in the Doppler group of this subset of patients, and it was related to maternal trauma. The study demonstrated the benefit of intervention because of the knowledge of Doppler velocimetry in patients with AEDV and in those with SGA even with end-diastolic velocity in the umbilical artery.

Nienhuis and associates performed a randomized trial to investigate whether hospitalization can safely be averted if the umbilical artery Doppler results were normal in women with singleton pregnancies and suspected fetal growth restriction (FGR) [14]. In the study group (74 patients), strong recommendations were made against hospitalization for suspected FGR if the Doppler findings were normal. In the control group (76 patients), the Doppler results were not revealed and the participants received the standard management. The endpoints included duration and frequency of hospitalization, perinatal outcome, neurological development, and postnatal growth. The duration but not the frequency of hospitalization was significantly shorter in the study group than in the control group. No significant differences were noted in the other outcome measures. The authors concluded that normal umbilical artery Doppler findings in suspected cases of IUGR may justify ambulatory management.

A collaborative multicenter French study investigated the efficacy of routine umbilical artery Doppler between 28 and 34 weeks of gestation in a low risk population of 4,187 women who were randomly assigned to the study and the control groups [15]. Apart from a significant increase in the frequency of subsequent ultrasonographic and Doppler examinations no significant differences were noted in the outcome. Although perinatal mortality was three times lower in the Doppler group (3 versus 9), this difference failed to achieve significance (OR 0.33; 95% CI 0.06–1.33).

Haley and coworkers [16] conducted a randomized trial on 150 mothers with the prenatal diagnosis of FGR. The objective was to compare the efficacy of umbilical artery Doppler sonography with that of fetal heart rate monitoring on resources utilization. In comparison with the fetal monitoring group, the Doppler group had the average hospital inpatient stay reduced from 2.5 days to 1.1 days ($p = 0.036$). Moreover, there was a reduction in monitoring frequency and fewer hospital prenatal ambulatory visits.

Ott and associates conducted a randomized trial to investigate the efficacy of the addition of the middle cerebral to umbilical artery systolic/diastolic ratios to the modified biophysical profile in 665 high risk pregnant patients [17]. The study group received the Doppler test in addition to the standard management of modified biophysical profile for fetal surveillance whereas the control group received only the standard management. Although no significant differences in the outcome were noted, a significant decline in cesarean deliveries in the Doppler tested patients was noted in a subgroup of patients at risk for uteroplacental insufficiency.

McCowan and colleagues performed a pilot randomized trial in 167 pregnant women between 24 and 36 weeks' gestation with small for gestational age fetuses to study whether the frequency of fetal surveillance could be safely reduced in the cases with normal umbilical artery Doppler [18]. In comparison with those who had fortnightly surveillance, those undergoing twice-weekly fetal surveillance were delivered 4 days earlier (264 vs 268 days; $p = 0.04$) and were more likely to have labor induced ($n = 70$, 82%, vs $n = 54$, 66%; $p = 0.02$). There were no differences in the neonatal outcome between the groups. Given the small sample size associated with preliminary nature of the study the authors prudently advised a larger trial for a more definitive recommendation.

Williams and associates [19] conducted a prospective randomized study where 1,360 at risk women at ≥ 32 weeks of gestation were randomized to either umbilical artery Doppler studies or nonstress testing. Women with umbilical artery S/D ratios $>90^{th}$ percentile or equivocal nonstress testing had the amniotic fluid index determined. Induction of labor and delivery were recommended when the amniotic fluid index was $<5^{th}$ percentile, the S/D ratio had ARDV or when the nonstress test was abnormal. In comparison with the control group, the Doppler group had more frequent induction of labor (4.8% versus 1.9%; $p < 0.005$), and lower incidence of cesarean section for fetal distress (4.6% versus 8.7%, $p < 0.006$). Those with hypertension (1.5% versus 13.6%) and FGR (2.4% versus 8.8%) experienced the greatest reduction in cesarean section for fetal distress. The neonatal morbidity between the two groups was similar.

A multicenter randomized controlled trial, the Growth Restriction Intervention Trial (GRIT), compared two strategies: the consequences of delivering within 48 hours for steroid administration (immediate delivery) with delaying for as long as the fetal status permitted to foster maturity (delay until the obstetrician is no longer uncertain) [20]. The population consisted of high risk pregnancies between 24 and 36 weeks. Over 90% of the population was complicated with fetal growth restriction. Cesarean deliveries were more frequent in the immediate delivery group (91%) compared to the delay group (79%) (OR 2.7, 95% CI 1.6–4.5). While there were more stillbirths in the delay group, more neonatal deaths were recorded in the immediate delivery group. However, the study failed to resolve the issue of optimal timing as no significant differences were noted in the deaths before discharge from the hospital between the two groups (10% in the immediate group versus 9% in the delay group).

In a continuation of the study for long term outcomes, death or disability at or beyond 2 years of age were investigated. Disability was assessed by Griffith's developmental quotient and the presence of severe motor or perceptual compromise [33]. No important differences in mortality or in the developmental assessment were seen. However, most of the difference in disability was observed in gestations below 31 weeks of gestation at randomization: 14 (13%) immediate versus five (5%) delayed deliveries. This prompted the investigators to caution against delivering before 30 weeks of gestation.

In the only randomized trial performed exclusively in twin gestations, Giles and coinvestigators [21] assigned randomly 526 women to receive either the standard sonographic biometry assessment or standard assessment and umbilical artery Doppler ultrasound at 25 weeks and again at 30 and 35 weeks. More intense fetal surveillance was instituted in the presence of any indicators of fetal compromise. No differences in the outcome was noted between the two groups although both groups showed a lower than expected fetal mortality probably resulting from the more intense fetal surveillance in general.

Doppler Randomized Trials: Cumulative Summary

The 21 studies described above encompass a total population of 25,279 pregnant mothers.

There was considerable clinical heterogeneity among the studies, including the characteristics of the population, study objectives and a predetermined measure of the primary outcome, Doppler sonographic technique, and management protocol.

Population Characteristics

Despite the risk categorization, there was no uniformity among the studies regarding their observed high-risk attributes. There were five trials conducted on populations of unselected pregnant mothers. Although presumed to be representative of the low-risk general obstetric population, not all of these studies appeared to be so qualified, as their site included university-based tertiary medical centers, which tend to attract complicated cases. This point is exemplified by the Utrecht study [11, 32], which was conducted on unselected cases but was found to include approximately 50% high-risk mothers. This study also had a perinatal mortality rate of 2.7%, which was higher than that of five studies in the high-risk group. Similarly, this study also had a 3.5% incidence of AEDV in comparison with an incidence of 1.9%–4.4% in the high-risk group. There is also some degree of heterogeneity in the stated objectives of the trials.

Objective and Primary Outcome

Considerable variation was also noted in the purpose of the trials and the measures of the primary outcome. Many of the studies measured various outcomes related to pregnancy management, fetal surveillance, management of labor and delivery, and perinatal morbidity and mortality. Lack of uniformity, however, was apparent with regard to the specific criteria of these measures. Among the rest, the objective of one was to assess physicians' use of Doppler information [9], and that of the other was to evaluate the effect of Doppler testing on the time required for fetal assessment [3]. Only half the studies reported a predetermined, specific primary outcome measure.

Doppler Sonographic Technique and Research Design

Although it may be difficult to expect a significant degree of dissimilarity in the instrumentation and procedure for Doppler interrogation of the umbilical arteries, there are some aspects of the method that can become critical sources of variance in results. They include the Doppler mode and the high-pass filter, a high level of which may produce false identification of AEDV. Many studies utilized continuous-wave Doppler ultrasound, while others used pulsed-wave Doppler mode, or did not specify the type of Doppler setup used for the study. One trial [12] utilized a 280-Hz high-pass filter setting; interestingly, this study reported the highest occurrence of AEDV. Five studies did not state the filter setting, and the rest utilized a threshold of 50–100 Hz. With regard to the use of Doppler sonography in the trial design, four studies [1, 4, 13, 32] used a Doppler technique in all patients, but the results were revealed to the obstetric care providers only for the study group. There is no measure, however, of the success rate for concealing Doppler information for the control group. In three studies [2, 3, 10] Doppler sonography was used in the control group in a selective manner, which was not uniform among the studies. In the remainder of the trials, Doppler sonography was not supposed to be performed in the control group of patients, although this "rule" was not universally implemented.

Management Protocol

Management protocol probably represents the most problematic source of clinical heterogeneity in these trials. Only seven of the studies had predefined treatment protocols [6, 11, 12]. The rest had limited or no set protocol for management; the results were given to the care providers, and it was anticipated that they would exercise their experience and knowledge to make the best use of this information. Others may have had some guidelines, but it was not apparent in the paper. This drawback severely limits the utility of these trials for formulating any evidence-based fetal surveillance policy utilizing Doppler ultasonography.

Doppler Randomized Trials: Meta-Analysis

Meta-Analysis: Brief Introduction

Although the traditional review of the published clinical trials of Doppler velocimetry as presented above is informative, it does not help to arrive at a definitive conclusion regarding its efficacy, nor does it provide us with a reasonable basis for developing a management plan. Even if Doppler sonography is highly effective, a traditional review fails to give us a measure of the magnitude of benefit that may result from its use in clinical practice for fetal surveillance. These problems can be significantly mitigated by performing a more systematic review by aggregating and statistically analyzing data from the various trials to derive a valid quantitative conclusion. The process is called meta-analysis, a term coined by Glass [34] to distinguish it from the primary analysis, which is the original process of analyzing the information from an individual research study, and from the secondary analysis, which is reanalysis of the original data to address new research questions. The concept is not entirely new, as quantitative statistical synthesis of past research data was described by several eminent statisticians decades before the origin of the term meta-analysis [35–37].

The technique has been used widely for systematic review of scientific research in the social sciences and was applied extensively later to clinical research in medicine. As the number of clinical trials has mushroomed, the need to depart from the more traditional subjective, often inconclusive review process has grown. The application of this type of quantitative systematic review of published data has been slow in the field of obstetrics. One of the key elements for popularizing this approach in obstetrics and gynecology has been the effort of the Oxford Perinatal Data Group and its inheritor, the Cochrane Perinatal Collaboration in the United Kingdom. An in-depth discussion of meta-analysis is beyond the scope of this chapter, but a brief review, specifically relevant to Doppler trials, is included here. It should be noted that this concise discussion is limited to the meta-analysis of experimental studies, such as randomized clinical trials, and excludes meta-analysis of non-experimental investigations or observational studies,

Table 26.2. Steps of conducting a meta-analysis

1. Formulate the research question.
2. Define the protocol for meta-analysis.
3. Define the criteria for selection of the target trials.
4. Comprehensive search and retrieval of information on trials.
5. Independent selection of trials as per the defined criteria.
6. Extract relevant information from the trials.
7. Aggregate the study results.
8. Analyze the data.
9. Interpret the results.
10. Report the results.

Table 26.3. Advantages and limitations of meta-analysis

Advantages

Provides a systematic quantitative review of all available data

Provides a quantitative estimation of the effect of a treatment from the cumulative data

Amplifies the statistical power of individual studies

Significantly less subjective and less biased than the traditional reviews

Assists in directing future research based on the strengths and weaknesses of all reviewed studies

Prevents redundant studies and saves resources

Allows continuous updating of the systematically reviewed information

Limitations

Retrospective analysis – limited by the quality of the constituent studies

Heterogeneity of the studies meta-analyzed – the "apples and oranges" issue

Pooling of many mediocre or poor studies does not necessarily yield better results

Oversimplifies the complex but critical etiologic and therapeutic relations

Obfuscates the reasons for the effect variability

Not entirely objective: publication bias, selection bias

which is not only a highly controversial issue but is not relevant to the Doppler clinical trials.

Meta-analysis is often regarded in a simplistic manner as a semiautomated process of collecting and feeding data from available past research into a computer program, which then provides simple quantitative aggregate measures of an effect. In reality, however, a proper meta-analysis consists of a rigorously systematic approach (Table 26.2). Moreover, it is important to consider the various methods of meta-analysis, which are based primarily on their manner of dealing with the heterogeneity of the studies included in the review.

The advantages and limitations of meta-analysis are summarized in Table 26.3. As mentioned earlier, the technique offers a vast improvement over the traditional review, which often is not comprehensive, does not produce a quantitative analysis of the existing information, and is highly susceptible to subjective biases. Moreover, the traditional review process cannot compensate for the loss of power of individual studies of inadequate sample size, nor is it subject to systematic updating, which is possible with a meta-analysis. Meta-analysis can offer great benefit when designing appropriate future trials based on the questions generated by the systematic review process so the limitations of the past trials are addressed. Moreover, if a well-conducted meta-analytic process demonstrates a significant benefit of a new diagnostic and therapeutic intervention, it may be introduced into clinical practice in a timely fashion without going through additional essentially redundant trials, thereby saving time and resources. Such a scenario highlights one of the principal beneficial contributions of the systematic review. Finally, meta-analysis is not a static process. As information on additional trials on a subject becomes progressively available, the results can be systematically and continuously updated and conclusions revised.

Meta-analysis, however, is not a panacea for all the inadequacies of individual trials; nor is it a replace-

ment for a large, well-designed, well-conducted primary clinical trial of sufficient power. Some of its essential attributes are often the potential sources of its limitations. It attempts to encompass all data within the scope of the defined objectives of the review process and the predetermined inclusion criteria for the trials. Indeed, to be comprehensive, the current recommendation is to enter all available information including abstracts, review articles, and unpublished data so subjective problems such as publication bias are minimized or eliminated. This approach, however, appears to be too nondiscriminatory, as data from potentially poorly conducted trials and unreliable sources are included. Meta-analysis is essentially a retrospective process limited by the quality of its constituent trials, which has given rise to the metaphoric criticism of meta-analysis as an alchemic process of converting "tons of garbage to a single diamond." There are scoring systems for assessing the quality of clinical trials, but these systems are often subjective, the score values may not be appropriately weighted, and there may be no clear guideline for dealing with the studies of low scores.

The validity of meta-analytic inference has been questioned on the basis of heterogeneity of constituent studies. The traditional response when dealing with heterogeneity has been to consider the objective of meta-analytic generalization. Glass [34] discussed this point metaphorically as the "apples and oranges" issue; if the objective is to generalize the apples and oranges to fruit, heterogeneity should not make much of a difference. The current trend, however, is not only to apply statistical methodology to minimize the impact of heterogeneity on the validity of the meta-analytic inference but also to analyze the sources of such heterogeneity in order to understand and improve therapeutic effectiveness.

There are several statistical methods for conducting meta-analysis. Traditionally, the method for deriving the average estimate of the effect size has been to use one of the fixed-effects models, which takes into account intrastudy but not interstudy variance. This model was developed by Mantel and Haentzel [38] and was subsequently modified by Yusuf et al. [39]. There is strong support for the use of this model for meta-analysis from many investigators [40, 41]. When the fixed-effects model is used, a separate statistical test (e.g. the χ^2 distribution) is usually performed to determine if the variations in the results can be explained by chance. However, it is a relatively insensitive tool to test for homogeneity [42]. Although the fixed-effects model is the most widely used method for meta-analysis in the medical field, there has been significant criticism of its exclusive use. The alternative method, the random-effects model, originally suggested by Cochran [43] and subsequently developed by DerSimonian and Laird [44], deals with study-to-study variations in the analytic process of generating the aggregate effect and the confidence intervals. There has been substantial support for this approach, particularly when one is aiming to apply the meta-analytic inference to the future application of the treatment rather than to the past trials under investigation [45, 46].

An in-depth discussion of statistical methodology for meta-analysis is well beyond the scope of this chapter. However, the choice between the fixed-effects model and the random-effects model is pertinent when considering the meta-analysis of Doppler trials. The issue here is more that of "oranges and tangerines" than of "apples and oranges". To be sure, there is great controversy among statisticians regarding the choice between the two models. The choice may be guided by the basic assumptions of these models. The fixed-effects model assumes that results of the analysis are applicable to the studies already performed and included in the systematic review process, whereas the random-effects model assumes that the results are applicable to all such studies in the future. Furthermore, if the studies are sufficiently homogeneous, the results do not differ between the models; however, the random effects model yields conservative results with wider confidence intervals. A pragmatic approach is first to avoid aggregating

obviously dissimilar studies and, in the absence of apparent heterogeneity, to use and report both models. If this practice reveals heterogeneity, one should systematically investigate its underlying reason. With this background information on meta-analysis, let us examine now its application to the Doppler trials.

Doppler Meta-Analysis

Alfirevic and Neilson [47] reported a meta-analysis of published and unpublished randomized Doppler trials in high-risk pregnancies. Of the 12 studies included, six were peer-reviewed original publications, two were unpublished (personal communication), two appeared to be abstracts published in conference proceedings, and two were review articles. The trials were subjected to a quality assessment program proposed by Chalmers and associates [48] and were found to be eligible for inclusion in the systematic review process. This report suggested a significant reduction in the perinatal deaths of normally formed fetuses consequent to the use of umbilical arterial Doppler surveillance (Fig. 26.2). The odds of perinatal mortality declined by 38%. A significant decrease was also noted in the number of antepartum admissions to the hospital (44%), inductions of labor (20%), and cesarean sections for fetal distress (52%). Moreover, significant declines were observed in elective delivery, intrapartum fetal distress, and hypoxic encephalopathy on post hoc analyses (Fig. 26.3). Obviously, the last group of benefits require additional investigation. It should also be noted that a meta-analysis does not replace the value of a randomized clinical trial based on a sufficient sample size. Depending on the choice of the outcome parameter and the effect size, it probably requires thousands of patients involving multiple centers. It would be a challenge to organize and obtain sufficient resources for a trial of this magnitude.

Noting that the statistical method utilized in this meta-analysis was based on the fixed-effects model, we undertook a random-effects model approach as described by DerSimonian and Laird [44] to reanalyze the data pertaining to perinatal deaths as collated by Alfirevic and Neilson [26]. The data are presented in Table 26.4, which confirms the results from the fixed-effects model analysis. The random-effects model analysis suggests that the use of umbilical artery Doppler velocimetry for fetal surveillance of complicated pregnancies may lead to a 36% decline in perinatal death (CI –54% to –10%). This figure is reassuring, although one may have reservations about the inclusion and exclusion criteria used in the Alfirevic and Neilson meta-analysis. Further refinement of our assessment of the benefits of Doppler velocimetry may be obtained by reexamining some of these issues.

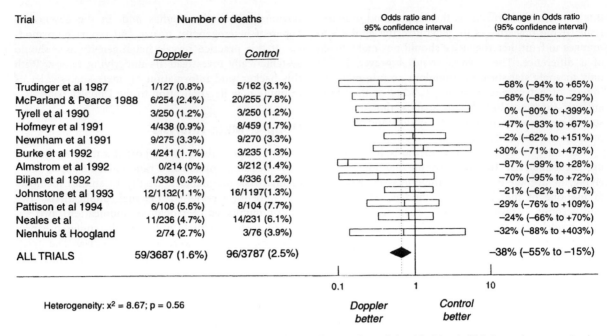

Fig. 26.2. Proportional effect of Doppler ultrasonography on the number of dead babies (stillbirths and neonates) when used for high-risk pregnancies. (Reprinted from [26] with permission)

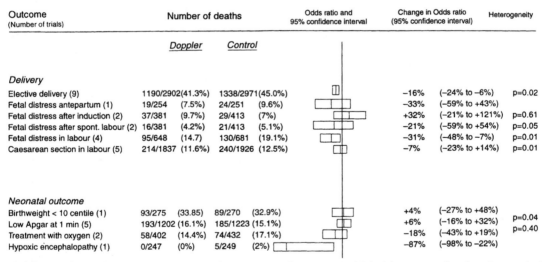

Fig. 26.3. Effects of Doppler ultrasonography on perinatal outcome in high-risk pregnancies. Post hoc analysis (Reprinted from [26] with permission)

Since the first systematic review of Alfirevic and Neilson [26] subsequent systematic reviews have been performed. Divon performed a meta-analysis of eight published and peer-review randomized trials of 6,838 patients [27]. Umbilical artery Doppler studies significantly decreased perinatal mortality (OR 0.66, CI 0.46–0.94). Divon concluded that there were enough data to show the benefit of umbilical artery Doppler velocimetry in high-risk patients and meta-analysis

of additional randomized controlled trials was unlikely to change these results.

In 1996, Neilson and Alfirevic [28] reviewed 11 randomized controlled trials of 7,000 high-risk pregnancies. The study by MacParland and Pearce [2] was removed from this meta-analysis because the veracity of the data presented was put into question. The use of Doppler ultrasound was associated with a trend toward a reduction in perinatal deaths (OR 0.71, 95%

Table 26.4. Meta-analysis of Doppler randomized clinical trials performed on high-risk pregnancies utilizing the random effects model of DerSimonian and Laird [44]. The analysis shows the effect on perinatal mortality

First author	Doppler	Control	Odds Ratio (95% CI)
Trudinger, 1987	1/127	5/162	0.25 (0.03–2.16)
McParland, 1988	6/254	20/255	0.28 (0.11–0.72)
Tyrrell, 1990	3/250	3/250	1.00 (0.20–5.00)
Hofmeyr, 1991	4/438	8/459	0.52 (0.16–1.74)
Newnham, 1991	9/275	9/270	0.98 (0.38–2.51)
Burke, 1992	4/241	3/235	1.31 (0.29–5.90)
Almstrom, 1992	0/214	3/212	0.14 (0.01–2.72)
Biljan, 1992	1/338	4/336	0.25 (0.03–2.22)
Johnstone, 1993	12/1,132	16/1,197	0.79 (0.37–1.68)
Pattinson, 1994	6/108	8/104	0.71 (0.24–2.11)
Neales, 1995	11/236	14/231	0.76 (0.34–1.71)
Nienhuis, 1995	2/74	3/76	0.68 (0.11–4.17)
Total	**59/3,687**	**96/3,787**	**0.64 (0.46–0.90)**

CI 0.50–1.01) especially in pregnancies complicated by hypertension or presumed impaired fetal growth. In addition, there were fewer inductions of labor (OR 0.83, 95% CI 0.74–0.93) and fewer hospital admissions (OR 0.56, 95% CI 0.43–0.72) without adverse perinatal effects. Moreover, there was no difference for fetal distress in labor (OR 0.81, 95% CI 0.59–1.13) or cesarean deliveries (OR 0.94, 95% CI 0.82–1.06). The investigators concluded that the use of Doppler ultrasound appeared promising in helping to reduce perinatal deaths.

Westergaard and colleagues [29] reanalyzed randomized controlled trials on the use of umbilical artery Doppler velocimetry in 8,633 high-risk pregnancies in order to determine which high-risk pregnancies benefit from the use of Doppler velocimetry. They divided 13 randomized controlled trials (including two unpublished studies) into "well-defined studies," when there was a strict definition of suspected intrauterine growth restriction or hypertensive disease of pregnancy, and "general risk studies." The "well-defined studies" showed a significant reduction in antenatal admissions (OR 0.56, 95% CI 0.43–0.72), inductions of labor (OR 0.78, 95% CI 0.63–0.96), elective deliveries (OR 0.73, 95% CI 0.61–0.88), and cesarean deliveries (OR 0.78, 95% CI 0.65–0.94). No significant difference was found in perinatal mortality (OR 0.66, 95% CI 0.36–1.22). The perinatal deaths were audited by a panel of 32 international experts who found that more perinatal deaths in the "well-defined studies" were potentially avoidable by use of Doppler velocimetry (50% controls versus 20% Doppler velocimetry group). The "general risk studies" did not show significant differences in the variables studied. These investigators concluded that only in pregnancies with suspected intrauterine growth re-

striction or hypertensive disease of pregnancy would the use of Doppler velocimetry reduce the number of perinatal deaths and unnecessary obstetric interventions.

Two other meta-analyses of trials of umbilical artery velocimetry in low-risk pregnancies have been performed. Goffinet and colleagues [30] conducted a meta-analysis of four randomized trials of umbilical Doppler in unselected or low-risk pregnancies with a total population of 11,375 women. Three other studies were not included because they did not meet the inclusion criteria or they had methodological problems. Screening Doppler umbilical artery velocimetry did not influence perinatal deaths (overall perinatal deaths OR 0.90, 95% CI 0.50–1.60) or stillbirth (overall stillbirths OR 0.94, 95% CI 0.42–1.98), antenatal hospitalization (OR 1.04, 95% CI 0.95–1.15), obstetric outcome, or perinatal morbidity.

A subsequent meta-analysis of five trials on routine Doppler ultrasound in unselected and low-risk pregnancies with a total population of 14,338 women also concluded that routine Doppler ultrasound examination in low-risk or unselected populations did not confer benefit on mother or infant [31]. Umbilical Doppler examination cannot be recommended as a routine test in low-risk or unselected populations.

Unfortunately, the many systematic reviews of trials on the effect of umbilical artery Doppler velocimetry have been based on essentially the same 12 trials that were evaluated in the first meta-analysis by Alfirevic and Neilson [26] with some modifications. Thornton has been critical of this pattern of repeated analysis, and believes that "repeated analysis of the same data set can at best only generate hypotheses for future researchers to test" [49]. He suggested the need for trials of the effect of umbilical artery Doppler velocimetry where there is a clearly defined group and a defined delivery timing policy to follow. Alternatively, trials with well-defined groups and different delivery timing policies should be addressed.

It is of interest to note that none of the existing modalities of fetal surveillance are based on affirmative evidence derived from clinical trials and systematic meta-analytic reviews. The benefit of the antepartum nonstress test was investigated in four randomized clinical trials [50–53]. None of the studies demonstrated any benefit. Moreover, a meta-analysis of these studies failed to show any benefit (Table 26.5). No randomized trial has ever been reported for the contraction stress test. There were two quasi-randomized trials on the fetal biophysical profile in the 1980s [55, 56]; neither demonstrated any difference in outcome after use of the test. Subsequent meta-analytic review also showed no benefit [57]. Two additional trials [58, 59] on the biophysical profile published in the 1990s were included in the meta-analysis by Al-

Table 26.5. Meta-analysis of randomized trials of antepartum nonstress cardiotocography for fetal surveillance [54]

	Cardiotocography	Control	Odds ratio (95% CI)
Delivery by cesarean	183/795	170/784	1.07 (0.84–1.36)
Fetal distress	172/631	140/613	1.27 (0.98–1.65)
Low Apgar score	38/380	38/369	0.91 (0.56–1.47)
Abnormal neonatal neurological signs	26/597	25/586	1.00 (0.57–1.77)
Admission to special care nursery	100/453	88/430	1.11 (0.80 1.54)
Perinatal deaths excl. lethal malformations	12/651	4/628	2.65 (0.99–7.12)

Table 26.6. Meta-analysis of controlled trials of biophysical profile for fetal surveillance [60]

	Biophysical profile	Control	Odds ratio (95% CI)
Perinatal mortality	13/1,405	11/1,434	1.30 (0.59–2.92)
Corrected perinatal mortality	3/1,122	2/1,058	1.42 (0.25–8.20)
Apgar score <7 after 5 min	37/1,400	32/1,428	1.21 (0.75–1.96)
Birthweight <10th percentile	9/279	17/373	0.71 (0.32–1.56)
Intrapartum fetal distress	14/279	25/373	0.74 (0.39–1.43)

firevic and Neilson [60]. These investigators concluded that the evidence was insufficient to evaluate the use of the biophysical profile as a test of fetal well-being in high-risk pregnancies (Table 26.6).

Management of High-Risk Pregnancy: A Proposal Based on Clinical Trials

If Doppler velocimetry is beneficial as a fetal surveillance tool, what is the optimal mode of its application for managing the fetus at risk? Regrettably, it is difficult to use the above reports to develop and recommend a specific management plan, as most of the trials did not seem to have any defined protocol to translate the Doppler surveillance findings into a clear plan for intervention.

A general approach can be developed from the studies reporting a management protocol and demonstrating an improved outcome after using the Doppler method [6, 11, 12]. The general approach may be described as follows. When the Doppler index remains within the normal limits or does not progressively rise, weekly testing should suffice. The nonstress test or the biophysical profile should be used either as a backup test or performed in conjunction with the Doppler. The latter approach is often used as a multimodal test for fetal well-being. If the fetal and maternal conditions remain assuring, allow the pregnancy to continue to maturity and assess the patient for delivery. In the presence of sonographically confirmed growth compromise, the pregnancy may not be allowed to become postdated.

A high or increasing Doppler index warrants more intense fetal surveillance consisting of weekly umbilical arterial Doppler, and once- or twice-weekly nonstress test and biophysical profile as warranted by the clinical condition until fetal maturity. If these tests indicate fetal compromise, or absent end-diastolic velocity develops, the likelihood of poor prenatal outcome is increased and urgent clinical response is indicated. The patient should be hospitalized and the management individualized depending on gestational age and fetal status.

The optimal timing for delivery in a preterm pregnancy with fetal growth restriction still remains uncertain. As discussed previously, the issue of a defined delivery timing policy for the compromised preterm fetus has been recently tested in the GRIT study, which failed to resolve the issue [19].

However, thanks to the recent impressive advances in neonatal care, a distinction can be made regarding the risks of prematurity between pregnancies beyond and before the 32nd completed week of gestation. In gestations less than 32 completed weeks, the absence of end-diastolic flow in the umbilical artery should prompt consideration for immediate delivery. Other ominous findings prompting delivery include (a) cessation of fetal growth on successive ultrasound examinations; (b) umbilical arterial absent or reversed end-diastolic flow; (c) nonreassuring fetal heart rate patterns including nonreactive nonstress test, poor fetal heart rate baseline variability, persistent variable or late decelerations; (d) oligohydramnios; and (e) biophysical profile score ≤4.

When absent end-diastolic flow develops in a preterm pregnancy (<32 weeks) with a significant risk of fetal lung immaturity, further assurance of fetal well-being is sought by daily surveillance with umbilical arterial Doppler sonography, nonstress test, and biophysical profile. Steroids should be administered to enhance fetal lung maturity. Delivery is indicated regardless of maturity when a single or combination of tests indicate imminent fetal danger (as described above) and the fetal risk from a hostile intrauterine environment is judged to be greater than that from pulmonary immaturity.

It should be noted that this management approach does not provide an answer for every contingency that may develop. The physician must individualize the care in the light of the myriad variations in the clinical situation. This recommendation should be used as a pragmatic guideline that integrates the new modality with the existing standards of fetal surveillance. As new evidence accumulates and our experience grows, these guidelines may contribute to the emergence of more effective standards of practice. Obviously, this plan of management requires refinement in the future so the issue of cost-effective integration of the various modalities of fetal monitoring in appropriate sequence and frequency may be addressed. Moreover, the utility of in-depth hemodynamic information, such as the middle cerebral arterial Doppler index and the cerebroplacental ratio, requires further investigation.

Conclusion

The development of Doppler sonography has made it feasible to assess the fetal and uteroplacental circulations. Numerous studies have established a significant association between abnormal Doppler indices and the various pregnancy disorders and adverse perinatal outcomes. Most clinical investigations suggest that, in high-risk pregnancies, umbilical arterial Doppler indices may be efficacious for predicting perinatal problems including fetal death. Many randomized trials on Doppler velocimetry have yielded positive results. Furthermore, systematic reviews of the trials by meta-analysis demonstrate a significant reduction in preventable fetal deaths. The current evidence mandates that Doppler velocimetry of the umbilical artery should be an integral component of fetal surveillance in pregnancies complicated with fetal growth restriction or preeclampsia. Obviously, no single testing modality should be regarded as the exclusive choice for fetal surveillance, as these tests reveal different aspects of fetal pathophysiology, often in a complementary manner.

References

1. Trudinger BJ, Cook CM, Giles WB, Connelly A, Thompson RS (1987) Umbilical artery flow velocity waveforms in high risk pregnancy. Lancet 1:188
2. MacParland P, Pearce JM (1988) Review article: Doppler blood flow in pregnancy. Placenta 9:427–450
3. Tyrrell SN, Lilford RJ, MacDonald HN et al (1990) Randomized controlled trial (RCT): clinical trial. Br J Obstet Gynaecol 97:909
4. Hofmeyr GJ, Pattinson R, Buckley D, Jennings J, Redman CW (1991) Umbilical artery resistance index as a screening test for fetal well-being. II. Randomized feasibility study. Obstet Gynecol 78:359–362
5. Newnham JP, O'Dea MA, Reid KP, Diepeveen DA (1991) Doppler flow velocity waveform analysis in high risk pregnancies: a randomized controlled trial. Br J Obstet Gynaecol 98:956–963
6. Alstrom H, Axelsson O, Cnattingius S et al (1992) Comparison of umbilical artery velocimetry and cardiotocography for surveillance of small for gestational age fetuses: a multi-center randomized controlled trial. Lancet 340:936–940
7. Davies JA, Gallivan S, Spencer JAD (1992) Randomised controlled trial of Doppler ultrasound screening of placental perfusion during pregnancy. Lancet 340:1299–1303
8. Mason GC, Lilford RJ, Porter J, Tyrrell S, Nelson E (1993) Randomised comparison of routine versus highly selective use of Doppler ultrasound in low risk pregnancies. Br J Obstet Gynaecol 100:130–133
9. Johnstone FD, Prescott R, Hoskins P et al (1993) The effect of introduction of umbilical Doppler recordings to obstetric practice. Br J Obstet Gynaecol 100:733–741
10. Newnham JP, Evans SF, Michael CA, Stanley FJ, Landau LI (1993) Effects of frequent ultrasound during pregnancy: a randomized controlled trial. Lancet 342:887–891
11. Omtzigt AMWJ, Reuwer PJHM, Bruinse HW (1994) A randomized controlled trial on the clinical value of umbilical Doppler velocimetry in antenatal care. Am J Obstet Gynecol 170:625–634
12. Pattinson RC, Norman K, Odendaal HJ (1994) The role of Doppler velocimetry in the management of high risk pregnancies. Br J Obstet Gynaecol 101:114–120
13. Whittle MJ, Hanretty KP, Primrose MH, Neilson JP (1994) Screening for the compromised fetus: a randomized trial of umbilical artery velocimetry in unselected pregnancies. Am J Obstet Gynecol 170:555–559
14. Nienhuis SJ, Vles JS, Gerver WJ, Hoogland HJ (1997) Doppler ultrasonography in suspected intrauterine growth retardation: a randomized clinical trial. Ultrasound Obstet Gynecol 9:6–13
15. Doppler French Study Group (1997) A randomised controlled trial of Doppler ultrasound velocimetry of the umbilical artery in low risk pregnancies. Br J Obstet Gynaecol 104:419–424
16. Haley J, Tuffnell DJ, Johnson N (1997) Randomised controlled trial of cardiotocography versus umbilical artery Doppler in the management of small for gestational age fetuses. Br J Obstet Gynaecol 104:431–435
17. Ott WJ, Mora G, Arias F, Sunderji S, Sheldon G (1998) Comparison of the modified biophysical profile to a "new" biophysical profile incorporating the middle cerebral artery to umbilical artery velocity flow systolic/diastolic ratio. Am J Obstet Gynecol 178:1346–1353
18. McCowan LM, Harding JE, Roberts AB, Barker SE, Ford C, Stewart AW (2000) A pilot randomized controlled trial of two regimens of fetal surveillance for small-for-gestational-age fetuses with normal results of umbilical artery doppler velocimetry. Am J Obstet Gynecol 182:81–86

19. The GRIT Study Group (2003) A randomised trial of timed delivery for the compromised preterm fetus: short term outcomes and Bayesian interpretation. Br J Obstet Gynaecol 110:27–32

20. Williams KP, Farquharson DF, Bebbington M, Dansereau J, Galerneau F, Wilson RD, Shaw D, Kent N (2003) Screening for fetal well-being in a high-risk pregnant population comparing the nonstress test with umbilical artery Doppler velocimetry: a randomized controlled clinical trial. Am J Obstet Gynecol 188:1366–1371

21. Giles W, Bisits A, O'Callaghan S, Gill A, DAMP Study Group (2003) The Doppler assessment in multiple pregnancy randomised controlled trial of ultrasound biometry versus umbilical artery Doppler ultrasound and biometry in twin pregnancy. Br J Obstet Gynaecol 110:593–597

22. Burke G, Stuart B, Crowley P, Scanelli S, Drumm J (1992) Does Doppler ultrasound alter the management of high risk pregnancy? In: Koppe JG, Eskes TKAB, van Geijn HP, Wiesenhaan PF (eds) Care, concern and Cure in Perinatal Medicine. Parthenon, Casterton Hall, pp 597–604

23. Almstrom H, Axelsson O, Cnattingius S et al (1991) Comparison of umbilical artery velocimetry and cardiotocography for surveillance of small for gestational age fetuses: a multi-center randomized controlled trial. J Matern Fetal Invest 1:127 [abstract]

24. Schneider KTM, Renz S, Furstenau U et al (1992) Doppler flow measurements as a screening method during pregnancy: is it worth the effort? J Matern Fetal Invest 2:125 [abstract]

25. Nimrod C, Yee J, Hopkins C et al (1991) The utility of pulsed Doppler studies in the evaluation of postdate pregnancies. J Matern Fetal Invest 1:127 [abstract]

26. Alfirevic Z, Nielson JP (1995) Doppler ultrasonography in high risk pregnancies: systematic review with meta-analysis. Am J Obstet Gynecol 172:1379

27. Divon MY (1995) Randomized controlled trials of umbilical artery Doppler velocimetry: how many are too many? Ultrasound Obstet Gynecol 6:377–379

28. Neilson JP, Alfirevic Z (2000) Doppler ultrasound for fetal assessment in high-risk pregnancies (Cochrane Review). The Cochrane Library, Issue 4

29. Westergaard HB, Langhoff-Roos J, Lingman G, Maršal K, Kreiner S (2001) A critical appraisal of the use of umbilical artery Doppler ultrasound in high-risk pregnancies: use of meta-analyses in evidence-based obstetrics. Ultrasound Obstet Gynecol 17:466–476

30. Goffinet F, Paris-Llado J, Nisand I, Breart G (1997) Umbilical artery Doppler velocimetry in unselected and low risk pregnancies: review of randomised controlled trials. Br J Obstet Gynaecol 194:425–430

31. Bricker L, Neilson JP (2000) Routine Doppler ultrasound in pregnancy. Cochrane Database Syst Rev 2:CD001450

32. Omtzigt AWJ (1990) Clinical Value of Umbilical Doppler Velocimetry. Doctoral thesis, University of Utrecht, The Netherlands

33. GRIT study group (2004) Infant well being at 2 years of age in the Growth Restriction Intervention Trial (GRIT): multicentred randomised controlled trial. Lancet 364:513–520

34. Glass GV (1976) Primary, secondary and meta-analysis of research. Educ Res 5:3–8

35. Fisher RA (1932) Statistical Methods for Research Workers (4th edn). Oliver & Boyd, London

36. Cochran WG (1937) Problems arising in the analysis of a series of similar experiments. J R Stat Soc 4:102

37. Pearson ES (1938) The probability integral transformation for testing goodness of fit and combining independent tests of significance. Biometrika 30:134

38. Mantel N, Haentzel W (1959) Statistical aspects of the analysis of data from retrospective studies of disease. J Natl Cancer Inst 22:719

39. Yusuf S, Peto R, Lewis J, Collins R, Sleight P (1985) Beta blockade during and after myocardial infarction: an overview of the randomized trials. Prog Cardiovasc Dis 27:335

40. Peto R (1987) Why do we need systematic overviews of randomized trials? Stat Med 6:233

41. Thompson SG, Pocock SJ (1991) Can meta-analysis be trusted? Lancet 338:1127

42. Chalmers TC, Buyse MEB (1988) Meta-analysis. In: Chalmers TC (ed) Data Analysis for Clinical Medicine: The Qualitative Approach to Patient Care in Gastroenterology. International University Press, Rome

43. Cochran WG (1954) The combination of estimates from different experiments. Biometrics 10:101

44. DerSimonian R, Laird N (1986) Meta-analysis in clinical trials. Controlled Clin Trials 8:177

45. Demets DL (1987) Methods for combining randomized clinical trials: strengths and limitations. Stat Med 6:341

46. Bailey KR (1987) Inter-study differences: how should they influence the interpretation and analysis of results? Stat Med 6:351

47. Neilson JP (1993) Doppler ultrasound (all trials). In: Enkin MW, Kierse MJNC, Renfrew MJ, Neilson JP (eds) Pregnancy and Childbirth Module. Update Software, Disk Issue 2, Review No. 07337. Cochrane Database of Systematic Reviews, Oxford

48. Chalmers TC, Smith H Jr, Blackburn M et al (1981) A method for assessing the quality of a randomized control trial. Controlled Clin Trials 2:31

49. Thornton J (2001) Systematic review of trials of umbilical artery Doppler: time for more primary research. Ultrasound Obstet Gynecol 17:464–465

50. Brown VA, Sawers RS, Parsons RJ, Duncan SLB, Cooke ID (1982) The values of antenatal cardiotocography in the management of high risk pregnancy: a randomized controlled trial. Br J Obstet Gynaecol 89:716

51. Flynn AM, Kelly J, Mansfield H et al (1982) A randomized controlled trial of non-stress antepartum cardiotocography. Br J Obstet Gynaecol 92:1156

52. Lumley J, Lester A, Renou P, Wood C (1983) A randomized trial of weekly cardiotocography in high risk obstetric patients. Br J Obstet Gynaecol 90:1018

53. Kidd LC, Patel NB, Smith R (1985) Non-stress antenatal cardiotocography: a prospective randomized clinical trial. Br J Obstet Gynaecol 89:716

54. Pattison N, McCowan L (2004) Cardiotocography for antepartum fetal assessment. In: The Cochrane Pregnancy and Childbirth Group Database. Volume 2. Cochrane Database of Systematic Reviews, Oxford, UK

55. Manning FA, Lange IR, Morrison I, Harman CR (1984) Fetal biophysical profile score and the non-stress test: a comparative trial. Obstet Gynecol 64:326

56. Platt LD, Walla CA, Paul RH et al (1985) A prospective trial of fetal biophysical profile vs the non-stress test in the management of high risk pregnancies. Am J Obstet Gynecol 153:624

57. Mohide P, Kierse MJNC (1989) Biophysical assessment of fetal well-being. In: Chalmers I, Enkins M (eds) Effective Care in Pregnancy and Childbirth. Oxford University Press, Oxford, p 477

58. Nageotte MP, Towers CV, Asrat T et al. (1994) Perinatal outcome with the modified biophysical profile. Am J Obstet Gynecol 170:1672–1676

59. Alfirevic Z, Walkinshaw SA (1995) A randomized controlled trial of simple compared with complex antenatal fetal monitoring after 42 weeks of gestation. Br J Obstet Gynaecol 102:638–643

60. Alfirevic Z, Neilson JP (2004) Biophysical profile for fetal assessment in high risk pregnancies. In: Cochrane Pregnancy and Childbirth Group Database. Volume 2. Cochrane Database of Systematic Reviews, Oxford, UK

Chapter 27

Doppler Investigation of the Fetal Inferior Vena Cava

Yoshihide Chiba, Toru Kanzaki, Zeev Weiner

Inferior vena cava (IVC) flow velocity waveforms represent both right atrial function and the blood flow pattern within the venous tree of the lower fetal body. Flow velocity waveforms obtained close to the venous entrance into the right atrium reflect mostly right atrial activity. Therefore the information obtained by studying blood flow patterns within the IVC includes (1) whether there is normal atrial filling; (2) detection of a fetal arrhythmia and the resulting blood flow pattern; and (3) estimation of hemodynamic disturbances in severely compromised fetuses.

In this chapter we describe the normal pattern of IVC blood flow and the various components of the IVC flow velocity waveforms. Typical alterations of the IVC flow velocity waveforms in hydropic fetuses, fetuses with arrhythmias, and severely compromised fetuses are discussed. Finally, special attention is devoted to the significance of umbilical vein pulsations.

Normal Blood Flow Pattern in Fetal IVC

A Doppler waveform in a fetal IVC under normal sinus rhythm shows a pulsating pattern synchronized with cardiac motions. There are three components in a cardiac cycle: the monophasic blood flow retrograding from the right atrium to the inferior vena cava, the initial forward flow, and the second forward flow. The reverse flow occurs during atrial contraction. The initial forward flow coincides with atrial diastole and ventricular systole, and the second forward flow coincides with ventricular diastole (Fig. 27.1) [1, 2].

Fetal movements, particularly fetal breathing movements, influence the blood flow, changing the pattern not only in the IVC but also in the umbilical vein. Blood flow in the IVC has a complicated pattern during fetal breathing movements [3].

Many studies have reported that blood flow in an adult vena cava has a pulsating pattern synchronized with cardiac movements [4–8]. The cause of each component of the blood flow in an adult vena cava has been analyzed from the viewpoint of the atrial pressure [7–9], with the conclusion that the cause of reverse flow is an increase in atrial pressure due to contraction of the right atrium. The cause of systole forward flow is controversial. Some authors have estimated it only for atrial dilatation [4, 5]. However, others have suggested that the cause of the forward flow is movement of the tricuspid annulus toward the

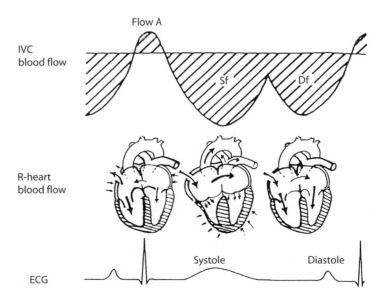

Fig. 27.1. Time relation of venous return in the inferior vena cava with a cardiac cycle. *A* reverse flow, *Sf* initial forward flow, *Df* second forward flow

apex at ventricular systole [9–11]. Some have suggested that both factors are responsible [6, 8, 12]. The cause of diastole forward flow is the decreased atrial pressure due to rapid ventricular filling.

Generally the blood flow pattern in the fetal IVC is similar to that in the adult, as is the cause. We believe, in addition, that the pressure of the left atrium and movement of the mitral annulus may influence flow in the fetal vena cava.

Changes of the IVC flow velocity waveforms throughout gestation were studied by Huisman et al. [13] and Wladimiroff et al. [14]. These authors described a significant increase in time-averaged velocity and a significant decrease in percent reverse flow with advancing gestational age. Such changes, which could be seen as early as 11–16 weeks' gestation, corresponded with the increasing peak E wave/A wave ratio. We may conclude therefore that the changes in the IVC flow velocity waveforms observed during pregnancy represent increased cardiac compliance during this period. Rizzo et al. studied the blood flow pattern in the umbilical vein during early gestation [15]. They reported pulsations in the umbilical vein in all cases until 8 weeks' gestation, after which the pulsations disappeared progressively until 13 weeks' gestation. The presence of umbilical venous pulsations correlated with reverse flow within the IVC during atrial contractions.

Doppler Evaluation of Preload Condition in the Fetal Vena Cava and the Umbilical Vein

Among 101 cases of nonimmune hydrops, 30 cases were complicated structural heart diseases. The prognosis of such cardiogenic hydrops is poor: the mortality was 86.7% [16]. To determine the best timing for delivery and the indications for intrauterine therapy of the fetus, one must understand the cardiac functions of the fetus with nonimmune hydrops.

The subjects for our study of cardiac function were divided into three groups according to diagnosis [3, 17]. The first group comprised those with structural heart disease associated with hydrops; the second had structural heart disease without hydrops; and the third contained those with hydrops but without heart disease.

We evaluated four parameters to establish the cardiac function of the three pathologic groups and that of normal fetuses. The first parameter, the cardiothoracic area ratio (CTAR), was the simplest and easiest to understand. The CTAR measures the dimensions of the heart with a four-chamber view. The next pa-

rameter was heart contractility, measured by Pombo's method. The third parameter was measurement of the peak systolic blood flow velocity in the descending aorta (U_{max}). The final parameter was the Doppler blood flow pattern in the IVC. We knew that fetuses with congenital heart disease associated with hydrops have high velocity of atrial reverse flow in the IVC, and based on that we defined two new indices, the preload index (PLI), which is calculated from the Doppler shift of the atrial reverse flow and that of systolic forward flow in a fetal IVC. During the evaluation of fetal cardiac functions using these four parameters, the PLI showed the highest sensitivity and specificity for the cardiogenic hydrops fetus versus the normal fetus. It also showed good resolution between the cardiogenic hydrops fetus and the fetus with structural heart disease not associated with hydrops.

Preload Index

The blood flow pattern in an IVC with normal sinus rhythm showed a pulsating pattern synchronized with the cardiac cycle. The Doppler waveform of the IVC includes three components: reverse flow (A), which occurs during atrial contraction; an initial forward flow (Sf), which coincides with atrial diastole and ventricular systole; and a second forward flow (Df), which is seen with ventricular diastole. A new index, the preload index (PLI), is defined as PLI = A/Sf. The PLI is independent of the angle between the Doppler beam incidence and the blood flow (Fig. 27.2) [3].

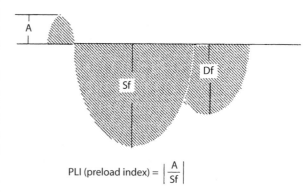

$$\text{PLI (preload index)} = \left| \frac{A}{Sf} \right|$$

Fig. 27.2. Definition of the preload index (*PLI*). *A* blood flow from the right atrium occurring at atrial contraction, *Sf* blood flow into the right atrium coinciding with ventricular systole, *Df* blood flow into the right atrium coinciding with ventricular diastole

Fig. 27.3. Chronological change of the preload index (*PLI*) after 20 weeks of gestation. (With permission from [18])

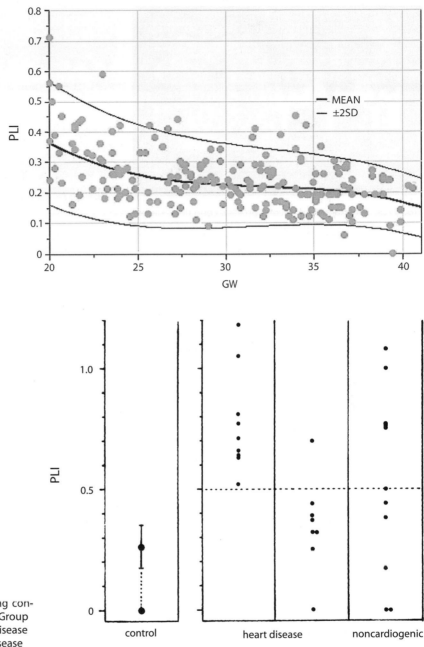

Fig. 27.4. Preload index (*PLI*) among controls and those with fetal disease. Group 1, hydrops associated with heart disease (*n* = 9); group 2, structural heart disease without hydrops (*n* = 8); group 3, hydrops without heart disease (*n* = 11)

Normal Fetuses

The PLI value of normal fetuses ranged from 0 to 0.37 (median 0.13). The PLI gradually decreased after 20 weeks (Fig. 27.3) [18]. The decrease was so slight after 24 weeks of gestation that the influence of age can be ignored on any analysis done beyond 24 weeks of pregnancy [3].

Fetuses with Hydrops and Heart Disease

The PLI values in the three groups of fetuses with disease are compared in Fig. 27.4. The PLI values for those with hydrops associated with heart disease (group 1) are significantly higher than those for normals and for the group with heart disease without hydrops (group 2). PLI values for group 1 ranged from 0.52 to 1.05. All PLI values in this group with cardiogenic hydrops were more than 0.5. PLI values

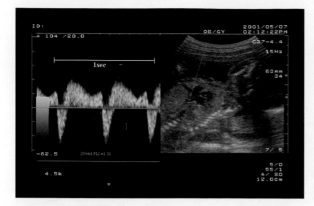

Fig. 27.5. An example of hyper preload condition. Higher preload index (*PLI*) in the recipient of twin-to-twin transfusion syndrome (*TTTS*)

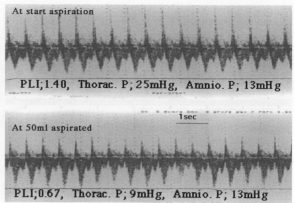

Fig. 27.6. Following aspiration of hydrothorax, the preload index (*PLI*) decreased from 1.40 to 0.67, the thoracic pressure also decreased from 25 mmHg to 9 mmHg. (With permission from [19])

for the third group (those with hydrops without heart disease) were in a wide range, from 0 to 1.08. According to the results of our studies [3, 17], cardiogenic hydrops is associated with less contractility of the heart, lower flow velocity in the descending aorta, and a significantly higher PLI in the IVC.

Another study has shown that umbilical venous pressure is higher in the presence of hydrops fetalis [19]. Thus it is logical to assume that excessive preload is present in the fetus with cardiogenic hydrops. Half of the fetuses with hydrops without heart disease had a higher PLI in our study. It is again reasonable to assume, then, that they might have secondary cardiac dysfunction, as their hydrops is not primarily cardiogenic. Thus we have assigned them a new designation: secondary cardiogenic hydrops (Fig. 27.5).

Blood Flow Change During Fetal Therapy

A high PLI in fetuses showing pleural effusion is always decreased in value by aspiration of the pleural effusion (Figs. 27.6, 27.7). This phenomenon suggests shunting surgery for hydrothorax (Fig. 27.8). In Japan between 1996 and 1999, 28 cases of hydrothorax underwent shunting surgery. In 20 of the 28 cases, surgery was judged effective by the committee on perinatal medicine of the Japan Society of Obstetrics and Gynecology [20].

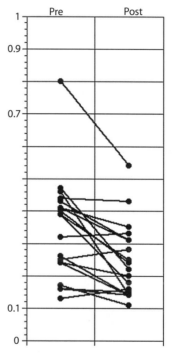

Fig. 27.7. Change in preload index (*PLI*) by the aspiration of hydrothorax, before and after

Blood Flow Dynamics in Fetal Central Veins During Labor

Our studies of venous blood flow during labor support the suggestion that high preload influences blood flow of the fetal central vein [22]. For example, during the recovering period from cord compression or during late deceleration, we recognize high reverse flow in the IVC. It is speculated that blood flow vol-

ume increases the total cardiac output during the recovering period due to cord compression. During late deceleration the blood flow volume may be relatively higher than the cardiac output. Pulsation of blood flow was observed in the umbilical vein under the same conditions during the recovering period from cord compression or during late deceleration (Fig. 27.9).

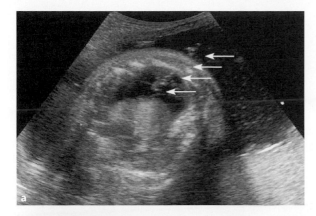

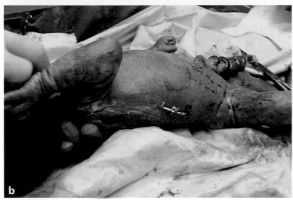

Fig. 27.8 a, b. Fetal therapy for hydrothorax using a double basket catheter. **a** During shunting surgery under ultrasound guidance and **b** immediately after birth

IVC Blood Flow at an Early Stage of Pregnancy

The high preload may present at an early stage of gestation in a normal fetus, an observation supported by our findings [23]. A statistical analysis was performed on the Doppler waveforms in the IVC during early pregnancy, as well as in the umbilical artery, middle cerebral artery, and descending aorta [23]. This study shows that the PLI values significantly increased from 9 to 12 weeks of gestation ($p < 0.05$). The PLI values decreased gradually after 13 weeks' gestation ($p < 0.05$) (Fig. 27.10). This study also shows that the resistance indices of the umbilical artery began to decrease at almost the same age (12 weeks' gestation). There was no end-diastolic component before 11 weeks of pregnancy (Fig. 27.11). It is logical to assume that at 12 weeks of pregnancy the compliance of the placental circulation may begin to decrease and the venous blood flow may tentatively increase [24].

Abnormal IVC Blood Flow Patterns with Fetal Arrhythmias

Many studies of the IVC in human adults [4–8] have contributed to our understanding of the mechanisms that cause variations of flow in a fetal vena cava. We have reported the characteristic blood flows associated with fetal arrhythmias elsewhere [1].

Fig. 27.9. Flow changes with fetal breathing movements before cord compression but begins to decrease with compression. Then, during the period of recovery from cord compression, blood flow pulsation is synchronized with cardiac motion, shown by the fetal electrocardiogram

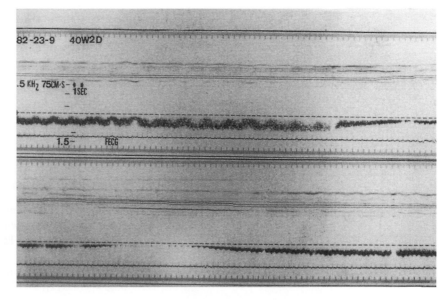

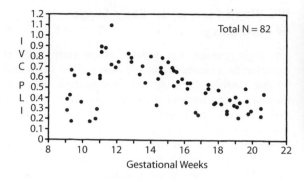

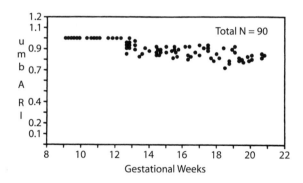

Fig. 27.10. Dynamics of preload index (*PLI*) from 9 to 20 weeks of normal pregnancy. *IVC* inferior vena cava

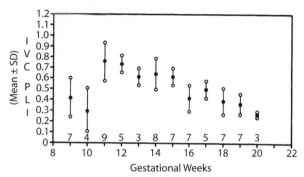

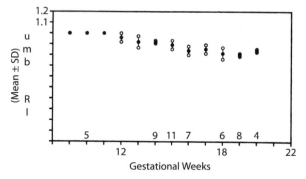

Fig. 27.11. Changes of resistance index (*RI*) from 9 to 20 weeks of normal pregnancy. *UmbA* umbilical artery

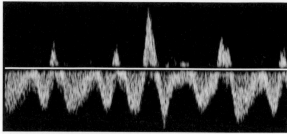

Fig. 27.12. Biphasic forward flow immediately after the dominant reverse flow in a case of premature atrial contraction of the fetus

Blood Flow Pattern of Premature Contractions

During premature atrial contractions (PACs), the systolic forward flow is suddenly interrupted by the reverse flow of the atrial contraction with a higher velocity than usual. The higher reverse flow is designated dominant A. The forward flow after dominant A has a biphasic pattern, with each phase corresponding to ventricular systole and diastole (Fig. 27.12) [1].

With premature ventricular contractions (PVCs), the dominant reverse flow suddenly interrupts the diastolic forward flow. This dominant reverse flow coincides with premature ventricular systole. The subsequent forward flow is monophasic, representing diastolic forward flow [1].

Bradycardic Arrhythmia

With bigeminy of a blocked PAC, the usual reverse flow (A) and dominant reverse flow (dominant A) appear alternately. The time from the preceding flow A to the dominant A is shorter than that from dominant A to the next flow A (Fig. 27.13) [1].

With complete atrioventricular block, reverse flow (including both normal reverse or flow and dominant reverse flow) appears regularly. The reverse flow coincides with the atrial contraction. Dominant reverse flow appears when an atrial contraction occurs during ventricular systole. The forward flow takes variable forms depending on the time relation between the P wave and the QRS complex on the fetal electrocardiogram (ECG) (Fig. 27.14) [1].

Tachyarrhythmias

With atrial flutters and 2:1 conduction, reverse flow appears twice as often as the QRS complex on the ECG. When the fetal ECG is not monitored, the Doppler waveform in a descending aorta may help to determine the rate of appearance of ventricular systole (Fig. 27.15) [1]. With supraventricular tachycardia,

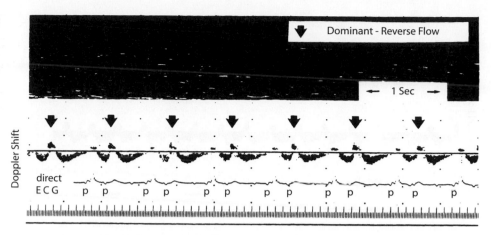

Fig. 27.13. Blood flow in an inferior vena cava during fetal bigeminy of a blocked premature atrial contraction

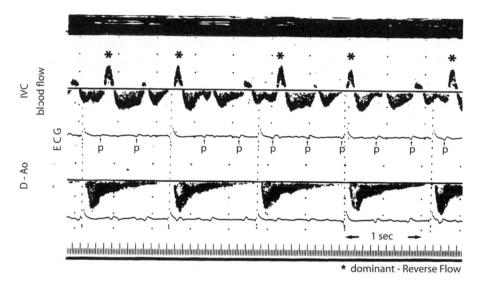

Fig. 27.14. Blood flow patterns of an inferior vena cava (*IVC*) and a descending aorta (*D Ao*) in a case of fetal complete atrioventricular block

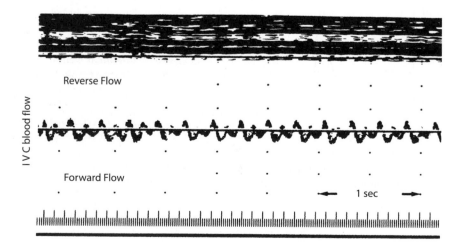

Fig. 27.15. Blood flow in an inferior vena cava (*IVC*) of a case of fetal atrial flutter with 2:1 conduction

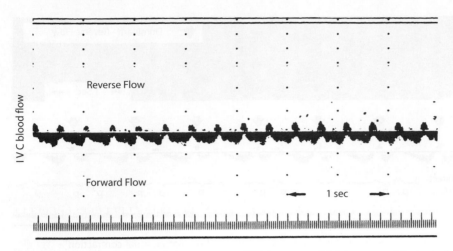

Fig. 27.16. Blood flow in an inferior vena cava (*IVC*) in a case of fetal supraventricular tachycardia

the blood flow pattern in an IVC is almost same as the normal sinus rhythm (Fig. 27.16).

Determination of Fetal Therapy According to the Type of Tachycardia

Some types of fetal tachycardia can be diagnosed by the Doppler waveform at the IVC. However, some conditions were difficult to diagnose, for example, Wolff-Parkinson-White Syndrome. It is necessary to establish the etiology of the tachycardia when we select an antiarrhythmic drug. We require a precise diagnosis to consider the type of intrauterine fetal therapy. We previously published some reports regarding the differential diagnosis of fetal tachycardia by magnetocardiography and direct fetal electrocardiography (Fig. 27.17) [25–29].

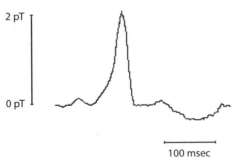

Fig. 27.17. Averaged fetal magnetocardiography of Wolff-Parkinson-White syndrome of the fetus

IVC and Umbilical Vein Blood Flow Patterns in High-Risk Fetuses

The occurrence of umbilical venous pulsations in abnormal and normal pregnancies has been described by several authors. Nakai et al. [30], Indik et al. [31], and Gudmundsson et al. [32] reported pulsatile flow in the umbilical vein with changes in the IVC blood flow pattern in hydropic fetuses. Arduini et al. [33] found that fetuses with absent end-diastolic velocity in the umbilical artery who present with umbilical venous pulsations deteriorate rapidly. In their study, fetuses with umbilical venous pulsations developed abnormal fetal heart rate patterns within a shorter time than did fetuses with normal umbilical venous flow.

As already mentioned, umbilical venous pulsations can be observed in normal pregnancies during the first trimester, and Nakai et al. [22] found such pulsations during the third trimester in normal fetuses. They concluded that umbilical venous pulsations in normal fetuses are due to pulsations of the umbilical artery. Their theory was supported by the fact that umbilical venous pulsations in normal fetuses were observed only transiently and only in the free loop of the umbilical vein.

We conclude that an abnormal blood flow pattern in the venous system represents hemodynamic deterioration in severely compromised fetuses.

References

1. Kanzaki T, Murakami M, Kobayashi H, Chiba Y (1991) Characteristic abnormal blood flow pattern of the inferior vena cava in fetal arrhythmias. J Matern Fetal Invest 1:35–39

2. Chiba Y, Utsu M, Kanzaki T, Hasegawa T (1983) Changes in venous flow and intratracheal flow in fetal breathing movements. Ultrasound Med Biol 11:43–49

3. Kanzaki T, Chiba Y (1990) Evaluation of the preload condition of the fetus by inferior vena caval blood flow pattern. Fetal Diagn Ther 5:168–174

4. Brawley RK, Oldham HN, Vasko JS, Henney RP, Morrow AG (1966) Influence of right atrial pressure pulse on instantaneous vena caval blood flow. Am J Physiol 211:347–353

5. Pinkerson AL, Luria MH, Feris ED (1966) Effect of cardiac rhythm on vena caval blood flows. Am J Physiol 210:505–508

6. Kalmanson D, Veyrat C, Chiche P (1970) Venous return disturbances induced by arrhythmia. Cardiovasc Res 4:279–290

7. Froysaker T (1972) Abnormal flow pattern in superior vena cava induced by arrhythmia. Scand J Cardiovasc Surg 6:140–148

8. Sivacian V, Ranganathan N (1978) Transcutaneous Doppler jugular venous flow velocity recording: clinical and hemodynamic correlates. Circulation 57:930–939

9. Brecher GA (1954) Cardiac variation in venous return studied with a new Bristle flowmeter. Am J Physiol 176:423–430

10. Eckstein RW (1946) Pulsatile changes in inferior cava flow of intrasvascular origin. Am J Physiol 148:740–744

11. Wexler L, Bergel DH, Gabe IT, Mrkin GS, Mills CJ (1968) Velocity of blood flow in normal human venae cavae. Circ Res 23:349–359

12. Kalmanson D, Veyrat C, Chiche P (1971) Atrial versus ventricular contraction in determining systolic venous return. Cardiovasc Res 5:293–302

13. Huisman TW, Stewart PA, Wladimiroff JW (1991) Flow velocity waveforms in the fetal inferior vena cava during the second half of normal pregnancy. Ultrasound Med Biol 17:679–682

14. Wladimiroff JW, Huisman TW, Stewart PA, Stijnen T (1992) Normal fetal Doppler inferior vena cava, transtricuspid, and umbilical artery flow velocity waveforms between 11–16 weeks' gestation. Am J Obstet Gynecol 166:921–924

15. Rizzo G, Arduini D, Romanini C (1992) Umbilical vein pulsations: a physiologic finding in early gestation. Am J Obstet Gynecol 167:675–677

16. Watanabe N, Hosono T, Chiba Y, Kanagawa T (2002) Outcome of infants with nonimmune hydrops fetalis born after 22 weeks' gestation – our experience between 1982 and 2000. J Med Ultrasound 10:80–85

17. Chiba Y, Kobayashi H, Kanzaki T (1990) Quantitative analysis of cardiac function in nonimmunological hydrops fetalis. Fetal Diagn Ther 5:175–188

18. Kanagawa T, Kanzaki T, Chiba Y (2002) Chronologic change in the PLI value at the fetal inferior vena cava in the Japanese fetus. J Med Ultrasound 10:94–98

19. Weiner CP, Heilskov J, Pelzer G et al (1989) Normal values for human umbilical venous and amniotic fluid pressure and their alteration by fetal disease. Am J Obstet Gynecol 161:714–717

20. Chiba Y (2000) Fetal intervention. Ultrasound in Med Biol 26[Suppl I]:S135–S136

21. Chiba Y (2001) Fetal therapy, today and future (Japanese). Acta Neonatologica Japonica 37:582–588

22. Murakami M, Kanzaki T, Utsu M, Chiba Y (1985) Changes in the umbilical venous flow of human fetuses in labor. Acta Obstet Gynecol Jpn 37:776–782

23. Itoh S, Chiba Y, Kanzaki T, Kobayashi H, Murakami N (1995) The dynamics of blood flow in fetal inferior vena cava in early pregnancy, evaluated with those in the umbilical artery, the middle cerebral artery and the descending aorta. J Matern Fetal Invest 5:20–24

24. Gunzman ER, Schulman H, Karmel B, Higgins P (1990) Umbilical artery Doppler velocimetry in pregnancies of less than 21 weeks' duration. J Ultrasound Med 9:655–659

25. Hosono T, Chiba Y, Shinto M, Kandori A, Tsukada K (2001) A fetal Wolff-Parkinson-White syndrome diagnosed prenatally by magnetocardiography. Fetal Diagn Ther 16:215–217

26. Kandori A, Miyashita T, Tsukada K, Hosono T, Miyashita S, Chiba Y, Horigome H, Shigemitsu S, Asaka M (2001) Prenatal diagnosis of QT prolongation by fetal magnetocardiogram – use of QRS and T-waves current-arrow maps. Physiol Meas 22:377–378

27. Kandori A, Hosono T, Kanagawa T, Miyashita S, Chiba Y, Murakami M, Miyashita T, Tsukada K (2002) Detection of atrial-flutter and atrial-fibrillation waveforms by fetal magnetocardiograms. Med Biol Eng Comput 40:213–217

28. Hosono T, Shinto M, Chiba Y, Kandori A, Tsukada K (2002) Prenatal diagnosis of fetal complete atrioventricular block with QT prolongation and alternating ventricular pacemakers using multi-channel magnetocardiography and current-arrow maps. Fetal Diagn Ther 17:173–176

29. Ishi K, Chiba Y, Sasaki Y, Kawamata K, Miyashita S (2003) Fetal atrial tachycardia diagnosed by magnetocardiography and direct fetal electrocardiography, a case report of treatment with propranolol hydrochloride. Fetal Diagn Ther 18:463–466

30. Nakai Y, Miyazaki Y, Matsuoka Y (1992) Pulsatile umbilical venous flow and its clinical significance. Br J Obstet Gynaecol 99:977–980

31. Indik JK, Chen V, Reed KH (1991) Association of umbilical venous with inferior vena cava blood flow velocities. Obst Gynecol 77:551–557

32. Gudmundsson S, Huhta JC, Wood DC et al (1991) Venous Doppler ultrasonography in the fetus with nonimmune hydrops. Am J Obstet Gynecol 164:33–37

33. Arduini D, Rizzo G, Romanini C (1993) The development of abnormal heart rate patterns after absent end-diastolic velocity in umbilical artery: analysis of risk factors. Am J Obstet Gynecol 168:43–50

Chapter 28

Ductus Venosus

Torvid Kiserud

The ductus venosus (venous duct, ductus Arantii) is one of the three physiological shunts responsible for the circulatory adaptation to intrauterine life. It is attributed to Giulio Cesare Aranzi (1530–1589), but the first written account dates back to his contemporary Vesalius in 1561 [1]. Its function was long recognized [2, 3] but of hardly any clinical importance until ultrasound techniques were introduced [4–6]. It is now widely used as an important part of the hemodynamic assessment of the fetus [7] and has been suggested for diagnostic use after birth as well [8].

Anatomy and Development

The ductus venosus is a thin, slightly trumpet-shaped vessel connecting the intra-abdominal umbilical vein with the inferior vena cava (IVC; Fig. 28.1). Its inlet, the isthmus, is on average 0.7 mm at 18 weeks and 1.7 mm at 40 weeks of gestation [9–11]. It leaves the umbilical vein (portal sinus) in a cranial and dorsal direction and reaches the IVC at the level of the hepatic venous confluence shortly below the atria. This section of the IVC is shaped as a funnel [12] but expands predominantly to the left side to receive blood from the ductus venosus and the left hepatic veins [13, 14]. Although variations in direction have been reported, the ductus venosus approaches the IVC at a fairly steep angle (on average 48°) [13]. In early pregnancy the ductus tends to be a straight continuation of the umbilical vein (Fig. 28.2). In late pregnancy a curvature after the isthmus is commonly observed. The relationship to the left and medial hepatic veins is close and sometimes their inlets into the IVC cannot be separated from that of the ductus venosus [15].

Topographically and functionally, the ductus venosus appears to be connected to the foramen ovale in the primate [16], fetal lamb [17, 18], and in the human fetus [2, 5, 19–21]. In the fetal sheep there is a valvular membrane that directs blood from the ductus venosus into the fairly long thoracic IVC to reach the foramen ovale [3]. Although this pattern is commonly presented in anatomical sketches of the human anatomy, it is quite different from the true human to-

pography. The thoracic IVC is short or non-existent in the human fetus and there is no valve developed at the ductus venosus outlet, the effect being that the ductus venosus projects the blood flow directly towards the foramen ovale from a short distance and is less dependent on laminar flow arrangement to avoid extensive blending with low oxygenated blood from the abdominal IVC [13].

During early gestation, the ductus venosus is formed as a confluence of hepatic sinuses, then devel-

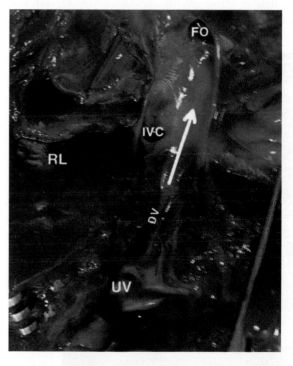

Fig. 28.1. Anterior anatomical view with the liver divided to expose the trumpet-shaped ductus venosus (*DV*) at 39 weeks of gestation. The DV leaves the abdominal portion of the umbilical vein (*UV*) in the direction of the foramen ovale (*FO*). The direction is slightly to the left of the abdominal inferior vena cava (*IVC*), which expands predominantly to the left side (*arrow*) as it reaches the liver confluence. This expansion represents also a continuation of the ductus venosus permitting umbilical blood to reach the FO without extensive blending with deoxygenated blood from the IVC. *RL* right lobe of the liver. (From [14])

ops into a separate channel [22–25], and is regularly recognized with ultrasound color Doppler in embryos of 8 weeks of gestation. Ultrasound visualization and volume flow calculations indicate that the ductus venosus has a more prominent role during early pregnancy than near term [11, 26].

A sphincter has been suggested to operate at the inlet [22, 27–30]. The scarcity of muscular and neuronal elements in the human ductus venosus have raised doubts as to whether such sphincter exists [21, 31–33]. Adrenergic nerves have been traced in the inlet area [34]. An α-adrenergic constriction and a β-adrenergic relaxation have been reported [33, 35, 36]. Both a prostaglandin and a peroxidase P-450 mechanism have been suggested to function in the ductus venosus in the same way as described for the ductus arteriosus [37–40]. The mechanisms could be responsible for the patency during fetal life and its closure in postnatal life; however, in contrast to the ductus arteriosus, oxygen does not seem to trigger the obliteration of the ductus venosus [41]. Recent studies indicate that it is the entire length of the ductus venosus that is active during regulation [33, 42, 43] and that the regulatory mechanism is less sensitive to

adrenergic stimuli than the portal venous branches in the liver tissue [33].

Physiological Background

Via Sinistra

The ductus venosus is an important part of the via sinistra, a classical concept still valid at present (Fig. 28.3). As a direct connection between the umbilical vein and the central venous system, it has the capacity to shunt well-oxygenated blood directly into the central circulation and feed the left atrium

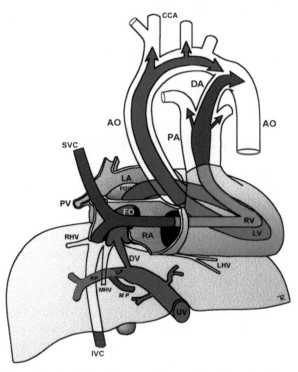

Fig. 28.3. Fetal circulatory pathways showing the three shunts, ductus arteriosus (*DA*), ductus venosus (*DV*), and the foramen ovale (*FO*). The via sinistra (*red*) directs blood from the umbilical vein (*UV*) through the DV and FO to reach the left atrium (*LA*), left ventricle (*LV*), and ascending aorta (*AO*) thus supplying the coronary and cerebral circuit with well-oxygenated blood before joining with the via dextra (*blue*) in the descending AO. The via dextra receives deoxygenated blood from the abdominal inferior vena cava (*IVC*) and superior vena cava (*SVC*) directed to the right atrium (*RA*), right ventricle (*RV*), and pulmonary trunk (*PA*) bypassing the pulmonary circuit through the DA. Splanchnic blood from the main portal stem (*MP*) is provided to the right liver lobe after blending with umbilical blood that reaches the right portal branch (*RP*) through the left branch (*LP*). *CCA* common carotid arteries, *FOV* foramen ovale valve, *LHV* left hepatic vein, *MHV* medial hepatic vein, *PV* pulmonary vein, *RHV* right hepatic vein. (Slightly redrawn from [11])

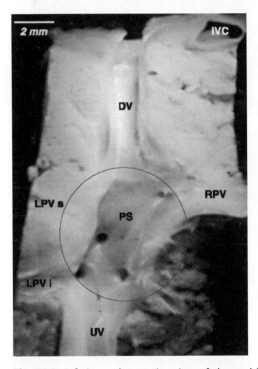

Fig. 28.2. Inferior and posterior view of the umbilical vein (*UV*), portal sinus (*PS*), and ductus venosus (*DV*) at 15 weeks' gestation. Note the considerable number of branches present in the area. Due to the preparation the main portal stem is not seen, but is expected to enter near the label for the right portal vein (*RPV*). *IVC* inferior vena cava, *LPV i* inferior left portal vein, *LPV s* superior left portal vein. (From [20])

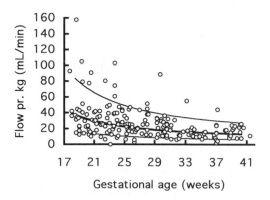

Fig. 28.4. Ductus venosus blood flow (ml/min per kg) in 193 low-risk fetuses presented with 10th, 50th, and 90th percentiles. The relative flow appears more prominent at mid-gestation than during the third trimester. (From [11])

Table 28.1. The fraction of umbilical blood shunted through the ductus venosus during the second half of the human pregnancy [11]

Gestational age (weeks)	Number	Degree of ductus venosus shunting (%)	
		50th percentile	(10th; 90th percentiles)
18–19	34	28	(14; 65)
20–24	45	25	(10; 44)
25–28	34	22	(10; 44)
29–32	32	19	(9; 46)
33–36	21	20	(10; 31)
37–41	27	23	(7; 38)

through the foramen ovale, thus ensuring oxygenated blood to the coronary and cerebral circuit. Animal studies have shown that around 50% of the umbilical blood bypassed the liver through the ductus venosus [16, 17, 44, 45]. In human fetuses it is around 30% at 20 weeks and 20% at 30–40 weeks of gestation when measured by Doppler ultrasound techniques [11, 26]; thus, the shunting through the ductus venosus seems more prominent at mid-gestation than at term (Fig. 28.4; Table 28.1).

During experimental hypoxemia and hypovolemia, the ductus venosus flow is maintained [16, 44, 46–49]; however, since the flow to the liver is reduced, it implies that the fraction of umbilical blood directed through the ductus venosus increases to 70% [16, 44, 46–50]. A similar effect seems to be present in growth-restricted human fetuses [50].

The size of the foramen ovale, the position, and the direction of the ductus venosus, and its high kinetic energy, are suggested to play a role to reduce degree of blending with de-oxygenated blood in the IVC and to force open the foramen ovale valve [13, 14]. Since the oxygen extraction in the liver tissue is

low, causing a reduction in saturation of 10–15% [51, 52], the hepatic venous blood flow from the left liver constitutes another important source of oxygenated blood directed towards the foramen ovale. In total, it is an abundant volume of oxygenated blood that predominantly fills the foramen ovale but additionally spills over to the right side. The result is a notably small difference in oxygen saturation between the left and the right ventricle, 10% under experimental conditions increasing to 12% during hypoxemic insults [3, 53].

Umbilical Liver Perfusion

Another aspect of the ductus venosus function is its role in the fetal liver circulation. Since 20%–30% of the umbilical blood is shunted through the ductus, it implies that 70%–80% of the umbilical blood perfuses the liver as the first organ in the fetus [11]. The pattern indicates the importance of the fetal liver during intrauterine development. Recent studies indicate that blood flow in the fetal liver regulates fetal growth (Fig. 28.5) [54, 55], and that this blood flow depends on external factors such as maternal nutritional state and dietary habits, at least during late pregnancy [56]. In addition to an active regulation of the ductus venosus influencing the distribution of umbilical blood to the liver, both passive regulation (blood pressure and viscosity) [17, 57, 58] and active regulation (vessel constriction) [33, 59, 60] tune the portal liver blood flow. This makes the liver a very delicate watershed area regulated at low pressures. In the long run, umbilical liver flow has a high priority in maintaining growth and development. During acute challenges (i.e., hypoxemia or hypovolemia) short-term responses with increased shunting through the ductus venosus ensures survival. If such challenges are main-

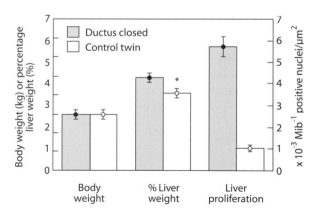

Fig. 28.5. Experimentally occluded ductus venosus in fetal lambs leads to an increased umbilical flow through the liver, increased signs of proliferative activity (*right ordinate*), and increased liver growth (*left ordinate*). (From [54])

tained over a longer period, adaptational mechanisms come into play, reducing the metabolic requirements, and the circulatory redistribution partially returns to normal patterns [61, 62].

Portal Watershed Area

Since blood from the umbilical vein and blood from the main portal stem both supply the liver, there is a watershed area in the liver between the two sources in the right liver. Conventionally umbilical blood supplies the left liver, the ductus venosus, and flows through the left portal branch to join with the blood from the main portal stem as the blood flows into the right portal branch (Fig. 28.3); thus, in the human fetus under physiological conditions in late pregnancy, the left half of the liver receives pure umbilical blood while the right half receives a 50% mixture of umbilical and splanchnic blood [26, 63]; however, during hypovolemia this distributional pattern is shifted to the left. During experimental hemorrhage, less umbilical blood is provided to keep up the pressure in the portal system with the perfusion of the liver and ductus venosus. An increasing component of splanchnic blood from the main portal stem fills up the left portal branch and an increasing proportion of the ductus venosus blood flow will be of splanchnic origin [44, 47, 48]. The phenomenon of shift of the watershed to the left has been observed in the human fetus as well [64, 65], but with no proof that the underlying cause was hypovolemia.

Porto-Caval Pressure Gradient

The position between the umbilical vein (i.e., portal sinus) and the IVC makes the blood flow in the ductus venosus an important indicator of the porto-caval pressure gradient that perfuses the liver tissue [10, 66]. The absolute blood velocity has been suggested as a marker of fetal portal hypertension seen during fetal liver diseases (e.g., lymphoproliferative infiltration, virus infections, mitochondrial diseases). The simplified Bernoulli equation is suggested for the estimation of the pressure gradient [10] (Δp; in mm Hg) based on the maximum trace of the ductus venosus blood velocity (V_{DV}) and the velocity in the umbilical vein (V_{UV}) measured in m/s:

$$\Delta p = 4\left((V_{DV})^2 - (V_{UV})^2\right)$$

It has been estimated that the energy dissipation at the isthmus does not exceed 30%, which makes the calculation a fairly reliable pressure estimate [67, 68] in spite of the possible pressure regain expected to occur during velocity retardation as the blood approaches the heart. Up to now, the diagnostic possibilities of this concept have not been explored to any extent.

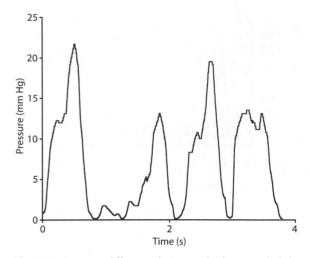

Fig. 28.6. Pressure difference between the lungs and abdomen during fetal respiratory activity at 39 weeks of gestation. It is based on the assumption that the close proximity to the diaphragm makes the ductus venosus blood velocity an indicator of the difference in pressure above and below the liver. The pressure is calculated from the velocities using the simplified Bernoulli equation. (From [10])

Fetal Respiratory Force

Since the liver and its venous confluence is situated just beneath the diaphragm, the ductus venosus blood flow velocity also reflects the abdomino-thoracic pressure gradient. This gradient varies during fetal respiratory movements and is calculated to reach more than 20 mmHg during maximal excursions (Fig. 28.6). The estimations are based on the Bernoulli equation in the same manner as above. The low velocities in the umbilical vein do not influence the calculations and can be left out. Again, this concept is another example of possible diagnostic ductus venosus examination hardly explored.

Postnatal Physiology

After birth, the ductus venosus is obliterated within 1–3 weeks (Fig. 28.7) [69, 70]. Interestingly, the high blood velocity seen prenatally seems to be maintained during that period [70], reflecting the fact that the portal perfusion pressure for the liver circulation is maintained. Observations of prematurely born neonates show that the ductus remains patent longer than in infants born at term [71, 72]. The hypothesis that a patent ductus venosus represents a bypass of the liver in the first weeks of postnatal life to the extent that it influences the clearance rate has been addressed by assessing the galactose concentration in prematurely born neonates [73]. No effect of the patent ductus was found, but the degree of shunting in the ductus venosus was not quantified. The ductus

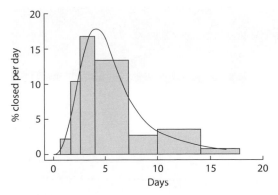

Fig. 28.7. Distribution of closing times of the ductus venosus in healthy neonates. The *bars* represent the percentage closure per day and the curve represents the fitted log logistic distribution. (From [70])

venosus stays open longer also in infants with congenital heart defects or persistent pulmonary hypertension [8], and the waveforms in these cases resemble those seen in abnormal cases prenatally; thus, the ductus venosus velocimetry has been suggested as a diagnostic adjuvant during the first weeks of postnatal life as well.

Ultrasound Imaging and Insonation

A sagittal anterior insonation offers the best visualization of the ductus venosus (Fig. 28.8) [5, 9]. To assess its course and diameters, the perpendicular insonation through the fetal liver suits best. An oblique

transverse section may be more convenient in some fetal positions but rarely offers visualization of the entire length of the vessel.

Color Doppler is an indispensable help in identifying the high velocity at the isthmus of the ductus (Fig. 28.9). With modern equipment the identification can be done from any direction but requires an appropriate setting of filters and ranges to distinguish the typical high velocity of the ductus venosus from velocities in neighboring vessels.

For the pulsed Doppler measurements the sagittal anterior or posterior insonation offers the best control of angle. The anterior insonation from below the fetal umbilicus (Fig. 28.9), or the posterior from the level of the chest, gives insonations that hardly require angle correction. If such insonations are not possible, then the oblique transverse section through the fetal abdomen will provide a good visualization of the ductus venosus inlet but less control of the insonation angle. For the measurement of waveforms this should suffice.

Sample volume should be kept wide to ensure the recording of the maximum velocity during the heart cycle. This holds true for the second half of pregnancy; however, during early pregnancy the sample volume has to be reduced to fit with the geometrical details in order to reduce interference of velocities of the umbilical vein, the proximal portion of the ductus, or neighboring veins and arteries. This is particularly important during the atrial contraction phase

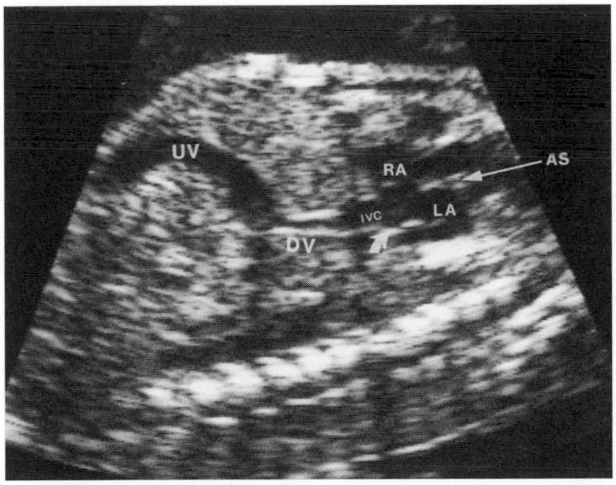

Fig. 28.8. Sagittal ultrasound insonation shows the ductus venosus (*DV*) connecting the umbilical vein (*UV*) to the proximal portion of the inferior vena cava (*IVC*) in a fetus of 18 weeks' gestation. Note how the continuation of the DV follows the posterior wall of the IVC and the foramen ovale valve (*curved arrow*) into the left atrium (*LA*) and behind the atrial septum (*AS; arrow*). *RA* right atrium

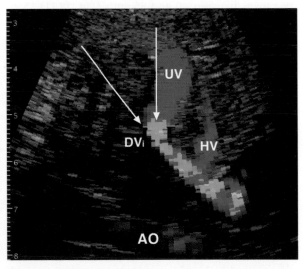

Fig. 28.9. Color Doppler helps identifying the isthmic inlet of the ductus venosus (*DVi*). The preferred insonation for Doppler recording is along or between the *arrows*. Note that the aliasing starts already in the umbilical vein (*UV*) in front of the inlet, the reason being that the blood starts to accelerate before reaching the isthmus. *AO* descending aorta, *HV* middle hepatic vein

since a zero velocity or inverted velocity, which is commonly used for diagnostic purposes [74–79], may be masked.

Angle of insonation and angle correction need particular attention. Transducers commonly used by obstetricians are broad with a flat or curved surface. Compared with sector scanners, these transducers make it harder to achieve an insonation along the ductus venosus with zero or near-zero angle correction. If the recording of absolute velocities has any diagnostic consequence, there is much to gain from getting accustomed to sector scanners so commonly used in cardiology. As mentioned, the sagittal insonation offers the best control of angle, but an oblique transverse interrogation may, in favorable positions, be a good alternative. The angle of insonation should always be documented. In case a curvature has developed centrally to the isthmus, a tangential insonation to this curvature ensures correct insonation and no need of angle correction.

Normal Ductus Venosus Blood Velocity

Typically, the ductus venosus blood flow has a high velocity during the entire cardiac cycle compared with neighboring veins at the corresponding gestational age (Fig. 28.10) [5, 6, 9, 80–82]. Starting in early pregnancy (e.g., 10 weeks of gestation) the velocity increases until reaching a plateau at 22 weeks [81, 82]. For the rest of the pregnancy the peak velocity ranges between 40 and 85 cm/s (Fig. 28.11) [5, 6, 80, 81]. Some variation in reference ranges is seen,

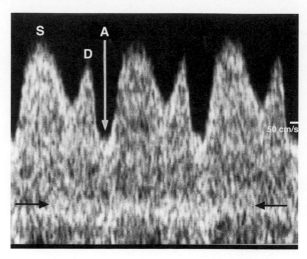

Fig. 28.10. Doppler recording of the blood velocity at the isthmus of the ductus venosus at 33 weeks of gestation. Typically there is high velocity during the entire cardiac cycle with a peak during systole (*S*), another peak during passive diastolic filling (*D*), and deflection (*white arrow*) during atrial contraction (*A*). The velocity of the interfering umbilical vein is faintly seen between *black arrows*

probably depending on equipment, insonation techniques, angle correction, and population.

The velocity pattern reflects the cardiac cycle with a peak during systole, another during passive diastolic filling and a nadir during active diastolic filling (atrial contraction; Fig. 28.10). Typically, the nadir during atrial contraction does not reach the zero line during the second half of pregnancy, in contrast to other precordial veins; however, below 15 weeks of gestation, an increasing number of zero or below-zero

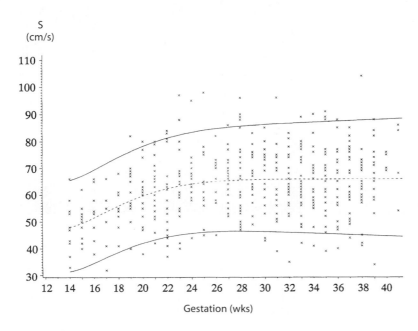

Fig. 28.11. Cross-sectional reference ranges for the systolic peak velocity (*S*) in the ductus venosus with the 5th, 50th, and 95th percentile. (From [81])

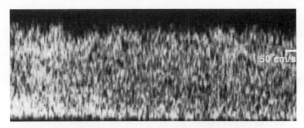

Fig. 28.12. Doppler recording of the blood velocity at the isthmus of the ductus venosus at 32 weeks of gestation shows no pulsation. The phenomenon occurs in 3% of all recordings in low-risk pregnancies. (See Chap. 5 for explanation)

velocities are observed in normal fetuses [14]. Reference ranges have been established for all the components of the wave as well as for the time-averaged maximum velocity during the entire cardiac cycle [5, 80–82]. The time-averaged weighted mean velocity is typically 0.7 of the maximum velocity. The relationship is established by mathematical modeling, and experimental and clinical observations, and is a quite useful information when calculating volume flow [68, 83–86].

It is important to acknowledge the wide normal variation of the waveform. Most reference ranges have not taken that into account, and some have. In 11% of the recording no second velocity peak will be found during the passive diastolic filling [9], and in 3% of all recordings there will be no well-defined nadir visible (Fig. 28.12) [9]. These patterns reflect the wide range of geometrical variation possible in the normal fetus. Squeezing of the ductus venosus outlet or the IVC at the level of the diaphragm will cause an increased wave reflection with less or no pulse wave

transmitted into the ductus venosus resulting in non-pulsatile velocity recording at the isthmus (see Chap. 5) [14, 87]. While this is a fairly common phenomenon in normal fetuses, there are no data on its occurrence in the compromised pregnancy; however, based on experience, it must be rare.

Absolute blood velocity thus has the advantage of directly reflecting both the porto-caval pressure gradient that drives the liver perfusion [10] and the cardiac events that modify the velocity waveform [5]; however, both the type of equipment used by the obstetrician and their tradition of examination technique have made the angle-independent waveform analysis the preferred method compared with the more demanding absolute velocity recording, but not without some loss in diagnostic information.

Waveform Analysis: Indices

To give an angle-independent evaluation, ratios of various components of the waveform during the heart cycle have been suggested (Table 28.2). Some of these ratios are used also for other fetal veins and in analysis of arterial blood velocities. The indices that include the entire heart cycle are more robust and are thus recommended for general use. The pulsatility index for veins (PIV) [80] is probably the most widely used index (Fig. 28.13).

The waveform reflects cardiac events, i.e., the intra-cardiac pressure variation, which is emitted into the precordial venous system as a pulse wave. As mentioned above, using the waveform as the only analysis of the velocity means disregarding the porto-caval pressure gradient reflected in the absolute

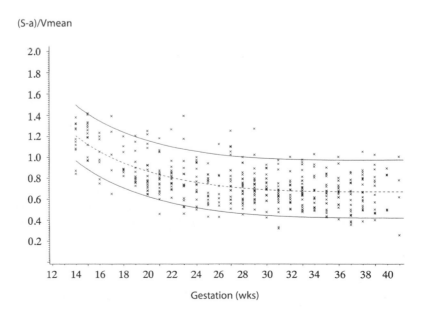

Fig. 28.13. Cross-sectional reference ranges for the pulsatility index for veins (($S-a$)/V_{mean}). (From [81])

Table 28.2. Indices suggested for the waveform analysis of the ductus venosus blood flow velocity. Some of the indices are suggested also for other veins. *A* minimum velocity during atrial contraction (a-wave), *D* peak velocity during ventricular diastole, *S* peak velocity during ventricular systole, V_{ta} time-averaged maximum velocity

Index	Author/date	Reference
$\dfrac{V_{ta}}{S}$	Kiserud et al. (1991)	[5]
$\dfrac{S}{D}$	Huisman et al. (1992)	[6]
$\dfrac{S}{A}$	Oepkes et al. (1993)	[128]
$\dfrac{S-A}{S}$	DeVore and Horenstein (1993)	[129]
$\dfrac{S-A}{D}$	Hecher et al. (1994)	[80]
$\dfrac{S-A}{V_{ta}}$	Hecher et al. (1994)	[80]

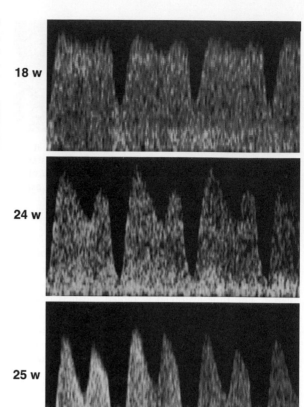

18 w

24 w

25 w

Fig. 28.14. A case of progressive placental compromise and growth restriction shows normal ductus venosus blood flow at 18 weeks with a normal a-wave (*upper panel*). At 24 weeks the augmented a-wave was apparent (*middle panel*). At 25 weeks a further deterioration was seen with a reversed a-wave and an increasing dichotomy between the systolic and diastolic peak (*lower panel*)

velocity. At a very acute angle of insonation an increased error assessing the lowest velocity during atrial contraction may make the waveform less reliable.

Interpretation of the Waveform

The Atrial Contraction Wave

The atrial contraction wave (a-wave) is the single most important part of the waveform from a diagnostic point of view. The augmented atrial contraction wave signifies an increased end-diastolic filling pressure in the heart, which may be induced by an increased distension of the atria leading to an augmented contraction (the Frank-Starling effect) commonly seen in cases with increased preload or congestive heart failure [88–94]. An increased afterload can also lead to a reinforced a-wave (Fig. 28.14) [95–99]. Experimentally imposed hypoxic insult has been shown to cause an increased a-wave in late pregnancy [86, 100, 101], but also at mid-gestation and in early pregnancy [102]. In case of the latter, the effect is believed to be primarily a direct hypoxic effect on the myocardium. In late pregnancy, the effect is predominantly orchestrated via immediate neural responses and secondary endocrine effects on cardiac rhythm and contractility as well as on peripheral vascular impedance [45, 103, 104].

Heart rate is an important determinant for the precordial venous waveforms [92]. A slowing of the heart rate permits a more pronounced venous filling and increased distension of the myocardium resulting

in augmented atrial contraction. The effect is seen in fetal bradycardic conditions.

An increased venous return causes a more pronounced myocardial distension, and a correspondingly augmented a-wave. Typically, this occurs in the twin–twin transfusion syndrome with one of the fetuses being overloaded through placental communications [105]. Arterio-venous malformations in the placenta, fetal liver, fetal brain, or the increased load due to cystic adenomatoid lung malformations are other examples of conditions causing an increased venous return.

Hyperkinetic circulation, such as in fetal anemia, also increases the preload, and the a-wave [106]. With the deterioration of cardiac function, i.e., congestive heart failure, the sign of augmented a-wave becomes more marked, with the minimum velocity reaching zero line or below, even in late pregnancy.

Compliance of the heart is reflected in the a-wave. The reduced compliance of the myocardium in cardio-myopathies, myocarditis (e.g., parvovirus B19 infection), hypoxemia, and acidosis is commonly associated with a deepened a-wave (Fig. 28.14). The compliance can also be influenced by extra-cardiac restrictions in the chest (see Chap. 5). Normally, the absence of free air during intrauterine life makes the entire vascular system, including the heart, less compliant than after birth. In addition, increased pressure in the fetal chest (e.g., large tumors, pleural effusions, or tracheal atresia) could lead to further restriction of the cardiac excursions and made visible in the a-wave.

A significant tricuspid or mitral regurgitation, or both, may contribute to a rapidly increasing volume and pressure in the atria thus causing an augmented a-wave.

Timing of the atrial contraction is also an important determinant for the magnitude of the a-wave. The various patterns found in arrhythmias are particularly instructive [107–109]. In its simplest form, the wave of a supraventricular extrasystole may hardly be visible in the ductus venosus Doppler recording, whereas the atrial contraction following the compensatory postictal pause has been given the extra time and load of volume to cause an augmented a-wave. An even more amplified version of the a-wave is seen in cases of atrioventricular block. When the atrial contraction coincides with the ventricular systole, the atrioventricular valves are closed and the compliance correspondingly reduced, the result being a stronger pulse-wave directed into the precordial veins, including the ductus venosus. During tachycardia the timing of the atrial contraction, the size of the atria, whether the atrioventricular valves are open, the momentary degree of filling, the functional condition of the myocardium itself, and probably details of where the contraction starts and how it propagates determine the details of the a-wave [109].

In recent years the a-wave has been the focus in the search for methods of surveillance of patients with placental compromise. Short-time variation of the computerized CTG and the a-wave (or its effect on the pulsatility indices) showed late changes compared with umbilical artery pulsatility and changes in the middle cerebral artery (Fig. 28.15) [110–112]. The sign seems easier to interpret in pregnancies before 32 weeks of gestation than after; thus, it has become a promising method for serial observations in order to determine timing of delivery of the growth-restricted fetus. Since the ductus venosus velocity pattern is an instantaneous reflection of the cardiac function, these changes are probably useful signs in other conditions where the fetus is at risk as well.

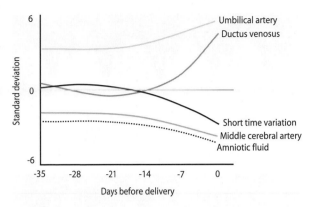

Fig. 28.15. Serial observations of cases with severe intrauterine growth restriction delivered 32 weeks of gestation. Changes in the pulsatility index of the umbilical and middle cerebral arteries and oligohydramnios are common findings 3–5 weeks before delivery. Alterations in the ductus venosus waveform and short time variation are notable during the last 2 weeks before delivery, indicating that these two parameters may be suitable for the final tuning of time of delivery. (Modified from [20])

Systolic Wave

Conventionally, the systolic peak during ventricular contraction is smooth and rounded (Fig. 28.16). Changes in myocardial function are reflected also in this part of the cardiac cycle. In conditions of reduced compliance, both of extracardiac and cardiac origin, the downstroke of the velocity becomes more acute (Fig. 28.16). This is particularly apparent during the deterioration seen in placental compromise [7, 113]. Increased afterload combined with an increased degree of hypoxemia and acidosis drives the myocardial function toward less compliance. The visible result is the acute up- and downstroke of the systolic peak and a corresponding dissociation between the systolic and diastolic peak (Fig. 28.16). A similar effect can be achieved by the externally increased pressure on the heart, and thus correspondingly reduced compliance (see Chap. 5). The increased blood volume and atrial pressure caused by a regurgitation of the atrioventricular valves causes an augmented a-wave; however, the more extensive the regurgitation is, the more rapid the atrial filling will be, and the earlier in the heart cycle the impact will come. In cases of Ebstein anomaly this may lead to an early downstroke during ventricular systole.

Pitfalls

For the beginner, sampling the velocity in a neighboring vein, or including interference from the IVC or other vessels, may falsely give the impression of an abnormal ductus venosus recording. The velocity in the hepatic veins tends to be more acute and, partic-

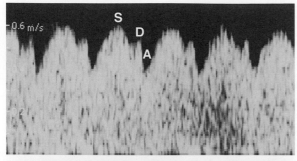

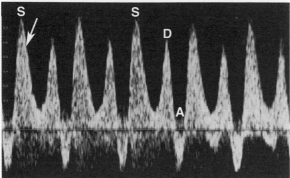

Fig. 28.16. Conventionally, the systolic peak (*S*) is smooth signifying good atrial compliance (*upper panel*). Increased stiffness of the myocardium due to hypoxia and acidosis, such as in advanced placental compromise, results in a rapid downstroke (*arrow*) of the S (*lower panel*). Typically the waveform is transformed into acute velocity changes and a dissociation between S and diastolic peak (*D*). The augmented a-wave (*A*) reaching below zero is a common part of the pattern

ularly during the second trimester, the veins have a zero or reversed velocity during atrial contraction. Before leaping to a conclusion, it is prudent to reproduce the recording in a renewed insonation. It is also helpful to know that the augmented pulsatility in the ductus venosus commonly has a corresponding pulsatile flow in the umbilical vein. If the insonation makes the identification of the ductus venosus less certain, the pulsatility and a-wave should be checked in more accessible precordial veins such as the IVC or hepatic veins.

The pulsatile flow in the left portal vein is the mirror image of the ductus venosus waveform [64]. One of the consequences is that the a-wave occurs not as a nadir but as a peak (see Chap. 5). The simultaneous sampling of the ductus venosus inlet and the left portal vein could then cause a masking of the true nadir in the ductus venosus. Masking may also be the case during simultaneous sampling at the isthmus of the ductus venosus and the umbilical vein where the pulsatility usually is less pronounced. This is a common problem in early pregnancy.

Local changes of no pathological significance may influence the waveform. The fetal position may be such a factor. A fetus bending forward, particularly in the extreme situations of oligohydramnios, may squeeze the IVC, the outlet, or the entire length of the ductus venosus to the extent that most of the wave is reflected and the recorded wave at the inlet has lost pulsation (see Chap. 5). In 3% of pregnancies this normal phenomenon may be observed. Usually, a change in fetal position within the next minutes is accompanied with the restoration of pulsatile flow velocity.

A normal ductus venosus does not exclude abnormal physiology. All the factors determining the waveform should be taken into consideration when interpreting the velocity recording, e.g., a metabolic error of the myocardium may not necessarily be reflected in an abnormal waveform in the ductus venosus if the heart has compensated for the increased stiffness of the muscle by increasing the cardiac volume and thus improving the compliance.

Increased vascular resistance in the fetal liver tissue may cause portal hypertension and ascites. Examining exclusively the waveform of the ductus venosus using indices may not reveal any abnormality since the waveform predominantly reflects cardiac function. It is a common error not to notice the absolute velocities, which may exceed 1 m/s and signify portal hypertension in such cases [66].

Reproducibility

In experienced hands a recording of the ductus venosus blood velocimetry is achieved in almost all women both in early and late pregnancy, even with substandard equipment. The limits of agreement for intra-observer variation are [–13; 12 cm/s] for the systolic peak, and [–15; 12 cm/s] during the a-wave [9]. The reproducibility is better for the indices than for the absolute velocity recordings [81]. That is due to the extra challenge it takes to record absolute velocities at a zero- or low angle of insonation, a less important detail when using the waveform analysis.

Doppler assessment of the ductus venosus during early pregnancy seems to have a reduced reproducibility, particularly for the peak systolic and the nadir during a-wave during transabdominal scanning at 10–14 weeks of gestation. The coefficient of variation for systolic and end-diastolic velocity was 19% and 29%, respectively [114]. The coefficient for the PIV was better, 9%. These results were reproduced in another study but with somewhat better numbers [115].

The normal ranges for absolute velocities were reasonably reproduced in the pioneering studies [5, 9, 80, 81]. When recording Doppler signals without the control of color Doppler, the velocities appeared to be slightly less, possibly due to less control of the correct insonation angle. For the pulsatility indices there is little variation from study to study.

Fetal movements and respiratory exercise could have a profound impact on the ductus venosus blood flow velocity and should carefully be avoided for the standard evaluation.

Agenesis of the Ductus Venosus

An increasing number of case reports link agenesis of the ductus venosus to fetal demise, hydrops fetalis, asphyxia, vascular and cardiac anomalies, and chromosomal aberrations [116–125]. This has led to the recommendation of an extended scan if the ductus venosus is not identified. It is likely that agenesis occurs more commonly in connection with chromosomal aberrations and anomalies, but so far there are no statistics to prove it. Some have taken the presence of ductus venosus agenesis in hydrops and intrauterine demise as an indication that a patent ductus venosus is vital for intrauterine development; however, it can be argued that the ductus venosus agenesis was discovered in these fetuses after a primary finding had made an extended ultrasound scan necessary or during post-mortem examination. In a recent study of 203 normal pregnancies one fetus had agenesis [11]. Perinatal outcome was uneventful for this fetus with a birth weight at the 39th percentile and a normal ponderal index.

Experimental occlusion of the ductus venosus in fetal sheep led to increased umbilical vein pressure and hepatic venous flow but otherwise had no impact on regional blood distribution [126]; however, such an occlusion has a considerable impact on liver cell proliferation and IGF-2 production, and thus growth [54, 55].

There is an interesting set of observations of agenesis in fetuses with porto-caval shunts, or similar shunts, draining umbilical venous blood directly to the central veins or heart [125]. These fetuses seem to be in the position of not being able to develop the ductus venosus or to close the ductus as a compensatory mechanism. Many of these fetuses have a hyperkinetic circulation, possibly in an attempt to keep up portal pressure and liver perfusion.

This is not in contradiction to the concept that the ductus venosus is an important fetal shunt. Instead, the story unfolds with the ductus venosus having at least two functions. In the long run, the regulation of the umbilical liver perfusion is crucial for fetal development and growth; however, during acute challenges of hypoxemia or hypovolemia, the priority of the liver is temporarily reduced to permit life-saving maneuvers of maintaining oxygenated blood to the heart and brain, or as some physiologists have put it: "The fetal dilemma: spare the brain and spoil the liver" [127].

References

1. Franklin KJ (1941) Ductus venosus (Arantii) and ductus arteriosus (Botalli). Bull Hist Med 9:580–584
2. Rudolph AM, Heymann MA, Teramo K, Barrett C, Räihä N (1971) Studies on the circulation of the previable human fetus. Pediatr Res 5:452–465
3. Rudolph AM (1985) Distribution and regulation of blood flow in the fetal and neonatal lamb. Circ Res 57:811–821
4. Chinn DH, Filly RA, Callen PW (1982) Ultrasonographic evaluation of fetal umbilical and hepatic vascular anatomy. Radiology 144:153–157
5. Kiserud T, Eik-Nes SH, Blaas H-G, Hellevik LR (1991) Ultrasonographic velocimetry of the fetal ductus venosus. Lancet 338:1412–1414
6. Huisman TWA, Stewart PA, Wladimiroff JW (1992) Ductus venosus blood flow velocity waveforms in the human fetus: a Doppler study. Ultrasound Med Biol 18:33–37
7. Kiserud T (2001) The ductus venosus. Semin Perinatol 25:11–20
8. Fugelseth D, Kiserud T, Liestøl K, Langslet A, Lindemann R (1999) Ductus venosus blood velocity in persistent pulmonary hypertension of the newborn. Arch Dis Child 81:F35–F39
9. Kiserud T, Eik-Nes SH, Hellevik LR, Blaas H-G (1992) Ductus venosus: a longitudinal Doppler velocimetric study of the human fetus. J Matern Fetal Invest 2:5–11
10. Kiserud T, Hellevik LR, Eik-Nes SH, Angelsen BAJ, Blaas H-G (1994) Estimation of the pressure gradient across the fetal ductus venosus based on Doppler velocimetry. Ultrasound Med Biol 20:225–232
11. Kiserud T, Rasmussen S, Skulstad SM (2000) Blood flow and degree of shunting through the ductus venosus in the human fetus. Am J Obstet Gynecol 182:147–153
12. Huisman TWA, Gittenberger-de Groot AC, Wladimiroff JW (1992) Recognition of a fetal subdiaphragmatic venous vestibulum essential for fetal venous doppler assessment. Pediatr Res 32:338–341
13. Kiserud T, Eik-Nes SH, Blaas H-G, Hellevik LR (1992) Foramen ovale: an ultrasonographic study of its relation to the inferior vena cava, ductus venosus and hepatic veins. Ultrasound Obstet Gynecol 2:389–396
14. Kiserud T (1999) Hemodynamics of the ductus venosus. Eur J Obstet Gynecol Reprod Biol 84:139–147
15. Champetier J, Yver R, Tomasella T (1989) Functional anatomy of the liver of the human fetus: application to ultrasonography. Surg Radiol Anat 11:53–62
16. Behrman RE, Lees MH, Peterson EN, de Lannoy CW, Seeds AE (1970) Distribution of the circulation in the normal and asphyxiated fetal primate. Am J Obstet Gynecol 108:956–969
17. Edelstone DI, Rudolph AM, Heymann MA (1978) Liver and ductus venosus blood flows in fetal lambs in utero. Circ Res 42:426–433

18. Edelstone DI, Rudolph AM (1979) Preferential streaming of ductus venosus blood to the brain and heart in fetal lambs. Am J Physiol 237:H724–H729

19. Lind J, Wegelius C (1949) Angiocardiographic studies on the human foetal circulation. Pediatrics 4:391–400

20. Mavrides E, Moscoso G, Carvalho JS, Campbell S, Thilaganathan B (2001) The anatomy of the umbilical, portal and hepatic venous system in the human fetus at 14–19 weeks of gestation. Ultrasound Obstet Gynecol 18:598–604

21. Mavrides E, Moscoso G, Carvalho JS, Campbell S, Thilaganathan B (2002) The human ductus venosus between 13 and 17 weeks of gestation: histological and morphometric studies. Ultrasound Obstet Gynecol 19:39–46

22. Chako AW, Reynolds SRM (1953) Embryonic development in the human of the sphincter of the ductus venosus. Anat Rec 115:151–173

23. Dickson AD (1957) The development of the ductus venosus in man and the goat. J Anat 91:358–368

24. Severn CB (1972) A morphological study of the development of the human liver. Am J Anat 133:85–108

25. Lassau JP, Bastian D (1983) Organogenesis of the venous structures of the human liver: a hemodynamic theory. Anat Clin 5:97–102

26. Bellotti M, Pennati G, Gasperi C de, Battaglia FC, Ferrazzi E (2000) Role of ductus venosus in distribution of umbilical flow in human fetuses during second half of pregnancy. Am J Physiol 279:H1256–H1263

27. Barron DH (1942) The "sphincter" of the ductus venosus. Anat Rec 82:389

28. Gennser G, Owman CH, Sjöberg N-O (1967) Histochemical evidence of an aminergic sphincter mechanism in the ductus venosus of the human fetus. In: Horsky J, Stembera ZK (eds) Intrauterine dangers to the foetus. Excerpta Medica Foundation, Amsterdam

29. Pearson AA, Sauter RW (1969) The innervation of the umbilical vein in human embryos and fetuses. Am J Anat 125:345–352

30. Pearson AA, Sauter RW (1971) Observations on the phrenic nerves and the ductus venosus in human embryos and fetuses. Am J Obstet Gynecol 110:560–565

31. Meyer WW, Lind J (1965) Über die struktur und den verschlussmechanismus des ductus venosus. Zeitsch Zellforschung 67:390–405

32. Meyer WW, Lind J (1966) The ductus venosus and the mechanism of its closure. Arch Dis Childh 41:597–605

33. Tchirikov M, Kertschanska S, Schroder HJ (2003) Differential effects of catecholamines on vascular rings from the ductus venosus and intrahepatic veins of fetal sheep. J Physiol 548:519–526

34. Ehinger B, Gennser G, Owman C, Persson H, Sjöberg N-O (1968) Histochemical and pharmacological studies on amine mechanisms in the umbilical cord, umbilical vein and ductus venosus of the human fetus. Acta Physiol Scand 72:15–24

35. Coceani F, Adeagbo ASO, Cutz E, Olley PM (1984) Autonomic mechanisms in the ductus venosus of the lamb. Am J Physiol 247:H17–H24

36. Coceani F (1993) The control of the ductus venosus: an update. Eur J Pediatr 152:976–977

37. Adeagbo ASO, Coceani F, Olley PM (1982) The response of the lamb ductus venosus to prostaglandins and inhibitors of prostaglandin and thromboxane synthesis. Circ Res 51:580–586

38. Adeagbo ASO, Breen CA, Cutz E, Lees JG, Olley PM, Coceani F (1989) Lamb ductus venosus: evidence of a cytochrome P-450 mechanism in its contractile tension. J Pharmacol Exp Ther 252:875–879

39. Adeagbo ASO, Bishai I, Lees J, Olley PM, Coceani F (1984) Evidence for a role of prostaglandine I2 and thromboxane A2 in the ductus venosus of the lamb. Can J Physiol Pharmacol 63:1101–1105

40. Morin FCI (1987) Prostaglandin E1 opens the ductus venosus in the newborn lamb. Pediatr Res 21:225–228

41. Coceani F, Olley PM (1988) The control of cardiovascular shunts in the fetal and perinatal period. Can J Pharmacol 66:1129–1134

42. Momma K, Ito T, Ando M (1992) In situ morphology of the ductus venosus and related vessels in the fetal and neonatal rat. Pediatr Res 32:386–389

43. Kiserud T, Ozaki T, Nishina H, Rodeck C, Hanson MA (2000) Effect of NO, phenylephrine and hypoxemia on the ductus venosus diameter in the fetal sheep. Am J Physiol 279:H1166–H1171

44. Itskovitz J, LaGamma EF, Rudolph AM (1983) The effect of reducing umbilical blood flow on fetal oxygenation. Am J Obstet Gynecol 145:813–818

45. Jensen A, Berger R (1993) Regional distribution of cardiac output. In: Hanson MA, Spencer JAD, Rodeck CH (eds) Fetus and neonate physiology and clinical application, vol 1. The circulation. Cambridge University Press, Cambridge

46. Edelstone DI, Rudolph AM, Heymann MA (1980) Effect of hypoxemia and decreasing umbilical flow on liver and ductus venosus blood flows in fetal lambs. Am J Physiol 238:H656–H663

47. Itskovitz J, LaGamma EF, Rudolph AM (1987) Effects of cord compression on fetal blood flow distribution and O2 delivery. Am J Physiol 252:H100–H109

48. Meyers RL, Paulick RP, Rudolph CD, Rudolph AM (1991) Cardiovascular responses to acute, severe haemorrhage in fetal sheep. J Dev Physiol 15:189–197

49. Jensen A, Roman C, Rudolph AM (1991) Effect of reduced uterine flow on fetal blood flow distribution and oxygen delivery. J Dev Physiol 15:309–323

50. Tchirikov M, Rybakowski C, Hünecke B, Schröder HJ (1998) Blood flow through the ductus venosus in singleton and multifetal pregnancies and in fetuses with intrauterine growth retardation. Am J Obstet Gynecol 178:943–949

51. Bristow J, Rudolph AM, Itskovitz J (1981) A preparation for studying liver blood flow, oxygen consumption, and metabolism in the fetal lamb in utero. J Dev Physiol 3:255–266

52. Bristow J, Rudolph AM, Itskovitz J, Barnes R (1982) Hepatic oxygen and glucose metabolism in the fetal lamb. J Clin Invest 71:1047–1061

53. Dawes GS, Mott JC (1964) Changes in O2 distribution and consumption in foetal lambs with variations in umbilical blood flow. J Physiol (Lond) 170:524–540

54. Tchirikov M, Kertschanska S, Schröder HJ (2001) Obstruction of ductus venosus stimulates cell proliferation in organs of fetal sheep. Placenta 22:24–31

55. Tchirikov M, Kertschanska S, Sturenberg HJ, Schröder HJ (2002) Liver blood perfusion as a possible instru-

ment for fetal growth regulation. Placenta 23:S153–S158

56. Haugen G, Godfrey K, Kiserud T, Shore S, Inskip HM, Hanson M (2003) Maternal pre-pregnancy subscapular skinfold thickness, parity and birthweight: influence on fetal liver blood flow in late pregnancy. Pediatr Res 53:12A

57. Edelstone DI (1980) Regulation of blood flow through the ductus venosus. J Dev Physiol 2:219–238

58. Kiserud T, Stratford L, Hanson MA (1997) Umbilical flow distribution to the liver and ductus venosus: an in vitro investigation of the fluid dynamic mechanisms in the fetal sheep. Am J Obstet Gynecol 177:86–90

59. Paulick RP, Meyers RL, Rudolph CD, Rudolph AM (1990) Venous and hepatic vascular responses to indomethacin and prostaglandin E1 in the fetal lamb. Am J Obstet Gynecol 163:1357–1363

60. Paulick RP, Meyers RL, Rudolph CD, Rudolph AM (1991) Umbilical and hepatic venous responses to circulating vasoconstrictive hormones in fetal lamb. Am J Physiol 260:H1205–H1213

61. Bocking AD, Gagnon R, White SE, Homan J, Milne KM, Richardson B (1988) Circulatory responses to prolonged hypoxemia in fetal sheep. Am J Obstet Gynecol 159:1418–1424

62. Bocking AD (1993) Effect of chronic hypoxaemia on circulation control. In: Hanson MA, Spencer JAD, Rodeck CH (eds) Fetus and neonate physiology and clinical application, vol 1. The circulation. Cambridge University Press, Cambridge

63. Haugen G, Godfrey K, Shore S, Kiserud T, Hanson M (2002) Fetal hepatic blood flow and liver size. J Soc Gynecol Invest 9:126A

64. Kiserud T, Kilavuz Ö, Hellevik LR (2003) Venous pulsation in the left portal branch: the effect of pulse and flow direction. Ultrasound Obstet Gynecol 21:359–364

65. Kilavuz Ö, Vetter K, Kiserud T, Vetter P (2004) The left portal vein is the watershed of the fetal venous system. J Perinat Med 31:184–187

66. Kiserud T (2001) Ductus venosus blood velocity in myeloproliferative disorders. Ultrasound Obstet Gynecol 18:184–185

67. Hellevik LR, Kiserud T, Irgens F, Ytrehus T, Eik-Nes SH (1998) Simulation of pressure drop and energy dissipation for blood flow in a human fetal bifurcation. J Biomech Eng 120:455–462

68. Pennati G, Redaelli A, Bellotti M, Ferrazzi E (1996) Computational analysis of the ductus venosus fluid dynamics based on Doppler measurements. Ultrasound Med Biol 22:1017–1029

69. Loberant N, Barak M, Gaitini D, Herkovits M, Ben-Elisha M, Roguin N (1992) Closure of the ductus venosus in neonates: findings on real-time gray-scale, color-flow Doppler, and duplex Doppler sonography. AJR 159:1083–1085

70. Fugelseth D, Lindemann R, Liestøl K, Kiserud T, Langslet A (1997) Ultrasonographic study of ductus venosus in healthy neonates. Arch Dis Child 77:F131–134

71. Fugelseth D, Lindemann R, Liestøl K, Kiserud T, Langslet A (1998) Postnatal closure of ductus venosus in preterm infants 32 weeks. An ultrasonographic study. Early Hum Dev 53:163–169

72. Loberant N, Herkovits M, Ben-Elisha M, Herschkowitz S, Sela S, Roguin N (1999) Closure of the ductus venosus in premature infants: findings on real-time gray-scale, color-flow Doppler, and duplex Doppler sonography. Am J Roentgenol 172:227–229

73. Fugelseth D, Guthenberg C, Hagenfeldt L, Liestøl K, Hallerud M, Lindemann R (2001) Patent ductus venosus does not lead to alimentary galactosaemia in preterm infants. Acta Paediatr 90:192–195

74. Montenegro N, Matias A, Areias JC, Barros H (1997) Ductus venosus revisited: a Doppler blood flow evaluation in first trimester of pregnancy. Ultrasound Med Biol 23:171–176

75. Borrell A, Antolin E, Costa D, Farre MT, Martinez JM, Fortuny A (1998) Abnormal ductus venosus blood flow in trisomy 21 fetuses during early pregnancy. Am J Obstet Gynecol 179:1612–1617

76. Matias A, Gomes C, Flack N, Montenegro N, Nicolaides KH (1998) Screening for chromosomal defects at 11–14 weeks: the role of ductus venosus blood flow. Ultrasound Obstet Gynecol 12:380–384

77. Matias A, Huggon I, Areias JC, Montenegro N, Nicolaides KH (1999) Cardiac defects in chromosomally normal fetuses with abnormal ductus venosus blood flow at 10–14 weeks. Ultrasound Obstet Gynecol 14:307–310

78. Matias A, Montenegro N, Areias JC, Leite LP (2000) Hemodynamic evaluation of the first trimester fetus with specific emphasis on venous return. Hum Reprod Update 6:177–189

79. Borrell A, Martinez JM, Seres A, Borobio V, Cararach V, Fortuny A (2003) Ductus venosus assessment at the time of nuchal translucency measurement in the detection of fetal aneuploidy. Prenat Diagn 23:921–926

80. Hecher K, Campbell S, Snijders R, Nicolaides K (1994) Reference ranges for fetal venous and atrioventricular blood flow parameters. Ultrasound Obstet Gynecol 4:381–390

81. Bahlmann F, Wellek S, Reinhardt I, Merz E, Welter C (2000) Reference values of ductus venosus flow velocities and calculated waveform indices. Prenat Diagn 20:623–634

82. Prefumo F, Risso D, Venturini PL, Biasio P de (2002) Reference values for ductus venosus Doppler flow measurements at 10–14 weeks of gestation. Ultrasound Obstet Gynecol 20:42–46

83. Pennati G, Bellotti M, Ferrazzi E, Rigano S, Garberi A (1997) Hemodynamic changes across the human ductus venosus: a comparison between clinical findings and mathematical calculations. Ultrasound Obstet Gynecol 9:383–391

84. Pennati G, Bellotti M, Ferrazzi E, Bozzo M, Pardi G, Fumero R (1998) Blood flow through the ductus venosus in human fetuses: calculation using Doppler velocimetry and computational findings. Ultrasound Med Biol 24:477–487

85. Kiserud T, Hellevik LR, Hanson MA (1998) The blood velocity profile in the ductus venosus inlet expressed by the mean/maximum velocity ratio. Ultrasound Med Biol 24:1301–1306

86. Tchirikov M, Eisermann K, Rybakowski C, Schröder HJ (1998) Doppler ultrasound evaluation of ductus venosus blood flow during acute hypoxia in fetal lambs. Ultrasound Obstet Gynecol 11:426–431

87. Kiserud T (2000) Fetal venous circulation: an update on hemodynamics. J Perinat Med 28:90–96

88. Reed KL, Appleton CP, Anderson CF, Shenker L, Sahn DJ (1990) Doppler studies of vena cava flows in human fetuses; insights into normal and abnormal cardiac physiology. Circulation 81:498–505

89. Reed KL, Chaffin DG, Anderson CF, Newman AT (1997) Umbilical venous velocity pulsations are related to atrial contraction pressure waveforms in fetal lambs. Obstet Gynecol 89:953–956

90. Kanzaki T, Chiba Y (1990) Evaluation of the preload condition of the fetus by inferior vena caval blood flow pattern. Fetal Diagn Ther 5:168–174

91. Gudmundsson S, Huhta JC, Wood DC, Tulzer G, Cohen AW, Weiner S (1991) Venous Doppler ultrasonography in the fetus with nonimmune hydrops. Am J Obstet Gynecol 164:33–37

92. Gudmundsson S, Gunnarsson G, Hökegård K-H, Ingmarsson J, Kjellmer I (1999) Venous Doppler velocimetry in relationship to central venous pressure and heart rate during hypoxia in ovine fetus. J Perinat Med 27:81–90

93. Tulzer G, Gudmundsson S, Rotondo KM, Wood DC, Cohen AW, Huhta J (1991) Doppler in the evaluation and prognosis of fetuses with tricuspid regurgitation. J Matern Fetal Invest 1:15–18

94. Tulzer G, Gudmundsson S, Wood DC, Cohen AW, Weiner S, Huhta JC (1994) Doppler in non-immune hydrops fetalis. Ultrasound Obstet Gynecol 4:279–283

95. Kiserud T, Eik-Nes SH, Blaas H-G, Hellevik LR, Simensen B (1994) Ductus venosus blood velocity and the umbilical circulation in the seriously growth retarded fetus. Ultrasound Obstet Gynecol 4:109–114

96. Hecher K, Snijders R, Campbell S, Nicolaides K (1995) Fetal venous, intracardiac, and arterial blood flow measurements in intrauterine growth retardation: relationship with fetal blood gases. Am J Obstet Gynecol 173:10–15

97. Hecher K, Campbell S, Doyle P, Harrington K, Nicolaides K (1995) Assessment of fetal compromise by Doppler ultrasound investigation of the fetal circulation. Circulation 91:129–138

98. Rizzo G, Capponi A, Rinaldo D, Arduini D, Romanini C (1995) Ventricular ejection force in growth-retarded fetuses. Ultrasound Obstet Gynecol 5:247–255

99. Rizzo G, Capponi A, Talone P, Arduini D, Romanini C (1996) Doppler indices from inferior vena cava and ductus venosus in predicting pH and oxygen tension in umbilical blood at cordocentesis in growth-retarded fetuses. Ultrasound Obstet Gynecol 7:401–410

100. Reuss ML, Rudolph AM, Dae MW (1983) Phasic blood flow patterns in the superior and inferior venae cavae and umbilical vein of fetal sheep. Am J Obstet Gynecol 145:70–76

101. Hasaart TH, de Haan J (1986) Phasic blood flow patterns in the common umbilical vein of fetal sheep during umbilical cord occlusion and the influence of autonomic nervous system blockade. J Perinat Med 14:19–26

102. Kiserud T, Jauniaux E, West D, Ozturk O, Hanson MA (2001) Circulatory responses to acute maternal hyperoxaemia and hypoxaemia assessed non-invasively by ultrasound in fetal sheep at 0.3–0.5 gestation. Br J Obstet Gynaecol 108:359–364

103. Giussani DA, Spencer JAD, Moor PD, Bennet L, Hanson MA (1993) Afferent and efferent components of the cardiovascular response to acute hypoxia in term fetal sheep. J Physiol 461:431–449

104. Giussani DA, Riquelme RA, Moraga FA et al. (1996) Chemoreflex and endocrine components of cardiovascular responses to acute hypoxemia in the llama fetus. Am J Physiol 271:R73–R83

105. Hecher K, Ville Y, Snijders R, Nicolaides K (1995) Doppler studies of the fetal circulation in twin–twin transfusion syndrome. Ultrasound Obstet Gynecol 5:318–324

106. Hecher K, Snijders R, Campbell S, Nicolaides K (1995) Fetal venous, arterial, and intracardiac blood flow in red blood cell immunization. Obstet Gynecol 85:122–128

107. Gembruch U, Krapp M, Baumann P (1995) Changes of venous blood flow velocity waveforms in fetuses with supraventricular tachycardia. Ultrasound Obstet Gynecol 5:394–399

108. Gembruch U, Krapp M, Germer U, Baumann P (1999) Venous Doppler in the sonographic surveillance of fetuses with supraventricular tachycardia. Eur J Obstet Gynecol Reprod Biol 84:187–192

109. Fouron JC, Fournier A, Proulx F et al. (2003) Management of fetal tachyarrhythmias based on superior vena cava/aorta Doppler flow recordings. Heart 89:1211–1216

110. Hecher K, Bilardo CM, Stigter RH, Ville Y, Hackelöer BJ, Kok HJ (2001) Monitoring of fetuses with intrauterine growth restriction: a longitudinal study. Ultrasound Obstet Gynecol 18:564–570

111. Baschat AA, Gembruch U, Harman CR (2001) The sequence of changes in Doppler and biophysical parameters as severe fetal growth restriction worsens. Ultrasound Obstet Gynecol 18:571–577

112. Ferrazzi E, Bozzo M, Rigano S et al. (2002) Temporal sequence of abnormal Doppler changes in peripheral and central circulatory systems of the severely growth-restricted fetus. Ultrasound Obstet Gynecol 19:140–146

113. Kiserud T (2003) Fetal venous circulation. Fetal Matern Med Rev 14:57–95

114. Mavrides E, Holden D, Bland JM, Tekay A, Thilaganathan B (2001) Intraobserver and interobserver variability of transabdominal Doppler velocimetry measurements of the fetal ductus venosus between 10 and 14 weeks of gestation. Ultrasound Obstet Gynecol 17:306–310

115. Prefumo F, De Biasio P, Venturini PL (2001) Reproducibility of ductus venosus Doppler flow measurements at 11–14 weeks of gestation. Ultrasound Obstet Gynecol 17:3001–3005

116. Jørgensen C, Andolf E (1994) Four cases of absent ductus venosus: three in combination with severe hydrops fetalis. Fetal Ther 9:395–397

117. Sivén M, Ley D, Hägerstrand I, Svenningsen N (1995) Agenesis of the ductus venosus and its correlation to hydrops fetalis and the fetal hepatic circulation. Pediatr Path Lab Med 15:39–50

118. Gembruch U, Baschat AA, Gortner L (1998) Prenatal diagnosis of ductus venosus agenesis: a report of two cases and review of the literature. Ultrasound Obstet Gynecol 11:185–189

119. Hofstaetter C, Plath H, Hansmann M (2000) Prenatal diagnosis of abnormalities of the fetal venous system. Ultrasound Obstet Gynecol 15:231–241

120. Achiron R, Hegesh J, Yagel S, Lipitz S, Cohen SB, Rotstein Z (2000) Abnormalities of the fetal central veins and umbilico-portal system: prenatal ultrasonographic diagnosis and proposed classification. Ultrasound Obstet Gynecol 16:539–548

121. Avni EF, Ghysels M, Donner C, Damis E (1997) In utero diagnosis of congenital absence of the ductus venosus. J Clin Ultrasound 25:456–458

122. Contratti G, Banzi C, Ghi T, Perolo A, Pilu G, Visenti A (2001) Absence of the ductus venosus: report of 10 new cases and review of the literature. Ultrasound Obstet Gynecol 18:605–609

123. Shih JC, Shyu MK, Hsieh MH et al. (1996) Agenesis of the ductus venosus in a case of monochorionic twins which mimics twin–twin transfusion syndrome. Prenat Diag 16:243–246

124. Brozot ML, Schultz R, Patroni LT, Lopes LM, Armbruster Moraes E, Zugaib M (2001) Trisomy 10: ultrasound features and natural history after first trimester diagnosis. Prenat Diagn 21:672–675

125. Jaeggi E, Fouron JC, Hornberger LK et al. (2002) Agenesis of the ductus venosus that is associated with extrahepatic umbilical vein drainage: prenatal features and clinical outcome. Am J Obstet Gynecol 187:1031–1037

126. Rudolph CD, Meyers RL, Paulick RP, Rudolph AM (1991) Effects of ductus venosus obstruction on liver and regional blood flows in the fetal lamb. Pediatr Res 29:347–352

127. Nathanielsz PW, Hanson MA (2003) The fetal dilemma: spare the brain and spoil the liver. J Physiol 548:333

128. Oepkes D, Vandenbussche FP, van Bel F, Kanhai HHH (1993) Fetal ductus venosus blood flow velocities before and after transfusion in red-cell alloimmunized pregnancies. Obstet Gynecol 82:237–241

129. DeVore GR, Horenstein J (1993) Ductus venosus index: a method for evaluating right ventricular preload in the second-trimester fetus. Ultrasound Obstet Gynecol 3:338–342

Chapter 29

Doppler Ultrasound Examination of the Fetal Coronary Circulation

Ahmet Alexander Baschat

Introduction

The coronary circulation provides blood to the myocardium. Matching myocardial blood flow and demand is critical to ensure cardiac function over a wide variety of physiologic and pathologic conditions. For this reason examination of coronary vascular dynamics in various fetal conditions is becoming increasingly relevant to the perinatal medicine specialist. Ultrasound examination of the fetal coronary circulation has become possible through advances in ultrasound technology and a better understanding of human fetal cardiovascular physiology. Although not yet standard clinical practice, continuing trends in ultrasound technology and spreading familiarity with the examination and interpretation is likely to expand clinical applications in the future [1].

Ultrasound examination of the fetal coronary system utilizes gray-scale, zoom and cine-loop techniques and requires optimal spatial and temporal settings of the Doppler modalities. A proper setup of the ultrasound system is therefore a necessary prerequisite. Traditional ultrasound planes used in cardiac scanning are modified to provide the best visualization of the coronary vessels. A comprehensive survey of extracardiac vascular dynamics is often necessary to provide the clinical context for interpretation of intracardiac and coronary flow dynamics. This chapter reviews embryology, functional anatomy, ultrasound technique, and clinical utility of ultrasound evaluation of the fetal coronary circulation.

Embryology and Functional Anatomy of the Coronary Circulation

Oxygenated blood is delivered to the myocardium through the right coronary artery (RCA) and left coronary artery (LCA) arising from the right anterior and left posterior aortic sinuses, respectively, and the left anterior descending branch (LAD) of the LCA [2, 3]. Venous return from the left ventricle drains mainly through a superficial system through the coronary sinus and anterior cardiac veins carrying ap-

proximately two-thirds of myocardial venous return. The deep system, consisting of arterioluminal vessels, arteriosinusoidal vessels, and thebesian veins, receives the remaining venous return and drains directly into the cardiac chambers [2–4].

In embryonic life endothelial cells migrate from the septum transversarium in the hepatic region of the embryo to form epicardial blood islands which eventually coalesce into vascular networks extending throughout the epicardium and myocardium [5, 6]. Concurrently, the RCA and LCA originate as microvessels that penetrate the outflow tracts and acquire a muscular coat in this process. The primitive coronary arterial circulation is established when main-stem coronary arteries and myocardial vascular channels connect. Venous drainage develops independently of the arterial system and becomes fully functional when the coronary sinus, as a remnant of the left horn of the sinus venosus, becomes incorporated into the inferior wall of the right atrium and thebesian veins gain access to the ventricular cavities. The coronary circulation is completely functional by the fifth to sixth week of embryonic life and ensures myocardial blood supply by the time the embryonic circulation is established.

Coronary vascular development can be modulated by various stimuli. Such stimuli include local oxygen tension, mechanical wall stress, and myocardial and vascular shear forces [6–9]. As a result, the coronary circulation is subject to great anatomic and functional variation that is manifested in several ways. Under physiologic conditions modulation of vascular growth enables matching coronary vascular development to myocardial growth [10]. This ensures a balanced relationship between ventricular mass and vascular density. Prolonged or progressive tissue hypoxemia may lead to an exaggeration of this physiologic process with a subsequent marked increase in vascular cross-sectional area in the coronary circulation [11–14]. Under these circumstances vascular reactivity to physiologic stimuli is also altered, often resulting in amplified responses [15]. Similarly, abnormal intracardiac pressure relationships, such as those found in outflow tract obstructive lesions, may force the development of accessory vascular channels between the coronary vessels and the ventricular cavity (ventriculo-coronary fistulae) [16]. The plasticity of the coronary circulation is responsible for the variation in myocardial vascular territories and blood flow found in various fetal conditions and illustrates the critical importance of myocardial oxygenation for proper cardiac function.

Myocardial metabolism is almost exclusively aerobic and in the presence of adequate oxygen various substrates, including carbohydrates, glucose, lactate, and lipids, can be metabolized [17–20]. In fetal life, myocardial glycogen stores and lactate oxidation constitute the major sources of energy while fatty acid oxidation rapidly becomes the primary energy source after birth. To maintain metabolism myocardial oxygen extraction is as high as 70%–80% in the resting state. Consequently, a coronary atrioventricular O_2 difference of 14 ml/dl exceeds that of most other vascular beds and allows little further extraction of O_2 unless blood flow is significantly augmented; therefore, coronary blood flow is closely regulated to match myocardial oxygen demands.

The regulation of myocardial perfusion operates at several levels and time frames. The unique parallel arrangement of the fetal circulation allows for delivery of well-oxygenated blood through the ductus venosus to the left ventricle and thus the ascending aorta. In the fetal lamb the coronary circulation receives approximately 8% of the left ventricular output at rest in this manner [21]. This proportion may be higher in the human fetus and may be further altered by modulating the degree of shunting through the ductus venosus [22]. Once blood enters the coronary vessels from the ascending aorta the pressure difference to the right atrium becomes the primary driving force for coronary blood flow. This perfusion pressure is further subjected to changes in vascular tone and extravascular pressure. Autonomic innervation of coronary resistance vessels regulates overall vascular tone [23, 24], but ventricular contractions are the main contributor to extravascular resistance with significant impact on the flow velocity waveform [25–27]. Myocardial perfusion predominantly occurs during diastole when the ventricles relax and pose little extravascular resistance. This diastolic timing of predominant perfusion is unique to the coronary circulation and distinguishes it from other vascular beds in the human body. In the adult, increases above a resting heart rate of 70 beats per minute result in a disproportional shortening of diastole. Fetal heart rates of 120–160 beats per minute place special demands on dynamic vascular mechanisms to regulate myocardial blood flow volume.

Efficiency of myocardial oxygen delivery is further enhanced by active autoregulatory control mechanisms ensuring optimal myocardial blood flow despite fluctuations in arterial perfusion pressure [28, 29]. This is achieved through caliber adjustment of precapillary resistance vessels allowing channeling of blood flow to areas of greatest oxygen demand [30, 31]. With maximal dilatation of these sphincters myocardial blood flow may be elevated four times above basal flow. The increase in blood flow volume that can be achieved under these circumstances is the myocardial blood flow reserve. If myocardial oxygenation cannot be sustained, long-term adaptation with formation of new blood vessels may be invoked thus increasing the myocardial blood flow reserve [32–34]. Such elevated myocardial blood flow reserve allows marked augmentation of blood flow during periods of acutely worsening hypoxemia or increased cardiac work and increases as high as 12 times the basal flow have been reported [15, 35, 36].

Ultrasound Examination Technique

Ultrasound Setup

The setup of the ultrasound system is of major importance for successful examination of the fetal coronary arteries. Gray-scale ultrasound, color-, and pulsed-wave Doppler are used in a complementary manner and machine settings need to be optimized to provide the best spatial and temporal resolution. Although visualization of coronary vessels can be achieved using 4-MHz transducers, higher frequencies are likely to improve resolution and therefore detection. The dynamic range of the gray-scale image should be set to an intermediate level that is generally used in cardiac setups. Zoom magnification of the area of interest limits the computing power that needs to be allocated to the generation of the gray-scale image. These two maneuvers will improve the frame repetition rate and should therefore be applied before adding color Doppler imaging. When adding color Doppler imaging the filter should be set to a high degree of motion discrimination and the color box and gate are kept as small as possible to optimize spatial and temporal resolution of this Doppler modality. The lateral dimension of the color box has the greatest impact on computing power and therefore frame rate. The color amplification gain is set to eliminate background noise on the screen. The persistence is set to a low level to minimize frame averaging. The color velocity scale is adjusted to a range that allows visualization of intra- and extracardiac flows without aliasing and suppression of wall-motion artifacts. A useful velocity range for coronary arteries is between 0.3 and 0.7 m/s for coronary arteries and between 0.1 and 0.3 m/s for the coronary sinus. Since initial detection of the coronary arteries relies on color Doppler, these aspects of the setup are essential preliminary steps. Once the coronary vessel is identified using these techniques the transducer position should be adjusted to provide an insonation angle close to 0° prior to obtaining pulsed-wave measurements. The pulsed-wave Doppler gate should be adjusted to exclude other cardiac and extracardiac flows and should be the only active display when measurements are taken. Concurrent activation of multiple image modalities (duplex or triplex mode) drastically increases computing requirements and affects the spatial and temporal resolution of the spectral Doppler waveform.

Examination of Coronary Arteries

Using gray-scale ultrasound the coronary ostia are discernable in late gestation (Fig. 29.1). Before this time, the size of the main-stem arteries is below 1 mm in diameter and thus frequently below the resolution threshold of current sonographic equipment in the majority of cases [37]. For this reason color and pulsed-wave Doppler ultrasound are necessary to detect and verify coronary artery blood flow. The Doppler examination of the fetal coronary vessels has been adopted from techniques developed for infants and neonates [38]. The main-stem right and left coronary arteries are best examined in a long-axis view of the left ventricular outflow tract and ascending aorta or a precordial short-axis view of the aorta. The LAD branch of the LCA is best identified from an apical short-axis view. In the standard precordial short-axis view the left coronary artery courses forward towards the transducer, whereas the right coronary artery runs more parallel. This view therefore facilitates examination of the LCA. In the lateral, or long-axis, view of the left ventricular outflow tract the RCA is more readily imaged if imaged from the right side of the fetus. In this view it may also be possible to visualize both coronary arteries (Fig. 29.2) [39, 40].

The LAD may be identified scanning from the apical four-chamber view. From this view the transducer is tilted towards the head until the level of the superior cardiac surface and interventricular groove is reached [41]. Cardiac wall motion, high blood flow velocities in the ventricles and ventricular outflow tracts and movement of pericardial fluid can all interfere with the relatively low coronary blood flow velocities on color Doppler imaging. Back and forward motion of pericardial fluid outlining the ventricular walls in particular may be mistaken for a coronary artery [42]. For these reasons identification of coronary artery blood flow by color Doppler imaging should always be followed by verification of the typical waveform pattern by pulsed-wave Doppler to provide assurance that the coronary arteries have indeed been identified.

Spectral Doppler measurement of coronary blood flow velocities is easiest proximally since vessel diameter is greatest and motion during the cardiac cycle is less than distally. After coronary vessels are identified by color Doppler, the pulsed-wave Doppler gate is positioned at the origin of the vessel. The gate may require adjustment to achieve continuous sampling of the waveform allowing for the movement of the aortic root in the cardiac cycle. The coronary artery flow velocity waveform has a biphasic pattern with systolic and diastolic peaks and antegrade flow throughout the cardiac cycle (Fig. 29.3). Predominant diastolic perfusion produces a unique waveform pattern with higher velocities during diastole than systole. In normal fetuses coronary blood flow has been visualized from 29 weeks onwards (median gestational age of 33±6 weeks). The median systolic and diastolic peak blood flow velocities are 0.21 and 0.43 m/s, respectively, and show little change during the latter part of gestation (Figs. 28.4, 28.5) [43]. Gestational age at visualization and coronary artery blood flow velocities are in part determined by the fetal condition (see below).

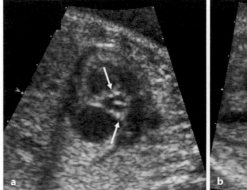
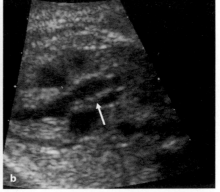

Fig. 29.1. The fetal heart is examined in a short-axis view of the aorta at 34±2 weeks gestation (**a**) and in a long-axis view of the left ventricular outflow tract at 35±5 weeks' gestation (**b**). The ostia of the left and right coronary arteries are discernible in **a** (*arrows*) in the area of the left posterior and right anterior aortic sinus. (From [87]). In **b** the ostium of the left coronary artery is discernible (*arrow*)

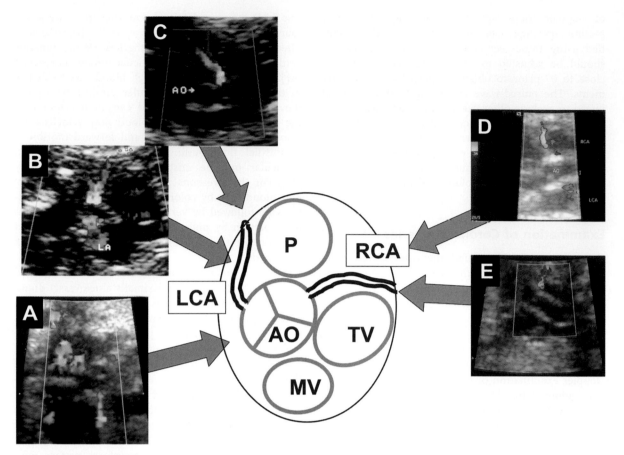

Short axis views

Long axis views

Fig. 29.2. The origin of the great vessels and the atrioventricular valves shows the course of the left and right coronary arteries (*RCA* and *LCA*, respectively) in relationship to the aorta (*AO*), pulmonary artery (*P*), mitral valve (*MV*), and tricuspid valve (*TV*). The angle of insonation and type of cardiac axis determines the orientation of the coronary arteries on the ultrasound image. Short-axis views facilitate examination of the left coronary artery (**B**) and may enable visualization of both coronary arteries (**C**) occasionally also allowing demonstration of the origin of the left anterior descending branch (**B, C**). Although the right coronary artery can be examined in the short-axis view (**A**), it is easier to identify this vessel in a right lateral long-axis view of the left ventricular outflow tract (**E**). This view also allows simultaneous visualization of both coronary arteries (**D**)

Examination of the Coronary Sinus

The larger size of the coronary sinus and its anatomic course greatly facilitate its ultrasound examination [44, 45]. The coronary sinus runs in the atrioventricular groove and enters the right atrium below the level of the foramen ovale just above the valve of the inferior vena cava. Because of its position, apical or basal four-chamber views provide the best opportunity for gray-scale biometry, whereas lateral four-chamber views provide a more favorable insonation angle for color- and spectral Doppler imaging (Figs. 29.6, 29.7).

Gray-scale and M-mode echocardiography have both been used to obtain normative data on the length and diameter of the coronary sinus. The caliber of the coronary sinus undergoes cyclic changes with the cardiac cycle being smallest at the beginning of diastole and largest in mid-systole with maximal descent of the arteriovenous ring. M-mode echocardiography allows precise documentation of caliber and dynamic changes (Fig. 29.8). The coronary sinus has a maximum diameter ranging from 1 to 3 mm with advancing gestation. The method utilized to obtain these measurements does influence the reference limits [45, 46]. Figures 29.9 and 29.10 show gestational reference ranges for the maximal diastolic and systolic dimensions that were measured using the M-mode technique. Appreciating the phenomenon of variations in coronary sinus diameter may call for

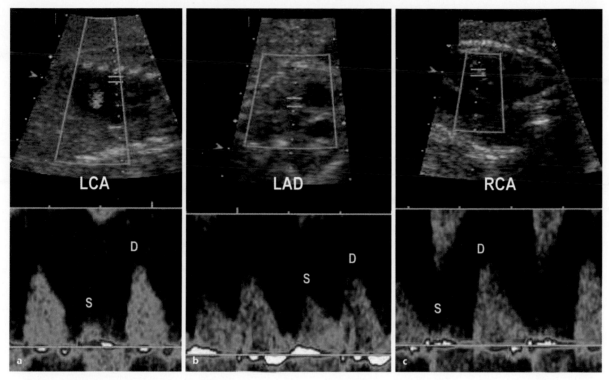

Fig. 29.3 a–c. Pulsed-wave Doppler images of the left coronary (*LCA*), left anterior descending (*LAD*), and right coronary arteries (*RCA*) obtained in a 29-week fetus. Of note is the predominance of blood flow during diastole that is observed in all three vessels. (From [87])

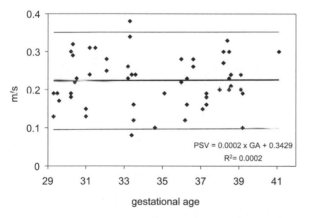

Fig. 29.4. The median and 95% confidence interval for the peak systolic velocity (*PSV*) in the coronary artery of appropriately grown fetuses in relation to gestational age (*GA*). (From [43])

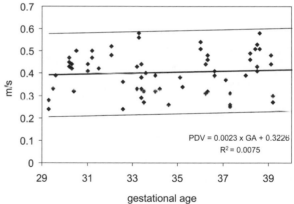

Fig. 29.5. The median and 95% confidence interval for the peak diastolic velocity (*PDV*) in the coronary artery of appropriately grown fetuses in relation to gestational age (*GA*). (From [43])

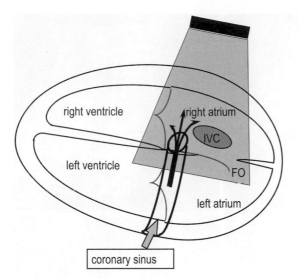

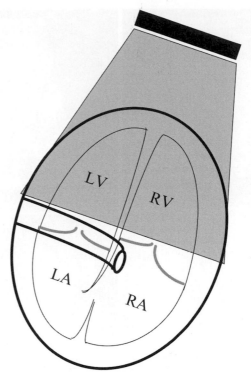

Fig. 29.6. The fetal heart shows the course of the coronary sinus in the right lateral four-chamber view. The coronary sinus runs in the atrioventricular groove and opens into the right atrium near the atrioventricular valve, in close proximity to the inferior vena cava (*IVC*) and foramen ovale (*FO*). In this imaging plane, the direction of blood flow is towards the transducer beam. (From [47])

Fig. 29.7. The fetal heart imaged in the apical four-chamber view shows the left and right ventricles (*LV* and *RV*) and the corresponding atria (*LA* and *RA*). The coronary sinus runs in the atrioventricular groove parallel to the mitral valve leaflets. The coronary sinus is visualized by tilting the transducer towards the inferior cardiac surface until the valve leaflets disappear. (From [45])

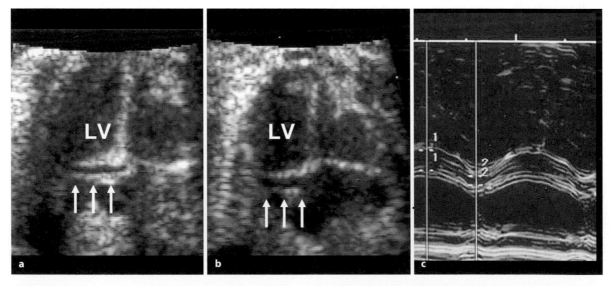

Fig. 29.8. The fetal heart imaged in an apical four-chamber view at 28±4 weeks' gestation. The coronary sinus (*arrows*) can be seen running in the atrioventricular groove between the left ventricle (*LV*) and atrium. Using the cine-loop technique a difference in diameter between end-systolic (**A**) and mid-systolic (**B**) diameters can be appreciated. M-mode tracing obtained from a normal coronary sinus at 29 weeks' gestation demonstrating fluctuations during systole and diastole (**C**). The cursors are placed on the anterior and posterior walls of the coronary sinus. (From [45])

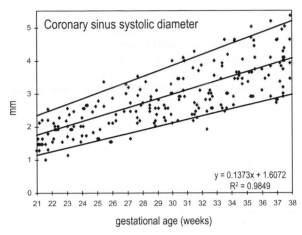

Fig. 29.9. Individual measurements, and the mean and 95% confidence interval of the maximum systolic diameter of the coronary sinus with respect to gestational age ($y = 0.1373x + 1.6072$; $r^2 = 0.9849$). (From [45])

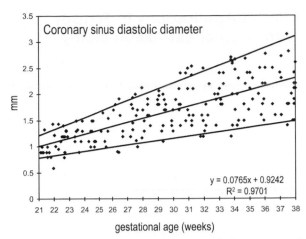

Fig. 29.10. Individual measurements, and the mean and 95% confidence interval of the maximum diastolic diameter of the coronary sinus with respect to gestational age ($y = 0.0765x + 0.9242$; $r^2 = 0.9701$). (From [45])

Fig. 29.11. The fetal heart is imaged in a lateral four-chamber view and coronary sinus blood flow towards the right atrium (*RA*) is identified with color Doppler imaging (**a**). Pulsed-wave Doppler shows a triphasic flow profile with a small systolic (*S*) and a larger diastolic peak (*D*) followed by brief reversal during atrial contraction (**b**). (From [87])

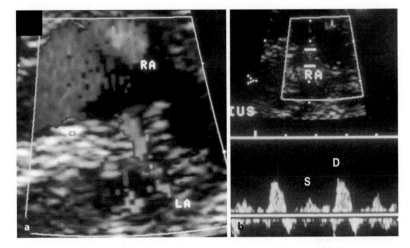

verification using this M-mode technique when dilatation of the coronary sinus is suspected.

Color Doppler identification of coronary sinus blood flow is successful in approximately 50% of normal fetuses. During diastole the direction of blood flow from the coronary sinus is towards the right atrium, whereas blood flow across the foramen ovale is directed towards the left atrium (Fig. 29.11) [47]. Despite its straight course, exact placement of the sample volume spectral Doppler measurements is only possible in approximately 10% of fetuses. This low success rate is partly due to lower coronary sinus blood flow velocities and interference caused by in-

tra-atrial blood flows and/or cardiac and atrioventricular valve movement. The coronary sinus flow velocity waveform has a triphasic pattern with systolic and diastolic antegrade flow and occasional reversal during atrial contraction (Fig. 29.11). Similar to the coronary arteries, diastolic forward velocities (median 0.38 m/s) exceed systolic velocities (median 0.18 m/s). These velocities are related to the periods of predominant myocardial blood flow. Methods to relate coronary sinus velocities to myocardial flow reserve have been described in neonates and adults [48, 49], but these are currently not practicable for validation in the human fetus.

Clinical Applications in Fetuses with Normal Cardiac Anatomy

In fetuses with normal cardiac anatomy disorders are frequently only apparent through alterations in cardiovascular status. Under these circumstances coronary blood flow dynamics may be altered to accommodate changes in myocardial oxygen requirements. Since spectral Doppler of the coronary sinus is rarely achieved, clinical observations revolve primarily around color- and pulsed-wave Doppler characteristics in coronary arterial vessels.

The "Heart-Sparing Effect" in Fetal Growth Restriction

Severe fetal growth restriction (IUGR) can progress to decompensation of cardiovascular status. Such deterioration can be documented through progressive deterioration of arterial and venous Doppler studies [50]. This progression often accompanies the deterioration of acid–base status from chronic hypoxemia to acidemia [51–54]. Under these circumstances the combination of elevated central venous pressure, elevated afterload, and worsening oxygenation places unique demands on myocardial oxygen balance. Elevated afterload increases myocardial oxygen demand because of an increase in cardiac work. Elevated central venous pressure and aortic pressures decrease the pressure difference across the coronary vascular bed and therefore diminish the driving force for coronary perfusion. The summation of these factors has detrimental effects on coronary perfusion at a time when myocardial oxygen balance and fetal metabolic state are critical. Consequently, adaptive mechanisms need to be evoked in order to maintain myocardial oxygen balance. The necessary augmentation of coronary blood flow can be achieved in two principal ways. One way is to increase the proportion of oxygenated left ventricular output available for myocardial delivery. The second way is through autoregulation-mediated coronary vasodilatation.

Several mechanisms operate in IUGR fetuses that increase the potential delivery of oxygenated blood to the myocardium. Under conditions of elevated placental resistance the relative proportion of left ventricular output increases [55–57]. Decreases in oxygen tension may further increase the proportion of oxygenated umbilical venous blood that is delivered through the ductus venosus to the left side of the heart [58, 59]. Prolonged chronic myocardial hypoxemia allows for angiogenesis and increases in vascular cross-sectional area and therefore myocardial flow reserve. These responses constitute chronic heart sparing in IUGR. When acute worsening of cardio-vascular status and/or oxygenation is superimposed the only mechanism to significantly augment myocardial blood flow is marked coronary vasodilatation with massive recruitment of coronary vascular reserve. This vascular response is more acute, often occurring over the course of 24 h, and is most consistently associated with severe elevation of precordial venous Doppler indices [60, 61].

The chronic initial phase of heart sparing can be implied by demonstrating certain Doppler abnormalities in the arterial and venous circulations. These include absent or reversed umbilical artery end-diastolic velocity and/or end-diastolic blood flow reversal in the aortic isthmus [62]. In the second trimester the magnitude of coronary blood flow may still be below the visualization threshold of ultrasound equipment; therefore, augmentation of coronary blood flow cannot be documented by spectral Doppler measurement of coronary arteries. With acute worsening of fetal cardiovascular and respiratory status color- and pulsed-wave Doppler measurement of coronary artery blood flow is readily achieved as a reflection of maximal augmentation of coronary blood flow – now exceeding the visualization threshold [40]. In IUGR both diastolic and systolic coronary artery peak blood flow velocities are significantly higher than in appropriately grown fetuses providing additional evidence of blood flow augmentation. There are no associated changes in the coronary sinus diameter as evidence of increased coronary venous return [63]. Since coronary artery blood flow may be visualized in normal and IUGR fetuses at overlapping gestational ages, concurrent examination of the arterial and venous circulations is mandatory to assess fetal status. Clinical management cannot be based on the evaluation of coronary vascular dynamics alone. In IUGR fetuses with abnormal arterial and venous Doppler, heart-sparing prognosis is poor with a high perinatal mortality and a high risk for acidemia and neonatal circulatory insufficiency requiring the highest level of neonatal care.

Fetal Anemia

Severe fetal anemia can result in reduction of oxygen-carrying capacity and subsequently impaired myocardial oxygenation. Fetal hydrops with tricuspid insufficiency and abnormal precordial venous flow is associated with elevated right-heart pressures and a decline in coronary perfusion pressure. Under these circumstances short-term augmentation of myocardial blood flow of four to five times basal flow can be achieved through autoregulation. Color- and spectral Doppler measurement of coronary artery blood flow velocities has been successful in circumstances of acute fetomaternal hemorrhage, non-immune hy-

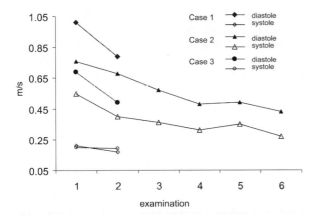

Fig. 29.12. Systolic and diastolic peak blood flow measurements in three cases of severe fetal anemia. In cases 1 and 3 velocities were obtained in hydropic fetuses prior to transfusion. In case 1 a hematocrit of 9% was corrected to 39.8% and in case 3 from 14% to 42.8%. In the second case of maternal trauma, repeated transfusions were necessary on days 1 and 5 for hematocrit levels of 21% and 24%, respectively. (From [43])

drops, and hemolytic disease [43, 64]. Peak diastolic velocities as high as 1 m/s and peak systolic velocities of 0.5 m/s may be observed, significantly exceeding those observed in any other fetal condition. Blood flow velocities are responsive to maternal oxygen therapy and fetal blood transfusion and fall below the visualization threshold after normalization of the fetal hematocrit (Fig. 29.12). With the development of fetal hydrops, a decrease in coronary sinus dynamics is observed. This finding is analogous to observations in adults with heart failure where coronary sinus caliber changes are attenuated presumably due to elevations in coronary venous pressures [45].

Ductus Arteriosus Constriction

Constriction of the ductus arteriosus is one of the reported fetal complications of maternal indomethacin therapy for preterm labor. As a conduit for the right ventricle to the systemic circulation, constriction of this vessel raises afterload and therefore cardiac work and oxygen requirement. In severe constriction tricuspid insufficiency and abnormal venous indices may develop. In such severe cases color- and pulsed-wave Doppler of coronary artery blood flow is possible. While the peak velocities are not significantly elevated, the gestational age at visualization is determined by the onset of the clinical condition. With resolution of ductus arteriosus constriction following discontinuation of indomethacin, coronary blood flow could no longer be visualized.

Other Fetal Conditions

Acute changes in fetal oxygenation and cardiac pre- and afterload also cause arterial and venous redistribution in favor of the organs essential for fetal life. These "heart-, brain-, and adrenal gland-sparing" phenomena have been described in different animal models. The few observations made by Doppler ultrasound in the human fetus support the presence of the same protective mechanisms. Transient "brain- and heart-sparing" phenomena were observed in a 30-week fetus following acute bradycardia after umbilical fetal blood sampling. Sudden visualization of coronary blood flow, "brain-sparing," and highly pulsatile precordial venous flow persisted for a long period after the 12-min bradycardia [65]. Changes in coronary sinus dynamics have been documented in a fetus with supraventricular tachycardia [45]. It is likely that more observations of alterations in coronary arterial and venous dynamics will be reported as familiarity with the examination technique and advances in ultrasound technology facilitate examination.

Clinical Applications in Fetal Cardiac Abnormalities

Due to the vascular properties of the coronary arterial circulation abnormalities frequently develop in cardiac lesions that are associated with disturbed intracardiac pressure/volume relationships during organogenesis. Owing to the embryologic development of coronary sinus abnormalities involving this vessel, anomalous central venous drainage (both systemic and/or pulmonary) is frequently present. Ultrasound biometry and assessment of coronary sinus dynamics has clinical relevance and may be the only apparent clue pointing in the direction of such anomalies.

Ventriculocoronary Connections in the Human Fetus

Ventriculocoronary connections are frequently noted in fetuses and newborns with pulmonary atresia, hypoplastic right ventricle, intact ventricular septum, or restrictive ventricular septal defect [66]. In cases of hypoplastic left heart with aortic atresia, intact ventricular septum and patent mitral valve ventriculocoronary connections may also be present but are less common. The genesis of these vascular abnormalities is discussed above. The abnormal coronary channels may provide a conduit to release intraventricular pressures and may partially avert hypoplasia and fibroelastosis; however, coronary blood flow dynamics may be significantly compromised, impacting on prognosis and approach to postpartum surgical man-

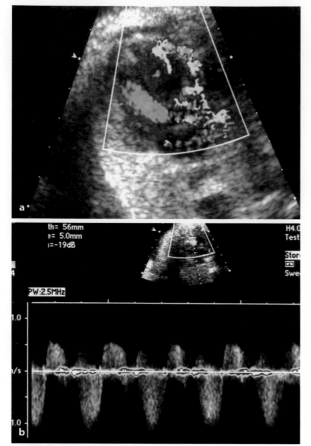

Fig. 29.13. The fetal heart is imaged in a lateral "five-chamber" view including the left ventricular outflow tract. A large tortuous vessel is seen originating from the aorta connecting into the right ventricular cavity, which is of moderate size (**a**). Pulsed-wave Doppler with the gate in the ventriculocoronary fistula shows the characteristic bidirectional flow pattern with systolic flow towards the aorta (below the baseline) and diastolic flow towards the right ventricle (above the baseline; **b**). (From [16])

phy. In cases of right ventricular outflow tract obstruction, diastolic flow from the aortic sinus is directed toward the hypoplastic right ventricle. Pressures are reversed during ventricular systole and blood flows from the right ventricle to the aorta (Fig. 29.13) [66, 70, 71].

Coronary Arteriovenous Fistula in the Human Fetus

Congenital coronary fistulae may occur occasionally if cardiac anatomy is otherwise normal; the majority of these involve a single coronary artery, less often multiple branches. Connections may involve the coronary arterial tree, right atrium, coronary sinus, caval veins, right ventricle, and the pulmonary trunk. Drainage into a low-pressure system can result in a large left-to-right shunt already causing symptoms in childhood such as congestive heart failure, myocardial ischemia from coronary artery steal, right-chamber enlargement, arrhythmia, thrombosis with consecutive embolization, and bacterial endocarditis [72]. In the majority of cases symptoms appear in the second and third decade of life. In a 20-week fetus prenatal detection of an isolated coronary fistula connecting to the right ventricle has been reported with demonstration of a progressive increase in size as well as tortuosity of the fistula during gestation [73]. A similar case with a fistula between the LCA and the right atrium has also been recently described [74]. The shunting blood caused a high-velocity flow in the dilated coronary sinus. In addition to the prenatal findings a persistent left superior vena cava and a small ventricle septum defect were also identified postnatally. Following coil embolization of the coronary fistula further clinical course was reported as uneventful.

Idiopathic Arterial Calcification in the Human Fetus

The idiopathic arterial calcification has an unknown etiology and is characterized by generalized arterial calcification and stenoses especially of the walls in the arterial trunk of the pulmonary artery and aorta [75, 76]. Most commonly the coronary arteries are also affected, but peripheral arteries of gastrointestinal tract, liver, kidneys, brain, extremities, and placenta may also be involved. Severe myocardial dysfunction may cause severe fetal hydrops, tissue ischemia, and fetal death in the late second or third trimester [77]. In less severe cases, especially in the absence of hydrops, palliative treatment post-partum may be started with steroids and bisphosphonates in order to stop or delay the progression of the disease [78]; however, most infants with idiopathic arterial

agement [67–69]. While coronary perfusion may be well maintained in utero, the situation may change after birth. Right ventricular dependent coronary circulation may occur and result in acute or chronic global myocardial ischemia or infarction due to coronary steal and segmental vascular obstruction. Because of these potential impacts, prenatally detected outflow tract obstructive lesions with relatively preserved ventricular architecture should prompt the search for ventriculocoronary fistula.

Prenatal diagnosis of ventriculocoronary fistula is achieved by demonstration of high-velocity bi-directional flow in the coronary artery by color Doppler flow mapping and verified by pulsed-wave Doppler examination. A severely dilated coronary artery may also be imaged by two-dimensional echocardiogra-

calcification die within the first year of life complicated by cardiac and pulmonary failure, severe hypertension, renal infarction, peripheral gangrene, and bowel infarction [76].

Critical Aortic Stenosis

Critical aortic stenosis in fetal life can be associated with a marked decrease in left ventricular output and reversal of shunting across the foramen ovale. Under these circumstances coronary perfusion pressure is affected by a decrease in arterial pressure and an elevation of right atrial pressure thereby decreasing the driving force across the coronary vascular bed. Concurrently, left ventricular work and therefore myocardial oxygen demand are increased. Development of acute heart sparing has been documented in a fetus presenting with severe left ventricular outflow tract obstruction and non-immune hydrops due to critical aortic stenosis. While these findings were ameliorated initially by transplacental digoxin therapy, visualization of coronary blood flow became visible at 39 weeks coinciding with shunt reversal across the foramen ovale [79].

Persistent Left Superior Vena Cava

While Doppler examination of the coronary sinus has limited utility in the human fetus, substantial dilatation may result from volume overload from a persistent left superior vena cava draining into the coronary sinus [80–82]. The frequency of a persistence of the left vena cava is 1–2 per 1000 but may be as high as 9% in the presence of congenital heart defects [83]. The degree of dilatation is often marked and lies appreciably above normal reference limits. This dilatation appears to be predominantly related to vascular volume changes and is independent of associated cardiac defects [63]. Other causes of coronary sinus dilatation in the human fetus may be a coronary arteriovenous fistula and anomalous pulmonary vein drainage into the coronary sinus. It is important to note that because of its close proximity to the insertion of the atrioventricular valve, a dilated coronary sinus has been mistaken for an atrial septal defect of ostium primum type and/or an atrioventricular septal defect, respectively [84–86]. Coronary sinus dynamics may be attenuated in fetal conditions associated with elevated right-heart pressures, severe fetal cardiac dysfunction, and hydrops. These alterations in dynamics may indicate elevated coronary sinus pressures or changes in coronary blood flow [45].

References

1. Abuhammad A (2003) Color and pulsed Doppler ultrasonography of the fetal coronary arteries: Has the time come for its clinical application? Ultrasound Obstet Gynecol 21:423–425
2. Williams PL, Warwick R (eds) (1983) Gray's anatomy. Churchill Livingstone, New York
3. McAlpine WA (1975) Heart and coronary arteries. Springer, Berlin Heidelberg New York
4. Ganong WF (1989) Review of medical physiology. Appleton Lange, Norwalk, Connecticut
5. Larsen WJ (1993) Human embryology. Churchill Livingstone, New York
6. Tomanek RJ (1996) Formation of the coronary vasculature: a brief review. Cardiovasc Res 31:E46–E51
7. Poole TJ, Coffin JD (1989) Vasculogenesis and angiogenesis: two distinct morphogenetic mechanisms establish embryonic vascular pattern. J Exp Zool 251:224–231
8. Hudlicka O, Brown MD (1996) Postnatal growth of the heart and its blood vessels. J Vasc Res 33:266–287
9. Skalak TC, Price RJ (1996) The role of mechanical stresses in microvascular remodeling. Microcirculation 3:143–165
10. Engelmann GL, Dionne CA, Jaye MC (1993) Acidic fibroblast growth factor and heart development. Role in myocyte proliferation and capillary angiogenesis. Circ Res 72:7–19
11. Banai S, Shweiki D, Pinson A, Chandra M, Lazarovici G, Keshet E (1994) Upregulation of vascular endothelial growth factor expression induced by myocardial ischaemia: implications for coronary angiogenesis. Cardiovasc Res 28:1176–1179
12. Levy AP, Levy NS, Loscalzo (1995) Regulation of vascular endothelial growth factor in cardiac myocytes. Circ Res 76:758–766
13. Ratajska A, Torry RJ, Kitten GT (1995) Modulation of cell migration and vessel formation by vascular endothelial growth factor and basic fibroblast growth factor in cultured embryonic heart. Dev Dyn 203:399–407
14. Scheel KW, Eisenstein BW, Ingram LA (1984) Coronary, collateral and perfusion territory responses to aortic banding. Am J Physiol 246:H768–H775
15. Reller MD, Morton MJ, Giraud GD (1992) Maximal myocardial flow is enhanced by chronic hypoxaemia in late gestational fetal sheep. Am J Physiol 263:H1327–H1329
16. Baschat AA, Love JC, Stewart PA, Gembruch U, Harman CR (2001) Prenatal diagnosis of ventriculocoronary fistula. Ultrasound Obstet Gynecol 18:39–43
17. Ascuitto RJ, Ross-Ascuitto NT (1996) Substrate metabolism in the developing heart. Semin Perinatol 20:542–563
18. Bartelds B, Knoester H, Beaufort-Krol GCM, Smid GB, Takens J, Zijlstra WG, Heymans HSA, Kuipers JRG (1999) Myocardial lactate metabolism in fetal and newborn lambs. Circulation 99:1892–1897
19. Fisher DJ, Heymann MA, Rudolph AM (1982) Fetal myocardial oxygen and carbohydrate consumption during acutely induced hypoxemia. Am J Physiol 242:H657–H661

440   A. A. Baschat

20. Spahr R, Probst I, Piper HM (1985) Substrate utilization of adult cardiac myocytes. Basic Res Cardiol 80 (Suppl 1):53–56

21. Rudolph AM (1985) Distribution and regulation of blood flow in the fetal and neonatal lamb. Circ Res 57:811–821

22. Kiserud T, Rasmussen S, Skulstad S (2000) Blood flow and the degree of shunting through the ductus venosus in the human fetus. Am J Obstet Gynecol 182:147–153

23. Bassenge E (1978) Direct autonomic control of the coronary system. Pflügers Arch Suppl 373:R6

24. Krajcar M, Heusch G (1993) Local and neurohumoral control of coronary blood flow. Basic Res Cardiol 88 (Suppl 1):25–42

25. Cannon PJ, Sciacca RR, Fowler DL, Weiss MB, Schmidt DH, Casarella WJ (1975) Measurement of regional myocardial blood flow in man: description and critique of the method using xenon-133 and a scintillation camera. Am J Cardiol 36:783–792

26. Mantero S, Pietrabissa R, Fumero R (1992) The coronary bed and its role in the cardiovascular system: a review and an introductor single-branch model. J Biomed Eng 14:109–116

27. Thornburg KL, Reller MD (1999) Coronary flow regulation in the fetal sheep. Am J Physiol 277:R1249–R1260

28. Guyton AC, Ross JH, Carrier OJ (1964) Evidence for tissue oxygen demand as the major factor causing autoregulation. Circ Res 14:60–69

29. Mosher P, Ross J, McFate PA (1964) Control of coronary blood flow by an autoregulatory mechanism. Circ Res 14:250–259

30. Barnea O, Santamore WP (1992) Coronary autoregulation and optimal myocardial oxygen utilization. Basic Res Cardiol 87:290–301

31. Hoffman JIE (1984) Maximal coronary blood flow and the concept of coronary vascular reserve. Circulation 70:153–159

32. Campbell SE, Kuo CJ, Hebert B, Rakusan K, Marshall HW, Faithfull NS (1991) Development of the coronary vasculature in hypoxic fetal rats treated with a purified perfluorocarbon emulsion. Can J Cardiol 7:234–244

33. Holmes G, Epstein ML (1993) Effect of growth and maturation in a hypoxic environment on maximum coronary flow rates of isolated rabbit hearts. Pediatr Res 33:527–532

34. Muller JM, Davis MJ, Chilian WM (1996) Integrated regulation of pressure and flow in the coronary microcirculation. Cardiovasc Res 32:668–678

35. Reller MD, Morton MJ, Giraud GD (1992) Severe right ventricular pressure loading in fetal sheep augments global myocardial blood flow to submaximal levels. Circulation 86:581–588

36. Thompson LP, Pinkas G, Weiner CP (2000) Chronic hypoxia inhibits acetylcholine induced vasodilatation in constant pressure perfused fetal guinea pig hearts (Abstract). J Soc Gynecol Invest 7 (Suppl 1):192a

37. Oberhoffer R, Land D, Feilen K (1989) The diameters of coronary arteries in infants without coronary disease. Eur J Pediatr 148:389–392

38. Meyer RA (1984) Kawasaki syndrome: coronary artery disease in the young. Echocardiography 1:75–86

39. Gembruch U, Baschat AA (1996) Demonstration of fetal coronary blood flow by color-coded and pulsed wave Doppler sonography: a possible indicator of severe compromise and impending demise in intrauterine growth retardation. Ultrasound Obstet Gynecol 7:10–15

40. Baschat AA, Gembruch U, Reiss I, Gortner L, Diedrich K (1997) Demonstration of fetal coronary blood flow by Doppler ultrasound in relation to arterial and venous flow velocity waveforms and perinatal outcome: the "heart-sparing effect". Ultrasound Obstet Gynecol 9:162–172

41. Mielke G, Wallwiener D (2001) Visualization of fetal arterial and venous coronary blood flow. Ultrasound Obstet Gynecol 18:407

42. Yoo SJ, Min JY, Lee YH (2001) Normal pericardial fluid in the fetus: color and spectral Doppler analysis. Ultrasound Obstet Gynecol 18:248–252

43. Baschat AA, Muench MV, Gembruch U (2003) Coronary artery blood flow velocities in various fetal conditions. Ultrasound Obstet Gynecol 21:426–429

44. Rein AJ, Nir A, Nadjari M (2000) The coronary sinus in the fetus. Ultrasound Obstet Gynecol 15:468–472

45. Abello KC, Stewart PA, Baschat AA (2002) Grey scale and M-mode echocardiography of the fetal coronary sinus. Ultrasound Obstet Gynecol 20:137–141

46. Chaoui R (1996) The fetal coronary system in prenatal diagnosis (Abstract). Ultrasound Obstet Gynecol 8 (Suppl):158

47. Baschat AA, Gembruch U (1998) Examination of fetal coronary sinus blood flow by Doppler ultrasound. Ultrasound Obstet Gynecol 11:410–414

48. Mundigler G, Zehetgruber M, Christ G (1997) Comparison of transesophageal coronary sinus and left anterior descending coronary artery Doppler measurements for the assessment of coronary flow reserve. Clin Cardiol 20:225–231

49. Zehetgruber M, Mundigler G, Christ G (1995) Estimation of coronary flow reserve by transesophageal coronary sinus Doppler measurements in patients with syndrome X and patients with significant left coronary artery disease. J Am Coll Cardiol 25:1039–1045

50. Hecher K, Campbell S, Doyle P (1995) Assessment of fetal compromise by Doppler ultrasound investigation of the fetal circulation. Circulation 91:129–138

51. Weiner CP (1990) The relationship between the umbilical artery systolic/diastolic ratio and umbilical blood gas measurements in specimens obtained by cordocentesis. Am J Obstet Gynecol 162:1198–1202

52. Nicolaides KH, Bilardo CM, Soothill PW (1988) Absence of end-diastolic frequencies in umbilical artery: a sign of fetal hypoxia and acidosis. Br Med J 297:1026–1027

53. Hecher K, Snijders R, Campbell S (1995) Fetal venous, intracardiac and arterial blood flow measurements in intrauterine growth retardation: relationship with fetal blood gases. Am J Obstet Gynecol 173:10–15

54. Rizzo G, Capponi A, Arduini D (1996) Doppler indices from inferior vena cava and ductus venosus in predicting pH and oxygen tension in umbilical blood at cordocentesis in growth-retarded fetuses. Ultrasound Obstet Gynecol 7:401–410

55. Al-Ghazali W, Chita SK, Chapman MG, Allan LD (1989) Evidence of redistribution of cardiac output in asymmetrical growth retardation. Br J Obstet Gynaecol 96:697–704

56. Reed KL, Anderson CF, Shenker L (1987) Changes in intracardiac Doppler flow velocities in fetuses with absent umbilical artery diastolic flow. Am J Obstet Gynecol 157:774–779

57. Rizzo G, Arduini D (1991) Fetal cardiac function in intrauterine growth retardation. Am J Obstet Gynecol 165:876–882

58. Tchirikov M, Eisermann K, Rybakowski C, Schröder HJ (1998) Doppler ultrasound evaluation of ductus venosus blood flow during acute hypoxemia in fetal lambs. Ultrasound Obstet Gynecol 11:426–431

59. Tchirikov M, Rybakowski C, Hunecke B, Schröder HJ (1998) Blood flow through the ductus venosus in singleton and multifetal pregnancies and in fetuses with intrauterine growth restriction. Am J Obstet Gynecol 178:943–949

60. Baschat AA, Gembruch U (1996) Triphasic umbilical venous blood flow with prolonged survival in severe intrauterine growth retardation: a case report. Ultrasound Obstet Gynecol 8:201–205

61. Baschat AA, Gembruch U, Reiss I, Gortner L, Weiner CP, Harman CR (2000) Coronary blood flow visualization indicates cardiovascular compromise in IUGR fetuses. Ultrasound Obstet Gynecol 16:425–431

62. Makikallio K, Jouppila P, Rasanen J (2002) Retrograde net blood flow in the aortic isthmus in relation to human fetal arterial and venous circulations. Ultrasound Obstet Gynecol 19:147–152

63. Chaoui R, Heling KS, Kalache KD (2003) Caliber of the coronary sinus in fetuses with cardiac defects with and without left persistent superior vena cava and in growth restricted fetuses with "heart sparing effect". Prenat Diagn 23:552–557

64. Baschat AA, Harman CR, Alger LS, Weiner CP (1998) Fetal coronary and cerebral blood flow in acute fetomaternal hemorrhage. Ultrasound Obstet Gynecol 12:128–131

65. Gembruch U, Baschat AA (2000) Circulatory effects of acute bradycardia in the human fetus as studied by Doppler ultrasound. Ultrasound Obstet Gynecol 15:424–427

66. Maeno YV, Boutin C, Hornberger LK, McCrindle BW, Cavallé-Garrido T, Gladman G, Smallhorn JF (1999) Prenatal diagnosis of right ventricular outflow tract obstruction with intact ventricular septum and detection of ventriculocoronary connections. Heart 81:661–668

67. Coles JG, Freedom RM, Lightfoot NE et al. (1989) Long-term results in neonates with pulmonary atresia and intact ventricular septum. Ann Thorac Surg 47:213–217

68. Giglia TM, Mandell VS, Connor AR, Mayer JEJ, Lock JE (1992) Diagnosis and management of right ventricle-dependent coronary circulation in pulmonary atresia with intact ventricular septum. Circulation 86:1516–1528

69. Hanley FL, Sade RM, Blackstone EH, Kirklin JW, Freedom RM, Nanda NC (1993) Outcomes in neonatal pulmonary atresia with intact ventricular septum. A multiinstitutional study. J Thorac Cardiovasc Surg 105:406–427

70. Arabin B, Aardenburg R, Schasfoort-van Leeuwen M, Elzenga N (1996) Prenatal diagnosis of ventriculocoronary arterial communications combined with pulmonary atresia (Letter). Ultrasound Obstet Gynecol 7:461–462

71. Chaoui R, Tennstedt C, Göldner B, Bollmann R (1997) Prenatal diagnosis of ventriculo-coronary communications in a second-trimester fetus using transvaginal and transabdominal color Doppler sonography. Ultrasound Obstet Gynecol 9:194–197

72. Liberthson RR, Sagar K, Berkoben JP, Weintraub RM, Levine FH (1979) Congenital coronary arteriovenous fistula: report of 13 patients, review of the literature and delineation of management. Circulation 59:849–854

73. Sharland GK, Tynan M, Qureshi SA (1996) Prenatal detection and progression of right coronary artery to right ventricle fistula. Heart 76:79–81

74. Mielke G, Sieverding L, Borth-Bruns T, Eichhorn K, Wallwiener D, Gembruch U (2002) Prenatal diagnosis and perinatal management of left coronary artery to right atrium fistula. Ultrasound Obstet Gynecol 19:612–615

75. Hajdu J, Marton T, Papp C, Hruby E, Papp Z (1998) Calcification of the fetal heart: four case reports and a literature review. Prenat Diagn 18:1186–1190

76. Crum AK, Lenington W, Jeanty P (1992) Idiopathic infantile arterial calcifications. Fetus 2:74781–74786

77. Juul S, Ledbetter D, Wright TN, Woodrum D (1990) New insights into idiopathic infantile arterial calcinosis. Am J Dis Child 144:229–233

78. Bellah RD, Zawodniak L, Librizzi RJ, Harris MC (1992) Idiopathic arterial calcification of infancy: prenatal and postnatal effects of therapy in an infant. J Pediatr 121:930–933

79. Schmider A, Henrich W, Dahnert I, Dudenhausen JW (2000) Prenatal therapy of non-immunologic hydrops fetalis caused by severe aortic stenosis. Ultrasound Obstet Gynecol 16:275–278

80. Snider AR, Ports TA, Silverman NH (1979) Venous anomalies of the coronary sinus: detection by M-mode, two-dimensional and contrast echocardiography. Circulation 60:721–727

81. Rostagno C, Diricatti G, Galanti G, Dabizzi RP, Dabizzi L, Giglioli C, Rega L, Gensini GF (1999) Partial anomalous venous return associated with intact atrial septum and persistent left superior vena cava: a case report and literature review. Cardiologia 44:203–206

82. Papa M, Camesasca C, Santoro F, Zoia E, Fragasso G, Giannico S, Chierchia SL (1995) Fetal echocardiography in detecting anomalous pulmonary venous connection: four false positive cases. Br Heart J 73:355–358

83. Nsah EN, Moore GW, Hutchins GM (1991) Pathogenesis of persistent left superior vena cava with a coronary sinus connection. Pediatr Pathol 11:261–269

84. Gembruch U, Knöpfle G, Bald R, Hansmann M (1993) Early diagnosis of fetal congenital heart diseases by transvaginal echocardiography. Ultrasound Obstet Gynecol 3:310–317

85. Allan LD, Sharland GK (2001) The echocardiographic diagnosis of totally anomalous pulmonary venous connection in the fetus. Heart 85:433–437

86. Park JK, Taylor DK, Skeels M, Towner DR (1997) Dilated coronary sinus in the fetus: misinterpretation as an atrioventricular canal defect. Ultrasound Obstet Gynecol 10:126–129

87. Baschat AA, Gembruch U (2002) Evaluation of the fetal coronary circulation. Ultrasound Obstet Gynecol 20:405–412

Chapter 30

Doppler Interrogation of the Umbilical Venous Flow

Enrico Ferrazzi, Serena Rigano

Introduction

The first reports about measurements of fetal umbilical venous blood flow in human fetuses go back to the early 1980s. Eik-Nes et al. in 1980 [1], Gill et al. in 1981 [2], and Eik-Nes et al. in 1982 [3] reported measurements obtained on the "intrahepatic" umbilical vein. It was not always certain whether these were sampled before the portal sinus, i.e., the origin of the portal veins. This pioneering era came to an end when Erskine and Ritchie [4] and Giles et al. [5] came to the conclusion that "The results obtained are in keeping with previous studies but indicate that, although the method is relatively simple, determination of absolute blood flow in these vessels has little clinical potential because of inherent measurement inaccuracies." Fortunately, over more than a decade, these statements on quantitative "measurement inaccuracies" and on "poor clinical potential" in the diagnosis of fetal growth restriction were challenged, among others by Gerson et al. [6], Reed et al. [7], Sutton et al. [8], Schmidt et al. [9], and Challis et al. [10].

In the past 20 years the potential role of the measurement of flow, in the umbilical vein, ductus venosus, and cardiac outflow tract, was perceived as a possible direct insight into the core of pathophysiology, not just how it looks, but how it works; however, the real limitation was set by expensive research ultrasound machines, and by the expertise of research sonologists, until high-technology digital instruments became the standard of quality in commercial ultrasound units.

Fetal Flow Volume Measurements in the Era of Digital Computing and Imaging

Sources of Inaccuracies

Even if all other hemodynamic variables were considered negligible, which is not the case, an error of 15% in diameter measurement could determine a major error in the calculation of flow itself since flow is determined according to the following equation:

$$\begin{aligned} \text{UV flow (ml/min)} \\ = \text{cross-sectional area} \left(\pi \times \text{radius}^2\right)\left(\text{mm}^2\right) \\ \times \text{mean velocity (mm/s)} \times 60, \end{aligned}$$

where linear measurements are squared and so is the error. Similar but more complex adjustment should be made for the error in the angle of interrogation of the Doppler beam, which at its best could be corrected on one plane, that of the plane of the image itself, but not within the thickness of the sonographic "slice" of the vessel. The third source of error is determined by the attempt to calculate the true mean velocity. Most sonographic software is designed to extract the mean velocity out of the instantaneous Doppler shift analysis, as an intensity-weighted mean velocity; however, when interrogated peak velocities are relatively slow (14–18 cm/s from 20 to 38 weeks of gestation) the amount of blood flow "cut" by high-pass filters becomes relevant, and in addition to this, each software operates on analog-to-digital conversion of the Doppler shift and on the signal-to-noise ratio which is largely dependent on the gain and on the software itself. The complex issue of precise assessment of mean velocity is also biased by the difference between two-dimensional imaging and three-dimensional reality. The ideal flow model is a perfect parabolic flow evenly distributed in the vessel in which the mean velocity is half that of the peak velocity (mean velocity = peak velocity × 0.5) measured in the cross-sectional area. Again we must underline that Doppler sample volumes are closer to a bi-dimensional sample volume more than to a whole cross-sectional sample volume. Peak velocity is a simple measurement, and that measured in a two-dimensional and a three-dimensional model are equal. The mean instantaneous velocity could be calculated by a simple coefficient which takes into account the shape of the flow in the cross-sectional area. Unfortunately, the conditions of perfect parabolic flow are seldom met in the umbilical vein. According to Pennati and co-workers [11] one should take into account the fact that close to the placenta the flow profile is closer to a flat profile in which the mean velocity and peak velocity differs by a coefficient of 0.74, whereas all along the free loops this coefficient is 0.61. This is higher than 0.5 and normative data derived from the formula reported above underestimate true flow by 18%.

Source of Accuracy

Imaging quality, color imaging quality, and pulsed Doppler velocimetry quality of today's technology are an obvious challenge to these limitations (Fig. 30.1).

In 1999 [12] we checked the intra- and inter-observer coefficients of variation of the umbilical vein diameter, mean velocity, and absolute flow. The diameter was calculated as the mean of three measurements on a magnified section of the cord. The brightest spot at low amplification was assumed as the best marker of true diameter. The brightest ultrasound echoes are in fact those reflected back by orthogonal

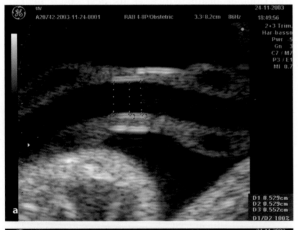

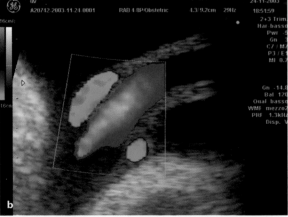

Fig. 30.1. a Magnified image of a straight section of the umbilical vein. **b** Magnified image of the color imaging of the umbilical vein. Note how the peak velocities are skewed toward the external wall of the curved vein

surfaces, which can be the case only when the ultrasound plane intersects the vessel at its true maximum diameter (Fig. 30.1). The ultrasound probe was tilted by 90° and the Doppler beam was spotted on the same section of the vessel where the diameter was measured. We considered that it was more reproducible, simpler, and probably more accurate, to assume for the given viscosity of blood, the diameter of the vessel and its length that an ideal parabolic flow truly occurs in those tracts of the umbilical vein where the lumen is linear for at least an approximate length of three times its diameter. The intra-observer coefficients of variation for the vein diameter, mean velocity, and absolute umbilical venous blood were 3.3%, 9.7%, and 10.9%, respectively. The inter-observer variabilities for the same parameters were 2.9%, 7.9%, and 12.7%, respectively. The same results were obtained by Lees and co-workers [13] and proved to be a little better for the intra-observer mean diameter calculated from four measurements of the UV (0.22 mm, respectively). Similar positive findings in reproducibility were reported by Boito et al. [14]. The coefficient of variation for the umbilical vein cross-sectional area was 6.6%, and for the time-averaged velocity it was 10.5%, resulting in a coefficient of variation of 11.9% for volume flow. The mean time required to obtain a complete set of measurements in our study was 3 min. These findings obtained in three different centers provide enough evidence to support the hypothesis that, as far as reproducibility and clinical feasibility are concerned, today's technology is able to achieve accurate measurements of the umbilical vein flow in the human fetus.

Volume Flow Values and Problems of Standardization

The specific umbilical vein flow we calculated from our findings [12] was 129 ml/min kg^{-1} at 20 weeks of gestation and 104 ml/min kg^{-1} at 38 weeks of gestation. Boito et al. reported similar, but lower values, 117.5 ± 33.6 ml/min kg^{-1} to 78.3 ± 12.4 ml/min kg^{-1} for the same gestational age span [14].

Di Naro, with a similar methodology, reported values of 126.0 ± 23.4 ml/kg per min at term [15]. Lees and co-workers reported [13], according to their methodology, values as high as 176 ml/min kg^{-1}, which are closer to the mean arterial values measured by Kunzel in 1992 (143 mm/kg min^{-1}) [16]. Actually, Lees et al. [13] was measuring an average of arterial and venous volume flow and Kunzel et al. [16] was measuring mean arterial flow. Accurate hemodynamic modeling of a pulsatile flow is quite complex, mostly because of problems in assessing the time-averaged mean velocity [17]. If we compare our present (108 ml/min kg^{-1} at 32–41 weeks of gestation) we appreciate the fact that these mean values are at the same level of umbilical volume flow measured by Eik-Nes in 1982 [3] (115 ml/min kg^{-1}). The only difference with these "historical" reports is the time required to obtain these measurements, and their reproducibility. Other methodologies had been tested for the same purpose by Kiserud [18] and Chantraine et al. [19]. This latter work represents newer technological possibilities and at the same time reminds us of the quest for standardization of non-invasive flow measurements. We still hold the opinion that given the limitations of Doppler technology, the true mean instantaneous velocity should be derived by the peak velocity times the coefficient derived by the general model of flow. According to Pennati et al. [20] this coefficient should be set at a value of 0.61. This report induced us to revise the values we reported in 1999 [12] just by increasing them by 18%. This means that the volume flow in the umbilical vein at 38 weeks of gestation is 123 ml/min kg^{-1} instead of 104 ml/min kg^{-1}. In this brief analysis we have met many methodologies that differ from our simple diameter-peak velocity interrogation: off-line measurement of cross-sectional area, software-dependent measurements of time-averaged mean velocity, mean values of venous and arterial flow measurements, and non-Doppler flow measurements. It is quite evident from published methodologies and results that the variability in measurements between centers is not stochastic; rather it is systematic, depending on the different methodologies adopted. So far, the simpler the better is our preferred choice.

Comparison Between Non-Invasive Doppler Volume Flow Values and Traditional Experimental Studies

The simple "diameter-peak velocity × 0.5" methodology was applied to the two veins of fetal lambs versus historical measurements of flow obtained with invasive technique [12]. Gestational age and fetal weights were not different between the animals studied by Doppler technique (129.6 ± 2.8 days, 2.75 ± 0.26 kg, respectively) and steady-state data (131.6 ± 4.1 days, 2.94 ± 0.68, respectively). Variability between the groups was similar (f test; $p = 0.138$). No significant differences were detected between the Doppler and diffusion technique groups for umbilical venous flow (210.8 ± 18.8 and 205.7 ± 38.5 ml/min kg^{-1}; $p = 0.881$).

A second study was then performed on the same set of seven animals [21]. Ultrasound Doppler and steady-state diffusion technique yielded virtually identical results (207 ± 9 vs 208 ± 7 ml/min kg^{-1}). A serendipitous result of that study was that the venous flow in each one of the two veins of the lamb was strictly correlated with the weight of the cotyledons

serving each vein. The accuracy of volume flow measurements was tested by Di Naro and co-workers [15] on human fetuses with different characteristics of the umbilical cord, normal coiled cord, and non-coiled lean cord, assuming and proving that the latter is a less favorable hemodynamic condition for umbilical circulation.

From Umbilical Flow Volume Measurements to Fetal Pathophysiology

The Relationship of Umbilical Vein Blood Flow to Growth Parameters in the Human Fetus

According to our reported study, umbilical blood flow increased exponentially throughout pregnancy from 63 ml/min at 20 weeks to 373 ml/min at 38 weeks [12]. By means of a different methodology, Boito and co-workers reported an increased volume flow from 33 ml/min at 20 weeks to 221 ml/min at 36 weeks of gestation [14]. When these absolute values are converted into weight-specific values, as reported above, the higher values become lower. In general, the estimation of fetal weight has a possible error of approximately ± 10% in 68% of cases. This error can even be larger in growth-restricted or macrosomic fetuses in which there is a change in the volumetric proportion between head and abdomen. As a result, expressing blood flow per kilogram estimated fetal weight introduces unnecessary errors and may obscure underlying pathophysiology. In contrast, the abdominal circumference as measured by ultrasound has been shown in many studies to serve as an early and sensitive biometric indicator of fetal growth restriction. Reporting data both as weight-specific values and abdominal or head circumference-specific values could help to compare "real measurements," and hopefully it could better serve the purpose of using flow volume in clinical practice.

Umbilical Vein Blood Flow and Abnormal Fetal Growth

The next step, which is relatively independent from systematic differences caused by various methodologies, is to observe what is happening under varied intrauterine conditions of the fetus and of the placenta. According to Kiserud and co-workers maternal hypoxemia on 12 pregnant sheep caused significantly reduced maximum and weighted mean blood velocity [22]. According to Padoan and co-workers at the University of Colorado Health Sciences Center, weight-specific umbilical venous flow is significantly reduced in fetal lambs affected by heath stress chronic growth

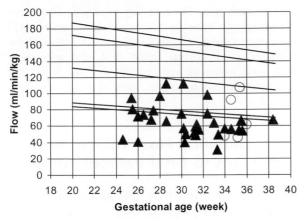

Fig. 30.2. Umbilical venous flow per unit weight (ml/min kg^{-1}). Growth-restricted fetuses with abnormal umbilical arterial pulsatility index (*triangles*). Growth-restricted fetuses with normal umbilical arterial pulsatility index (*circles*). The 2nd, 5th, 50th, 95th, and 98th percentiles of normal reference values

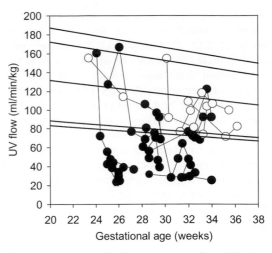

Fig. 30.3. Longitudinal assessment of umbilical venous flow per unit weight (ml/min kg^{-1}). Growth-restricted fetuses with abnormal umbilical arterial pulsatility index (*full circles*). Growth-restricted fetuses with normal umbilical arterial pulsatility index (*empty circles*). The 2nd, 5th, 50th, 95th, and 98th percentiles of normal reference values

restriction compared with normal fetuses of comparable gestational age (129.4 ± 14.8 vs 176.4 ± 13.3 ml/min kg^{-1}; $p < 0.05$) and is correlated to pO_2 (10.9 ± 1.2 vs 19.1 ± 0.7; $p < 0.001$) [23].

Obviously, when comparing normal fetuses to growth-restricted fetuses, it is important that the flow be related to some index of tissue mass, and not to gestational age, as is the case for qualitative waveform indices in the human "small" fetuses. This can be done by calculating an estimated fetal weight or from some other anthropomorphic measurement directly derived by ultrasound images. In our experience [24] umbilical volume flow in growth-restricted fetuses is reduced on a weight basis (Fig. 30.2). If we consider only those growth-restricted fetuses delivered without ominous heart rate signs (mean gestational age 32 ± 4; mean weight 1265 ± 424 g) weight-specific umbilical flow (ml/min kg^{-1}) was significantly lower than controls of comparable gestational age (98.4 ± 19.1 vs 117.1 ± 29.9; $p < 0.001$). A much larger difference was observed when flow measurements were obtained on growth-restricted fetuses with an abnormal heart rate, just before elective delivery (mean gestational age 29 ± 3 weeks; mean weight 962 ± 334 g; 63.0 ± 22.1 vs 124.0 ± 30.3 ml/min kg^{-1}; $p < 0.001$). Boito and co-workers reported umbilical volume flows per kilogram fetal weight below the normal range in 21 of 33 growth-restricted fetuses [14]. These findings were replicated by the same group on a second series [25] of 23 growth-restricted fetuses who showed a significant lower weight-specific flow compared with controls (59.6 vs 104.7 ml/min kg^{-1}; $p < 0.001$).

A broader impact on the understanding of fetal physiology under a condition of growth restriction

due to poor placental development can be derived by umbilical flow volume measurements when cross-sectional measurements obtained at a late stage of growth restriction, i.e., just before elective premature delivery, are highlighted by longitudinal observation from the early stage of the disease. The findings reported by Rigano and co-workers [26] showed that UV weight-specific flow (ml/min kg^{-1}) was reduced at the time of patient enrolment in 71.4% (15 of 21 IUGR fetuses) of the study population. By the time of delivery, 76.2% of the IUGR fetuses had UV weight-specific flow less than the 10th percentile. Figure 30.3 shows longitudinal umbilical flow volumes in growth-restricted fetuses per unit fetal weight with abnormal umbilical pulsatility index (PI), and with normal umbilical PI. These longitudinal observations suggest that this reduction is present weeks before heart rate abnormalities, this means that fetal–placental flow has its main impact on fetal metabolism. These data were replicated by Di Naro and co-workers [27]. Despite the different methodology and slightly different absolute value, the same message of early reduction was confirmed.

Diagnostic Usage of Umbilical Vein Blood Flow in Growth-Restricted Fetuses

Differences between normal and growth-restricted fetuses could be more reproducibly assessed if the head or the abdominal circumference were used directly instead of ultrasound assessment of fetal weight. Figure 30.4 shows the same volume flow measurements as Fig. 30.3. In this analysis absolute flow values are

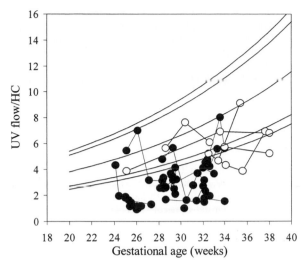

Fig. 30.4. Longitudinal assessment of umbilical venous flow per head circumference (ml/min mm⁻¹). Growth-restricted fetuses with abnormal umbilical arterial pulsatility index (*full circles*). Growth-restricted fetuses with normal umbilical arterial pulsatility index (*empty circles*). The 2nd, 5th, 50th, 95th, and 98th percentiles of normal reference values. *HC* head circumference

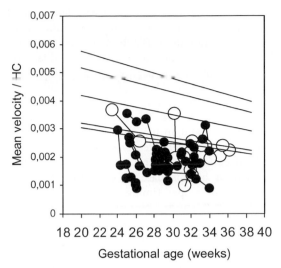

Fig. 30.5. Umbilical venous mean velocity per unit head circumference (ml/min mm⁻¹). Growth-restricted fetuses with abnormal umbilical arterial pulsatility index (*full circles*). Growth-restricted fetuses with normal umbilical arterial pulsatility index (*empty circles*). The 2nd, 5th, 50th, 95th, and 98th percentiles of normal reference values. *HC* head circumference

normalized by the head circumference (ml/min mm⁻¹). The advantage of this simplified normalization stems also from the fact that fetal head is an area of preferential distribution of flow and growth in the deprived fetus [28]; therefore, the use of this part of the fetal body as an index of fetal body mass improves the sensitivity of flow assessment in asymmetrically growth-restricted fetuses.

The increase in flow volume throughout gestation in normal fetuses is accounted for mainly by growth of the umbilical fetal vessels. The diameter of the vein increases from 4.1 to 8.3 mm, which would lead to a fourfold increase in cross-sectional area, whereas the velocity increased only 20% from 0.08 m/s at 20 weeks to 0.10 m/s at 38 weeks [12]. When blood velocity and diameter is normalized for fetal mass, an interesting result that can be observed in growth-restricted fetuses is that the diameter in small fetuses is not narrower than that of normal fetuses of comparable mass, whereas the main variable to decrease is blood velocity (Fig. 30.5). According to these data velocity itself could be used as a simple diagnostic test in growth-restricted fetuses. According to fetal sheep experiments [29] pressures and flow velocities are inversely related in the venous in-flow tract from the umbilical vein to the ductus venosus and inferior vena cava, this finding brings in both a diagnostic potential and a pathophysiological variable of interest.

In the same paper by Boito and co-workers, elsewhere quoted [25], a complex set of ultrasound volumetric measurements was performed on the head and

on the abdomen of restricted and normal fetuses and a significant ($p < 0.001$) inverse relationship was observed between fetal weight-related umbilical venous volume flow and fetal brain/liver volume ratio. The same diagnostic-oriented usage of umbilical venous flow was adopted by Tchirikov and co-workers [30]. In their reported experience the ratio between weight-specific umbilical vein blood volume (ml/min kg⁻¹) and umbilical artery PI was a better predictor of poor fetal outcome than umbilical arterial PI alone.

Redistribution of Umbilical Flow in Fetal Liver

Umbilical arterial qualitative velocimetry has probably reached its maximum clinical value. Its usage in fetal medicine is now a key criterion to differentiate severe growth-restricted fetuses from less severe forms and other diseases causing growth restriction. Umbilical volume flow measurements help us to better understand the pathophysiology of growth restriction. What happens under conditions of chronic hypoxia in the human fetus? From animal experimental studies we know that ductal dilatation sustained by the presence of an active sphincter regulation is the hypothesized mechanism allowing the fetal adaptation to the hypoxia [31]. This interpretation was confirmed in a recent experimental study in fetal sheep by Kiserud and co-workers [32]. Their data showed that induced hypoxemia determined a significant dilatation of the isthmus of DV. In 1998 our group reported the first suggestion of in vivo ductal dilatation in two IUGR human fetuses examined for a prolonged period of time [33] and more recently such findings were confirmed on a larger series of growth-restricted fetuses [11, 34, 35]. Reduction in umbilical vein flow volume and an increase in the ductal shunting determines a severe deprivation of substrate in the right liver lobe initiating a severe organ failure, the prevention of this damage can prove to be of great impact on proper timing of delivery in severe growth-restricted fetuses.

For clinical usage this set of knowledge can be used with a criteria of feasibility: the simpler the better. Since the reduction of flow in the umbilical vein is determined by a reduction in velocity and not by the diameter of the vessel [24], only the measurement of velocity only could be used. If volume flow per unit fetal weight is influenced by errors in weight estimation, why do we not use volume flow per unit head circumference? If we know that the ductal a-wave is determined by dilatation of the inlet [11, 33, 34], the diameter of the ductus only could be checked when qualitative indices change without resorting to complex velocity measurements.

References

1. Eik-Nes SH, Brubak AO, Ulstein M (1980) Measurement of human fetal blood flow. Br Med J 280:283–284
2. Gill RW, Trudinger BJ, Garrett WJ, Kossoff G, Warren PS (1981) Fetal umbilical venous flow measured in utero by pulsed Doppler and B-mode ultrasound. I. Normal pregnancies. Am J Obstet Gynecol 139:720–725
3. Eik-Nes SH, Maršál K, Brubak AO, Kristofferson K, Ulstein M (1982) Ultrasonic measurement of human fetal blood flow. J Biomed Eng 4:28–36
4. Erskine RL, Ritchie JW (1985) Quantitative measurement of fetal blood flow using Doppler ultrasound. Br J Obstet Gynaecol 92:600–604
5. Giles WB, Lingman G, Maršál K, Trudinger BJ (1986) Fetal volume blood flow and umbilical artery flow velocity waveform analysis: a comparison. Br J Obstet Gynaecol 93:461–465
6. Gerson AG, Wallace DM, Stiller RJ, Paul D, Weiner S, Bolognese RJ (1987) Doppler evaluation of umbilical venous and arterial blood flow in the second and third trimesters of normal pregnancy. Obstet Gynecol 70:622–626
7. Reed KL, Meijboom EJ, Sahn DJ, Scagnelli SA, Valdes-Cruz LM, Shenker L (1986) Cardiac Doppler Flow velocities in human fetuses. Circulation 73:41–46
8. Sutton MS, Theard MA, Bhatia SJ, Plappert T, Saltzman DH, Doubilet P (1990) Changes in placental blood flow in the normal human fetus with gestational age. Pediatr Res 28:383–387
9. Schmidt KG, Tommaso M di, Silverman NH, Rudolph AM (1991) Doppler echocardiographic assessment of fetal descending aortic and umbilical blood flows. Validation studies in fetal lambs. Circulation 83:1731–1737
10. Challis DE, Warren PS, Gill RW (1995) The significance of high umbilical venous blood flow measurements in a high-risk population. J Ultrasound Med 14:907–912
11. Pennati G, Bellotti M, Ferrazzi E, Rigano S, Garberi A (1997) Hemodynamic changes across the human ductus venosus: a comparison between clinical findings and mathematical calculations. Ultrasound Obstet Gynecol 9:383–391
12. Barbera A, Galan HL, Ferrazzi E, Rigano S, Jzwik M, Battaglia FC, Pardi G (1999) Relationship of umbilical vein blood flow to growth parameters in the human fetus. Am J Obstet Gynecol 181:174–179
13. Lees C, Albaiges G, Deane C, Parra M, Nicolaides KH (1999) Assessment of umbilical arterial and venous flow using color Doppler. Ultrasound Obstet Gynecol 14:250–255
14. Boito S, Struijk PC, Ursem NT, Stijnen T, Wladimiroff JW (2002) Umbilical venous volume flow in the normally developing and growth-restricted human fetus. Ultrasound Obstet Gynecol. 19:344–349
15. Naro E di, Ghezzi F, Raio L, Franchi M, D'Addario V, Lanzillotti G, Schneider H (2001) Umbilical vein blood flow in fetuses with normal and lean umbilical cord. Ultrasound Obstet Gynecol 17:224–228
16. Kunzel W, Jovanovic V, Grussner S, Colling T (1992) Blood flow velocity in the fetal abdominal aorta and in the umbilical artery in uncomplicated pregnancies. Eur J Obstet Gynecol Reprod Biol 23:31–40
17. Kiserud T, Rasmussen S (1998) How repeat measurements affect the mean diameter of the umbilical vein and the ductus venosus. Ultrasound Obstet Gynecol 11:419–425
18. Kiserud T (2003) Umbilical venous blood flow and reference ranges. Acta Obstet Gynecol Scand 82:1061
19. Chantraine F, Reihs T, Henrich W, Tutschek B (2003) Measurement of volume flow by "colour velocity imaging (CVI)": technique of measurement in the intrahepatic fetal umbilical vein. Zentralbl Gynäkol 125:179–182
20. Pennati GC, Bellotti M, de Gasperi C, Rognoni G (2004) Spatial velocity profile changes along the cord in normal human fetuses:Can these affect Doppler measurements of umbilical blood flow? Ultrasound Obstet Gynecol 23:131–137
21. Galan HL, Jozwik M, Rigano S, Regnault TR, Hobbins JC, Battaglia FC, Ferrazzi E (1999) Umbilical vein blood flow determination in the ovine fetus: comparison of Doppler ultrasonographic and steady-state diffusion techniques. Am J Obstet Gynecol 181:1149–1153
22. Kiserud T, Jauniaux E, West D, Ozturk O, Hanson MA (2001) Circulatory responses to maternal hyperoxaemia and hypoxaemia assessed non-invasively in fetal sheep at 0.3–0.5 gestation in acute experiments. BJOG 108:359–364
23. Padoan A, Regnault TRH, Limesand SW, Russell AV, Enrico Ferrazzi A, Wilkening RB, Galan HL (2004) Endothelial nitric oxide synthase in uteroplacental vasculature in an ovine model of IUGR. Am J Obstet Gynecol Suppl

24. Ferrazzi E, Rigano S, Bozzo M, Bellotti M, Giovannini N, Galan H, Battaglia FC (2000) Umbilical vein blood flow in growth-restricted fetuses. Ultrasound Obstet Gynecol 16:432–438

25. Boito S, Struijk PC, Ursem NT, Fedele L, Wladimiroff JW (2003) Ultrasound fetal brain/liver volume ratio and umbilical volume flow parameters relative to normal and abnormal human development. Ultrasound Obstet Gynecol 21:256–261

26. Rigano S, Bozzo M, Ferrazzi E, Bellotti M, Battaglia FC, Galan HL (2001) Early and persistent reduction in umbilical vein blood flow in the growth-restricted fetus: a longitudinal study. Am J Obstet Gynecol 85:834

27. di Naro E, Raio L, Ghezzi F, Franchi M, Romano F, Addario VD (2002) Longitudinal umbilical vein blood flow changes in normal and growth-retarded fetuses. Acta Obstet Gynecol Scand 81:527–533

28. Lngman G, Maršál K (1989) Noninvasive assessment of cranial blood circulation in the fetus. Biol Neonate 56:129–135

29. Schroder HJ, Tchirikov M, Rybakowski C (2003) Pressure pulses and flow velocities in central veins of the anesthetized sheep fetus. Am J Physiol Heart Circ Physiol 284:H1205–H1211

30. Tchirikov M, Rybakowski C, Huneke B, Schoder V, Schröder HJ (2002) Umbilical vein blood volume flow rate and umbilical artery pulsatility as "venous-arterial index" in the prediction of neonatal compromise. Ultrasound Obstet Gynecol 20:580–585

31. Gennser G (1992) Fetal ductus venosus and its sphincter mechanism. Lancet 339:132

32. Kiserud T, Ozaki T, Nishina H, Rodeck C, Hanson M (2000) Effect of NO, phenylephrine, and hypoxemia on ductus venosus diameter in fetal sheep. Am J Physiol Heart Circ Physiol 279: H1166–H1171

33. Bellotti M, Pennati G, Pardi G, Fumero R (1998) Dilatation of the ductus venosus in human fetuses: ultrasonographic evidence and mathematical modeling. Am J Physiol 275:H1759–H1767

34. Ferrazzi E, Bellotti M, Galan H, Pennati G, Bozzo M, Rigano S, Battaglia FC (2001) Doppler investigation in intrauterine growth restriction: from qualitative indices to flow measurements: a review of the experience of a collaborative group. Ann NY Acad Sci 943:316–325

35. Bellotti M, Pennati GC, de Gasperi C, Bozzo M, Battaglia FC, Ferrazzi E (2004) Simultaneous measurements of umbilical venous, fetal hepatic and ductus venosus blood flow in growth restricted human fetuses. Am J Obstet Gynecol 190:1347–1358

Chapter 31

Doppler Examination of the Fetal Pulmonary Venous Circulation

Rabih Chaoui, Franka Lenz, Kai-Sven Heling

Introduction

The assessment of the pulmonary venous system in the fetus has evolved dramatically in the past decade due to the routine use of spectral and color Doppler ultrasound. Besides checking the normal connection of pulmonary veins during fetal echocardiography, the interest in these veins has increased recently in order to get insight into the mystery of the pulmonary circulation in the human fetus in vivo. Physiologic conditions and changes during pregnancy have been assessed and have allowed the comparison with data under abnormal conditions. This chapter briefly reviews the clinical value of Doppler assessment of pulmonary veins.

Visualization of Pulmonary Veins Using Real-Time and Color Doppler Ultrasound

There are four pulmonary veins, inferior and superior on the right and left sides. All these veins enter the left atrium separately and have their own ostium. Using high-resolution real-time equipment and a perpendicular approach to the site of connection, the echolucent veins may then be recognizable in the surrounding gray lung (Fig. 31.1). It is generally difficult to visualize all four pulmonary veins in the fetus, but in the four-chamber view the two inferior veins can be visualized. Pulmonary veins in the fetus have a diameter of approximately 1 mm or less and are therefore difficult to identify routinely on screening ultrasound. This is also the reason why pulmonary volume flow is analyzed quantitatively on the arterial side.

In our examination technique we seek one right pulmonary vein (inferior) along a fictive line prolonging the intra-atrial septum. In real-time this is best visualized from the right transverse or slight dorsoanterior approach (Fig. 31.1). Using color Doppler this vein can be visualized either by an apical approach when (red) flow is seen toward the left atrium at the site where the inter-atrial septum inserts (Fig. 31.2) or by a dorsoanterior approach (flow in blue; Fig. 31.3).

The left pulmonary vein (inferior) is found as a vessel directly pointing toward the foramen ovale flap (Figs. 31.4, 31.5). It can be visualized in real-time when the heart is examined from the left transverse side (Fig. 31.4). Using color Doppler the same plane can be used to visualize flow in blue (Fig. 31.4), or a transverse right side to visualize blood flow in red toward the transducer (Figs. 31.2, 31.5). An apical approach slightly more from the right thoracic side may allow the visualization of two veins from the right and the left coursing into the left atrium (Fig. 31.2). New color Doppler techniques, such as power Doppler ultrasound or dynamic flow, can be very helpful tools in visualizing pulmonary veins especially when insonation angle is more perpendicular to the vessels of interest (Fig. 31.6).

Real-time visualization of the pulmonary veins was facilitated in the past few years by using new contrasting techniques, such as harmonic imaging or compound imaging (SonoCT, CRI, etc.; Figs. 31.1,

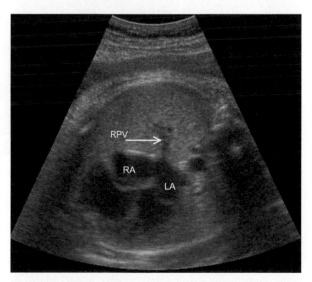

Fig. 31.1. Third-trimester fetus in dorsoanterior position. One right pulmonary vein (*RPV*) is visualized as the prolongation of the intraatrial septum. In this case we used harmonics imaging and a 5-MHz transducer. *RA* right atrium, *LA* left atrium

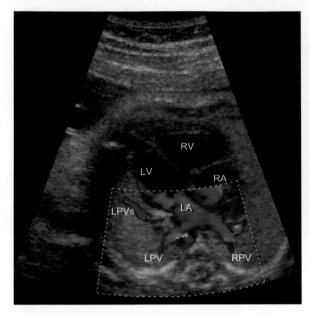

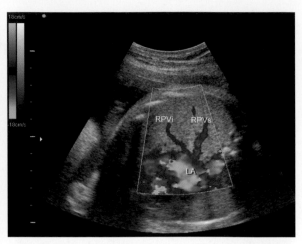

Fig. 31.3. Basal visualization of the heart in a dorsoanterior fetal position. Both inferior and superior right pulmonary veins (*RPVi*, *RPVs*) are seen in *blue* entering the left atrium (*LA*). Note the color presetting as seen on the color bar with +18 cm/s

Fig. 31.2. Apical four-chamber view in color in a 30-week fetus demonstrates both inferior left and right pulmonary veins (*LPV*, *RPV*) entering the left atrium (*red*). Flow toward the transducer is visualized in *red*. On the left side the superior left pulmonary vein is seen in *blue*. (*LA*, *RA* left and right atrium, *LV*, *RV* left and right ventricle)

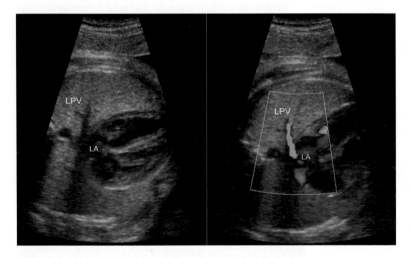

Fig. 31.4. Left approach to the four-chamber view with one left pulmonary vein seen in real-time image (in harmonic mode). The flow is parallel to the insonation angle and this plane is ideal for visualizing pulmonary flow, here seen in *blue*. *LA* left atrium

31.4). When using color Doppler, velocity range should be reduced to a range of 15–25 cm/s (Figs. 31.3, 31.7) with low filter and high persistence as we have described elsewhere [1]. The visualization of pulmonary veins using color Doppler is possible from the late first trimester by optimizing color Doppler presets (Fig. 31.8). Whether this contributes to increased diagnosis accuracy is not yet known. We include this visualization in first trimester mainly in

cases with suspected isomerism or in targeted examination, e.g., when totally anomalous pulmonary venous connection (TAPVC) was present in a previous child.

Usually it is sufficient to identify one pulmonary vein on each side during a routine study [2]. If, however, there is a heart defect detected, it is advisable to demonstrate at least three of the veins [2]. The examiner has, however, to be careful when assuming that

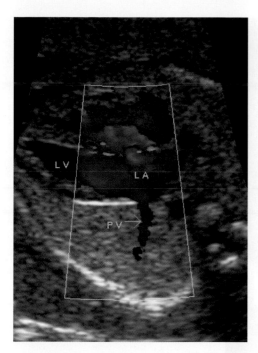

Fig. 31.5. Left pulmonary vein is visualized from a right lateral view of the heart. Here also the insonation angle is ideal for a color setting and flow is visualized in *red*

color Doppler confirmed the correct connection of the veins in a heart defect [3] as explained later in this chapter. In these cases we recommend a combination of color Doppler with pulsed Doppler of the pulmonary vessels, since flow velocity waveforms are often abnormal in TAPVC.

Pulsed Doppler Ultrasound of Lung Veins

Physiologic Conditions

Conversely to postnatal life, where whole blood passes through the pulmonary vessels to be oxygenated, the pulmonary circulation in the fetus is only a small part of cardiac output. Whereas animal experiments in fetal sheep found that pulmonary flow is around 8% of combined cardiac output [4], Doppler studies on human fetuses in vivo suggested that this flow is larger, being 13% at 20 gestational weeks and increasing to 20%–25% during the last trimester [5].

Doppler studies of volume flow were performed mainly on the arterial side where vessel diameter is easily measurable, whereas Doppler examination of the pulmonary venous system focused mainly on the study of velocity waveform. Pulmonary venous flow patterns in the adult were demonstrated to be influenced by dynamic changes in left atrial pressure created by contraction and relaxation of the atrium and ventricle [6]. Systolic peak (S) is caused by left atrial pressure reduction that results from the relaxation of the left atrium and the downward move of the mitral valve in systole. Diastolic peak (D) is caused by rapid emptying of the left atrium during left ventricular relaxation. During atrial contraction (A) there is a rise in left atrial pressure which causes in the adult a reversed flow into the pulmonary vein, i.e., a negative A-wave [7] which is not present [8, 9] (or occasionally present [10, 11]) in the fetus.

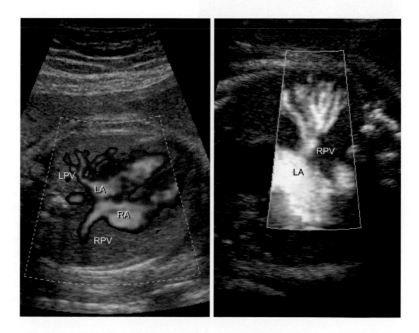

Fig. 31.6. *Left:* Power Doppler ultrasound in a lateral four-chamber view. With this technique pulmonary veins and the atria and ventricles are visualized at the same time. *Right:* Dynamic flow is very sensitive and arterial and venous flow are visualized

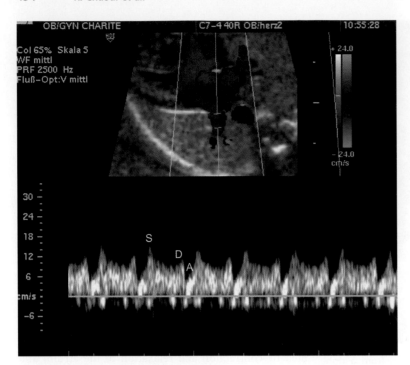

Fig. 31.7. Spectral Doppler of a pulmonary vein with a triphasic envelope characterized by the systolic (*S*) and diastolic (*D*) waves, and the A-wave as nadir during the atrial contraction

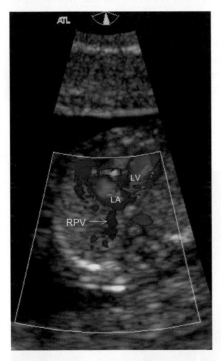

Fig. 31.8. A 13-week fetus examined transvaginally with visualization of a right pulmonary vein (*RPV*) entering the left atrium (*LA*). In a previous pregnancy there was a right isomerism with totally anomalous pulmonary venous connection

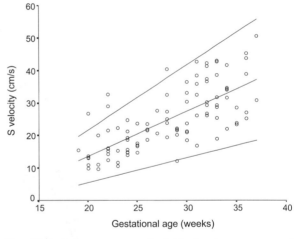

Fig. 31.9. Reference range (individual values, mean and 95% data intervals) for peak systolic velocity in the pulmonary veins plotted against gestational age. (From [9])

The fetal pulmonary vein velocity waveform is therefore very similar to that of the venous duct, with a forward triphasic flow throughout the heart cycle (Fig. 31.7). Parameters of blood flow velocity waveforms have been examined in several studies in recent years and similar results were reported [8–11]. Peak systolic (Fig. 31.9), diastolic velocities (Fig. 31.10), and time velocity integral (TVI) increase significantly during the second half of pregnancy, whereas pulsatility index decreases (Fig. 31.11) [9]. The rise in

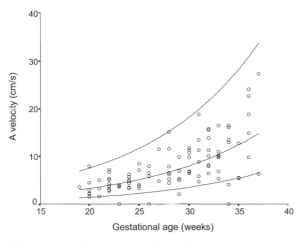

Fig. 31.10. Reference range (individual values, mean and 95% data intervals) for velocities during atrial contraction in the pulmonary veins plotted against gestational age. (From [9])

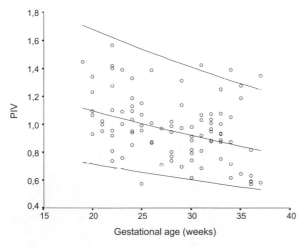

Fig. 31.11. Reference range (individual values, mean and 95% data intervals) for pulsatility index of the pulmonary veins plotted against gestational age. (From [9] with permission)

peak velocities and TVI is compatible with the increase in pulmonary blood flow during gestation.

Given that the fetal pulmonary vein waveform reflects changes in the left atrium, studies have been performed to analyze indirectly the impact of left atrial pressure changes on the waveform. The pulmonary venous velocity pattern can be influenced by following determinants [12]:

1. Pulmonary volume flow
2. Foramen ovale size and flow
3. Left atrial compliance (size and muscle distensibility)
4. Atrial contraction, end-diastolic pressure (e.g., adrenergic drive, hypoxemia)

5. Left ventricular size and performance
6. Mitral valve size and function (e.g., regurgitation).

Abnormal Patterns of Flow Velocity Waveforms

If we assume that left atrial pressure is a major determinant of the pulmonary vein velocity waveform, an obstruction of the left atrium should lead to typical changes in the waveform envelope. This was confirmed for fetuses with hypoplastic left heart syndrome, for example, where a distinct reversed flow during atrial contraction was demonstrated (Fig. 31.12) [13–15]. When the mitral valve is closed or severely dysplastic, left atrial blood can only escape during atrial contraction by passing across the foramen ovale from left to right or by returning to the lung. The larger the interatrial communication, the less blood will return into the lung during atrial contraction, and vice versa. Better et al. [14] reported an increase in systolic velocity and a reversal in A-velocity in such fetuses that correlated with the degree of restriction of the atrial septum after birth. This was

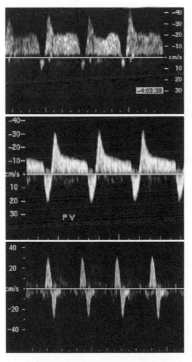

Fig. 31.12. Three types of an obstructed left atrium as reflected in the pulmonary vein flow velocity waveforms. The *upper wave* is a mild obstruction with a slight reverse A-wave, the *middle wave* is a serious obstruction with a pronounced reversed A-wave. The *lower wave* is severely abnormal and indicates an obstructive left atrium, often associated with thickened pulmonary veins and congestive lungs

supported by a recent observation we reported in two different cases of hypoplastic left heart [15], one showing a wide patent and the other a sealed foramen ovale. In the patent interatrial communication, the pulmonary venous velocity waveform was normal with a positive A-wave. In the sealed foramen ovale, however, the waveform showed a nearly to-and-fro pattern (Fig. 31.12), since all blood flow coming from the lung returns back into the lung. This is associated with congested pulmonary veins. This chronic high pressure leads to vascular damage as observed at autopsy, with arterialization of pulmonary veins as well as the development of lymphangiectasia of the lung as we observed in other cases.

In a further study we examined changes of the velocity waveforms in other heart anomalies ($n=96$) and were not able to find any changes depending on the heart anomaly, mainly due to the interatrial conditions of obstruction [16].

Besides obstructed left atrium conditions (e.g., hypoplastic left heart, mitral atresia), we also found abnormal waveform patterns in TAPVC. In this severe malformation pulmonary veins are not connected to the left atrium and interestingly velocity waveforms reflect the site of connection. When connecting to a descending channel into the liver, infradiaphragmatic blood flow in the pulmonary veins was shown to be continuous [3]. Connection directly to the right atrium or indirectly via a vertical vein may show pulsations but not with the typical shape of a pulmonary vein [12]; therefore, it has been suggested that the routine use of pulsed Doppler of lung veins may help in diagnosing TAPVC in the fetus.

In summary, it can be emphasized that left atrial obstruction as seen in hypoplastic left heart syndrome or mitral atresia can be associated in most cases with an increased pulsatile flow due to the reversal of flow during atrial contraction. A to-and-fro pattern is suggestive for a sealed foramen ovale and associated with severe impairment of lung development, showing a poor prognosis. Flow pulsations are decreased or absent in TAPVC with infradiaphragmatic connection, or show an atypical pattern resembling inferior vena cava or a more dumped pattern in cardiac or supracardiac connections.

Other Fields of Interest Assessing Pulmonary Vein Doppler

The relationship of pulmonary venous flow with systolic and diastolic cardiac times assessed at the level of the mitral valve are used in cardiology to assess diastolic function. Brezinka and coworkers [17] analyzed this relationship in 28 healthy fetuses in the second half of pregnancy and found that pulmonary venous inflow into the left atrium occurs predomi-

nantly during the filling and ejection phases of the cardiac cycle. Absolute cardiac diastolic and systolic time intervals as well as the distribution of pulmonary venous flow velocity integrals between these cardiac time intervals remained unchanged with advancing gestational age.

Macklon and coworkers [18] examined the influence of fetal behavioral states on venous blood flow velocity waveforms in ten normally grown fetuses at term. The examinations were performed either during quiet (state 1F) or active (state 2F) sleep. Whereas no changes were observed on the arterial side, venous pulmonary blood flow velocity waveforms demonstrated a significant increase in time-averaged peak diastolic and end-diastolic velocity during active sleep, suggesting an increase of pressure gradient between the pulmonary venous system and the left atrium in these behavioral states.

DeVore and Horenstein [19] described a new technique for the evaluation of fetal arrhythmia by simultaneous recording of the intraparenchymal pulmonary artery and vein. Since both vessels are adjacent to each other within the lung showing opposite flow directions, a simultaneous spectral Doppler sampling will demonstrate waveforms on both sides of the baseline (Fig. 31.13): the peak of the pulmonary artery reflects the ventricular systole, whereas the atrial

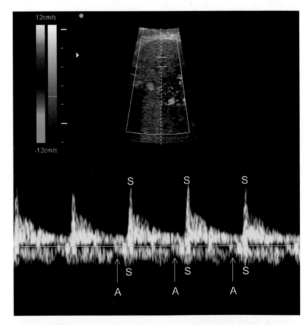

Fig. 31.13. Simultaneous pulmonary artery and vein Doppler tracing in a normal fetus. Sampling is performed in lung parenchyma where peripheral pulmonary artery and veins are adjacent to each other. Peak velocity on the arterial side indicates systole (*S*) and is observed on the venous side as well. The nadir on the venous side indicates the atrial contraction (*A*)

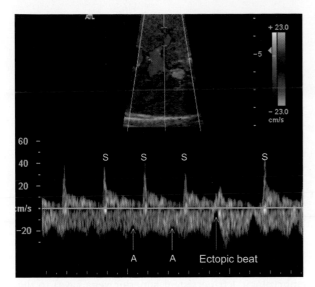

Fig. 31.14. Simultaneous pulmonary artery and vein Doppler tracing in a fetus with ectopic beat. The ectopic beat originating from the atrium is seen as a notching on the venous side with a reversal flow

contraction is identified by an interruption or a nadir in venous flow (Fig. 31.13). Using this technique the examiner is able to easily assess qualitatively the relationship of atrial to ventricular contraction and to quantify the arteriovenous time as well. The method seems to be helpful in differentiating arrhythmias (Figs. 31.14, 31.15).

Malformations of Pulmonary Veins and Their Diagnosis

Embryology in Summary

Understanding embryologic development facilitates the comprehension of different anomalies involving the pulmonary system.

Embryology of the fetal venous system is complex and has been reviewed several times in the past few years [20–22] to facilitate the understanding of detected (mainly intrahepatic) venous anomalies by the use of color Doppler. The development of the pulmonary vein system is better examined, since the anomalies are known entities in pediatric cardiology.

The sinus venosus is incorporated at the end of the fourth week into the posterior wall of the right and left atria. The right part of the sinus venosus encircles the superior and inferior vena cava and becomes part of the dorsal wall of the right atrium. The left part becomes remnant and builds the coronary sinus of the left atrium.

Separately from the development of the left atrium, the pulmonary veins develop as part of the splanchnic venous bed. During further development pulmonary veins differentiate into the individual veins but still connect to the systemic venous circulation. At a certain stage these pulmonary veins connect to the left atrium where a "common" pulmonary vein arises as a bud and they lose their connection to the central circulation. It is still debated whether the pulmonary veins from the lung connect with the bud resulting from the invagination of the dorsal wall of the left atrium or with remnants of the coronary sinus [23].

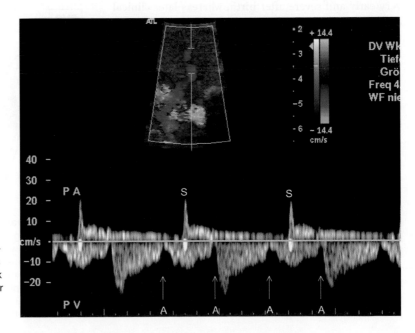

Fig. 31.15. Simultaneous pulmonary artery and vein Doppler tracing in a fetus with second-degree arteriovenous block in connective disease of the mother. For every second atrial contraction there is one ventricular systole recorded

Anomalies of the Pulmonary Venous Connections

Failure of the meeting of the common pulmonary vein and its splanchnic components results in various forms of anomalous venous connections. In the case of a complete failure to connect there is a total bilateral anomalous pulmonary venous connection. This is the embryologic persistence of the connection to the systemic veins, since this remains the only pathway for lung blood to return to the heart. According to their site of connection, there are four forms of TAPVC: at supracardiac, cardiac, and infracardiac levels, and mixed connections [2]. In partial anomalous venous drainage there is a failing of one, two, or three pulmonary veins to connect to the common pulmonary vein and the vein(s) remain connected to a systemic vein, either the superior caval, the brachiocephalic vein, or the coronary sinus. The right pulmonary veins are more often involved than the left.

The postnatal hemodynamic consequence of anomalous pulmonary venous connection is that oxygenated blood from the lung reaches directly or indirectly together with the systemic veins into the right instead of the left atrium. If arterialized blood does not reach the left atrium, the neonate may present with cyanosis. The obstruction can be at cardiac level, if the atrial communication is small, or at more proximal stages either at the level of the pulmonary veins themselves, within the course of the confluence or at their connection with a systemic vein [2]. The most severe form of obstruction is assumed to be the infradiaphragmatic connection. When a TAPVC with obstruction is present, the clinical presentation is very early and severe after birth, whereas later clinical appearance is observed in cases with no obstruction and may present first late in childhood in cases with partial anomalous pulmonary venous connection (PAPVC).

Prenatal Diagnosis of Anomalous Pulmonary Venous Connection

Total or partial anomalous pulmonary venous connections occur in 2% of all live births. They can occur as an isolated incidence or as a part of complex heart anomalies, mainly right atrial isomerism (asplenia syndrome; see review in [24]). Despite the "theoretical" ease of visualization of pulmonary veins during fetal echocardiography, diagnosis of TAPVC has been, however, reported prenatally only in case reports or very small series [3, 25]. In large series on fetal echocardiography this condition was among the missed diagnoses; therefore, clues for diagnosis are probably indirect signs, on one hand, and the tar-geted examination for this condition when typical associated heart anomalies are suspected, on the other [25]. The diagnosis can be assisted by the use of pulsed Doppler sampling of the pulmonary veins [25].

The diagnosis of partial anomalous pulmonary vein connection is very difficult prenatally but can occasionally be made. We focus on the total anomalous venous connections. The prenatal clues for diagnosis depend mainly on the site of connection and we discuss it according to this classification.

Supracardiac TAPVC

Supracardiac TAPVC is the most common form of anomalous connection. In most cases the four pulmonary veins form a confluence posterior to the left atrium and connect via a vertical vein (which is the embryologic left persistent superior vena cava) to the brachiocephalic vein, which drains into the superior vena cava (Fig. 31.16). This condition is rarely detected by visualizing the confluence behind the left atrium, but by visualizing the left persistent superior vena cava as a fourth vessel in the three-vessel-trachea view in the upper thorax (Fig. 31.17, right). Since an LVCS is a common anomaly seen in the fetus as well, the differentiation from an isolated LVCS is mandatory. This is achieved by means of color Doppler (Fig. 31.17). In isolated LVCS, blood from the jugular vein continues via the LVCS toward the heart, which means that flow in the LVCS goes in the direction of the heart. In supracardiac TAPVC with connection to LVCS blood flow goes the opposite way,

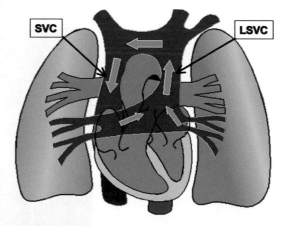

Fig. 31.16. Supracardiac total anomalous pulmonary vein connection. Lung veins are connecting to a left persistent superior vena cava (*LSVC*) which drains the blood to the anonymous vein and then to the right superior vena cava (*SVC*). Blood flow in the left vena cava is toward the head and the right superior cava in the opposite direction (compare with Fig. 31.17). (Courtesy of Philippe Jeanty from www.thefetus.net)

Fig. 31.17. Supracardiac totally anomalous pulmonary venous connection (TAPVC). *Left:* Longitudinal view of the upper left thorax with a left persistent superior vena cava (*LSVC*) with blood flow is seen with a perfusion toward the fetal head (*in red*). *Right:* In the three-vessel view the pulmonary trunk is antegrade perfused (*blue*), and the aorta is hypoplastic and cannot be seen. On both sides of the pulmonary trunk the left persistent (LSVC) and right SVC are perfused in opposite directions which is typical for a supracardiac TAPVC

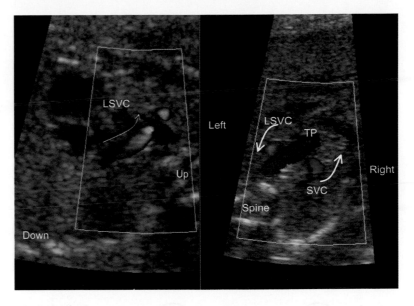

upward toward the upper thorax (Fig. 31.17, left). A longitudinal visualization of the LVCS may therefore help enormously (Fig. 31.17, left). Furthermore, blood flow in the innominate vein appears increased compared with other conditions, since in addition to blood coming from the left side of the upper extremity, blood flow of the lungs will pass through it. Even by using a cardiac setting of color Doppler with high velocities, the innominate vein will appear very clearly with high flow. Pulsed Doppler of pulmonary veins may be of help in these conditions, especially in cases with obstruction of these veins.

The supracardiac type of TAPVC connecting directly to the superior vena cava is difficult to detect unless the superior vena cava is dilated.

A common feature in both conditions could be the discrepant size of the right and left heart [25]. In supracardiac and cardiac TAPVC the left side of the heart is more narrow due to lack of blood flow to the left and the right side is dilated due to the increased flow; therefore, it has to be borne in mind that conditions suspicious for size discrepancy, such as right ventricular dysfunction suggesting tricuspid insufficiency or aortic coarctation, should be suspicious for supracardiac or cardiac TAPVC as well.

Cardiac TAPVC

In cardiac TAPVC pulmonary veins connect directly to the coronary sinus, which becomes dilated, or less commonly the connection is directly into the posterior wall of the right atrium (Fig. 31.18).

The first condition can be detected when a dilated coronary sinus is found. Generally, the best plane to visualize a coronary sinus is a cross section just below the four-chamber view as we recently described

in an article on normal and abnormally dilated coronary sinus [26].

The direct connection of pulmonary veins with the right atrium can be visualized by means of color Doppler or power Doppler (Fig. 31.19). This is rarely detected primarily on screening ultrasound but mainly when there is a suspicious sign. The two clues for suspicion are either the small size of the left side of the heart compared with the right or the presence of right atrial isomerism (asplenia) as detected from upper abdomen anatomy (juxtaposition of aorta and inferior vena cava) [24]. In Fig. 31.19 one can recognize the sampling vein behind the right atrium where the pulmonary veins drain. Pulsed Doppler demonstrates the continuous rather than the typical pulsatile flow.

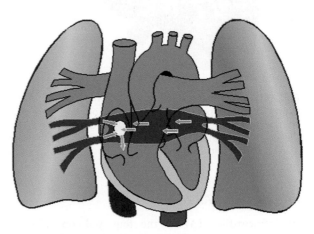

Fig. 31.18. Cardiac TAPVC. All pulmonary veins are connected to the right atrium. (Courtesy of Philippe Jeanty from www.Thefetus.net)

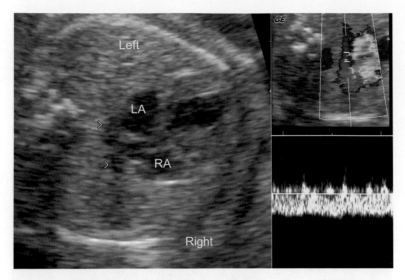

Fig. 31.19. Cardiac TAPVC in a fetus with right isomerism. *Left:* Pulmonary veins drain into the right atrium (*RA*) after coursing behind the left atrium (*LA*; compare with Fig. 31.18). *Right:* Color Doppler shows the vessel behind the left atrium with a course toward the right atrium (*blue* with sample volume). Spectral Doppler demonstrates the continuous flow instead of the pulsatile flow

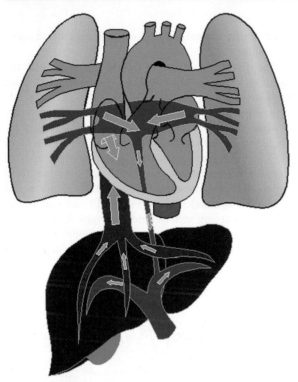

Fig. 31.20. Infracardiac (or infradiaphragmatic) TAPVC shows the four pulmonary veins draining into a vertical vein which courses across the diaphragm and ends in the liver vasculature. (Courtesy of Philippe Jeanty from www.Thefetus.net)

Infracardiac TAPVC

In infracardiac TAPVC the four pulmonary veins form a confluence which is localized behind the atria. This confluence is connected to an anomalous descending vein which passes the diaphragm accompa-

nying the esophagus and drains into the portal veins in most cases but occasionally into the hepatic veins or into the ductus venosus (Fig. 31.20). In isolated cases a discrepant size of the ventricles is not typical and the main suspicion can only be made in cases with right isomerism. The confluence and the descending veins are, according to our experience, so tiny that on real-time and color Doppler examination they appear to be part of the left atrium and are not easily recognizable.

Three diagnostic clues can be of help:

1. The proper use of color Doppler by changing the settings in order to visualize the proper connection of the veins may help in detecting the confluence (Fig. 31.21). Interestingly, in contrast to normal connecting pulmonary veins, where a certain distance is found between the connecting sites of the right and the left inferior pulmonary veins, in this condition the veins connect in the same place – the confluence vein (Fig. 31.21).
2. Pulsed Doppler of pulmonary veins shows a continuous flow [3] as demonstrated in Fig. 31.22.
3. Of further help is the longitudinal view of the upper abdomen and heart using color Doppler, which can demonstrate a vessel with the opposite color to the hepatic veins and entering the liver from cranially (Fig. 31.23). At a time where in IUGR conditions and most cardiac anomalies the ductus venosus is examined routinely, the examiner could shift the transducer slightly to the left and the right to recognize such an abnormal vessel. This should of course not be confused with the hepatic artery showing an increased flow in fetuses with severe IUGR, which is again easy to differentiate by means of pulsed Doppler.

Fig. 31.21. Infracardiac TAPVC. *Left:* At first sight analysis of pulmonary venous connection may suggest a normal connection. *Right:* Increasing velocity range demonstrates that both veins are draining into a vessel behind the atrium (*arrows*). In another plane this vein is seen crossing the diaphragm (see Fig. 31.23)

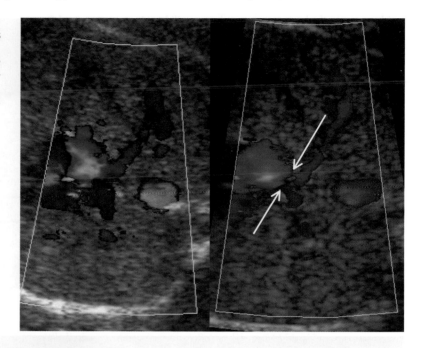

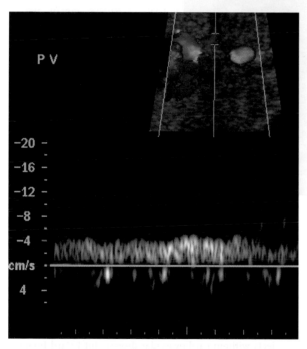

Fig. 31.22. Infracardiac TAPVC. Spectral Doppler of the intrathoracic vein shows a continuous flow instead of the pulsatile flow as sign of a abnormal connection (compare with Figs. 31.7 and 31.19)

Rare Anomalies of the Pulmonary Veins

Other anomalies of the pulmonary venous system are the presence of arteriovenous fistulae within the lung. In the past few years there have been some case reports of such conditions leading prenatally to volume overload [27, 28]. The hint for detection was sonolucent echoes in the lung showing a high turbulent flow on color Doppler (Fig. 31.24). Another rare condition is the direct connection of the pulmonary artery branch directly to the left atrium bypassing the vein as we described in a case report within a series of different cases of cardiomegaly [29].

Table 32.2. Echocardiographic planes

Apical four chamber
Basal four chamber
Lateral four chamber
Ventricular long axis
    Aortic outflow
    Pulmonic outflow
Ventricular short axis
    Ventricular apex
    Ventricular chamber
    Mitral-tricuspid plane
    Ventricular base
Aortic arch
Pulmonic-ductal arch

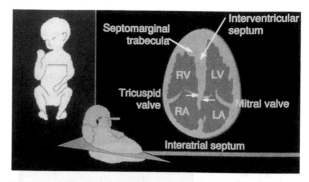

Fig. 32.4. Method for obtaining an apical four-chamber view of the fetal heart. *Far left*: Orientation of the transducer plane in relation to the fetal thorax. *Bottom left*: Echocardiographic plane in relation to the fetal heart

Table 32.3. Information content of fetal echocardiographic examination

Location of the heart in the thorax
Cardiac size: normally one-third of the thoracic cross-sectional area
Number of cardiac chambers
Comparability of right and left atrial sizes
Comparability of right and left ventricular sizes
Aortic and pulmonary outflow tracts and their crossover relation
Integrity of the atrial and ventricular septa
Location and movement of the tricuspid and mitral valves
Location and movement of the valve of the foramen ovale in the left atrium
Abnormal flow patterns
Abnormal rhythm
Presence of effusion, pericardial and pleural

and reliability of the procedure for general application. The views of the fetal heart at various echocardiographic planes are described below. These views offer a comprehensive evaluation of the fetal heart, although they do not constitute all the available approaches to cardiac imaging. The minimal information to be derived from the 2D fetal echocardiographic examination is listed in Table 32.3.

Four-Chamber View

As the fetal heart lies horizontally in the thorax, a cross-sectional scan of the fetal thorax just above the level of the diaphragm reveals the four-chamber view of the fetal heart (Fig. 32.4). It is an apical four-chamber view when the fetal spine is posterior, as encountered in the occipitoposterior position (Fig. 32.5 A). When the fetus is in the occipitoanterior position with the fetal spine directed anteriorly, the cardiac apex is directed toward the maternal spine and the base faces the maternal anterior (Fig. 32.5 B). This position constitutes the basal four-chamber view. When the fetus lies on its side in the occipitolateral position, the lateral four-chamber view is visualized with the cardiac apex directed laterally (Fig. 32.5 C).

The four-chamber view is one of the most important approaches for fetal cardiac assessment. It is readily obtainable, does not require in-depth expertise in the echocardiographic technique, and yields an immense body of information regarding the functional integrity of the fetal heart. Although it constitutes an essential component of the screening examination of the fetus, it should be clearly recognized that this view in itself is not sufficient for ruling out fetal cardiac malformations and cannot act as a surrogate for comprehensive systematic sonographic examination of the fetal heart.

The four-chamber view allows assessment of the following components of the fetal cardiac anatomy: atria, interatrial septum, foramen ovale and its valve, eustachean valve, tricuspid and mitral valves, ventricles, and interventricular septum. The right and left ventricles appear to be of comparable size. The right ventricle is nearer the anterior abdominal wall, whereas the left ventricle faces the posterolateral abdominal wall and is nearer the spine. The septomarginal trabeculum, or moderator band, can be seen near the apex in contiguity with the interventricular septum. The right ventricular cavity is irregular, whereas the left cavity is smooth. The tricuspid and mitral orifices and the respective valves are clearly imaged in this plane. The former is situated more toward the apex than the latter. The right and left atria appear to be of similar size. The superior and inferior vena caval entry into the right atrium and the pulmonary venous entry into the left atrium may also be seen in this or a similar plane. The interatrial septum can be visualized separating the at-

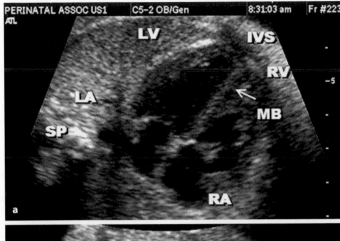

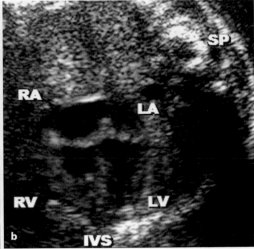

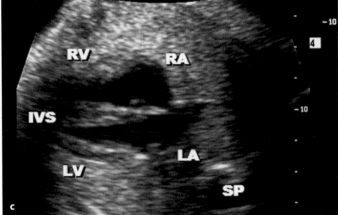

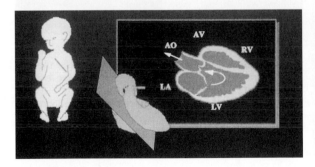

Fig. 32.5 a–c. Two-dimensional echocardiogram of the fetal heart. **a** Apical four-chamber view. **b** Basal four-chamber view. **c** Lateral four-chamber view. *LA* left atrium, *LV* left ventricle, *RA* right atrium, *RV* right ventricle, *IVS* interventricular septum, *SP* Spine, *MB* moderator band

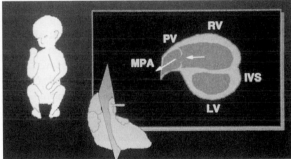

Fig. 32.6. Method for obtaining the left ventricular long-axis view of the fetal heart. *Far left*: Orientation of the transducer plane in relation to the fetal thorax. *Middle*: Echocardiographic plane in relation to the fetal heart. *AO* aorta, *AV* aortic valve, *LA* left atrium, *LV* left ventricle, *RV* right ventricle

Fig. 32.7. Method for obtaining the right ventricular long-axis view of the fetal heart. *Far left*: Orientation of the transducer plane in relation to the fetal thorax. *Middle*: Echocardiographic plane in relation to the fetal heart. *MPA* main pulmonary artery, *PV* pulmonary valve, *RV* right valve, *IVS* interventricular septum, *LV* left ventricle

ria, although the apical or basal four-chamber view may not offer the best acoustic exposure for the septum, which may be better imaged in the lateral four-chamber view. The foramen ovale can be visualized in the septum, and its valve can be seen in the left atrial cavity. The pulmonary veins entering the left atrium may be identified in the image.

Pulmonic and Aortic Outflow Tracts: Long-Axis Crossover Views

From the four-chamber plane, rotational movement of the transducer of approximately 45° (clockwise with the fetal spine posterior and counterclockwise

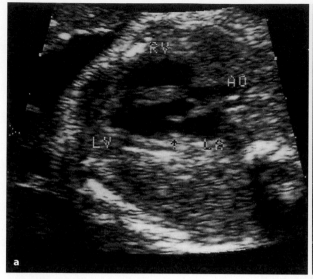

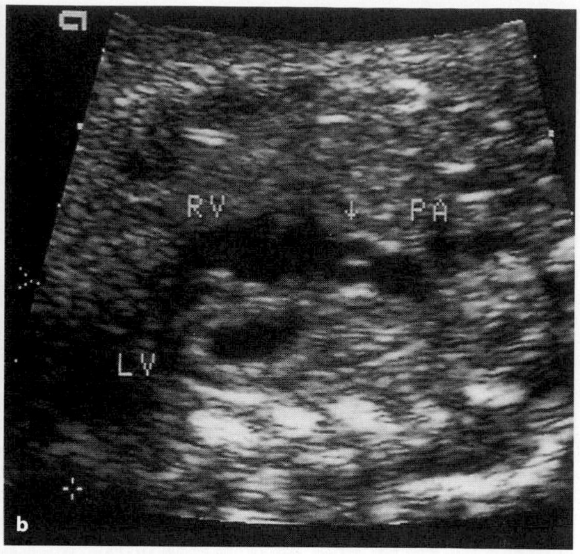

Fig. 32.8. Two-dimensional echocardiogram of the fetal heart. *Left*: Long-axis view of the left ventricular outflow. *AO* aorta, *LA* left atrium, *LV* left ventricle, *RV* right ventricle.

Right: Long-axis views of the right ventricular outflow. *PA* main pulmonary artery, *LV* left ventricle, *RV* right ventricle

with the spine anterior) along its central axis with slight fanning motion cephalad toward the left shoulder of the fetus reveals the left parasternal long-axis view of the left ventricle and the aortic outflow tract (Fig. 32.6). The transition from the four-chamber plane to this view is swift, requiring only minimal transducer manipulation. Further slight rotation and fanning motion of the beam in the longitudinal plane in the left parasternal area reveals the right ventricle and the pulmonic outflow tract (Fig. 32.7).

These views allow assessment of the right and left ventricular outflow tracts (Fig. 32.8). Particularly noteworthy is the aortic-pulmonary crossover relationship, which is characteristic of normal cardiac anatomy. Absence of this feature is pathognomonic of great artery transposition.

Parasternal Short-Axis View

Ventricular short-axis views may be obtained by rotating the transducer approximately 90° from the four-chamber view and moving the beam plane perpendicular to and along the long axis of the ventricles, starting at the cardiac apex and concluding at the cardiac base (Fig. 32.9). This maneuver generates cross-sectional images of the ventricles at the apex, midcavity, atrioventricular junctions, and the root of the great vessels (aortic short-axis pulmonic outflow view). These approaches allow assessment of the ventricles, the mitral and tricuspid valves and orifices, and the ventricular outflow tracts, especially the pulmonary arteries (Fig. 32.10).

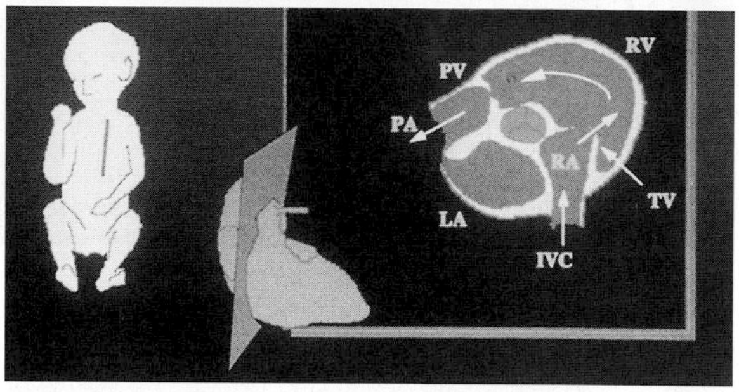

Fig. 32.9. Method for obtaining ventricular short-axis (parasternal) view of the fetal heart at the level of the cardiac base and the origin of the great arteries. *Far left*: Orientation of the transducer plane in relation to the fetal thorax. *Middle*: Echocardiographic plane in relation to the fetal heart. *PA* pulmonary artery, *PV* pulmonary valve, *RV* right ventricle, *TV* tricuspid valve, *IVC* inferior vena cava, *LA* left atrium, *RA* right atrium

Ductal and Aortic Arch: Long-Axis View

From the four-chamber plane, the transducer should be rotated (clockwise with fetal spine posterior) to align the imaging plane to the left of the fetal midline sagittal plane (Fig. 32.11). This maneuver reveals the long-axis view of the pulmonic artery-ductal arch (Fig. 32.12). With fine manipulation and slight tilting motion of the transducer, the imaging plane can be projected slightly oblique in reference to the sagittal plane, traversing from the right anterior thorax to the left of the fetal spine with an occipitoposterior position (Fig. 32.13), or from the left of the spine to the right

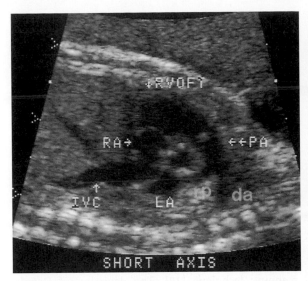

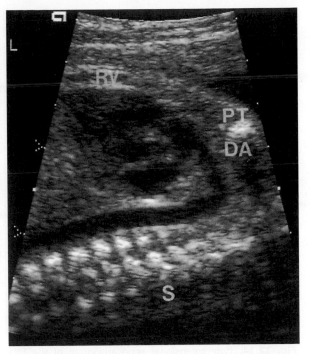

Fig. 32.10. Two-dimensional echocardiogram of the basal short-axis view of the fetal heart. *RVOFT* right ventricular outflow tract, *LA* left atrium, *RA* right atrium, *PA* pulmonary artery, *RV* right ventricle, *da* ductus arteriosus, *rp* right pulmonary artery, *IVC* inferior vena cava

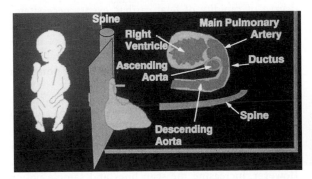

Fig. 32.12. Two-dimensional echocardiogram of the fetal heart depicting the ductal arch. Note the wider curve. *RV* right ventricle, *PT* pulmonary trunk, *DA* ductus arteriosus, *S* fetal spine

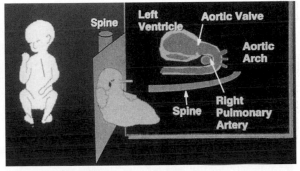

Fig. 32.11. Method for obtaining the ductal arch view of the fetal heart. *Far left*: Orientation of the transducer plane in relation to the fetal thorax. *Middle*: Echocardiographic plane in relation to the fetal heart

Fig. 32.13. Method for obtaining the aortic arch view of the fetal heart. *Far left*: Orientation of the transducer plane in relation to the fetal thorax. *Middle*: Echocardiographic plane in relation to the fetal heart

anterior thorax with an occipitoanterior position. This maneuver reveals the aortic arch (Fig. 32.14).

Spectral Doppler Sonographic Examination

Whereas 2D imaging provides information on the structural integrity of the fetal heart, the addition of Doppler ultrasonography provides information on the cardiac circulatory state, which may reflect the presence of fetal cardiac disease. Thus Doppler ultrasonography may be of adjunctive diagnostic value. Spectral Doppler sonographic interrogation of the fetal heart can be performed only with a pulsed-wave duplex Doppler technique in which imaging provides guidance for the Doppler sample volume placement. Continuous-wave Doppler ultrasonography has lim-

ited use for assessing fetal cardiac flow because it lacks range discrimination.

Once a detailed anatomic examination of the heart has been performed, the Doppler cursor is moved across the plane of the 2D cardiac image, and the Doppler sample volume is then placed at the desired intracardiac or outflow locations. The ultrasound mode is then changed to pulsed-wave spectral Doppler sonography and the frequency shift signals are obtained (Fig. 32.15). Because of fetal movement and consequent unpredictable changes in the fetal posi-

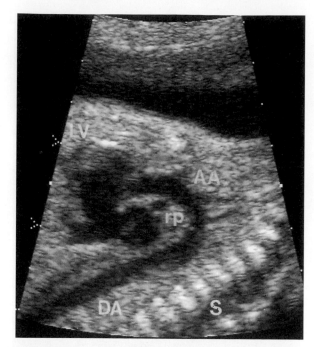

Fig. 32.14. Two-dimensional echocardiogram of the fetal heart depicting the aortic arch. Note the tight curvature of the aortic arch and the origin of the arteries supplying the head and neck. Compare it with the curvature of the ductal arch shown in Fig. 32.12. *LV* left ventricle, *AA* aortic arch, *rp* right pulmonary artery, *S* fetal spine, *DA* descending aorta

short interval during which spectra are interpolated; and (3) time-sharing algorithms that produce simultaneous display of spectral Doppler images and 2D images by sharing the available pulses during a given time interval between the two modes. Unfortunately, all of these approaches have trade-offs and therefore do not provide an ideal solution.

Finally, duplex pulsed-wave Doppler ultrasonography can be used to determine fetal cardiac output. The principle of this technique is briefly described later in the chapter.

Color Doppler Flow Mapping

The introduction of color Doppler echocardiographic technique represents one of the major advances in noninvasive cardiac diagnosis [17, 18]. Fetal cardiac hemodynamics have been imaged using the color mapping technique [19]. The depiction of Doppler mean frequency shifts by 2D flow mapping requires a balanced compromise between spatial resolution, Doppler accuracy, and temporal resolution. The normal range of the fetal cardiac cycle in 0.375–0.545 s (corresponding to a heart rate of 120–160 bpm). This degree of rapidity of fetal cardiac events necessitates an adequate processing speed to maintain temporal resolution. The small size and deep location of the fetal heart and the inability to ensure its favorable orientation impose further restrictions on obtaining adequate signals.

With Doppler color flow mapping for a given sector size, the more numerous the scan lines, the better the spatial resolution of the color (see Chap. 6). Furthermore, the more profuse the samples per scan line, the more accurate the mean velocity estimation. However, increasing the scan lines and sample points

tion, repeated verification of the location of the Doppler sample volume is essential. Various approaches may be used, including (1) display of a frozen 2D image that is updated at predetermined intervals, verifying the Doppler sample volume location; (2) interpolation techniques that produce a 2D image during a

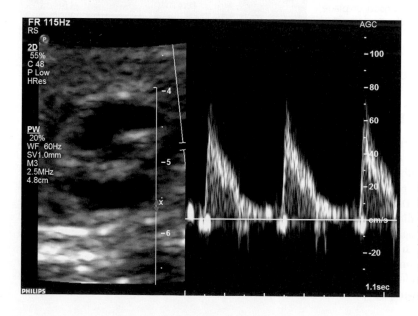

Fig. 32.15. Spectral Doppler interrogation. *Left panel*: Pulmonary outflow. The Doppler path is indicated by the *cursor line*. The Doppler sample volume (*horizontal lines*) is placed in the outflow tract. *Right panel*: Spectral Doppler waveforms from the ductus. As the flow is towards the transducer, the waveforms deflect upward from the baseline

leads to greater processing time, which in turn leads to a slower frame rate and therefore a consequent loss of temporal resolution, especially in a hyperdynamic situation with a shorter cardiac cycle as is encountered in the fetus. The small size of the fetal heart compensates for this problem to some extent by allowing an adequate anatomic exposure with a relatively smaller scan area. Limiting the scanned area of interrogation can substantially improve both color sensitivity and temporal resolution. Another important consideration is the device's ability to distinguish between the various types of motion detected by the Doppler mode within the interrogated area. Doppler shift signals are generated not only by blood flow but also by tissue motions, such as fetal cardiac wall movements or during fetal breathing, which result in color artifacts. Although these artifacts can be eliminated by a high-pass filter, the latter also eliminates low-velocity flow information. Many devices now minimize this problem by utilizing advanced filtering technology that processes multiple parameters including velocity and amplitude. These issues are discussed in detail in Chap. 6.

The methodology is similar to the pulsed-wave Doppler technique described above. Appropriate 2D views of the fetal heart are first obtained by 2D echocardiography. The mode of operation is then changed to color Doppler sonography, which results in the depiction of 2D color-coded flow patterns superimposed on real-time gray-scale images of the heart. Manipulation of the transducer allows interrogation of various cardiac chambers, orifices, and outflow tracts. The presence of the color flow patterns facilitates identification of cardiac anatomy, particularly of those components that often are not amenable to ready recognition by 2D echocardiographic imaging. This method, however, has limitations for fetal application, some of which have been briefly discussed above. An additional problem may arise from the relatively high-velocity fetal cardiac wall movement, which results in color artifacts of "ghosting". This problem can be eliminated by increasing the high-pass filter, but this step also eliminates low-velocity flow components. The problem is compounded if the fetal position is such that the fetal heart is oriented perpendicular to the beam axis. In this situation, because of the high angle, Doppler frequency shifts are significantly attenuated. In contrast, the ventricular wall movement is in the beam axis, thus enhancing ghosting. Finally, color flow depiction in high-velocity flow areas such as the ductus arteriosus, aortic root, or pulmonary root frequently demonstrates velocity ambiguity or the Nyquist effect, so color directionality of the flow is depicted as reversed.

Spectral and Color Doppler M-Mode Echocardiography

The designation M-mode represents motion mode, or time-motion mode, as it displays unidimensional moving images of tissues and organs. A single line of ultrasound is transmitted, and the echoes returning from the tissue reflectors along the line of transmission are displayed in the intensity modulation mode. If the display is now swept across, the motion changes in the image are displayed or recorded as a function of time (Fig. 32.16, see color insert). It is customary to display and record M-mode images with the vertical axis representing the tissue depth from the transducer and the horizontal axis representing the time. Usually the former is marked at 1-cm intervals and the latter at 0.5-s intervals. Both spectral and color Doppler sonography can be used in conjunction with M-mode sonography. For fetal applications it is obvious that duplex mode sonography must be used so the M-mode cursor can be precisely aligned with the target. Such a combined approach can offer substantial benefit when identifying abnormal hemodynamics with high temporal accuracy. Maulik et al. [10] demonstrated the utility of using spectral pulsed-wave Doppler sonography with M-mode sonography when they reported fetal tricuspid regurgitation. With the Doppler color M-mode

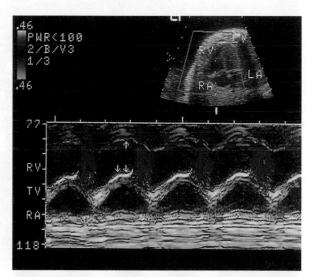

Fig. 32.16. Color M-mode echocardiogram of the fetal heart. *Top:* Color Doppler image of the apical four-chamber view with the M-line cursor passing through the right ventricle (*RV*) and right atrium (*RA*). *LV* left ventricle, *RV* right ventricle. *Bottom:* color M-mode tracing. The atrioventricular flow across the tricuspid orifice is depicted in *red*. Note the motion of the tricuspid valve. The *down arrows* show the valve leaflets prior to their opening at the beginning of the ventricular diastole. The *up arrow* indicates the moderator band movement

technique, multigated Doppler sampling is performed on a single scan line, which is sampled 1,000 times a second, and the unidimensional tissue and color flow images are scrolled (usually from right to left on the video screen) and therefore displayed as a function of time. Because of the high sampling rate from a single line, the color M-mode technique provides a high Doppler sonographic sensitivity and temporal resolution and allows reliable timing of the flow with the events of the cardiac cycle. For these reasons, color M-mode sonographic technique is useful for fetal echocardiographic examination.

Tissue Doppler Echocardiography

Tissue Doppler sonography comprises processing and analyzing Doppler frequency shift generated by tissue movement. The physical and technical principles of tissue Doppler imaging of the heart are similar to those of Doppler sonography of blood flow with the exception of the approach to filtering. Doppler insonation of the heart generates signals from cardiac blood flow and myocardial movement. However, the Doppler signals generated by blood flow are of substantially lower amplitude and higher frequency than those from myocardial movement. In depicting flow, the high-pass filter system eliminates the high-amplitude and low-frequency myocardial Doppler signals so that only flow signals are displayed. In contrast, tissue Doppler echocardiography utilizes filtering that eliminates the low-amplitude high-frequency flow signals permitting tissue Doppler signals being displayed (Fig. 32.17). There are three types of tissue Doppler: pulse-wave tissue Doppler mode, color flow tissue Doppler mode, and color tissue Doppler M-mode.

In the adult, tissue Doppler echocardiography has been used for assessing cardiac systolic and diastolic functions [20–22]. Such assessments can be performed by measuring myocardial velocity, myocardial velocity gradient, myocardial strain, and strain rate. Myocardial strain is its deformation during systole and diastole. Strain implies differential velocities in the cardiac wall and does not reflect overall movement of the heart including its translational motion within the thorax in relation to the other structures. Detailed reviews of these concepts may be found elsewhere [23].

More recently the feasibility of tissue Doppler sonography for fetal cardiac assessment has been reported. Harada and associates measured motion

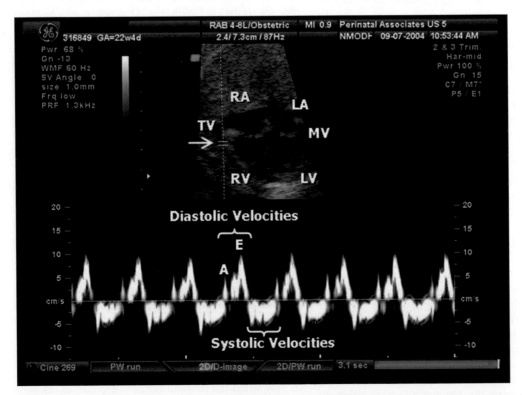

Fig. 32.17. Tissue Doppler velocity waveforms from the right ventricular wall below the parietal insertion of the tricuspid valve. The sampling site is indicated by the *horizontal arrow* pointing to the Doppler sample volume (*two horizontal lines*). The diastolic and systolic velocity waveforms are indicated on the *lower panel*. *A* indicates arterial systole and *E* indicates end diastole. *RA* right atrium, *LA* left atrium, *MV* mitral valve, *TV* tricuspid valve, *RV* right ventricle, *LV* left ventricle

velocities of the left ventricular posterior wall, right ventricular anterior wall, and interventricular septum along the longitudinal axis in normal fetuses aged 19–38 weeks' gestation and observed gestational age-specific increases in the peak myocardial velocities during early diastole and atrial contraction in the left and the right ventricular walls [24]. The authors speculated that such changes in tissue Doppler velocities may indicate maturational changes in the diastolic function. Tutschek and colleagues performed fetal tissue Doppler echocardiography with a high-resolution ultrasound system by changing the Doppler settings optimized for low-velocity motion assessment and observed increasing longitudinal contraction velocities of the fetal heart with the progression of gestation [25].

The limitations of the technique include angle dependency which may compromise the accuracy of measuring myocardial motion. Moreover, translational movements of the heart within the thorax will also generate Doppler shift. However, this effect can be reduced by restricting the velocity measurements within the cardiac wall rather than in relation to the transducer. Such assessments include determination of myocardial velocity gradient and myocardial strain rate imaging as briefly noted above.

Tissue Doppler echocardiography offers a potentially powerful tool for assessing fetal cardiac function in utero. Future studies will demonstrate to what extent this potential will be realized for both investigational and clinical use of this technique.

Doppler Depiction of Fetal Cardiac Circulation

Color flow mapping and directed pulsed-wave spectral Doppler sonography allow characterization of normal and abnormal fetal cardiac flow dynamics,

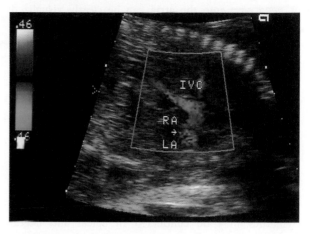

Fig. 32.18. Color Doppler flow mapping of the inferior vena caval (*IVC*) inflow into the right atrium (*RA*) and then to the left atrium (*LA*) through the foramen ovale (*arrow*)

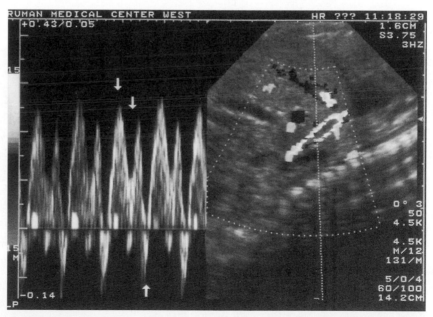

Fig. 32.19. Spectral Doppler interrogation of the inferior vena caval flow. *Right*: Color flow imaging of the inferior vena cava and placement of the Doppler sample volume. *Left*: Inferior vena caval Doppler waveforms. Note the triphasic waveform, two positive peaks (*down arrows*) and a negative peak (*up arrow*), reflecting the events of the cardiac cycle. The first positive peak coincides with ventricular systole and the second positive peak with ventricular diastole. The negative peak is associated with atrial systole

which may assist in the diagnosis of congenital cardiac disease. Doppler examination thus supplements 2D echocardiographic findings. The technique and Doppler flow characteristics of fetal cardiac hemodynamics are described below.

Atrial Flow

Doppler flow mapping of atrial circulatory dynamics using a color flow duplex system offers an impressive depiction of the atrial flow. The flow from the inferior vena cava into the atria can be clearly visualized (Fig. 32.18). Spectral Doppler waveforms from this vessel exhibit a triphasic flow pattern (Fig. 32.19). Doppler investigation of vena caval hemodynamics is presented in Chap. 27. The superior vena caval flow entering the right atrium can be visualized separately from the inferior vena caval return. These two inflows become confluent in the right atrial chamber. Regarding the left atrial inflow, the pulmonary veins can be investigated using color and spectral Doppler systems. The left pulmonary veins are more readily accessible. Doppler waveforms from the pulmonary veins reflect atrial and ventricular cycles (Fig. 32.20).

Spectral Doppler investigation of fetal atrial hemodynamics may be conducted in apical and lateral four-chamber and other views. Such interrogation demonstrates complex flow patterns (Fig. 32.21) consistent with multiple inflows in the atria, two outflows of the right atrium, and a single outflow of the left at-

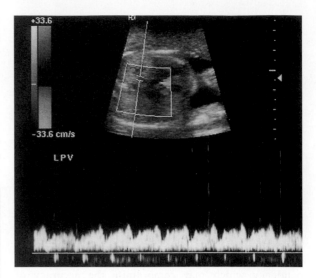

Fig. 32.20. Doppler interrogation of pulmonary venous return. *Top*: Lateral four-chamber view of the fetal heart, with the Doppler sample volume placed at the upper left pulmonary vein. *Bottom*: Pulmonary venous Doppler waveforms. The trough coincides with atrial systole

rium. A higher Doppler frequency shift is observed in the right atrium than in the left atrium. This description of the Doppler flow characteristics of the atria further elucidates the previously reported observations in previable human fetuses using acute radioangiographic studies [26] and in fetal sheep [27].

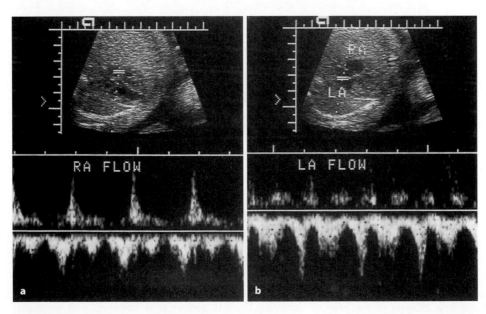

Fig. 32.21 a, b. Doppler waveforms from the atria. **a** *Top panel* shows interrogation of the right atrium. *Bottom panel* shows the complex pattern of the right atrial Doppler waves.

b *Top panel* shows the complex interrogation of the left atrium. *Bottom panel* shows the complex pattern of the left atrial Doppler waves. *RA* right atrium, *LA* left atrium

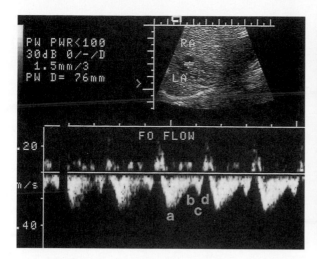

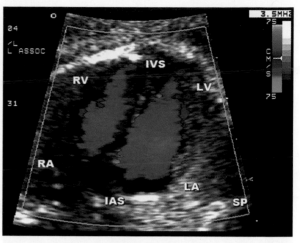

Fig. 32.22. Doppler insonation of the foramen ovale flow. *Top*: Placement of the Doppler sample volume at the foramen ovale. *RA* right atrium, *LA* left atrium. *Bottom*: Interatrial Doppler waves. *FO* foramen ovale, *a* ventricular peak systole, *b* ventricular end-systole, *c* atrial passive filling, *d* atrial systole

Fig. 32.23. Color Doppler echocardiogram of the mitral and tricuspid flow. The fetal heart is viewed in the apical (oblique) four-chamber plane. As flow is directed toward the transducer, it is coded in red. *RA* right ventricle, *LV* left venctricle, *IVS* interventricular septum, *RA* right atrium, *LA* left atrium, *IAS* interatrial septum, *SP* fetal spine

Interatrial Flow

The foramen ovale valve movement is associated with changes in the Doppler frequency shift in the left atrium; a higher frequency shift is observed when the valve is open than when it is closed [5]. Flow across the foramen ovale is optimally investigated with the lateral four-chamber view or a short-axis view, which allows angle-appropriate alignment of the Doppler cursor with flow direction across the foramen. Spectral Doppler investigation of the flow across the foramen shows a biphasic flow velocity pattern (Fig. 32.22). Ventricular systole is associated with a sharp rise in the frequency shift, reaching a peak coinciding with peak systole, following which the shift decelerates to a nadir at end-systole. With passive atrial filling the shift rises again, reaching a second peak that is lower than the first peak. This phase is followed by a rapid decline that coincides with atrial systole. These changes are influenced by the fetal behavioral state. The ventricular end-systolic and atrial passive filling phases demonstrate a significantly higher-frequency shift when the fetus actively sleeps (state 2F) than when it sleeps quietly (state 1F). It is reflective of flow redistribution and increased right-to-left shunt during active sleep.

Tricuspid and Mitral Flow

The color Doppler flow technique vividly portrays the flow patterns across the atrioventricular flow channels (Fig. 32.23). Color imaging may facilitate acquisition of the Doppler signals from the various areas of the atrioventricular flow jets.

Spectral Doppler insonation demonstrates a biphasic flow pattern across the tricuspid and mitral orifices, reflecting the contributions of ventricular relaxation and atrial contractions to the atrioventricular flow. The peak flow velocity due to contraction of the atrium (A wave) is significantly greater than the peak flow velocity caused by ventricular diastole (E wave) (Fig. 32.24 A). However, in the left heart, the A wave is less than, equal to, or only marginally greater than the E wave (Fig. 32.24 B). These findings suggest a physiologically lower compliance of the right ventricle than of the left ventricle and are similar to the pulsed-wave Doppler echocardiographic observations in neonates and infants.

Takahashi et al. [14] investigated mitral and tricuspid flows using pulsed-wave Doppler sonography in 23 fetuses of 30–38 weeks gestational age. They noted that the peak velocity across the mitral orifice was 52.1 ± 9.9 cm/s (mean $\pm$ SD) and that across the tricuspid orifice was 56.1 ± 8.7 cm/s. They also reported that the velocity patterns of the right ventricle and left ventricle inflow demonstrated two peaks consistent with the rapid filling phase and the atrial contraction phase, and the peak velocity of the atrial contraction phase was slightly greater than that of the rapid filling phase. Kenny et al. [28] investigated E and A waves comprehensively in 80 normal human fetuses at 19–40 weeks' gestation. They identified clearly defined E and A waves from the tricuspid orifice in 48% of the fetuses and from the mitral orifice in 60%. The ratio for both atrioventricular orifices increased during gestation.

These gestational age-related changes in the atrioventricular flow velocities were confirmed by Reed et

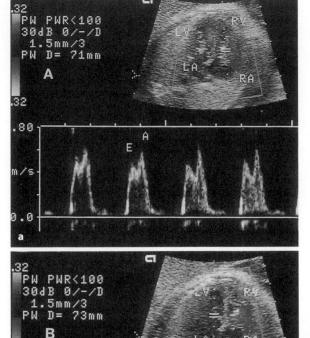

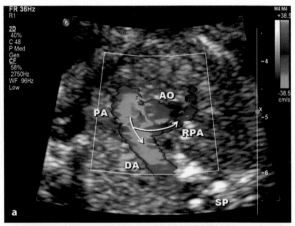

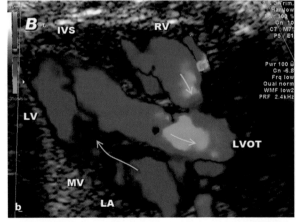

ing) and the A velocity (active ventricular filling during atrial contraction) increased progressively and significantly ($p < 0.01$) during pregnancy in both transmitral and transtricuspid waveforms, approaching 1.0 at term. These changes suggest progressive structural and functional maturation of the ventricles resulting in age-related increases in myocardial compliance. Romero et al. [30] studied the pressure-volume relation in fetal, neonatal, and adult hearts and demonstrated low compliance of the fetal heart. These changes may also be related to the known fetal hemodynamic changes with the progression of gestation, including the significant fall in fetoplacental vascular impedance [30].

Fig. 32.24 a, b. Doppler interrogation of the tricuspid and mitral flow. **a** *Top panel* presents the Doppler echocardiogram in the apical four-chamber plane. Note the location of the Doppler sample volume in the right ventricular chamber just distal to the tricuspid orifice. *Bottom panel* presents the biphasic tricuspid Doppler waveforms. *E* peak velocity related to forward flow during the ventricular diastole, *A* peak velocity related to forward flow during the atrial systole. **b** Doppler interrogation of the mitral flow. *Top panel* shows the Doppler echogram of the fetal heart in the apical four-chamber plane. Note the location of the Doppler sample volume in the left ventricular chamber just distal to the mitral orifice. *Bottom panel* presents the biphasic mitral Doppler waveforms. *E* peak velocity related to forward flow during the ventricular diastole, *A* peak velocity related to forward flow during atrial systole

al. [19] and Rizzo et al. [29]. The latter group prospectively studied 125 normally grown fetuses and 35 small-for-gestational-age (SGA) fetuses longitudinally at 27–42 weeks' gestation. In normal fetuses the ratio between the E velocity (early passive ventricular fill-

Fig. 32.25. a Right ventricular outflow tract is shown in the aortic short axis plane of the fetal heart. Note aliasing in the outflow tracts. **b** Left ventricular outflow is shown in the oblique long axis view of the fetal heart. The *lighter color* at the beginning of the aorta is indicative of higher velocity. The *arrows* depict flow direction. *AO* aorta, *IVS* interventricular septum, *DA* ductus arteriosus, *LV* left ventricle, *RV* right ventricle, *LVOT* left ventricular outflow tract, *MV* mitral valve, *PA* pulmonary artery, *RPA* right pulmonary artery, *SP* fetal spine

Pulmonary and Aortic Outflows

The right and left ventricular outflow can be imaged in the ventricular long-axis plane (Fig. 32.25). This plane allows clear assessment of the aortic-pulmonary cross-over relation (Fig. 32.26). Color flow imaging facilitates recognition of this important normal characteristic of the heart. The main pulmonary arterial flow can be conveniently seen in the parasternal short-axis plane at the base of the heart, which demonstrates the aortic cross section surrounded by the right atrium, right ventricle and pulmonary trunk, and right pulmonary

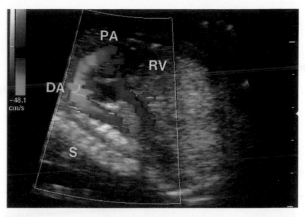

Fig. 32.28. Color Doppler echocardiogram of the ductal arch. Note the wider curve of the arch and color aliasing at the ductal level. *DA* ductus arteriosus, *PA* pulmonary artery, *RV* right ventricle, *S* fetal spine

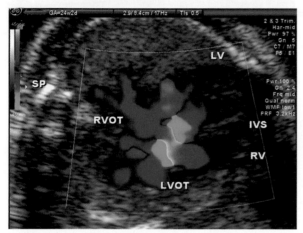

Fig. 32.26. Color Doppler imaging of the cross over relation between the origins of the great arteries. *SP* fetal spine, *LV* left ventricle, *RV* right ventricle, *IVS* interventricular septum, *RVOT* right ventricular outflow, *LVOT* left ventricular outflow

artery. The orientation of the main pulmonary artery in this plane often facilitates alignment of the Doppler beam along the pulmonary blood flow axis, ensuring an optimal angle of insonation. Aortic and pulmonary arterial hemodynamics can also be readily investigated in the aortic arch (Fig. 32.27) and ductal arch (Fig. 32.28) planes, respectively. Doppler frequency shift waveforms from the main pulmonary artery are characterized by rapidly accelerating and decelerating slopes, with sharp peaks during right ventricular systole (Fig. 32.29). In comparison with the maximal aortic velocity wave, however, the immediate postpeak deceleration slope is less acute in the pulmonary waveform. The peak velocity values from the pulmonary artery and the aorta, measured longitudinally in 27 normal pregnancies from 18 weeks to term, are presented in Table 32.4 (D. Maulik and P. Ciston, unpublished data).

In a longitudinal study, Rizzo et al. [31] showed significant increases in the pulmonic peak velocity ($p \leq 0.001$) and in the aortic peak velocity ($p \leq 0.05$) during early pregnancy between the end of the first trimester (11–13 weeks) and midgestation (20 weeks). Hata et al. [32] performed a cross-sectional investigation of 54 normal fetuses at 16–40 weeks of pregnancy and noted increases in transpulmonic peak velocity ($r = 0.39$, $p < 0.05$) and transaortic peak velocity ($r = 0.61$, $p < 0.001$) throughout the gestation. The transpulmonary peak velocity/transaortic peak velocity ratio was 1:1 in 45% of the instances. In contrast, Reed et al. [33], in a cross-sectional study of 87 fetuses at 17–41 weeks' gestation, did not note any changes in the peak aortic velocity with advancing gestational age ($p < 0.001$). Moreover, peak Doppler flow velocities were greater in the aorta than in the pulmonary artery ($p < 0.001$).

Imaging by Doppler color flow mapping in the main pulmonary artery produces a graphic depiction

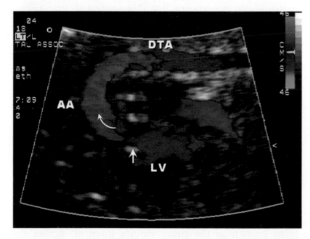

Fig. 32.27. Color Doppler echocardiogram of the aortic arch. Note the tighter curve of the arch and the change in the color depiction of flow, reflecting the changes in the flow direction in relation to the transducer. The *curved arrow* indicates flow direction at the root of the aorta. *Vertical arrow* indicates root of aorta. *AA* aortic arch, *LV* left ventricle, *DTA* descending thoracic aorta

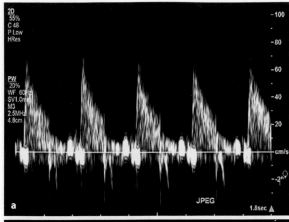

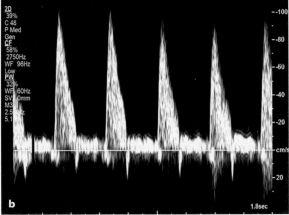

Fig. 32.29. Spectral Doppler waveforms from the pulmonary artery (**a**) and aorta (**b**). Both waves show rapid accelerations. The deceleration slope of the pulmonary artery, however, is slightly less step than that of the aorta

Table 32.4. Peak velocity in fetal pulmonary artery and aorta

Site	Peak velocity (cm/s) at three gestational ages (mean ± SD)		
	18–23 weeks	24–31 weeks	32–40 weeks
Pulmonary artery	51±7	59±9	61±11
Aorta	55±10	63±12	73±11

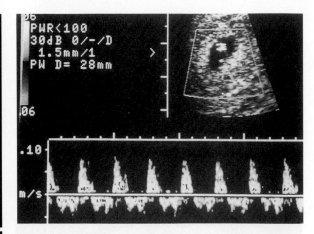

Fig. 32.30. Doppler depiction of the fetal cardiac circulation during the early first trimester. *Top*: Embryo and flow of the primitive heart. *Bottom*: Simultaneous interrogation of the atrioventricular flow and ventricular outflow

Doppler Echocardiography During Early Pregnancy

Although it has been customary to initiate fetal echocardiography at 16–20 weeks' gestation, advances in imaging resolution and color Doppler sonography and the introduction of transvaginal sonography have made it possible to image cardiac hemodynamics in the embryonic heart during the first trimester. These developments have raised the possibility of early echocardiographic diagnosis in certain cases of congenital heart disease. Figure 32.30 shows the spectral Doppler interrogation of the embryonic heart and the atrioventricular and great arterial Doppler waveform. Preliminary experience has demonstrated that transvaginal echocardiography is feasible [34]. This approach may prove useful in the future.

Determination of Fetal Cardiac Output

The theoretic basis, technical implementation, and limitations of Doppler sonographic flow quantification are discussed in Chap. 4. The methodology for fetal cardiac output measurement was first described by Maulik et al. [5]. Briefly, the stroke volume is determined by integrating the temporal average velocity (also known as the time-velocity integral) across the valvular orifice or vascular lumen with the cross-sectional area of the vascular tract. The cardiac output is obtained by multiplying the stroke volume by the fetal heart rate. The combined cardiac output is the sum of the right and left cardiac outputs. The various measures of the fetal cardiac output are presented in

of the pulmonic flow entering the descending thoracic aorta via the ductus arteriosus (Fig. 32.15). With color Doppler imaging the flow in the ductus arteriosus often appears to be of higher intensity because of the greater velocity of ductal flow. In our experience, color Doppler sonography assists in quickly identifying the ductus and confidently aligning the Doppler beam along the direction of pulmonary flow.

Table 32.5. Measures of fetal cardiac output

Stroke volume (ml) = temporal mean velocity (cm/s) × cross-sectional area (cm^2)

Cardiac or ventricular output (ml/min) = stroke volume (ml) × fetal heart rate (bpm)

Left cardiac output = cardiac output measured at the aortic or mitral orifice

Right cardiac output = cardiac output measured at the pulmonic or tricuspid orifice

Combined cardiac output (ml/min) = sum of the right and left cardiac outputs

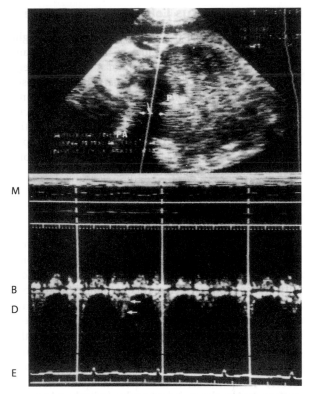

Fig. 32.31. Doppler characterization of pulmonary artery (PA) flow and measurement of right ventricular stroke volume in a normal fetus. *Top:* Doppler sample volume, indicated by a short transverse bar (*oblique arrow*), was placed along an M-line cursor in the midlumen of the PA imaged by two-dimensional echocardiography. Maximal inner PA diameter (*d*) (*horizontal arrows*) at the level of the Doppler sample volume measured 0.9 cm. The cross-sectional area at this level was calculated as 0.636 cm^2 (3.14 d^2/4). *PV* pulmonary valve. *Bottom:* Doppler frequency shifts (*D*) obtained from the PA. Deflection above the baseline (*B*) represents flow toward the transducer and that below the baseline denotes flow away from the transducer. As would be expected, the predominant flow is directed away from the transducer toward the distal PA and is characterized by sharp peaks with rapidly accelerating and decelerating slopes. The maximal area under the flow curve for one cardiac cycle was measured in kilohertz-seconds (vertical distance between the two horizontal arrows = 0.5 kHz) and was converted to the maximum velocity curve area (s-cm/s) (*A*) using the instrument calibration factor K = 25.667 cm/s-kHz. Multiplying *A* by the PA cross-sectional area gave a stroke volume of 3.76 ml. Cardiac output was then calculated by multiplying the stroke volume by the fetal heart rate. The *vertical lines* represent 1-s time markers. *M* M-mode tracing, *E* maternal electrocardiogram

Table 32.5. In the fetus the right and the left sides of the heart work in parallel. Therefore fetal cardiac output must be determined separately for each side. The measurements may be performed either at the root of the great vessels [5, 29, 35, 36] or across the atrioventricular orifices [31, 38]. The right heart output may be measured either across the tricuspid orifice or at the root of the main pulmonary artery just distal to the pulmonary semilunar valves (Fig. 32.31). Similarly, the left cardiac output may be measured across the mitral orifice or at the root of the aorta immediately distal to the aortic semilunar valves. The precision of the technique in terms of reproducibility depends on the site of measurement, the parameters measured, the imagability of the patient in a given instance, and operator skill. In our experience, the roots of the great vessels provide a more reliable measure than the atrioventricular channels. Groenenberg et al. [38] investigated this question and noted high reproducibility of peak systolic velocity and average velocity measured in the ductus arteriosus, pulmonary artery, and ascending aorta. The coefficients of variation between tests within individual patients were less than or equal to 7%.

Cardiac Output: Normative Data

Maulik et al. [5], in a preliminary report, noted a right ventricular output range of 148 ml/min in a 28-week fetus to 451 ml/min in a near-term fetus. Reed et al. [37] observed a tricuspid flow rate of 307 ± 30 ml·kg^{-1}·min^{-1} and a mitral flow rate of 232 ± 25 ml·kg^{-1}·min^{-1} in fetuses of 26–30 weeks gestational age. In a comprehensive longitudinal study, De Smedt and coworkers [39] performed echocardiographic examinations on 28 normal fetuses at 4-week intervals from 15–18 weeks to term. The fetal cardiac output was measured from the tricuspid and mitral orifices. They observed that with advancing gestation the mean temporal blood flow velocities increased linearly, whereas the area of blood flow and calculated right and left ventricular output increased exponentially. The combined ventricular output at term was noted to be 1,735 ml/min and 553 ± 153 ml·kg^{-1}·min^{-1} when corrected for sonographically estimated fetal weight.

Chapter 33

Doppler Echocardiography for Managing Congenital Cardiac Disease

Dev Maulik

Introduction

Fetal cardiac development is regulated by various genetic and environmental influences. Aberrations in these developmental mechanisms result in structural and functional abnormalities of the fetal heart. There has been a greater recognition of the need for antepartum diagnosis of these disorders in recent years. Perinatal diagnosis and management of congenital cardiac disease in conjunction with advances in pediatric cardiac surgery has led to remarkable improvements in the outcome in these infants. An essential component of this approach is the reliable prenatal diagnosis, which permits planning and implementation of appropriate perinatal management. Although high-resolution two-dimensional (2D) dynamic imaging remains the foundation of fetal echocardiographic assessment, the Doppler modality constitutes an essential component of this process by providing hemodynamic insight into the morphologic and functional aberrations of the fetal heart. With the advent of real-time three-dimensional (3D) echocardiography, there are exciting possibilities for prenatal cardiac assessment including Doppler echocardiography.

In the previous chapter, we reviewed the scope and technique of Doppler echocardiography and normative information on fetal cardiac hemodynamics, while the next chapter, which is a new addition to this edition, deals with real-time 3D echocardiography of the human fetus. In this chapter, we review the risk factors for congenital cardiac disease, the common indications for fetal cardiac evaluation, and the application of Doppler echocardiography in managing malformations and dysrhythmias of the fetal heart.

Risk Factors and Indications for Fetal Cardiac Evaluation

Congenital cardiac disease, as diagnosed clinically, has a prevalence of approximately 8 cases per 1,000 live births [1]. The rate of critical cardiac malformations requiring early therapeutic and surgical intervention has been reported to be 3.5 per 1,000 live births [2]. The risk of cardiac malformations is increased in many conditions (Table 33.1). When these risk factors are present, prenatal counseling and diag-

Table 33.1. Risk factors for congenital heart disease

Familial
History of congenital cardiac disease
Genetic syndromes (Mendelian)
  Noonan
  Tuberosus sclerosis
  Marfan
  Holt-Oran
  TAR (thrombocytopenia with absent radii)

Maternal
Congenital heart disease
Teratogenic exposure
  Anticonvulsants – phenytoin, trimethadione, valproic acid
  Lithium
  Amphetamines
  Retinoic acid
  Alcohol
Nonteratogenic exposure
  Indomethacin
Maternal infection
  Viral – rubella, cytomegalovirus, coxsackievirus, mumps
  Parasitic – toxoplasmosis
Metabolic disease
  Diabetes mellitus
  Phenylketonuria
Autoimmune disease
Obstetrical
  Polyhydramnios

Fetal
Suspicion of cardiac malformation in basic fetal scan
Abnormal fetal cardiac rhythm
Extracardiac malformation
Increased nuchal translucency
Chromosomal disorders
  Down's syndrome
  Trisomy 13, 18
  Turner's syndrome
Genetic syndromes
Fetal growth restriction
Nonimmune hydrops
Situs inversus and ambiguous

Table 33.2. Approximate risk of cardiac anomalies for selected high risk conditions

Anomaly	Risk (%)
Isolated cardiac anomalies (multifactorial)	
Overall	3–5
Mother	10
Father	3–5
Sibling	3
Left heart anomalies	10–15
Environmental	
Maternal rubella infection	35
Pregestational diabetes	3–5
Phenylketonuria (phenylalanine > 16 mg/dl)	18
Alcohol consumption	25–30
Trimethadone	15–30
Retinoic acid	4
Genetic	
Overall	25
Marfan syndrome	60–80
Holt-Oram syndrome	100
Chromosomal	
Overall	25
Trisomy 21	50
Trisomy 18	100

Data are derived from the literature.

Table 33.3. Indications for fetal echocardiographic assessment

- Non-reassuring fetal cardiac image during obstetrical sonography
- Extracardiac malformations
- Fetal cardiac arrhythmia
- Increased nuchal translucency
- Insulin-dependent diabetes mellitus in pregnancy
- History of congenital cardiac disease
- Teratogenic exposure
- Maternal viral infection
- Nonimmune hydrops
- Nonlethal aneuploidy

Benefits of Fetal Echocardiographic Assessment

Fetal echocardiographic examination allows prenatal diagnosis of congenital heart disease so that appropriate perinatal management can be planned and implemented. An accurate diagnosis of the cardiac lesion will obviously lead to more reliable prognostication and informed management choices. The process involves participation by a multidisciplinary perinatal cardiology team which should include primary obstetricians, maternal-fetal medicine specialists, neonatologists, pediatric cardiologists, cardiac surgeons, and other relevant support personnel. In addition, the parents must be an integral part of this process so that they are appropriately counseled regarding the fetal condition and prognosis, and are able to participate in the decision-making process. In early gestation, severe cardiac anomalies with poor prognosis may prompt the parents to opt for a termination of pregnancy. If this is not an option, a multidisciplinary medical team can develop optimal plans for surveillance, delivery, and perinatal intervention. Table 33.4 summarizes the prognostic factors for survival. Depending on the complexity of the fetal cardiac problem, the site for delivery and neonatal management can be carefully selected. This is particularly important as not all medical centers may have adequate medical or surgical resources to deal effectively with the complexities of congenital heart disease. In this context, one should also note that recent progress in surgical management of certain malformations has improved the chances of survival in cases previously considered hopeless [7]. The reported mortality rate following pediatric cardiac surgery in one of the prominent centers is given in Table 33.5. As noted during the 32nd Bethesda Conference, "Care Of The Adult With Congenital Heart Disease", the survival rate has continued to improve over the last few decades and the estimated cumulative survivors of con-

nostic procedures should be offered to the mother. Recently, increased nuchal translucency at 10–14 weeks of gestation in chromosomally normal fetuses has emerged as an indication because of its association with cardiac malformations. The extent of this association varies between 7% and 9% [3, 4]. Controversy, however, exists on whether polymorphisms of 5,10-methylenetetrahydrofolate reductase (MTHFR) lead to a higher risk of congenital cardiac defect [5, 6], and it therefore remains uncertain whether this abnormality should indicate fetal cardiac evaluation. Although a precise measure of the increased risk is not available for all the conditions listed in Table 33.1, a summary of risk quantification for selected conditions is presented in Table 33.2. Such information should be an essential part of informed counseling of patients. More detailed information may be obtained from the standard texts on pediatric cardiology. Fetal echocardiography is indicated whenever a higher probability of fetal cardiac malformation exists. It is also indicated for the precise diagnosis and follow-up of fetal cardiac arrhythmias and fetal heart failure. Furthermore, a suspicious fetal cardiac image during general obstetrical ultrasonography mandates more focused assessment. In many centers, a non-reassuring fetal cardiac image is the most common reason for echocardiographic referral. Frequency of these indications varies from center to center. Common indications for fetal echocardiography are listed in Table 33.3.

Table 33.4. Survival after surgery in the presence of congenital heart disease: Boston Children's Hospital

Anomaly	Time of surgery	Early mortality %	Late mortality %
AV canal defect	1976–1987	2.9	
Ventricular septal defect	1984–1990	0	0
Fallot's tetralogy	1985–1990	2.5	0
Ebstein's anomaly	1982–1990	17.0	11
Left heart hypoplasia syndrome	1984–1985	24.0	17
D-Transposition of great vessels	1989–1992	0.5	0
Truncus arteriosus	1987–1991	18.0	

Compiled from [3].

Table 33.5. Prognostic factors for congenital heart disease

- Type and severity of the malformation
- Presence of cardiac failure
- Abnormal cardiac rhythm
- Extracardiac malformations
- Chromosomal abnormalities
- Fetal growth restriction
- Level of expertise

Table 33.6. Advantages and disadvantages of spectral and color Doppler echocardiography

Advantages
  Corroborates anatomic diagnosis
  Defines normal and abnormal cardiac hemodynamics
  Provides functional definition of a cardiac lesion
  Elucidates complex malformations
  Potentially reduces imaging time

Disadvantages
  More expensive instrumentation although increasingly less expensive
  Requires personnel with advanced skills

genital heart disease to the year 2000 in the United States approached almost 800,000 [8]. An additional emerging benefit of prenatal diagnosis of congenital heart disease may be the potential for in utero intervention for congenital structural cardiac disease, which has been investigated in animal models [9, 10]. Preliminary anecdotal accounts of human fetal cardiac interventions have been reported in the medical press [11]. Although they are still experimental approaches at present, future advances may transform these approaches into clinical realities. Obviously fetal echocardiography including Doppler sonography will continue to play a critical role in any such development. This is further discussed below.

Utility of Fetal Doppler Echocardiographic Assessment

The importance of Doppler echocardiography lies in the fact that it allows noninvasive assessment of cardiovascular hemodynamic function. Both modalities of Doppler ultrasound offer significant advantages in supplementing the diagnostic information obtained from the 2D echocardiography. However, the operators should be appropriately trained to use the device optimally. The advantages and disadvantages of Doppler echocardiography are summarized in Table 33.6.

Spectral Doppler insonation, used in conjunction with the other ultrasound modalities, allows the measurement of peak or mean velocity, which may be utilized to define the normal and the abnormal blood flow characteristics. Almost two decades ago, the diagnostic potential of duplex spectral pulsed Doppler and color Doppler echocardiography was demonstrated in recognizing fetal cardiac abnormalities such as pulmonary arterial aneurysm and tricuspid regurgitation [12, 13]. As reviewed in this chapter, numerous extensive investigations subsequently confirmed the utility of these approaches. Chiba and associates [14] noted the usefulness of color flow mapping for identifying congenital cardiac malformations in 107 high-risk mothers, about a third of whom had cardiac disease. Fetal cardiac malformations were present in 19 cases and included complex disorders. Copel and associates [15] used color Doppler in 45 of 48 fetuses with cardiac anomalies and noted that color flow mapping was essential for making correct anatomical diagnoses in almost a third of the cases. Over time, the technique has proved useful in defining structural, functional, and hemodynamic anomalies of the fetal heart. Color Doppler facilitates the recognition of anomalies, especially when they are not clearly defined in 2D imaging, and may reduce the examination time. Furthermore, spectral and color Doppler modes are essential for identifying abnormal flow patterns associated with valvular incompetence or stenotic lesions of the vascular channels.

In Utero Evolution of Cardiac Malformations

Experience with fetal echocardiographic examination over the years has revealed the dynamics of in utero evolution of fetal cardiac disease [16]. In addition to the structural defects, functional changes in the fetal heart can also be observed secondary to various disorders including viral infection and rhythm disturbances. Allan and associates were one of the first groups [17] to report in utero worsening of cardiac anomalies; they observed discrete coarctation with a normal aortic arch noted first at 21 weeks deteriorating to a markedly hypoplastic aortic arch by 34 weeks. Subsequently, a multiplicity of reports appeared. These include (a) development or progression of pulmonary stenosis in the fetus with advancing gestation [18–21]; (b) development of dilated cardiomyopathy later in pregnancy when no abnormalities were observed at 20 weeks [22]; (c) development of left heart hypoplasia syndrome despite normal echocardiographic scan in early pregnancy [23–25]; (d) intrauterine closure of foramen ovale [26]; and (e) development of right ventricular hypoplasia [27]. In contrast to deterioration, there are infrequent reports of improvement of cardiac lesions in utero; these include: (a) improvement of left heart hypoplasia because of progressive growth of the left heart during gestation [21]; and (b) in utero closure of ventricular septal defect [28]. There are important practical implications of these observations. It is apparent that cardiac assessment performed at midpregnancy may not ensure the absence of cardiac malformation later in pregnancy or at birth. In a pregnancy at a higher risk of cardiac malformation, it may be prudent to repeat the examination at mid third trimester. However, the cost-effectiveness of a policy of cardiac scanning twice during pregnancy in all cases referred for fetal echocardiographic assessment remains undetermined.

Doppler Characterization of Congenital Cardiac Malformations

Doppler echocardiographic examination constitutes a component of the overall assessment of the fetal heart. This integrated approach is described in Chap. 32. Doppler ultrasonography provides a range of hemodynamic information (see Chap. 4) that should be interpreted in terms of normal and abnormal cardiac function and anatomy. An understanding of the morphologic correlates of abnormal cardiac Doppler flow patterns is helpful for diagnosing congenital heart disease. These correlates are discussed below and summarized in Table 33.7.

1. *Absence of flow in expected locations.* As discussed in Chap. 4, some of the primary hemodynamic information offered by Doppler insonation regards the presence or absence of flow. The reliability of this function depends on the instrumental characteristics and setting and on the circumstances of the examination. For example, the transducer frequency, gain setting, and angle of insonation affect the ability of the operator to identify and reliably conclude that there is or is not flow. Thus one may spuriously fail to note flow even when it exists because of an unfavorable angle or low gain. Similarly, low-flow states may not

Table 33.7. Anatomic correlates of Doppler hemodynamic information

Hemodynamic information	Anatomic correlates
Presence of normal flow in expected location	Corroborative of normal anatomic image
Presence of flow in an unexpected location	Anatomic lesions: septal defects, aneurysms
Absence of flow in an expected location	Nonfunctioning chamber; hypoplasia; severe vascular stenosis
Abnormally high-velocity flow	Stenotic lesion, functional constriction
Abnormal flow direction	Regurgitant flow – valvular incompetence; redirected flow in vascular lesion

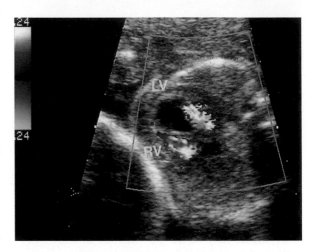

Fig. 33.1. Doppler color flow mapping of left ventricular dilation preceding hypoplastic change. *LV* left ventricle, *RV* right ventricle. Color Doppler shows flow in RV extending to the ventricular apex. In contrast, flow could not be demonstrated in most of the LV chamber, which shows marked dilation and poor contractility. This condition developed into left ventricular hypoplasia

be identified unless the device is optimized for such function. Assuming that these factors have been taken into consideration, color and spectral Doppler demonstration of the absence of flow in an expected location is helpful for diagnosing an existing or evolving cardiac problem. The most remarkable example is the absence of flow in one of the ventricles, which in conjunction with the observation (by 2D imaging) of the absence of an echo-lucent space in the ventricle is diagnostic of left or right ventricular hypoplasia (see below). We have also seen examples of progressive ventricular developmental failure starting as a dilated ventricular chamber with no discernible flow culminating in left ventricular hypoplasia (Fig. 33.1). There are other instances where Doppler depiction of the absence of flow is suggestive of structural anomalies

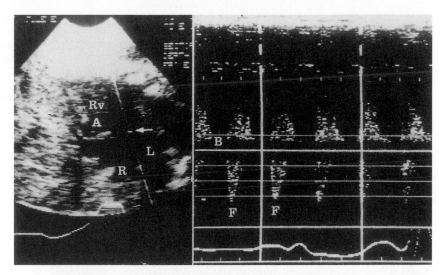

Fig. 33.2. Fetal Doppler echocardiographic examination of tetralogy of Fallot and aneurysmal dilatation of the main pulmonary artery. The large echo-free space present on the left of the aorta on real-time two-dimensional examination (*left*) was demonstrated by pulsed Doppler to be vascular in nature, as pulsatile flow similar to that obtained in the pulmonary artery could be demonstrated within it (*right*). This Doppler finding helped to make a confident diagnosis of aneruysmal dilatation of the main pulmonary artery. *Arrow* indicates the location of the Doppler sample volume. *A* aorta, *B* Doppler baseline, *F* Doppler waveforms, *L* left branch of the pulmonary artery, *RV* right ventricle. (Reprinted from [12] with permission)

of the heart. Thus the diagnosis of tricuspid atresia may be facilitated by color Doppler insonation demonstrating no recognizable flow across the tricuspid orifice [13].

2. *Presence of flow in unexpected locations.* Visualizing flow in an expected or an unexpected vascular location may significantly enhance our ability to identify and define congenital cardiac lesions. Identifying the presence of flow in an expected location may be helpful for establishing structural integrity when the imaging appearance is uncertain. The color or spectral Doppler recognition of flow in an unexpected location may, on the other hand, assist in diagnosing a malformation. For example, the demonstration of spectral Doppler flow patterns in a large echo-lucent area adjacent to the aorta helped us to make the prenatal diagnosis of pulmonary arterial aneurysm [2] (Fig. 33.2). Similarly, demonstration of a flow jet across the interventricular septum indicates a septal defect. It should be noted, however, that large defects may be recognizable by imaging alone without the added benefit of color Doppler flow depiction, whereas small defects may not be recognizable even by color flow mapping unless there is a demonstrable flow jet through the septal defect. As the right and left ventricular intracavitary pressures are approximately equal in the fetus, there is no flow across the defect unless there are additional malformations, such as outflow tract stenosis altering the interventricular pressure equilibrium. The presence of a flow jet across a ventricular septal defect (VSD) therefore should alert the observer about the existence of ad-

ditional cardiac lesions. Although atrial septal defects (ASDs) are more difficult to recognize in the fetus, large defects are easily identifiable by the clear demonstration of confluence of flow between the two atria without a visible intervening septal structure (see below).

3. *Abnormal flow direction.* Spectral Doppler depiction of directionality of flow offers a unique opportunity to detect abnormal cardiac hemodynamics. Demonstration of aberrant flow patterns, such as regurgitant flow across a valvular orifice or abnormal flow direction in a vessel, significantly enhances our ability to define fetal cardiac lesions (Fig. 33.3). Atrioventricular regurgitant flow has been identified using spectral and color Doppler [2, 7, 27]. Isolated semilunar valve incompetence of the pulmonary trunk or the aorta is rare and is often difficult to detect, even when present in association with other cardiac anomalies.

Doppler echocardiography can significantly assist in assessing the severity of valvular incompetence. Several approaches have been described in relation to pediatric and adult echocardiographic applications. They include assessment of: (1) the duration of the regurgitant flow in relation to the cardiac cycle; (2) the magnitude of the length of the regurgitant jet into the atrial cavity as measured by pulsed-wave Doppler interrogation; and (3) measurement of the regurgitant jet as a proportion of the area of the atrial cavity.

If the regurgitant flow is minimal and occupies only a fraction of the total duration of the cardiac cycle, it may be considered relatively benign in the absence of associated cardiac anomalies. Pansystolic

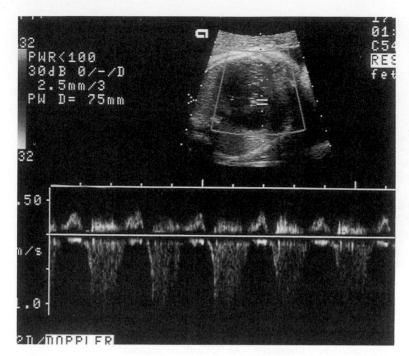

Fig. 33.3. Spectral Doppler depiction of severe tricuspid regurgitation in a case of Ebstein's anomaly. *Top*: Doppler echocardiogram shows placement of the Doppler sample volume in the regurgitant jet in the dilated right atrial chamber immediately proximal to the tricuspid valve. *Bottom:* Spectral Doppler waveforms showing regurgitant jet projecting downward from the baseline

leakage, on the other hand, signifies severe incompetence. The length of jet backflowing into the atrial cavity has been used as an indicator of the severity of the atrioventricular valvular incompetence. This technique, however, is not reliable, as the pulsed-wave Doppler interrogation may not fully recognize the direction and extent of the regurgitant flow jet in the atrial chamber. Color Doppler flow mapping of the jet area in relation to the atrial area has been shown to correspond well to angiographic grading in adults with cardiac lesions [29, 30].

There is a paucity of reports on the utilization of these techniques in the fetus. Gembruch and colleagues [31] reported on the prenatal diagnosis of 14 cases of atrioventricular (A-V) canal malformation (A-V septal defect) utilizing 2D imaging and color and spectral Doppler sonography. In nine fetuses the A-V regurgitant jet area was compared with the atrial area using planimetry. Hydropic fetuses exhibited a proportionately larger jet area and pansystolic insufficiency. Analysis of the regurgitant jet has also been used to assess ventricular function for fetal prognostication. Tulzer and associates [32] investigated right ventricular function in 20 fetuses with pansystolic tricuspid regurgitation associated with either indomethacin-induced ductal constriction (10 cases) or nonimmune hydrops fetalis (10 cases). They determined right ventricular pressure rise over time (dP/dt) from spectral Doppler tracing of the regurgitation jet (Fig. 33.4). Color Doppler-directed continuous-wave Doppler sonography was used. The right ventricular shortening fraction (RVSF), determined by

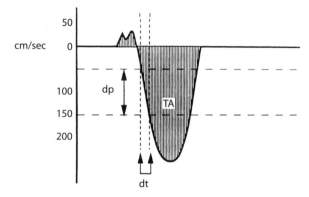

Fig. 33.4. From a tricuspid regurgitation Doppler tracing (*TR*). The time interval (*dt*) is measured on the TR upstroke between 50 cm/s (correlating to a 1 mmHg gradient between the right ventricle and right atrium) and 150 cm/s (correlating to a 9 mmHg gradient). *dp* pressure. (Reprinted from [32]. with permission)

M-mode echocardiography, did not correlate with the dP/dt. It was observed that right ventricular dP/dt values were consistently lower in the nonimmune hydrops group (Fig. 33.5). Similarly RVSF values were lower in the nonimmune hydrops group. All fetuses with indomethacin-induced ductal constriction recovered completely within 48 h of medication cessation and survived. In contrast, three fetuses with nonimmune hydrops who died had a significantly higher right ventricular dP/dt than those who survived (275 ± 140 versus 718 ± 151 mmHg/s; $p < 0.01$). This study demonstrated the potential utility of echocar-

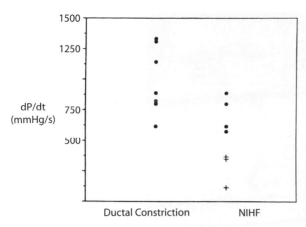

Fig. 33.5. Doppler-derived right ventricular dP/dt in fetuses with ductal constriction compared to fetuses with nonimmune hydrops (*NIHF*). *Filled circles* survivors, *crosses* nonsurvivors. (Reprinted from [32] with permission)

diographic assessment of the fetal cardiac function as a tool of prognostication.

Demonstration of abnormal direction of blood flow in the central vascular channels may assist in defining complex cardiac lesions. For example, the presence of reverse flow in the ductus arteriosus in cases where the pulmonary outflow is difficult to image is diagnostic of pulmonary atresia. Chiba and associates [14] reported the utility of color flow mapping, including the depiction of abnormal flow directionality for identifying intricate malformations.

4. *High velocity and turbulent flow.* Abnormal magnitude of flow velocity is pathognomonic of cardiac pathology. As a general principle, flow velocity is increased in the alternative flow paths as they accommodate the flow diverted from hypoplastic chambers and atretic flow channels. Thus with tricuspid atresia flow velocity is increased in the mitral orifice and the aorta. In contrast, flow velocities across the atretic channels and in the hypoplastic chambers are absent or decreased (during the initial phase of the lesion). With fetal congenital heart block, the aortic and pulmonic flow velocity and flow are significantly increased. Stenotic lesions present a different problem. If there are no alternative circulatory paths, inflow in a vascular system equals outflow.

Doppler Echocardiographic Assessment of Specific Cardiac Anomalies

Color flow and spectral Doppler modes can substantially assist 2D echocardiography in defining various congenital cardiac malformations. This section pre-

sents the Doppler characterization of anomalous hemodynamic patterns for commonly encountered congenital heart diseases in the fetus. The categorization used here is imperfect and somewhat arbitrary, as many of these conditions are characterized by multiple lesions. Furthermore, this review is brief, as a comprehensive discussion of these conditions is beyond the scope of this chapter.

Cardiac Position

Anomalies of the cardiac position are rare. Fetal cardiac malposition may be intrathoracic or extrathoracic. Intrathoracic malposition may result from (1) secondary displacement of the heart due to a thoracic mass or fluid collection, which may lead to pseudo-dextrocardia; or (2) visceral malrotation resulting in dextrocardia. Extrathoracic malposition results from defective development of the anterior thoracic wall or the diaphragm causing ectopia cordis. Although these conditions are recognized by 2D echocardiography, color and spectral Doppler modes assist in defining altered vascular connections and associated cardiac malformations.

Intrathoracic Cardiac Displacement

The most common malposition of the heart is probably related to a mediastinal shift caused by a space-occupying intrathoracic lesion such as a left diaphragmatic hernia (Fig. 33.6). With this condition, although the heart is displaced to the right hemithorax, the cardiac apex remains oriented to the left. The diagnosis is established by sonographic demonstra-

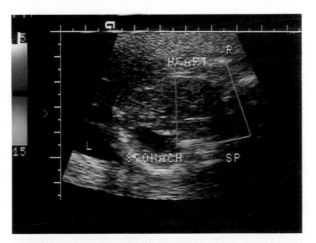

Fig. 33.6. Color Doppler depiction of pseudo dextrocardia secondary to left diaphragmatic hernia. *SP* fetal spine, *L* left, *R* right. The fetal heart is located on the right side of the thorax; its normal position on the left is occupied by the stomach. Note that despite the left displacement the cardiac apex remains directed to the left

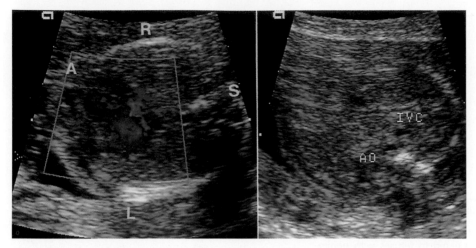

Fig. 33.7. Color Doppler imaging of dextrocardia. *Left:* Intrathoracic displacement of the fetal heart to the right with the cardiac apex directed to the right. The fetal heart exhibited ventricular inversion, left ventricular hypoplasia, and transposition of the great arteries. *Right:* The situs was solitus as indicated by the normal orientation of the inferior vena cava (*IVC*), aorta (*AO*), and other viscera

tion of the primary thoracic abnormality, cardiac displacement and levo-orientation, and normal visceral situs. Dextrocardia is a rare anomaly (Fig. 33.7). A detailed discussion of the features is not relevant here. The condition is diagnosed by echocardiographic examination demonstrating the presence of the heart on the right side of the fetal thorax. The direction of the cardiac apex in dextrocardia is toward the right. The condition should be distinguished from the situation in which the heart is displaced to the right because of a diaphragmatic hernia, left pleural effusion, or a mediastinal mass. Although 2D imaging is sufficient for recognizing the malposition, color and spectral Doppler echocardiography may assist in defining abnormalities of ventricular organization or ventriculoarterial connection, which are commonly encountered with dextrocardia [33]. The most common abnormal connection is the complete and corrected transposition of the great arteries. In addition, abnormalities of visceral situs are seen, including situs inversus, incomplete visceral lateralization, and atrial isomerism syndromes.

Extrathoracic Cardiac Displacement

Ectopia cordis may be thoracic, abdominal, or cervical; the thoracic type is encountered most frequently. The characteristics include cephalad orientation of the cardiac apex, a sternal defect, varying degrees of deficiency of the pericardium, diminished intrathoracic space, and omphalocele [34]. Intracardiac anomalies are frequent, as are associated anomalies that involve the central nervous system, skeletal system, and ventral wall. Although the condition can be

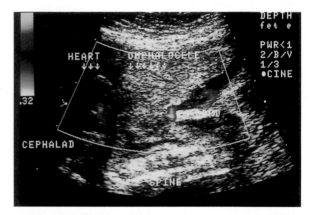

Fig. 33.8. Ectopia cordis with omphalocele. Note the hypoechogenicity of the fetal heart

identified by 2D sonographic imaging, detailed identification of the intracardiac anatomy may be difficult because of poor echogenicity of the cardiac structures, and color Doppler may be of significant assistance. An example of ectopia cordis is shown in Fig. 33.8. The image also demonstrated the presence of an anterior abdominal wall defect associated with an omphalocele. Defining cardiac structural integrity was difficult with 2D echocardiographic examination; Doppler color flow images, however, suggested a univentricular chamber, which was confirmed at autopsy after pregnancy termination.

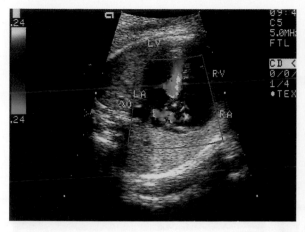

Fig. 33.9. Color Doppler depiction of an ostium secundum atrial septal defect. It is noteworthy that the condition may not be distinguishable from physiologic flow through the foramen ovale

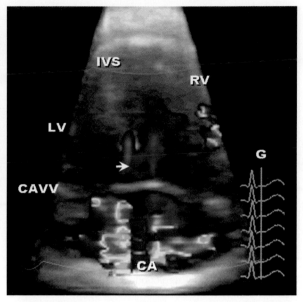

Fig. 33.10. Color flow depiction of atrioventricular septal defect. The image is a two-dimensional frame from a real-time three-dimensional duplex color flow image. Note the flow across the ventricular septal defect (*horizontal arrow*). The interatrial septum is absent and the flow in the common atrial cavity is turbulent. External simulated fetal heart rate gating (*G*) was used to combine the sub-volumes. *RV* right ventricle, *LV* left ventricle, *IVS* interventricular septum, *CA* common atrium, *CAVV* common atrioventricular valve

Atrial, Atrioventricular, and Ventricular Anomalies

Atrial Septal Defects

Recognition of defects in the interatrial septum is challenging as physiologic flow exists across the foramen ovale, the septum is less echogenic than the interventricular septum, and the valve of the foramen ovale is not always recognizable. The ASD may be located (1) in the fossa ovalis in the central septum, where it is known as an ostium secundum defect; (2) in the upper septum, where it is known as a sinus venosus defect, often associated with anomalous venous return; and (3) in the posterior septum, where it is known as an inferior vena caval defect. Of the three, the ostium secundum defect is the most common and the inferior vena caval defect the least common. It is difficult to identify an ASD unless the deficiency is a large one. Figure 33.9 shows a large ostium secundum defect that was almost indistinguishable from the normal foramen ovale, except the valve of the foramen could not be seen even with careful high-resolution imaging.

Atrioventricular Septal Defect

In contrast to the deficiencies of the ASD, defects involving the atrioventricular septum (AVSDs) are more easily identifiable in the fetus because of their large size and associated structural and hemodynamic anomalies. Variously known as A-V canal defect, endocardial cushion defect, and ostium primum defect, the AVSD is characterized by complete absence of the interatrial septum and the presence of a common A-V orifice (Fig. 33.10). The A-V flow direction is regulated by a five-leaflet valve. Occasionally there are two A-V orifices separated by a straddling A-V valve, known as

the double-outlet atrium. AVSD variations exist in which the malalignment of the septum may lead to right or left atrial outflow obstruction. Hemodynamic abnormalities associated with AVSD may be recognizable by prenatal Doppler echocardiographic examination. Of specific relevance is the A-V flow regurgitation caused by the valvular incompetence. The condition has a high association with trisomy 21: Approximately 80% of infants with AVSD have trisomy 21 and approximately 40% of infants with Down syndrome suffer from AVSD [35]. Therefore when fetal echocardiographic examination leads to the prenatal diagnosis of AVSD, fetal karyotyping should be offered.

Ventricular Septal Defect

The VSD is the most frequently occurring congenital cardiac lesion, accounting for about one-third of all cardiovascular malformations [36]. An isolated VSD carries an excellent prognosis, and most VSDs close spontaneously within 5 years of life [37]. Prenatal diagnosis of the defect depends on the size of the defect and the presence of associated cardiac malformations causing hemodynamic disturbance. However, isolated VSDs of moderate or small size may not be easily recognizable during Doppler echocardiographic examination, as they are not associated with detect-

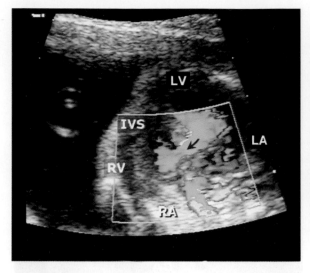

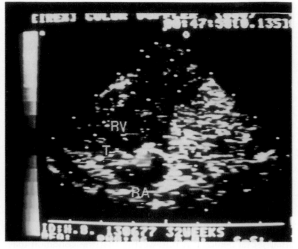

Fig. 33.11. Color flow depiction of ventricular septal defect. Flow away from the transducer is coded in *blue* and toward the transducer in *red*. Flow from the left ventricle (*LV*) across the defect in the interventricular septum (*IVS*) into the right ventricle (*RV*) is indicated by the *black arrow*. *LA* left atrium, *RA* right atrium

Fig. 33.12. Fetal Doppler color flow mapping. Apical right ventricular two-chamber view. The *blue area* in the right atrium underneath the close tricuspid valve represents tricuspid regurgitation in this fetus. *RA* right atrium, *RV* right ventricle, *T* tricuspid valve. (Reprinted from [13] with permission)

able flow shunting between the ventricles (which may be attributable to the pressure equilibrium that presumably exists between the two ventricles in the fetus). The presence of obstructive lesions in conjunction with a VSD alters this equilibrium, and shunting may be seen across a defect that itself may not be detectable by 2D imaging. Figure 33.11 demonstrates a flow jet from the left ventricle to the right ventricle across a defect in the membranous part of the interventricular septum in a fetus with aortic stenosis.

Tricuspid and Mitral Valvular Incompetence

The conditions associated with intracardiac regurgitant flow are listed in Table 33.8. Significant tricuspid regurgitation is associated with structural and functional cardiac pathology. Approximately 9% of infants with cardiac malformations demonstrate tricuspid incompetence [15]. Congenital tricuspid regurgitation is seen mostly in association with other malformations of the fetal heart, including Ebstein's anomaly and AVSD. Hornberger and associates [38] reported 27 fetuses with significant tricuspid regurgitation and tricuspid valvular disease: 17 with Ebstein's anomaly and 7 with poorly developed dysplastic, normally inserted valves. The perinatal outcome was severely compromised, with 48% stillborn and 35% dying during the neonatal period. We have encountered an occasional fetus with mild tricuspid regurgitation without demonstrable cardiac pathology. Figure 33.12 illustrates the Doppler echocardiographic demonstra-

Table 33.8. Intracardiac regurgitant flow and congenital malformations

Congenital tricuspid regurgitation
Physiologic
Ebstein's anomaly
Atrioventricular septal defect
Pulmonary stenosis without ventricular septal defect
Congenital cardiomyopathies including subendocardial fibroelastosis
Isolated malformations of the tricuspid valve
Congenital mitral regurgitation
Atrioventricular septal defect
Corrected transposition of the great arteries
Aortic stenosis
Congenital cardiomyopathies including subendocardial fibroelastosis
Isolated malformations of the mitral valve

tion of tricuspid regurgitation in the presence of apparently normal cardiac anatomy [13]. This observation was consistent with the postnatal findings. Martin and colleagues [39] observed tricuspid regurgitation in 3% of normal children. "Physiologic tricuspid regurgitation" has been reported in adults, especially in women with intense athletic training (93% of long distance runners and 57% of women with moderate athletic training) [40].

In contrast to tricuspid regurgitation, congenital mitral regurgitation is not encountered in healthy subjects. Its presence implies that there are mostly

Fig. 33.13 A, B. Duplex pulsed Doppler echocardiographic demonstration of mitral and tricuspid regurgitation in a fetus with cardiomyopathy. **A** *Top*: Apical four-chamber view of the fetal heart with the Doppler sample volume placed at the mitral orifice. **A** *Bottom*: Mitral waveforms with flow from the left atrium to the left ventricle as upward defections and the regurgitant flow as downward defections (*arrows*). **B** *Top*: Apical four-chamber view of the fetal heart with the Doppler sample volume placed at the tricuspid orifice. **B** *Bottom.: Tricuspid Doppler waveforms. Right atrium to ventricle flow is shown as upward deflections and the ventriculoatrial regurgitant flow as downward deflections*

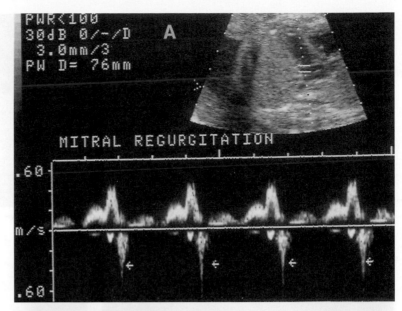

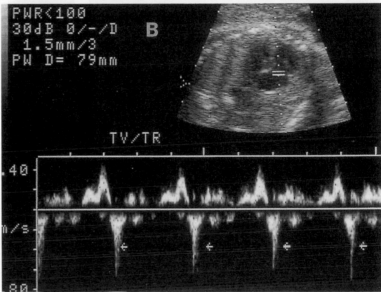

complex and occasionally isolated cardiac structural malformations or cardiomyopathy (Table 33.8). Figure 33.13 shows mitral and tricuspid regurgitation in a fetus with cardiomyopathy.

Ebstein's Anomaly

An uncommon malformation, Ebstein's anomaly is identifiable in the fetus with relative ease by 2D and Doppler echocardiographic scans. The defining malformation is apical displacement of the tricuspid valve leaflets from the annulus, affecting the septal and posterior leaflets and occasionally the anterosuperior leaflet. In addition to the displacement, the valves are dysplastic and have varying degrees of dis-

tal attachment [41]. As a result of valvular displacement, the superior or proximal part of the right ventricular chamber is incorporated into the functional right atrial chamber. This situation is known as atrialization of the right ventricle. The inferior or distal part of the ventricular chamber retains the pumping role. The tricuspid valves also demonstrate incompetence of varying severity, and the resulting regurgitant flow contributes to the right atrial dilation. These features are recognizable by 2D imaging and can be corroborated by Doppler insonation. The latter is essential for detecting and assessing the severity of valvular incompetence (Fig. 33.14). There are associated anomalies of the heart, the prenatal diagnosis of which may be facilitated by use of Doppler sonog-

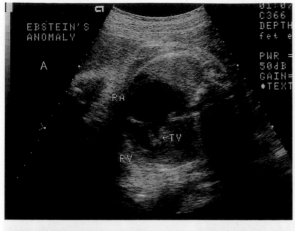

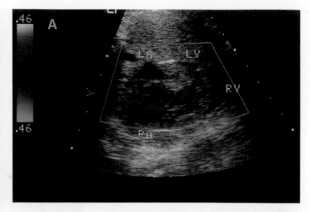

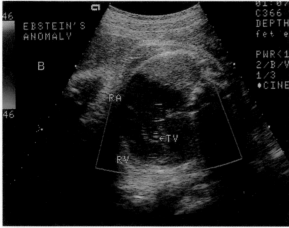

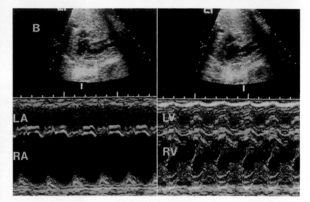

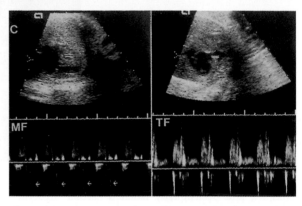

Fig. 33.14 A, B. Fetal echocardiographic assessment of Ebstein's anomaly. *RA* right atrium, *RV* right ventricle, *TV* tricuspid valve. **A** Two-dimensional image shows four-chamber view of the fetal heart. Note the apical displacement of the septal leaflet of the tricuspid valve with an enlarged right atrium and a diminutive right ventricle. **B** Color flow mapping of Epstein's anomaly. Note the impressive regurgitant flow projecting retrograde into the right atrium across the thickened tricuspid valve

raphy. They include ASD, pulmonary stenosis, absence of semilunar valves resulting in regurgitant flow, AVSD, and other malformations. The prognosis depends on the severity of the malformations. Severe dysplasia and abnormal distal tethering directly contribute to the functional and hemodynamic abnormalities. In general, neonatal survival has been poor. Advances in pediatric cardiac surgery have contributed to the relatively improved outcome.

Hypoplastic Left Heart Syndrome

Hypoplastic left heart syndrome is characterized by a hypoplastic or completely obliterated left ventricular chamber, mitral atresia, and aortic valvular atresia or

Fig. 33.15 A–C. Fetal echocardiogram shows the sonographic characteristics of the hypoplastic left heart syndrome. *LA* left atrium, *RA* right atrium, *LV* left ventricle, *RV* right ventricle. **A** Lateral four-chamber view of the fetal heart shows virtual absence of the left ventricular chamber and a small left atrial chamber. Flow in the right heart extends from the atrium to the apex of the ventricle. **B** M-mode depiction of the hypoplastic left atrium, a relatively enlarged right atrium (*left*), and a grossly hypoplastic left ventricle. **C** *Top left:* Doppler sample volume in the ventricle just distal to the valve. **C** *Bottom left:* Mitral Doppler waveform. **C** *Top right:* Doppler interrogation of the tricuspid flow. **C** *Bottom right:* Tricuspid Doppler waveforms

stenosis. The left atrium is small, with the foramen ovale usually patent. The right ventricle and atrium are enlarged because of hypertrophy and dilation. The condition may evolve with advancing gestation, so early echocardiographic examination may not detect the problem. Although 2D and M-mode echocardiographic examination can establish the diagnosis, addition of color and spectral Doppler interrogation is invaluable for defining the malformation (Fig. 33.15). The cause of left heart hypoplasia is obscure, but it is noteworthy that a similar malformation can be created in animals by decreasing the interatrial blood flow. Such an aberrant hemodynamic phenomenon may be responsible in the human fetus because of the secondary effect of aortic atresia or herniation of the foramen ovale valve. Once the lesion is developed, the right ventricle supplies the lower body and lungs through the pulmonary trunk, pulmonary arteries, ductus, and descending aorta. Retrograde flow with a right-to-left shunt across the transverse aortic arch supplies the subclavian-innominate system and the coronary arteries. This altered flow pattern may be recognized by careful color flow mapping. Without surgical intervention the condition is fatal during neonatal life. Progress in pediatric cardiac surgery, especially introduction of the Norwood procedure staged with the Fontan operation [42], has substantially improved the outcome (Table 33.4). Because the condition is associated with neonatal crisis and the staged surgical repair requires prior preparation, prenatal diagnosis is essential for developing an appropriate, timely management plan.

Pulmonary Atresia, Intact Ventricular Septum, Right Heart Hypoplasia Syndrome

Pulmonary atresia with an intact ventricular septum and right heart hypoplasia is a common variant of pulmonary atresia/intact ventricular septum syndrome and is related to the atretic condition of the tricuspid valve. The latter is associated with underdevelopment of the right ventricular chamber. In the absence of atresia, the tricuspid valve is incompetent and the right ventricular chamber, instead of being hypoplastic, becomes enlarged. The right atrium shows varying degrees of hypertrophy and dilation and often demonstrates a secundum-type septal defect. Hemodynamic adjustment includes diversion of flow from the right atrium to the left atrium and retrograde flow via the ductus into the pulmonary vessels. Echocardiographic diagnosis, in most cases, can be performed with relative ease by demonstrating the diminutive right ventricular cavity with scant or absent flow (Fig. 33.16). In addition, pulmonary vascular atresia may be recognized in the long-axis and arch views. The prognosis without intervention is

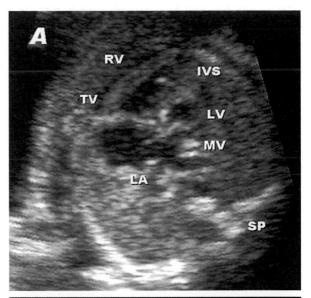

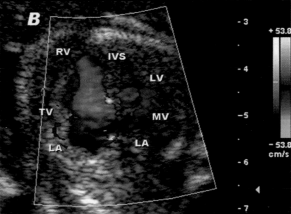

Fig. 33.16 A, B. B-mode and Color Doppler flow depiction of hypoplastic left heart. B-mode gray-scale echocardiogram. **A** Diminutive left atrium (*LA*) and left ventricle (*LV*). This is reconfirmed by color flow depiction of markedly decreased atrioventricular flow on the left side. **B** The right atrium (*RA*) and the right ventricle (*RV*) demonstrate compensatory increase in size and flow. Flow away from the transducer is coded in *blue* and toward the transducer in *red*

poor, although the outcome has improved with the introduction of medical management with prostaglandin to maintain ductal patency and advanced surgical interventions, such as balloon atrial septostomy and systemic-to-pulmonary artery anastomosis.

Outflow Tract Anomalies

Tetralogy of Fallot

The tetralogy of Fallot involves a perimembranous VSD, pulmonic stenosis, aortic root overriding the ventricular septum, and a hypertrophic right ventricle. The anomalous development is attributable to

of the cardiac sarcolemmal membrane, suggesting a molecular mechanism for the pathogenesis of the heart block [53]. A high titer of anti-Ro antibody (>1:16) [54] and the concurrent presence of anti-La antibodies increase the risk of congenital heart block.

Compared with other commonly encountered fetal arrhythmias, congenital heart block generally carries a substantially poorer prognosis, with an overall mortality ranging from 50% to 60% [55, 56]. The prognosis is worse when (1) fetal cardiac malformation is present; (2) the ventricular rate is <60 bpm; (3) the atrial rate is below the normal range of the fetal heart rate (<110–120 bpm); and (4) fetal heart failure supervenes as evidenced by the presence of pericardial effusion or hydrops. One of the early reports observed 75% mortality among fetuses with isolated heart block, compared with 15% mortality when the heart block was complicated by cardiac malformations [47].

Although the initial diagnosis is made by auscultation and electronic monitoring of the fetal heart, fetal echocardiography is indispensable for a precise diagnosis. This situation contrasts with that during postnatal life, when electrocardiography is the standard technique for diagnosing arrhythmic conditions. An initial 2D echocardiographic examination is essential for establishing the integrity of the fetal cardiac anatomy and identifying fetal cardiac failure. The 2D echocardiographic examination is also needed for guiding specific M-mode and pulsed-wave Doppler interrogation. M-mode echocardiography is the standard approach for establishing the discordance of the A-V rhythm. It is achieved by simultaneous interrogation and synchronous recording of atrial and ventricular activities. When pericardial effusion is present, M-mode sonography is also useful for assessing any changes in its severity. Finally, Doppler echocardiography is invaluable for recognizing hemodynamic abnormalities such as valvular incompetence, which may complicate these cases. The Doppler mode may also be used to determine A-V rates (see above) and to assess fetal cardiac function in terms of ventricular output, which is illustrated by our reported experience [7]. Figure 33.27, an M-mode recording from a fetus suffering from complete congenital heart block, demonstrates A-V discordance. The M-mode technique was also employed to further assess the pericardial effusion, which was recognized during 2D imaging. Figure 33.28 demonstrates tricuspid incompetence recognized in this case utilizing duplex pulsed-wave Doppler interrogation, which was used in conjunction with M-mode sonography for timing the events of the fetal cardiac cycle. These tests were undertaken prior to the introduction of color flow mapping, which can now be employed for effective elucidation of hemodynamic aberrations. As discussed in Chap. 32, color flow M-mode sonography is particularly useful in this regard. Because of the poor perinatal prognosis, a serial ultrasound examination is required to follow the development and progression of fetal cardiac decompensation. It is noteworthy that the utility of Doppler velocimetry of the umbilical or other fetal arteries is severely limited in this condition because of the undue prolongation of the diastolic phase. M-mode and Doppler echocardiography may be beneficial for intermittent monitoring of the atrial and ventricular rates and for evaluating fetal cardiac status.

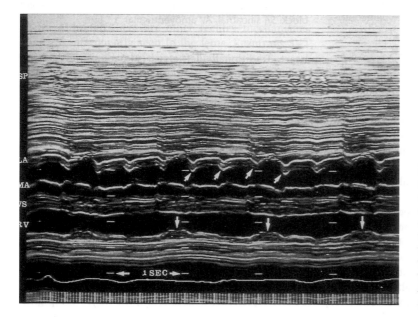

Fig. 33.27. M-mode echocardiogram shows a relatively rapid left atrial rate of approximately 120 bpm and a ventricular rate of 50 bpm. *Oblique arrows* indicate the contractions of the left atrial wall; *vertical arrows* denote systolic inward motion of the right ventricular wall. *LA* left atrium, *MA* mid-atrium, *VS* ventricular septum, *RV* right ventricle, *SP* fetal spine. (Reprinted from [12] with permission)

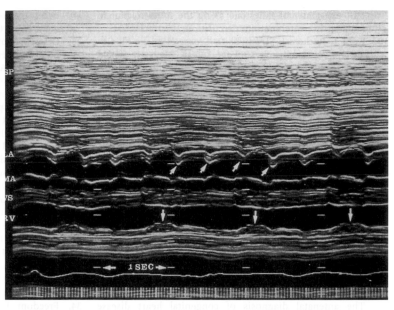

Fig. 33.28. Doppler identification of tricuspid regurgitation in a fetus with complete heart block and heart failuee. *Left:* The Doppler sample volume (*oblique arrow*) was placed in the right atrium (*RA*) imaged in the aortic (*AO*) short axis plane. *Right:* Doppler tracing shows prominent reversed flow (*R*) during systole indicative of tricuspid incompe tence. Normal flow patterns were seen during diastole (*D*). M-mode echocardiogram (*oblique arrow*) was used to time the diastolic and systolic phases of the fetal cardiac cycle. *Horizontal arrow* denotes the position of the Doppler sample volume for the M-mode system. *B* Doppler baseline, *TV* tricuspid valve. (Reprinted from [12] with permission)

Summary

Recent years have witnessed significant progress in the technique of fetal echocardiography and perinatal management of fetal cardiac disease. Although 2D cardiac imaging remains the major tool for this evaluation, its diagnostic efficacy is significantly enhanced by the other ultrasound modalities. Specifically, spectral pulsed Doppler, 2D Doppler color flow mapping, and color M-mode provide essential tools for elucidating hemodynamic abnormalities associated with structural and functional congenital cardiac disease. This hemodynamic information plays a crucial role in enhancing the efficacy of investigating these complex problems. It is not surprising, therefore, that Doppler echocardiography now plays such a critical role in the diagnosis, treatment, and surveillance of fetal cardiac disorders. Future developments in this area will certainly encompass 3D Doppler flow evaluation, which has been addressed in Chaps. 7 and 34.

References

1. Mitchell SC, Korones SB, Berendes HW (1971) Congenital heart disease in 56,109 births: incidence and natural history. Circulation 43:323–332
2. Benson Jr DW (1989) Changing profile of congenital heart disease. Pediatrics 83:790–791
3. Zosmer N, Souter VL, Chan CS, Huggon IC, Nicolaides KH (1999) Early diagnosis of major cardiac defects in chromosomally normal fetuses with increased nuchal translucency. Br J Obstet Gynaecol 106:829–833
4. Galindo A, Comas C, Martinez JM, Gutierrez-Larraya F, Carrera JM, Puerto B, Borrell A, Mortera C, de la Fuente P (2003) Cardiac defects in chromosomally normal fetuses with increased nuchal translucency at 10–14 weeks of gestation. J Matern Fetal Neonatal Med 13:163–170
5. Junker R, Kotthoff S, Vielhaber H, Halimeh S, Kosch A, Koch HG, Kassenbohmer R, Heineking B, Nowak-Gottl U (2001) Infant methylenetetrahydrofolate reductase 677TT genotype is a risk factor for congenital heart disease. Cardiovasc Res 51:251–254
6. McBride KL, Fernbach S, Menesses A, Molinari L, Quay E, Pignatelli R, Towbin JA, Belmont JW (2004) A family-based association study of congenital left-sided heart malformations and 5,10 methylenetetrahydrofolate reductase. Birth Defects Res Part A Clin Mol Teratol 70:825–830
7. Castaneda AR, Jonas RA, Mayer Jr HE, Hanley FL (1994) Cardiac surgery of the neonate and the infant. Saunders, Philadelphia
8. Warnes CA, Liberthson R, Danielson GK, Dore A, Harris L, Hoffman JI, Somerville J, Williams RG, Webb GD (2001) Task force 1: the changing profile of congenital heart disease in adult life. J Am Coll Cardiol 37:1170–1175
9. Kohl T, Strumper D, Witteler R, Merschhoff G, Alexiene R, Callenbeck C, Asfour B, Reckers J, Aryee S, Vahlhaus C, Vogt J, Van Aken H, Scheld HH (2000) Fetoscopic direct fetal cardiac access in sheep: an impor-

true real-time 4D echocardiography of the fetal heart [8]. The other is the motor-driven unidimensional linear-array transducer mentioned above but significantly enhanced with the development of the spatio-temporal image correlation technique [9]. These two approaches are discussed further in this chapter.

Basic Principles of Three- and Four-Dimensional B-Mode and Doppler Sonography

There are three fundamental sequential steps of 3D sonography: image acquisition; image processing; and image display. Real-time implementation of these sequential processes constitutes 4D sonography (Fig. 34.1).

Three-dimensional images are acquired either by direct scanning with 3D ultrasound beam produced by 2D matrix array transducers or reconstructed from a series of 2D ultrasound images as discussed in the previous section. Color Doppler interrogation which is based on mean Doppler angular frequency shift can be performed in both these approaches; however, the inherent limitations of Doppler sonography, such as angle dependence, are valid in these modalities. Power Doppler can be used without this limitation; however, the loss of flow directional information significantly restricts the utility of this approach. Three-dimensional color Doppler flow depiction can be used to quantify abnormal flow conditions such as regurgitant jets. Potential also exists to quantify volumetric flow. Many of these functions can be performed now to a variable degree with dedicated off-line processing. Future technological advances may permit real-time hemodynamic assessments, including flow quantification, with greater reliability than has been possible up to now.

Three-dimensional image processing requires defining the spatial location of a point in 3D space from the digital graphic information. The unit of 3D spa-

Steps of 4D Sonography

3D data acquisition
3D image reconstruction
3D image display
All of the above in real time

$$3D \rightarrow 4D$$

Fig. 34.1. Steps of four-dimensional sonography. *3D* three dimensional, *4D* four dimensional

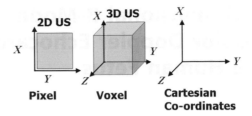

Fig. 34.2. Image processing in three-dimensional ultrasound. A pixel is the smallest definable unit of the two-dimensional (2D) image and defines the location in a 2D plane. A voxel is the counterpart of a pixel in three-dimensional (3D) imaging and defines the location in 3D space. *X*, *Y*, and *Z* represent the orthogonal planes of Cartesian co-ordinates for spatial location of a voxel

tial graphic information is known as a voxel. The term stands for volume pixel and constitutes the smallest definable unit of a 3D image. A voxel is the 3D counterpart of a pixel which defines location in a 2D plane. Geometrically, the relative spatial locations of a voxel are represented by the Cartesian co-ordinates x, y, and z (Fig. 34.2). The location is defined by the point's distances from three orthogonal planes determined by these co-ordinates. This is a fundamental concept that is crucial for 3D ultrasound image processing and interpretation. Each voxel can be digitally quantified to represent objective properties such as opacity, density, color, velocity, or even time. The ability to modify the opacity of a voxel is critical for 3D imaging. This is known as opacity transformation which allows visualization of internal morphology of an image which would otherwise be obscured by more opaque surface voxels.

Three-dimensional images can be displayed by (a) surface rendering with identification of various structures, (b) multiplanar reconstruction with dynamic orthogonal display, or (c) as a texture mapped block, such as a pyramidal 3D object, which can be rotated and cropped to reveal internal structures or flow.

Reconstructed 3D images are subject to motion artifacts which may be generated by fetal movements, patient movements including breathing, or inadvertent transducer movement; however, direct 3D imaging employing the 2D matrix transducers is not subject to similar motion artifacts except when two or more images are combined to produce a wide angle view.

Two-Dimensional Matrix Array

The 2D matrix array technology essentially consists of a phased-array transducer with 3,000 piezoelectric elements all of which transmit and receive ultrasound (Fig. 34.3; Sonos 7500 with X4 transducer, Philips Medical Systems, Andover, Mass.). The enormous vol-

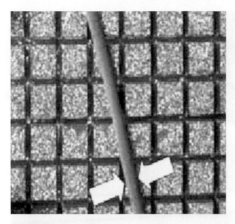

Fig. 34.3. Microscopic view of a matrix array transducer. Each *small square* is an active ultrasound element. The size of a human hair is shown for comparison (*arrows*). (From [9])

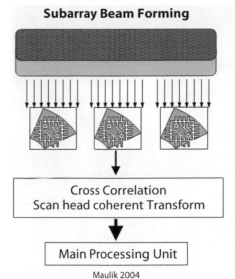

Subarray Beam Forming

Cross Correlation
Scan head coherent Transform

Main Processing Unit

Maulik 2004

Fig. 34.4. Graphic depiction of the concept of subarray beam forming

ume of data thus generated offer a formidable challenge in real-time processing; however, the system resolves this issue by devising a highly innovative technological solution known as subarray beam forming (Fig. 34.4). The elements are connected via layers of wiring to several custom integrated circuits. The currently marketed device uses many such circuits which are located in the handle of the transducer which itself still remains very modest in size. These circuits perform the initial processing of the ultrasound signals which are then transmitted to the main computer system of the device where further fast processing results in the real-time on-line generation of moving cardiac images. The system allows color Doppler flow depiction in real time in conjunction with the 4D depiction of cardiac anatomy.

The system generates a 3D pyramid-shaped volumetric sector restricted to an angle of about 30°–50° (Fig. 34.5). No gating is needed for this volume. A wider pyramidal sector image measuring 90×90° can also be produced. This is accomplished by swift automatic acquisition and integration of four sectors in real time during consecutive cardiac cycles with each sector measuring approximately 23×90°; however, generation of the extended sector requires some form of cardiac gating which in the adult or pediatric patient is provided by a modified type of electrocardiographic trigger. Although this is not feasible to accomplish in the fetus, an external electronic periodic trigger, which

Fig. 34.5. Two-dimensional matrix array: the sector size. **a** On-line 3D scanning. The sector size depends on chosen image resolution or line density, and is about 30×50°. **b** Wide-angle scanning. An *arrow sector* is scanned during each of four consecutive heart beats. The four sectors (shown with different color coding) are integrated automatically within a fraction of second. (From [9])

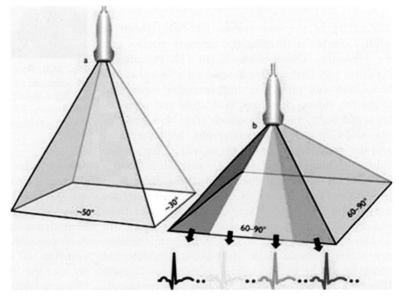

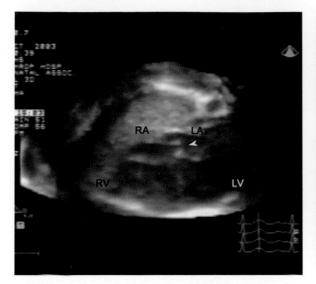

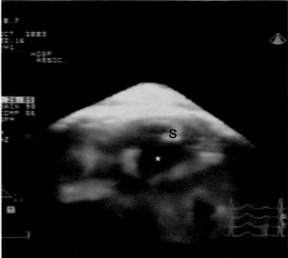

Fig. 34.6. Two-dimensional matrix array: the sector size. Pyramid-shaped wide-angle sector image of the fetal heart. Fetal back is toward the apex of the pyramid. Fetal spine can be seen at the right upper corner of the apex. The *arrowhead* points to the foramen ovale. *RA* right atrium, *LA* left atrium, *RV* right ventricle, *LV* left ventricle. (From [12])

Fig. 34.7. Four-dimensional echocardiography in a fetus with complete atrioventricular septal defect. En face view of the defect (*asterisk*) from the inferior aspect. *S* ventricular septum. (From [12])

can approximate the fetal heart rate, has been used successfully to produce a reliable full volume data set of the fetal heart (Fig. 34.6) [12].

Brightness and contrast can be adjusted to optimize the 3D image quality. The images can be cropped using the Cartesian co-ordinate x, y, and z planes as well as oblique planes to obtain the 3D perspective.

Two-Dimensional Matrix Array: Fetal Application of the Technique

The utility of the new system has been shown in adult patients for imaging the coronary arteries and for evaluating mitral stenosis [10, 11]. Preliminary experience in fetal cardiac assessment shows that this technology can provide a comprehensive assessment of cardiac valves, chambers, both atrial and ventricular septal walls, and great vessels [12]. Moreover, unlike real-time 2D echocardiography, both the atrial and the ventricular septal walls as well as the cardiac valves can be visualized as if the examiner is directly facing these structural surfaces in three dimensions in real time (also known as *en face* view) for any abnormalities (Fig. 34.7). Three-dimensional color Doppler allows comprehensive assessment of regurgitant and shunt lesions (Figs. 34.8, 34.9). In normal fetuses, the foramen ovale with right-to-left physiological shunting can be well visualized by 4D color Doppler (Fig. 34.8). In a 36-week-old fetus with complete at-

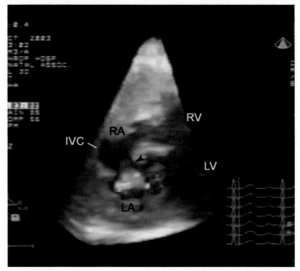

Fig. 34.8. Four-dimensional echocardiography in a normal 31-week-old fetus. Color Doppler image shows physiological right-to-left shunting (*arrowhead*). *RA* right atrium, *LA* left atrium, *RV* right ventricle, *LV* left ventricle, *IVC* inferior vena cava. (From [12])

rioventricular septal defect, we could fully visualize the septal defect from any desired angulation including en face views (Figs. 34.10, 34.11). Four-dimensional color Doppler allowed depiction of abnormal hemodynamics of the lesion with clarity (Fig. 34.12). Such comprehensive assessment is not possible using real-time 2D echocardiography because of its inability to view the defect using cross sections taken at different levels and angulations.

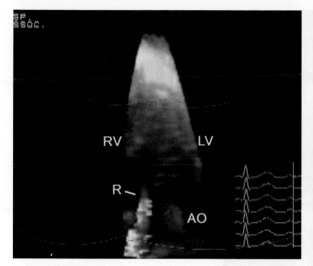

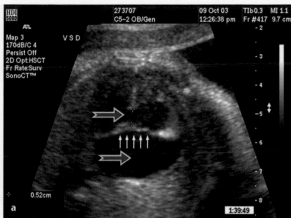

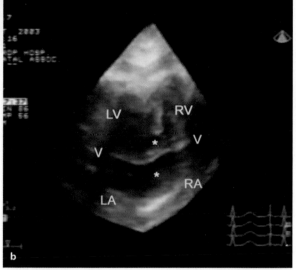

Fig. 34.9. Four-dimensional echocardiography in a fetus with complete atrioventricular septal defect. The pyramidal section has been cropped to show regurgitation (*R*) from the right-sided component of *V. AO* aortic cross section. (From [12])

One of the apparent limitations of the technique in our preliminary assessment is the inability to use fetal electrocardiography signals to trigger the volume acquisition which is the approach utilized in assessing the adult heart; however, as mentioned above, a simulated heart rate can be used within the range of the normal fetal heart rate with no visually detectable artifacts. The other potential challenge in any fetal imaging is related to fetal movements which may also interfere with live 3D imaging; however, this is not a significant problem in this system because of the very fast volume acquisition in both B- and color Doppler modes.

Motorized Curved Linear-Array System and Spatio-Temporal Image Correlation

This is an advanced system essentially based on 3D image reconstruction from sequentially acquired 2D images (Voluson 730 Expert System, General Electric Medical Systems, Kretztechnik, Zipf, Austria). The transducer assembly encases a curved linear array of transducer elements and a motor drive. The drive mechanism allows an automated sweep of the target area to generate 2D images sequentially constituting the volume data set. This method is inherently inadequate for fetal echocardiography because of fetal cardiac motion. Development of the spatio-temporal correlation technology (STIC), however, has resolved this issue.

An integral part of the 3D volume acquisition system, STIC processing, determines the fetal heart rate

Fig. 34.10. Four-dimensional echocardiography in a fetus with complete atrioventricular septal defect. **a** Two-dimensional B-mode image of the lesion. The *upper horizontal arrow* shows the ventricular septal defect; the *lower horizontal arrow* shows the absence of the atrial septum. **b** Four-chamber view cropped to show the common atrioventricular valve (*V*) and the defect (*asterisks*). *RA* right atrium, *LA* left atrium, *RV* right ventricle, *LV* left ventricle. (From [12])

from the systolic peaks of the fetal cardiac motion and immediately reorganizes the 2D images with spatial and temporal coherence so that images from the same cardiac cycle are collated together to form a single volume data set for that cardiac cycle (Fig. 34.13). Many such volumes are produced during a single sweep, and the actual number depends on the duration of the sweep and the heart rate. The images can be displayed as orthogonal multiplanar, volume-rendered, or single-plane displays either as cine loops or still images. The images can be gray scale or color B mode, color Doppler, or a combination of B mode and color Doppler with variable translucency, the so-called glass-body display. The

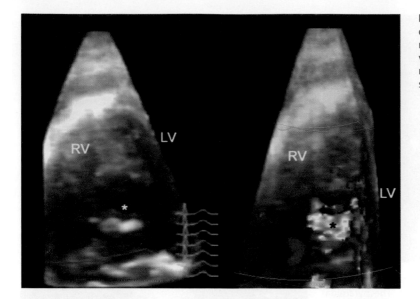

Fig. 34.11. Four-dimensional echocardiography in a fetus with complete atrioventricular septal defect. En face view of the defect (*asterisk*) from the right side. Turbulent color flow can be seen across the defect. (From [12])

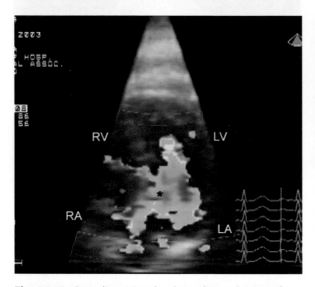

Fig. 34.12. Four-dimensional echocardiography in a fetus with complete atrioventricular septal defect. Four-chamber view cropped to show the color Doppler depiction of shunt across the septal defect. *RA* right atrium, *LA* left atrium, *RV* right ventricle, *LV* left ventricle. (From [12])

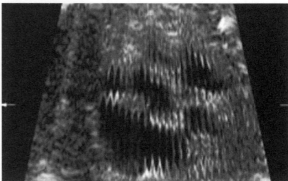

Fig. 34.13. Raw data volume showing a beating fetal heart during a slow 3D sweep. This information is used to calculate the fetal heart rate. (From [8])

STIC processing is very fast so that the images are produced in real time. Moreover, B-mode resolution has continued to improve. The 3D image volume data set can be archived and reexamined comprehensively later which may improve the efficacy of the prenatal diagnosis of congenital heart defects.

The STIC approach is sensitive to movements. Fetal body movements, or sometimes even fetal breathing, will produce artifacts rendering the images uninterpretable. Maternal breathing or transducer movement may also create this problem.

Fetal Echocardiography with STIC Technology

Introduction of this technique represents a significant advance in prenatal cardiac diagnosis. Several investigators have reported the use of this approach for fetal echocardiography [13–15]. These studies demonstrate the feasibility of using the STIC approach to obtain not only the traditional views of the fetal cardiac anatomy but also the ability to view the cardiac structures in an innovative manner. Our own preliminary experience corroborates these reports. A single sweep was able to produce four-chamber and outflow tract images with the color Doppler demonstrating the cross-over relationship between the pulmonary and the aortic outflows (Figs. 34.14, 34.15). It is apparent that this approach and its future evolution

Fig. 34.14. Spatio-temporal image correlation 4D echocardiography in the color Doppler mode. Multiplanar view of the fetal heart simultaneously showing four-chamber view and the outflow tracts. *RA* right atrium, *LA* left atrium, *RV* right ventricle, *LV* left ventricle, *AO* aortic cross section, *PA* pulmonary artery, *SP* fetal spine

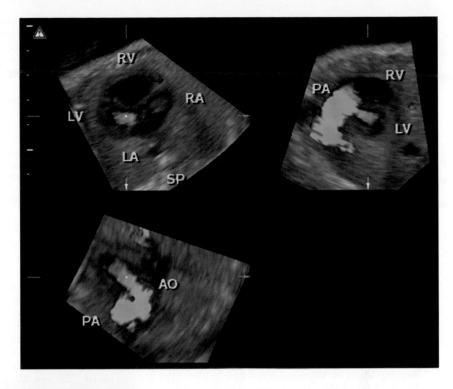

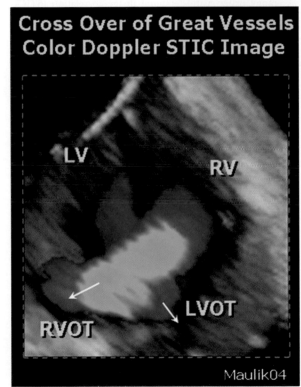

Fig. 34.15. Spatio-temporal image correlation 4D echocardiography in the color Doppler mode. Single-plane view of the fetal heart showing cross-over relationship of the great vessels and the outflow tracts. *RV* right ventricle, *LV* left ventricle, *RVOT* right ventricular outflow tract, *LVOT* left ventricular outflow tract. The *arrows* depict directionality of the flow

could substantially increase the ease of fetal echocardiography and improve its diagnostic efficacy.

Conclusion

Development of 4D ultrasound represents a major advance in non-invasive diagnostic technology and its introduction in clinical practice has initiated a significant paradigm shift in medical ultrasound imaging. Four-dimensional echocardiography allows a more comprehensive assessment of the fetal cardiac anatomy and hemodynamics than has been achievable in any of the current or legacy systems. It has the real potential of significantly expanding the scope of in utero diagnosis of congenital heart diseases and other abnormalities of the fetal heart. This is a very new technology and there is a real dearth of investigations critically evaluating its promises and limitations in the fetal application. This is especially relevant for extending its use outside the domain of experts and enthusiasts. At present, traditional 2D B-mode and Doppler sonography will continue to be the standard of practice for fetal cardiac assessment with substantial supplemental assistance from the 4D echocardiography which, however, has the strong potential to become the mainstream approach in the future.

References

1. Dekker DL, Piziali RL, Dong E Jr (1974) A system for ultrasonically imaging the human heart in three dimensions. Comput Biomed Res 7:544–553
2. Ghosh A, Nanda NC, Maurer G (1982) Three-dimensional reconstruction of echocardiographic images using the rotation method. Ultrasound Med Biol 8:655–661
3. Matsumoto M, Inoue M, Tamura S, Tanaka K, Abe H (1981) Three-dimensional echocardiography for spatial visualization and volume calculation of cardiac structures. J Clin Ultrasound 9:157–165
4. Pandian NG, Roelandt JRTC, Nanda NC et al (1994) Dynamic three dimensional echocardiography: methods and clinical potential. Echocardiography 11:237–259
5. Ramm OT von, Smith SW, Pavy HG Jr (1991) High speed ultrasound volumetric imaging system. Part II. Parallel processing and image display. IEEE Trans Ultrason Ferroelec Ferq Contr 38:109–115
6. Downey DB, Fenster A, Williams JC (2000) Clinical utility of three dimensional ultrasound. Radiographics 20:559–571
7. Deng J, Sullivan ID, Yates R, Vogel M, McDonald D, Linney AD, Rodeck CH, Anderson RH (2002) Real-time three-dimensional fetal echocardiography: optimal imaging windows. Ultrasound Med Biol 28:1099–1105
8. Franke A, Kuhl HP (2003) Second generation real time 3D echocardiography: a revolutionary new technology. Medicamundi. Philips Ultrasound 47:34–40; http://www.medical.philips.com
9. Falkensammer P, Brandl H (2003) Ultrasound technology update: 4D fetal echocardiography; spatio-temporal image correlation. GE Medical Systems, Kretz Ultrasound http://www.gemedicalsystems.com
10. Vengala S, Nanda NC, Agrawal G, Singh V, Dod HS, Khanna D, Chapman G, Upendram S (2003) Live three-dimensional transthoracic echocardiographic assessment of coronary arteries. Echocardiography 20:751–754
11. Singh V, Nanda NC, Agrawal G, Vengala S, Dod HS, Misra V, Narayan V (2003) Live three-dimensional echocardiographic assessment of mitral stenosis. Echocardiography 20:743–750
12. Maulik D, Nanda NC, Singh V, Dod H, Vengala S, Sinha A, Sidhu MS, Khanna D, Lysikiewicz A, Sicuranza G, Modh N (2003) Live three-dimensional echocardiography of the human fetus. Echocardiography 20:715–721
13. Goncalves LF, Lee W, Chaiworapongsa T, Espinoza J, Schoen ML, Falkensammer P, Treadwell M, Romero R (2003) Four-dimensional ultrasonography of the fetal heart with spatiotemporal image correlation. Am J Obstet Gynecol 189:1792–1802
14. DeVore GR, Polanco B, Sklansky MS, Platt LD (2004) The 'spin' technique: a new method for examination of the fetal outflow tracts using three-dimensional ultrasound. Ultrasound Obstet Gynecol 24:72–82
15. Chaoui R, Hoffmann J, Heling KS (2004) Three-dimensional (3D) and 4D color Doppler fetal echocardiography using spatio-temporal image correlation (STIC). Ultrasound Obstet Gynecol 23:535–545

Chapter 35

Doppler Echocardiographic Assessment of Fetal Cardiac Failure

William J. Ott

Introduction

In the fetus heart failure is the end stage of many pathological events that may lead to significant neonatal morbidity or mortality. In the adult heart failure is defined as *"the pathophysiological state in which an abnormality of cardiac function is responsible for the failure of the heart to pump blood at a rate commensurate with the requirements of the metabolizing tissues and/or to be able to do so only from an elevated filling pressure"* [1, 2]. In many instances this definition also applies to the fetus, but differences in the anatomy and physiology of the fetal heart, when compared with the adult or neonatal heart, may not allow this definition to be fully applicable to the fetus.

Fetal Cardiac Anatomy and Physiology

Anatomical and physiological differences between the fetal and neonatal or adult heart call into question the ability to translate the knowledge of the pathophysiological events occurring during heart failure in the adult or neonate to the fetus. In the adult the two ventricular chambers of the heart work in series, with the right ventricle pumping deoxygenated venous blood into the pulmonary circuit and the left ventricle supplying oxygenated blood to the systemic circulation. The fetal heart, however, works in parallel with little of the right ventricular output going to the pulmonary circuit. Figures 35.1–35.3 review the normal fetal intra-cardiac circulation.

Although there is some venous return to the fetal left atria via the pulmonary veins, the majority of venous return to the heart is through the superior and inferior vena cava and associated vessels [3–8]. Deoxygenated blood from the fetal head returns to the right atria from the superior vena cava and directly passes through the tricuspid valve into the right ventricle. Studies in the fetal lamb and other animal models have shown that oxygenated venous blood from the umbilical vein passes through the ductus venosus and preferentially enters the left heart via the foramen ovale [3–

8]. Studies on chronically instrumented fetal lambs have shown that, in physiological conditions, 50%–60% of the umbilical venous blood bypasses the hepatic circulation and enters directly into the inferior vena cava via the ductus venosus [8]. From the inferior vena cava, this highly oxygenated blood preferentially streams through the foramen ovale to the left atrium, left ventricle, and ascending aorta. Figure 35.4 shows venous return in a 22-week fetus. Doppler flow (Fig. 35.4b) shows that, under normal conditions, there is always forward flow throughout the cardiac cycle in the ductus venosus.

Although there may be many anatomical variations in the venous return to the fetal heart, the following general anatomical relationships are noted [9]:
1. The inferior vena cava widens in the proximal portion and enters the atria in a slightly anterior direction. An extension of the inferior vena cava continues into the atria itself as a short tube-like

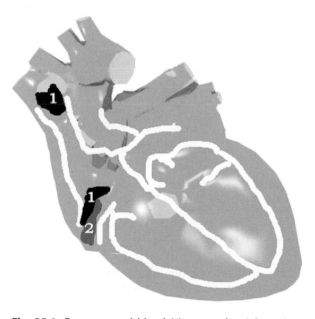

Fig. 35.1. Deoxygenated blood (*1*) enters the right atrium from the superior and inferior vena cava. Oxygenated blood (*2*) enters the right atrium primarily from the ductus venosus

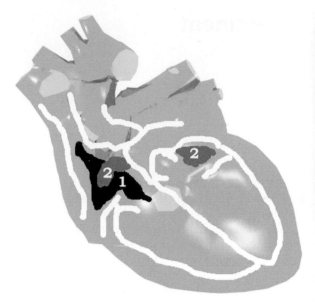

Fig. 35.2. The oxygenated blood (*2*) is directed through the foramen ovale into the left atria, while the deoxygenated blood (*1*) passes into the right ventricle

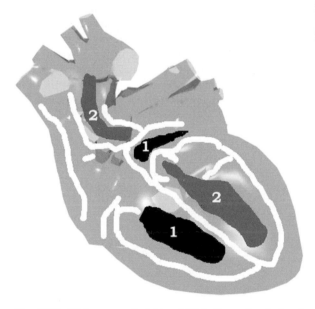

Fig. 35.3. Well-oxygenated blood (*2*) is then directed out the left ventricular outflow tract to the head and brain; while the deoxygenated blood (*1*) is directed via the ductus arteriosus down the aorta to the umbilical arteries for oxygenation in the placenta

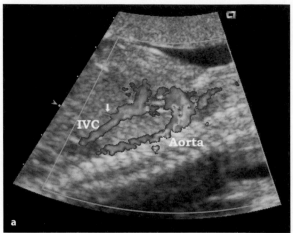

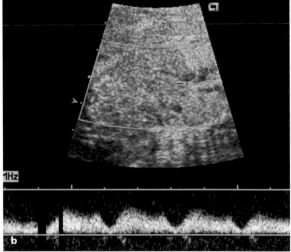

Fig. 35.4. a Gray-scale image of parasagittal scan of a 22-week fetus using color Doppler. The aorta and inferior vena cava (*IVC*) are shown. The *arrow* points to a segment of the ductus venosus as it enters the inferior vena cava just proximal to the right atria. **b** Doppler velocity flow in the ductus venosus of the fetus in **a**. Note the triphasic pattern, but that the flow is always forward throughout the cardiac cycle

structure bounded on the right side by the Eustachian valve (or valve of the inferior vena cava) and on the left side by the foramen ovale flap. The atrial septum lies above the middle of the inferior vena cava in a crest-like structure known as the crista dividens (or septum secundum or limbus fossae ovalis). The inferior vena cava/foramen ovale complex can be described as a Y-shaped unit with a long branch to the left atrium and a short branch to the right atrium.

2. This anatomical relationship results in two venous pathways for blood return to the fetal heart from the placental and lower body circulations. (a) A right inferior vena cava/right atrium pathway: blood flow from the right hepatic vein and right portion of the proximal inferior vena cava is directed along this pathway. (b) A left ductus venosus/foramen ovale pathway: blood flow from the umbilical sinus, ductus venosus, and left portion of the proximal inferior vena cava is directed along this pathway. The left and medial hepatic

veins connect to this pathway. Blood flow in these two pathways has the proximal inferior vena cava in common but travels in different directions.

These anatomical and physiological relationships result in different pathways for oxygenated and deoxygenated blood returning to the fetal heart. Distal inferior vena cava blood with low oxygen saturation passes through pathway "a" together with the right hepatic venous flow and is directed into the right atria where it joins the deoxygenated blood from the superior vena cava and passes into the right ventricle. Oxygenated blood from the umbilical vein passed through the ductus venosus with some mixing with blood from the left and medial hepatic veins and is directed towards the foramen ovale and the left atria and hence to the left ventricle. These studies in normal human fetuses are, in the main, consistent with previous studies in animal models.

The fetal anatomical shunt of the ductus arteriosus allows the fetal heart to function in parallel rather than in series, as in the adult heart [3]. The deoxygenated blood from the superior vena cava and the "a" pathway blood from the inferior vena cava passes through the tricuspid valve and is ejected out the pulmonary artery. Because of the ductus arteriosus shunt, this poorly oxygenated blood is directed into the descending aorta to the lower carcass, and to the umbilical arteries for oxygenation in the placental circulation. The left ventricle outflow is directed through the ascending aorta to the head and neck to supply the fetal brain with better oxygenated blood derived primarily from the "b" pathway via the foramen ovale. In the normal fetus right ventricular output is significantly greater than the left ventricular output in a ratio of 1.3 to 1.

A detailed evaluation of cardiac anatomy should always be undertaken in cases of suspected fetal heart failure. Normally the two ventricles should be of relatively similar size. Significant differences in ventricular size can be related to structural anomalies (such as hypoplastic left or right heart) or heart failure. Cardiomegaly is a common finding in fetal heart failure. Figure 35.5 shows cardiomegaly in a 24-week fetus with both chronic and acute abruption. An evaluation of cardiac size can be made by comparing the anterior–posterior (AP) and transverse (trans.) diameters of the thorax with the AP and the transverse diameters of the heart in the axial view:

$$Ratio = \{[AP(Hrt) + Trans.(Hrt)]/2\}/$$

$$\{[AP(Th) + Trans.(Th)]/2\}$$

This ratio ranges from 45% to 55% and is independent of gestational age [10]. Using M-mode, measurements of the pulmonary and aortic root diameters

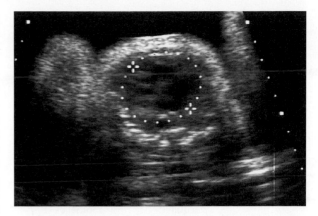

Fig. 35.5. Cardiomegaly in a 24-week fetus with acute and chronic abruption

can be obtained. Deng et al. have shown a consistent ratio between the pulmonary and aortic diameters of 1.09 (SD = 0.06) with 5th and 95th percentile values of 1.06 and 1.11, respectively [11–13].

Fetal Cardiac Response to Stress

Because of the anatomical and physiological differences between fetal and adult circulations, the development of heart failure in the fetus may follow slightly different pathways than in the adult. In the adult alterations in myocardial function, and subsequent decrease in cardiac output, can be caused by alterations in one (or a combination) of three basic mechanisms: (a) preload, or ventricular filling pressure; (b) myocardial contractility and heart rate; and (c) afterload or peripheral resistance [1, 2]. Alterations in any of these mechanisms can lead to decreased cardiac output and eventually to cardiac failure.

In the fetus the development of chronic stress and hypoxia results in alterations in fetal cardiovascular function. Both animal experimentation and Doppler evaluation of the human fetus have shown that chronic stress causes an alteration in the right/left heart dominance. During conditions of acute stress the primary fetal response is increased fetal heart rate. During conditions of chronic stress, however, alterations in ventricular function lead to redistribution of cardiac output and preferential perfusion of the fetal brain and coronary arteries.

Rizzo et al. have postulated the theoretical response of the fetal cardiovascular system to increasing fetal stress: a decrease in fetal oxygenation or substrate supply leads to a redistribution of cardiac output, the so-called brain-sparing effect [14]. Eventually the impairment of cardiac function causes an increase in the atrioventricular gradient and an abnormal cardiac filling which causes increased periph-

Table 35.1. Causes of heart failure: comparison of adult and fetal causes

Cause	Adult	Fetus
Cardiac arrhythmia	Disorders of arrhythmia	Congenital arrhythmias
		Maternal collagen vascular disease
Decreased contractility	Metabolic disorders	Maternal ketoacidosis
	Anoxia/ischemia	Intrauterine growth restriction
	Myocarditis	Myocarditis
Cardiac anomalies	Congenital or acquired	Congenital anomalies
Increased peripheral demand	Myocarditis	Myocarditis
	Systemic infection	Chorioamnionitis Systemic infection
	Anemia	Anemia
	AV shunts	Fetal tumors Chorioangioma
Increased afterload	Hypertension	Uteroplacental insufficiency?
	Valvular stenosis	Congenital heart disease
Increased preload	Valvular regurgitation	Recipient twin Indomethacin?
Decreased venous return	Hemorrhage	Hemorrhage (abruption, vasa previa, fetomaternal, other)
	Vena cava obstruction	Venous obstruction (tumor, hydrops, other)
Iatrogenic	Drug effects	Indomethacin, tocolytics, others

Table 35.2. Causes of fetal death: SJMMC Stillbirths 1988–1992

Category	Number	Percentage (%)
Placental		
Abruption	13	9
Other	27[a]	17
Infection	32[b]	21
Anomalies	19	13
Twin complications		
Mono/Mono	3[c]	2
Twin–twin transfusion	10[d]	6
Unknown	2	1
Cord accident		
Nuchal	7	5
True knot	2	1
Vasa previa	1	1
Fetal heart failure	4	3
Maternal		
Liver rupture	2	1
Ketoacidosis	1	1
Aortic aneurysm	1	1
Unknown	27	18
Fetal trauma:	–	–
Rh:	–	–
Total	151	100

[a] Includes two sets of twins with three stillbirths.
[b] Includes one set of twins with two stillbirths.
[c] Two sets of twins with one survivor.
[d] Includes one set of triplets with a single survivor.

eral venous pressure and fetal decompensation and cardiac failure. Table 35.1 compares the causes of cardiac failure in the adult with known or postulated causes in the fetus.

The Scope of Fetal Cardiac Failure

Changes in obstetrical management, the development of new and more accurate methods of fetal surveillance, and a better understanding of the pathogenesis of fetal demise has led to changes in the distribution of the causes of stillbirths. Table 35.2 shows the distribution of stillbirths from a review at the author's institution for the years 1988 through 1992. There were four fetal deaths directly caused by fetal heart failure: one premature closure of the foramen ovale; one case of non-immune hydrops caused by tachyarrhythmia; one case of significant increase in cardiac afterload caused by prune-belly syndrome; and one case of myocardial hypertrophy with heart failure in

a fetus of a diabetic mother. Although only 3% of fetal deaths were directly caused by fetal heart failure, it most likely played a significant role in many other fetal deaths: heart failure was the most likely terminal event in the cases of intrauterine infection (21%), twin–twin transfusion (6%), cord accidents (7%), and acute maternal problems (3%); and may have play a role in many of the cases of placental failure (17%). It is, therefore, likely that fetal heart failure plays a significant role in at least 40%–50% of stillbirths.

Duplex Doppler Evaluation of the Fetal Cardiovascular System

Evaluation of fetal cardiac status includes measurements of velocity parameters in both peripheral vessels and the heart itself. In peripheral vessels angle-independent indices, such as the pulsatility index, resistance index, and systolic/diastolic (S/D) ratio, are most commonly used. The peripheral vessel most commonly evaluated is the umbilical artery. Changes in the velocity indices in this vessel reflect alterations in placental perfusion that may precede evidence of heart failure in situations of uteroplacental insufficiency. Additional peripheral fetal vessels, such as the aorta, renal arteries, and carotid and middle cerebral vessels, have also been studied. Alterations in the velocity indices of these vessels, especially in the carotid and cerebral vessels, have been reported to be a sensitive indication of fetal well-being. Velocity measurements at the cardiac level are all absolute values. Measurements of absolute flow velocities require knowledge of the angle of insonation and vessel diameter, each of which maybe difficult to obtain with accuracy. The following formula can be used to calculate volume flow per minute:

Volume flow(ml/min)

$$= \pi/4 \times D^2 \times 1/\cos 0 \times FVI \times HR$$

where D is the diameter (in centimeters) of the vessel studied, 0 is the angle between the ultrasound beam and the vessel, FVI is the flow velocity integral (area under the velocity waveform), and HR is the heart rate in beats per minute [12]. The error in the estimation of the absolute velocity depends on the magnitude of the angle itself and the diameter of the vessel being interrogated. For angles $<20°$, the error is low. With larger angles, the cosine term in the Doppler equation changes the small uncertainty in the measurement of the angle to a large error in velocity equations. In addition, small errors in the measurement of the vessel diameter is magnified by the Doppler equation [12].

The parameters most commonly used to describe the cardiac velocity waveforms are: (a) peak velocity, the maximum velocity at a given moment (e.g., systole, diastole); (b) time-to-peak velocity, or acceleration time, expressed by the time interval between the onset of the waveform and its peak; (c) time–velocity integral, calculated by planimetry of the area underneath the Doppler spectrum; and (d) volume flow (see above) [12]. Velocity flow measurements can be obtained from a number of sites in or near the fetal heart.

Umbilical Venous Pulsations

During pathologic situations, increased reverse flow in the inferior vena cava may result in venous pulsations in the umbilical vein [14–21]. Indik et al. postulated that it may be possible to distinguish subgroups of fetuses with abnormal umbilical artery S/D ratios by evaluating fetal vena cava flow [21]. They described five sub-groups of fetuses with abnormal umbilical venous pulsations:

1. Tachycardia, which shortens ventricular filling and leads to increased end-diastolic pressure. During atrial contraction the increased end-diastolic pressure causes increased reverse flow in the inferior vena cava.
2. Sinus bradycardia also increases reverse flow by increased ventricular or atrial filling during pro-

longed diastole, leading to increased pressure during atrial contraction.
3. Complete heart block may cause increased reverse caval flow during ventricular systole, most likely due to independent atrial contractions against closed atrioventricular valves.
4. Premature atrial contractions were also noted to cause increased reversed caval flow during the pause following a premature atrial contraction. The mechanism was postulated to be similar to that seen with sinus bradycardia.
5. Abnormal filling of the ventricles is thought to be another etiology for increased reverse flow in the inferior vena cava.

Clinical situations associated with abnormal ventricle filling were congenital heart disease, infants of diabetic mothers, chorioangioma, nonimmune hydrops, and intrauterine growth restriction (IUGR). Umbilical venous pulsations therefore appear to be a significant pathologic event that requires careful fetal evaluation, especially of the fetal cardiovascular system.

Other Studies

Animal investigations have produced results similar to those seen by Doppler interrogation in the human fetus. Reuss et al. evaluated superior and inferior vena cava and umbilical vein blood flow patterns in fetal sheep using electromagnetic flow transducers [18]. The patterns of velocity flow were similar to those noted above for the human fetus. They were also able to manipulate the circulation of the fetal sheep to study the effects of afterload differences and hypoxia on venous dynamics. Administration of acetylcholine caused a reduction in afterload associated with peripheral vasodilatation, which allowed greater ventricular emptying with increased diastolic peak flow. Hypoxia was associated with an increase in superior vena caval blood flow through the foramen ovale to the left atrium and ventricle. Rizzo et al. postulated the pathophysiological steps leading to changes in biophysical parameters during fetal decompensation [14]: (a) increased resistance in the umbilical artery (S/D ratio); (b) increasing resistance in fetal peripheral vessels with a concomitant decrease in the resistance of vessels in the central nervous system (brain-sparing effect); (c) change in the ratio of right/left ventricular cardiac output with a shift to left ventricular dominance; (d) a decrease in the peak systolic velocities of the outflow tracts with a decrease in combined cardiac output; (e) increase in reverse flow in the inferior vena cava during atrial contractions leading to (f) umbilical venous pulsations and eventually (g) abnormal fetal heart rate tracings.

Velocity Measurements Across the Atrioventricular Valves

Blood flow across the atrioventricular valves can easily be seen with Doppler sonography (Fig. 35.6) [14, 22–26]. Blood flow velocity can be studied at the level of the mitral or tricuspid valves by placing the Doppler sample volume immediately distal to the valve leaflets in the right or left ventricle. In addition to

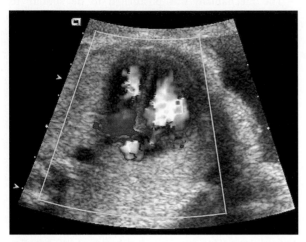

Fig. 35.6. Gray-scale image of a color Doppler axial scan through the fetal chest at 25 weeks showing flow across the AV valves

obtaining diastolic velocities across the atrioventricular valves, the presence of valvular insufficiency can be ascertained by moving the Doppler gate retrograde through the valve opening. Valvular stenosis has been reported to be associated with increased velocity flow through the affected valve. The waveforms recorded at the level of the mitral and tricuspid valves are characterized by two diastolic peaks: an early ventricular filling peak (E wave) and a second filling peak corresponding to the active ventricular filling phase during atrial contraction (A wave; Figs. 35.7, 35.8). These waveforms can be recorded as early as 12 weeks' gestational age [27].

The ratio between the A and E waves (A/E) is an index of ventricular diastolic function and is related to both cardiac compliance and preload conditions. The A/E ratio shows a significant decrease with advancing gestational age but remains above unity (Figs. 35.7, 35.8). This picture is the converse of that seen in the adult and suggests that ventricular compliance is less in the fetus than the neonate but improves with advancing gestational age. Reed [23] and Reed et al. [25] have shown that in most of the fetuses studied, tricuspid flow velocities during both early and late diastole were greater than those across the mitral valve. This confirms the impression of right heart dominance in the fetus that is seen when evaluating ventricular outflow.

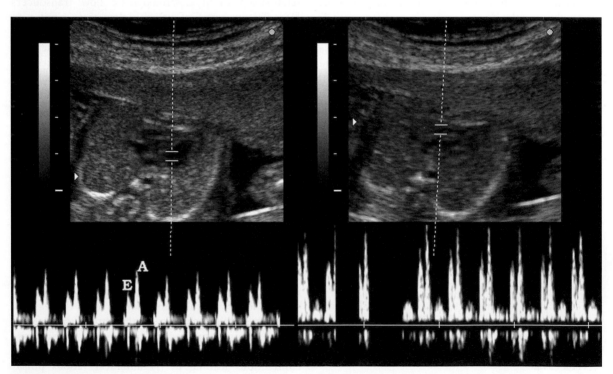

Fig. 35.7. Doppler blood flow across the mitral (*left*) and tricuspid (*right*) valves of a 20-week fetus. Note that the A/E ratio is greater than one

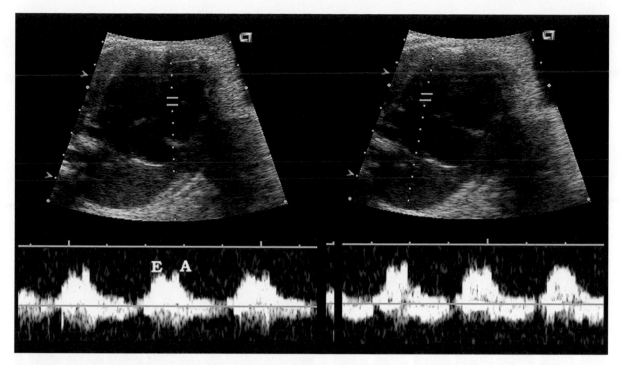

Fig. 35.8. Doppler blood flow across the mitral (*right*) and tricuspid (*left*) valves of a 34-week fetus. Although the A/E ratio is still greater than one, the ratio is less than that at 20 weeks

There is disagreement in the literature concerning the effects of gestational age on the maximal velocity across the atrioventricular valves. Allan et al. [22] and Reed [23] thought that there was no significant change in maximum or mean velocity flow across the valves throughout gestation, although van der Mooren et al. [26] showed a small but significant increase in velocity parameters with advancing gestational age. The decrease in inferior vena cava reverse flow and the A/E ratio with advancing gestational age is consistent with the increased ventricular compliance seen during that time.

Ventricular Outflow Velocities

Velocity flow and volume flow measurements have been reported for the right and left ventricular outflows (pulmonary artery and aorta, respectively; shown in Fig. 35.9) [14, 22–26]. The aortic outflow tract can be visualized as it leaves the left ventricle through a slightly rotated, angled four-chamber view, the "five-chamber" view. The pulmonary artery outflow tract as it leaves the right ventricle can be seen from a modified two-chamber view. A number of studies have shown that right cardiac output is greater than left cardiac output throughout gestation, and that beginning at 20 weeks the right/left cardiac output ratio remains constant with a mean value of 1.3, indicating right heart dominance in the human fetus, which has also been reported for the fetal lamb [28, 29].

Ductus Arteriosus

Ductus arteriosus velocity waveforms can be recorded from a parasagittal short-axis view of the fetus that shows the ductal arch. There is continuous forward flow throughout the cardiac cycle. Ductal peak velocity increases with gestation, and its values represent the highest velocity in fetal circulation occurring under normal conditions. Premature closure of the ductus, which has been reported in patients undergoing indomethacin therapy for premature labor, markedly increases right ventricular afterload and leads to tricuspid regurgitation and eventual cardiac failure. Tulzer et al. confirmed this finding with experimental ductal occlusion in fetal lambs [30].

Errors in Doppler Blood Flow Velocity Measurements

Doppler velocity flow measurements are prone to error [14, 24]. The most critical factor that affects the accuracy of the measurements is the angle of insonation. Measurement errors increase rapidly if the angle of insonation is greater than 20°. Rizzo et al. reported a coefficient of variation of less than 10% for Doppler velocity flow indices (except for volume flow) when the angle is kept at less than 20° [14]. In addition, the location of the volume flow gate should be frequently checked with duplex or color flow Doppler sonography to confirm the accurate placement of the interrogation site.

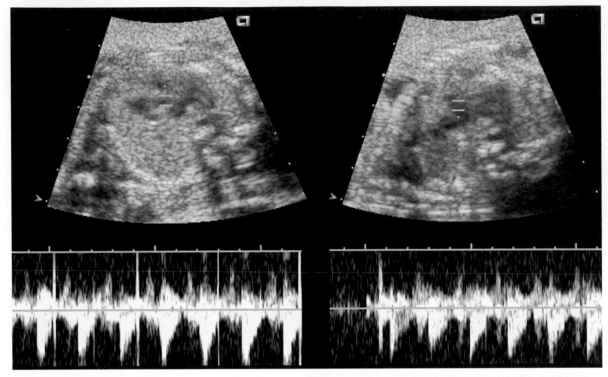

Fig. 35.9. Doppler blood flow across the aortic (*left*) and pulmonary (*right*) outflow tracts at 24 weeks of gestation

Calculation of volume flow introduces an additional error: measurement of vessel or valve diameter. Because the diameter term is squared in the formula for calculating volume flow, any error in the measurement is significantly magnified. Alverson reported a study of 33 pediatric patients who were scheduled for cardiac catheterization where in the Doppler-calculated volume flow and volume flow measured by the Fick principle during catheterization were directly compared [31]. He demonstrated an excellent correlation between the two methods, with a correlation coefficient (*r*) of 0.981. Fillinger and Schwartz studied Doppler flow measurements in an in vivo canine pulsatile flow model and found good correlation between Doppler-calculated and actual flow rates when laminar flow was seen [32]. They expressed caution about the accuracy of Doppler calculations, however, when flow was non-laminar, and they stressed the importance of the angle of insonation. In addition to the above measurement techniques, care must be taken to record velocity flow measurements during periods of fetal rest.

Clinical Conditions Associated with Fetal Heart Failure

Experience in obstetrical duplex Doppler examinations of the fetus have identified a number of clinical conditions where fetal heart failure is the cause of fetal death or a significant contributor to it.

Congenital Heart Disease

Structural fetal heart disease is the most common congenital anomaly seen at birth with an incidence of 7–10 per 1,000 live births. Although congenital heart disease is the most common birth defect seen in the neonatal period, there is strong evidence that it is even more common during the fetal period. Two reports have shown that 24% of fetuses with diagnosable congenital heart disease died in utero, most likely from fetal heart failure [33, 34].

Ultrasound has been used extensively for the diagnosis and evaluation of structural congenital heart disease [35–42]. Many structural anomalies can be visualized using only conventional ultrasound; however, the use of color flow Doppler can significantly enhance the diagnostic accuracy in suspected congenital heart disease [33, 34, 38, 43–47]. Color Doppler flow studies, coupled with velocity flow measurements,

Table 35.3. Changes in Doppler flow velocities with cardiac anomalies. *I* increased, *D* decreased, *A* absent, *U* unchanged, *R* possible regurgitation, *V* variable. (From [45])

Anomaly	Velocity flow			
	Tricuspid valve	Mitral valve	Pulmonary artery	Aorta
Hypoplastic right heart	D	I	D	I
Hypoplastic left heart	I	A	I	A
Tricuspid atresia	A		I	D
Ebstein's anomaly	I or R	I	D	I
Pulmonary atresia	I or R	I	A	I
Tetralogy of Fallot	U	U	D	I
Transposition	U	U	U	U
Double-outlet right ventricle	I	D	V	V
Atrioventricular canal	I or R	I or R	V	V

can (a) confirm the presence or absence of normal flow patterns in cardiac structures, (b) note the presence of abnormal flow patterns such as valvular regurgitation, absence of normal chamber filling (which might be seen in valvular atresia), or increased peak velocity (which may be seen in cases of valvular stenosis), and (c) identify reversal of normal flow direction (such as in the foramen ovale and aortic arch in the case of mitral atresia or in the ductus arteriosus with pulmonary atresia). In cases of fetal ventricular septal defect (VSD), however, there is little flow across the VSD since the pressure gradient between the two ventricles is minimal during intrauterine life. Table 35.3, modified from an article by Reed, shows the alterations in velocity flow that are frequently seen in many cases of congenital heart disease [45]. Umbilical and middle cerebral artery flow in fetuses with congenital heart disease was evaluated by Meise et al., who found little change in arterial blood flow velocities compared with normal fetuses [46]. Only in fetuses with severe outflow tract obstructions were there significant changes in arterial flow. They felt that abnormal arterial Doppler waveforms reflected uteroplacental dysfunction rather than alterations caused by the congenital heart disease.

A number of authors have reported hydrops fetalis and fetal heart failure associated with congenital heart disease. Sahn et al. reported a case of trisomy 13 with hypoplastic left heart syndrome that developed hydrops fetalis [44]. Interrogation of the tricuspid valve revealed high-velocity flow, 1.5 times greater than the normal values for their laboratory. Blake et al. reviewed a series of twenty fetuses with hypoplastic left heart syndrome [33]. Three of the 11 (27%) fetuses that were not terminated died in utero, most likely secondary to fetal cardiac failure. These authors also point out the importance of antenatal diagnosis of congenital heart disease. It allows (a) timely cytogenetic studies to be done, (b) early diagnosis and intervention in the neonatal period and planning for definitive therapy, and (c) additional time for parents to plan and discuss various treatment options for the fetus and obtain sufficiently informed consent.

Additional reports of fetal heart failure in infants with congenital heart disease have also been published in the literature. Respondek et al. reported a case of heart failure in a fetus with left atrial isomerism (common atrium) associated with complete heart block [47]. Color Doppler flow showed abnormal, turbulent flow in the regions of both the pulmonary artery and the aortic valve and increased flow velocity across the atrioventricular valves. Pericardial effusion and hepatomegaly were also noted. The infant died shortly after birth and an autopsy also disclosed unsuspected vegetation close to the thickened atrioventricular valves. The endocardium also showed evidence of endocarditis. Guntheroth et al. [48] and DeVore et al. [49] have reported abnormal flow studies in cases of pulmonary valve stenosis or atresia. Tricuspid regurgitation was felt to be a key sign of impending fetal heart failure. Rustico et al. reported a case of endocardial fibroelastosis associated with critical aortic stenosis and abnormal outflow track flow diagnosed at 15 weeks' gestation.

An excellent review of the use of color Doppler flow studies for the diagnosis of congenital heart disease can be found in two articles by DeVore et al. [49] and DeVore [51]. They describe abnormal Doppler flow findings in some of the more common cardiac anomalies:

1. Aortic stenosis: retrograde flow into the left atrium during ventricular systole.
2. Ventricular septal defect (VSD): since the pressure in the left and right ventricle are almost identical in the fetus, there is frequently no flow disturbance across the septum. Flow disturbances may be seen, however, when there is an associated abnormality of the outflow tract with increased resistance to the flow of blood leaving the ventricle.
3. Atrioventricular canal defect (AV canal): the presence of AV valvular regurgitation has been found to be a sign of developing hydrops fetalis and heart failure.
4. Atrial septal defect (ASD): reverse flow (left–right shunt) across the ASD may lead to right ventricular dilatation and heart failure.

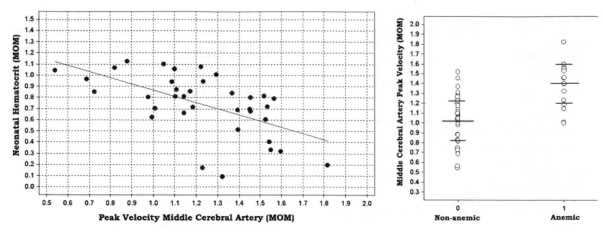

Fig. 35.10. Regression of the peak velocity of the middle cerebral artery [converted to multiples of the mean (MOM) for gestational age] against the fetal/neonatal hematocrit (converted to MOM for gestational age) at cordocentesis or delivery. The *right side* of the figure shows the peak velocity in the middle cerebral artery in anemic vs non-anemic fetuses or neonates

crease in the A/E ratio at both atrioventricular valves [60]. The increased cardiac output seen in these anemic fetuses my be due to a decrease in blood viscosity which, in turn, leads to increased venous return and cardiac preload; and/or to peripheral vasodilatation caused by a fall in blood oxygen content and therefore reduced cardiac afterload. There is no evidence for a redistribution of cardiac output similar to that described in hypoxic IUGR fetuses [60].

The traditional method of evaluating fetal anemia in sensitized patients is the serial determination of amniotic fluid changes in optical density at 450 nm [61, 62]. The use of Doppler ultrasound to measure peak velocity in the fetal middle cerebral artery has been shown to be an accurate, non-invasive method of evaluating fetal anemia [63–65]. Figure 35.10 shows the correlation between fetal/neonatal hematocrit and peak velocity in the fetal middle cerebral artery in 36 patients with suspected fetal anemia (primarily due to isoimmunization) followed at the author's institution. Doppler ultrasound appears to be as accurate as serial amniocentesis in evaluating suspected fetal anemia, and has the important advantage of being a non-invasive test [66].

Non-Immune Hydrops

As has been mentioned previously non-immune fetal hydrops may be secondary to a multitude of different causes. The first step, therefore, in the evaluation and management of fetuses with suspected non-immune hydrops is to attempt to determine its etiology. Some of the more common causes of non-immune fetal hydrops include chromosomal abnormalities, mass lesions that affect fetal blood flow, lymphatic abnormalities, metabolic diseases of the fetus, and infection

Table 35.5. Evaluation of non-immune fetal hydrops. *TORCH* toxoplasmosis, other, rubella, cytomegalovirus, herpes. (From [57])

Evaluation	Test	Etiology?
Maternal	Antibody screen	Rule out isoimmunization
	Complete blood count and indices	Hematological disorders
	Electrophoresis	Thalassemia
	Kleihauer-Betke stain	Fetal–maternal hemorrhage
	VDRL and TORCH titers	Fetal infection
	Glucose tolerance test	Maternal diabetes
Fetus	Level II ultrasound and color Doppler	Anatomical or physiological abnormalities of the fetus
	Cordocentesis	Karyotype (chromosomal anomalies)
	Amniocentesis Paracentesis Thoracenteses	Cultures/immunology (infection)

[67–72]. Table 35.5, modified from a review by Holzgreve et al., lists many of the tests necessary to appropriately evaluate cases of non-immune hydrops [57].

A study by Saltzman et al. reviewed the ultrasonic differences seen in anemic and non-anemic fetuses with hydrops [60]. The lack of a thickened placenta, and the presence of pleural effusions and/or marked edema, was more frequently associated with non-anemic causes of fetal hydrops. Doppler echocardiography may be useful in the additional differentiation between cardiac and non-cardiac causes of non-immune hydrops [45, 71]. Increased velocity in the middle cerebral artery correlates with fetal anemia. Low-peak velocity in the outflow tracts, exaggerated pulsations in the inferior vena cava, or an increase in the percentage of reverse flow in the inferior vena cava during atrial contractions, pulsations in the umbilical vein, and tricuspid regurgitation are all developing signs of fetal heart failure. Pulsations in the umbilical vein appear to be a sign of significant fetal compromise.

The outcome for fetal non-immune hydrops depends on the cause of the condition and the gestational age at diagnosis. Diagnosis before 20 weeks carries a worse prognosis, but even with aggressive therapy the mortality rate for non-immune hydrops is 40%–60% [73–75]. As has been mentioned previously, there are multiple causes of non-immune hydrops and a discussion of even some of its major causes is beyond the scope of this chapter; however, two specific causes of non-immune hydrops should be mentioned since they are directly related to fetal heart failure: fetal cardiac arrhythmia and fetal anemia.

Fetal Cardiac Arrhythmia

Persistent alterations in the rate or rhythm of the fetal heart can lead to heart failure, non-immune hydrops, and significant neurological morbidity after delivery [76–84]. A number of excellent review articles on the diagnosis and treatment of fetal cardiac arrhythmia have been published [77]. Arrhythmia tachycardia is the most common pathological anomaly noted and the one that most frequently leads to hydrops.

Doppler echocardiographic evaluation of the fetal heart can be an important adjunct in the proper classification of fetal cardiac arrhythmia and in the evaluation of fetal therapy. Chan et al. reported the use of simultaneous recordings of the Doppler waveforms from the inferior vena cava and aorta for the precise diagnosis of the type of arrhythmia seen [82]. Intermittent or non-persistent tachycardia can be managed by careful observation [85–88]. In many situations, spontaneous resolution of fetal tachycardia has been noted, leading some investigators to recommend a conservative approach to fetal tachycardia if there is no evidence of fetal cardiac compromise (no evidence of chamber dilatation, valvular regurgitation, hydrops, or decreased ventricular systolic function) [89].

If there are any signs of fetal cardiac compromise or if the tachyarrhythmia is persistent, intrauterine therapy may be necessary. Table 35.6, modified from the work of a number of investigators, lists the dosage of maternally administered oral drugs frequently used in the treatment of in utero fetal arrhythmias [77–80]. Careful monitoring of both fetus and mother is necessary in the pharmacological treatment of fetal arrhythmia, and consultation with a cardiologist is essential.

Table 35.6. In utero therapy of fetal arrhythmia

Arrhythmia	Drug	Dosage (maternal)
Supraventricular tachycardia	Digoxin	0.25–0.75 mg q 8 h
(may be added if no response)	(Verapamil)	80–120 mg q 6–8 h
	(Flecainide)	100 mg three to four times a day

Persistent fetal bradycardia is a much less frequent problem. Congenital heart block, which may be associated with maternal systemic lupus or with some congenital heart defects (transposition of the great vessels or AV canal defects), can usually be managed conservatively [84]. The use of M-mode for diagnosis and evaluation of fetal arrhythmias has also been reported [86].

Fetal Anemia

Fetal anemia can develop from a number of causes, with isoimmunization leading to fetal hemolysis being a classical case. Alpha-thalassemia 1 (Bart's disease), caused by an inherent deficiency in the alpha-globin hemoglobin chain, leads to severe fetal anemia, hydrops and fetal death [90]. Cardiomegaly, increasing velocities in the middle cerebral artery, and eventual fetal hydrops are ultrasonic hallmarks of the disease [90, 91].

Significant fetal–maternal hemorrhage can be a cause of stillbirth or neonatal anemia [92]. The diagnosis is usually made after delivery by finding significant fetal blood in the maternal circulation using the Kleihauer-Betke test. The use of Doppler ultrasound to measure the peak velocity in the middle cerebral artery has provided an accurate, non-invasive method of evaluating suspected fetal anemia. Figure 35.11 shows the graph of the peak velocity in the middle cerebral artery of a fetus that was evaluated for decreased movement at 32 weeks of gestation. The marked increase in peak velocity together with a non-reactive NST led to an emergency Cesarean delivery. The neonate was anemic with a hemoglobin/hematocrit of 10.2/29. A Kleihauer-Betke test on the mother's blood showed evidence of greater than 120 cc of fetal blood, confirming the diagnosis of fetal–maternal bleeding.

A number of other causes of fetal bleeding and subsequent anemia have been reported. Cases of intracranial hemorrhage secondary to trauma, thrombocytopenia, or preeclampsia has been published [93–95]. Fetal hemorrhage into cystic tumors or fetal bleeding secondary to abruption or ruptured vasa previa can also cause severe fetal anemia.

walls in fetuses of diabetic mothers even in infants of mothers who were under good glucose control [117]. The hemodynamic effects of these morphological changes may lead to impairment of cardiac diastolic function and eventual heart failure. Infants of diabetic mothers, even in those situations where tight glucose control has been obtained, have a significantly higher incidence of sudden fetal death [117–122]. An increased thickness in the ventricular walls, particularly in the interventricular septum, has been noted in these infants. Hypertrophy and disorganization of the myofibrils of the fetal heart have also been found at time of autopsy.

Doppler studies have shown evidence that the disproportional thickening of the intraventricular septum results in functional left ventricular outflow tract obstruction which may lead to cardiac failure. Increased A/E ratios at the level of both atrioventricular valves and higher peak velocity values at the outflow tracts were found in such fetuses. Weiner et al. felt that this was due to an increasing A wave during the later part of gestation suggesting increased cardiac contractility and output in fetuses of diabetic women [121]. Polycythemia, which is frequently present at birth in infants of diabetic mothers, results in increased blood viscosity which may alter preload and affect ventricular filling. The high peak velocity values in the aorta and pulmonary artery may be due to increased contractility, or secondary to an increased intra-cardiac flow volume, due to the fetal macrosomia frequently seen in infants of diabetic mothers.

Other Causes of Fetal Heart Failure

A wide variety of other known, and probably unknown, conditions can lead to fetal heart failure [122–129]. Primary myocarditis of viral etiology has been reported in the fetus. Blood-borne transplacental infection or ascending chorioamnionitis may cause significant systemic fetal infection which, in turn, may cause fetal cardiac failure. High output failure in the fetus has been reported in association with rare fetal tumors, such as fetal teratoma, goitrous hypothyroidism, hemangiomas, or rhabdomyosarcomas [122–129]. In most of these cases the high output failure is due to arterial–venous shunts within the tumor itself or secondary to vascular compression by an expanding mass.

Morine et al. described a case of high-output failure in a fetus (cardiomegaly, pleural effusion, and increased velocity in the carotid artery) diagnosed with goitrous hypothyroidism [127]. The symptoms reversed after intrauterine treatment with levothyroxine. Arterial–venous malformations in the fetus, such as an aneurysm of the vein of Galen, have also been reported to cause fetal hydrops [128]. Chorioangio-

mas of the placenta are benign hemangiomas that can be seen in 1% of all placentas. Usually they cause no problems, but when large (> 5 cm), they can cause polyhydramnios and, occasionally, high-output failure in the fetus secondary to arterial–venous shunts [129]. Cardiomegaly and abnormal venous flow in the fetus are typical signs of developing heart failure [130].

Iatrogenic causes of fetal heart failure may be associated with maternal drug use, especially indomethacin, which has been reported to cause premature closure of the fetal ductus arteriosus resulting in fetal heart failure. Indomethacin has been shown to cause transient constriction of the ductus arteriosus, resulting in an increase in both systolic and diastolic velocity in the ductus. As a consequence, tricuspid regurgitation and heart failure may occur. Beta-agonists have an inotropic effect on the fetal heart which may lead to an increase of both peak velocity in the aorta and pulmonary artery and an increase of the stroke volume. Levy et al. have reported that the combined use of indomethacin and corticosteroids may have additive effects on ductal constriction [131]. The long-term effects of these drugs is still unknown.

Fisher has reviewed many of the causes of cardiomyopathies that may affect the fetus [132]. Hypoxia and acidemia, metabolic abnormalities, such as hypocalcemia, or congenital metabolic diseases, such as Pompe's disease or endocardial fibroelastosis, have all been reported to cause fetal cardiac failure.

Summary and Conclusion

A large number of clinical conditions have been found that may lead to intrauterine cardiac failure. Pulsed and color Doppler techniques have improved our knowledge of fetal cardiovascular response to structural and functional heart diseases. Key features of developing fetal heart failure that may be seen include:
1. Valvular regurgitation
2. Altered velocities
3. Chamber dilatation
4. Fluid collections: ascites, edema, pericardial
5. Reverse flow: vena cava, umbilical pulsations.

Doppler blood flow studies have enabled investigators and clinicians to better understand the pathological processes involved in developing fetal heart failure and to plan appropriate treatments or interventions. We can expect that further study and experience with the use of Doppler blood flow studies will lead to increased improvement in perinatal morbidity and mortality.

References

1. Braunwald E, Grossman W (1992) Clinical aspects of heart failure. In: Braunwald E (ed) Heart disease: a textbook of cardiovascular medicine. Saunders, Philadelphia, pp 444–449

2. Friedman R (1987) Congestive heart failure. In: Kravis T, Warner C (eds) Emergency medicine: a comprehensive review. Aspen, Rockville, Maryland, pp 1005–1011

3. Kiserud T, Eik-New H, Blaas H et al. (1992) Foramen ovale: an ultrasonography study of its relation to the inferior vena cava, ductus venosus and hepatic veins. Ultrasound Obstet Gynecol 2:389–396

4. Dawes GS (1982) Physiological changes in the circulation after birth. In: Fishman AP, Richards DW (eds) Circulation of the blood. Men and ideas. American Physiological Society, Bethesda, pp 743–816

5. Barclay AE, Franklin KJ, Prichard MM (1942) Further data about the circulation and about cardiovascular system before and just after birth. Br J Radiol 15:249–256

6. Barcroft J (1946) Researches on pre-natal life, vol 1. Blackwell, Oxford, pp 211–225

7. Lind J, Wegelius C (1949) Angiographic studies on the human fetal circulation. Pediatrics 4:391–400

8. Peltonen T, Hirvonen L (1965) Experimental studies on fetal and neonatal circulation. Acta Pediatr 44 (Suppl 161):1–55

9. Hofstaetter C, Plath H, Hansmann M (2000) Prenatal diagnosis of abnormalities of the fetal venous system. Ultrasound Obstet Gynecol 15:231–241

10. Filkins KA, Brown TI, Levine OR (1981) Real time ultrasonic evaluation of the fetal heart. Int J Gynaecol Obstet 19:35–39

11. Deng J, Cheng P, Gao S et al. (1992) Echocardiographic evaluation of the valves and roots of the pulmonary artery and aorta in the developing fetus. J Clin Ultrasound 20:3–9

12. Shiraishi H, Silverman N, Rudolph A (1993) Accuracy of right ventricular output estimated by Doppler echocardiography in the sheep fetus. Am J Obstet Gynecol 168:947–953

13. Ott WJ (1988) The diagnosis of altered fetal growth. Obstet Gynecol Clin North Am 15:237–264

14. Rizzo G, Arduini D, Romanini C (1992) Doppler echocardiographic assessment of fetal cardiac function. Ultrasound Obstet Gynecol 2:434–445

15. Wladimiroff J, Huisman T, Stewart P (1991) Normal fetal arterial and venous flow-velocity waveforms in early and late gestation. In: Jaffe R, Warsof S (eds) Color Doppler imaging in obstetrics and gynecology. McGraw-Hill, New York, pp 155–173

16. Reed K (1991) Venous flow velocities in the fetus. In: Jaffe R, Warsof S (eds) Color Doppler imaging in obstetrics and gynecology. McGraw-Hill, New York, pp 175–181

17. Appleton C, Hatle L, Popp R (1987) Superior vena cava and hepatic vein Doppler echocardiography in healthy adults. J Am Coll Cardiol 10:1032–1039

18. Reuss M, Rudolph A, Dae M (1993) Phasic blood flow patterns in the superior and inferior venae cavae and umbilical vein of fetal sheep. Am J Obstet Gynecol 145:70–78

19. Huisman T, van den Eijnde S, Tweart P (1993) Changes in inferior vena cava blood flow velocity and diameter during breathing movements in the human fetus. Ultrasound Obstet Gynecol 3:26–30

20. Reed K, Appleton C, Anderson C (1990) Doppler studies of vena cava flows in human fetuses. Circulation 81:498–505

21. Indik J, Chen V, Reed K (1991) Association of umbilical venous with inferior vena cava blood flow velocities. Obstet Gynecol 77:551–557

22. Allan L, Chita S, Al-Ghazali W et al. (1987) Doppler echocardiographic evaluation of the normal human fetal heart. Br Heart J 57:528–533

23. Reed K (1987) Fetal and neonatal cardiac assessment with Doppler. Semin Perinatol 11:347–356

24. Kurjak A, Alfirevic Z, Miljan M (1988) Conventional and color Doppler in the assessment of fetal and maternal circulation. Ultrasound Med Biol 14:337–354

25. Reed K, Shan D, Scagnelli S et al. (1986) Doppler echocardiographic studies of diastolic function in the human fetal heart: changes during gestation. J Am Coll Cardiol 8:391–395

26. Van der Mooren K, Barendregt L, Waldimiroff J (1991) Fetal atrioventricular and outflow tract flow velocity waveforms during normal second half of pregnancy. Am J Obstet Gynecol 165:668–674

27. Leiva MC, Tolosa JE, Binotto CN, Weiner S, Huppert L, Denis AL, Huhta JC (1999) Fetal cardiac development and hemodynamics in the first trimester. Ultrasound Obstet Gynecol 14:169–174

28. Anderson DF, Bissonnette JM, Faber JJ et al. (1981) Central shunt flows and pressures in the mature fetal lamb. Am J Physiol 241:H60

29. Daws GS, Mott JC, Widdicombe JG (1954) The fetal circulation in the lamb. J Physiol (Lond) 126:563–566

30. Tulzer G, Gudmundsson S, Rotondo K et al. (1991) Acute fetal ductal occlusion in the fetal lamb. Am J Obstet Gynecol 165:775–778

31. Alverson D (1985) Neonatal cardiac output measurements using pulsed Doppler ultrasound. Clin Perinatol 12:101–127

32. Fillinger M, Schwartz R (1993) Volumetric blood flow measurement with color Doppler ultrasonography: the importance of visual clues. J Ultrasound Med 3:123–130

33. Blake D, Copel J, Kleinman C (1991) Hypoplastic left heart syndrome: prenatal diagnosis, clinical profile and management. Am J Obstet Gynecol 165:529–534

34. Chiba Y, Kanzaki T, Kobayashi H et al. (1990) Evaluation of fetal structural heart disease using color flow mapping. Ultrasound Med Biol 16:221–229

35. DeVore G (1985) The prenatal diagnosis of congenital heart disease: a practical approach for the fetal sonographer. J Clin Ultrasound 13:229–245

36. DeVore G, Saissi B, Platt L (1988) Fetal echocardiography: VIII. Aortic root dilatation: a market for Tetralogy of Fallot. Am J Obstet Gynecol 159:129–136

37. DeVore G, Saissi B, Platt L (1985) Fetal echocardiography: V. M-mode measurements of the aortic root and aortic valve in second- and third-trimester normal human fetuses. Am J Obstet Gynecol 152:543–550

38. Huhta J, Rotondo K (1991) Fetal Echocardiography. Semin Roentgenol 26:5–11

39. Sharf M, Abinader E, Shapiro I et al. (1983) Prenatal echocardiographic diagnosis of Ebstein's anomaly with pulmonary atresia. Am J Obstet Gynecol 147:300–303

40. Jackson G, Ludmir J, Castelbaum A et al. (1991) Intrapartum course of fetuses with isolated hypoplastic left heart syndrome. Am J Obstet Gynecol 165:1068–1072

41. McGahan J, Choy M, Parrish M et al. (1991) Sonographic spectrum of fetal cardiac hypoplasia. J Ultrasound Med 10:539–546

42. Sandor G, Farquarson D, Wittmann B et al. (1986) Fetal echocardiography: results in high-risk patients. Obstet Gynecol 67:358–364

43. Maulik D, Nanda N, Perry G (1987) Application of Doppler echocardiography in the human fetus. In: Maulik D, McNellis D (eds) Doppler ultrasound measurement of maternal–fetal hemodynamics. Perinatology Press, Ithaca, New York, pp 167–184

44. Sahn D, Shenker L, Reed K (1982) Prenatal ultrasound diagnosis of hypoplastic left heart syndrome in utero associated with hydrops fetalis. Am Heart J 104:1368–1372

45. Reed K (1989) Fetal Doppler echocardiography. Clin Obstet Gynecol 32:728–737

46. Meise C, Germer U, Gembruch U (2001) Arterial Doppler ultrasound in 115 second- and third-trimester fetuses with congenital heart disease. Ultrasound Obstet Gynecol 17:398–402

47. Respondek M, Kaluzynski A, Alwasiak J et al. (1993) Fetal endocarditis in left atrial isomerism: a case report. Ultrasound Obstet Gynecol 3:45–47

48. Guntheroth W, Cyr D, Winter T et al. (1993) Fetal Doppler echocardiography in pulmonary atresia. J Ultrasound Med 5:281–284

49. DeVore G, Horenstein J, Saissi B et al. (1987) Fetal echocardiography. VII. Doppler color flow mapping: a new technique for the diagnosis of congenital heart disease. Am J Obstet Gynecol 156:1054–1064

50. Rustico MA, Benettoni A, Bussani R, Maieron A, Mandruzzato G (1995) Early fetal endocardial fibroelastosis and critical aortic stenosis: a case report. Ultrasound Obstet Gynecol 202–205

51. DeVore G (1991) The use of color Doppler imaging to examine the fetal heart: normal and pathologic anatomy. In: Jaffe R, Warsof S (eds) Color Doppler imaging in obstetrics and gynecology. McGraw-Hill, New York, pp 121–154

52. Paladini D, Calabro R, Palmieri S et al. (1993) Prenatal diagnosis of congenital heart disease and fetal karyotyping. Obstet Gynecol 81:679–682

53. Birnbacher R, Salzer-Muhar U, Kurtaran A, Marx M et al. (2000) Survival after intrauterine myocardial infarction: noninvasive assessment of myocardial perfusion with ^{99m}Tc-sestamibi scintigraphy Am J Perinatol 17:309–331

54. Bernstein D, Finkbeiner W, Soifer S, Teitel D (1986) Perinatal myocardial infarctions: a case report and review of the literature. Pediatr Cardiol 6:313–317

55. Boulton J, Henry R, Roddick LG, Rogers D et al. (1991) Survival after neonatal infarction. Pediatrics 88:145–150

56. Balbul ZR, Rosenthal DN, Kleinman CS (1994) Myocardial infarction in the perinatal period secondary to maternal cocaine abuse: a case report and literature review. Arch Pediatr Adolesc Med 148:1092–1096

57. Holzgreve W, Holzgreve B, Curry C (1985) Nonimmune hydrops fetalis: diagnosis and management. Semin Perinatol 9:52–67

58. Hutchison A (1990) Pathophysiology of hydrops fetalis. In: Long W (ed) Fetal and neonatal cardiology. Saunders, Philadelphia, pp 197–210

59. Lingman G, Legarth J, Rahman F et al. (1991) Myocardial contractility in the anemic human fetus. Ultrasound Obstet Gynecol 1:266–268

60. Saltzman D, Frigoletto F, Harlow B et al. (1989) Sonographic evaluation of hydrops fetalis. Obstet Gynecol 74:106–111

61. Sikkel E, Vandenbussche FPHA, Oepkes D, Meerman R et al. (2002) Amniotid fluid delta OD 450 values accurately predict severe fetal anemia in D-alloimmunization. Obstet Gynecol 100:51–57

62. Moise KJ (2002) Management of rhesus alloimmunization in pregnancy. Obstet Gynecol 100:600–611

63. Mari G (2000) Noninvasive diagnosis by Doppler ultrasonography of fetal anemia due to maternal red-cell alloimmunization. N Engl J Med 342:9–14

64. Bahado-Singh RO, Oz AU, Hsu CD et al. (2000) Middle cerebral artery Doppler velocimetric deceleration angle as a predictor of fetal anemia in Rh-alloimmunized fetuses without hydrops. Am J Obstet Gynecol 183:746–751

65. Detti L, Oz U, Guney I et al. (2001) Doppler ultrasound velocimetry for timing the second intrauterine transfusion in fetuses with anemia from red cell alloimmunization. Am J Obstet Gynecol 185:1048–1051

66. Hajdu J (2002) Non-invasive diagnosis and follow-up of fetal anemia. Ultrasound Rev Obstet Gynecol 2:73–82

67. Hill LM (2001) Non-immune hydrops. Ultrasound Rev Obstet Gynecol 1:248–255

68. Jauniaux E, Hertzkovitz R, Hall JM (2000) First-trimester prenatal diagnosis of a thoracic cystic lesion associated with fetal skin edema. Ultrasound Obstet Gynecol 16:74–77

69. Thibeault DW, Black P, Taboada E (2002) Fetal hydrops and familial pulmonary lymphatic hypoplasia. Am J Perinatol 19:323–331

70. Schmider A, Henrich W, Reles A, Vogel M, Dudenhausen JW (2001) Isolated fetal ascites caused by primary lymphangiectasia: a case report. Am J Obstet Gynecol 184:277–278

71. Sergi C, Beedgen B, Kopitz et al. (1999) Refractory congenital ascites as a manifestation of neonatal sialidosis: clinical, biochemical and morphological studies in a newborn Syrian male infant. Am J Perinatol 16:133–141

72. Levine Z, Sherer DM, Jacobs A, Rotenberg O (1998) Nonimmune hydrops fetalis due to congenital syphilis associated with negative intrapartum maternal serology screening. Am J Perinatol 15:233–236

73. Kleinman C, Donnerstein R, DeVore G et al. (1982) Fetal echocardiography for evaluation of in utero congestive heart failure. N Engl J Med 306:568–575

74. Iskaros J, Jauniaux E, Rodeck C (1997) Outcome of nonimmune hydrops fetalis diagnosed during the first half of pregnancy. Obstet Gynecol 90:321–325

75. Wy CAW, Sajous CH, Loberiza F, Weiss MG (1999) Outcome of infants with a diagnosis of hydrops fetalis in the 1990s. Am J Perinatol 16:561–567

76. Kleinman C, Copel J (1992) In utero cardiac therapy. In: Kleinman C, Copel J (eds) Medicine of the fetus and mother. Lippincott, Philadelphia, pp 800–814

77. Lingman G, Maršál K (1987) Fetal cardiac arrhythmias: Doppler assessment. Semin Perinatol 11:357–361

78. Pinsky W, Rayburn W, Evans M (1991) Pharmacologic therapy for fetal arrhythmias. Clin Obstet Gynecol 34:304–309

79. Kleinman C, Copel J (1991) Electrophysiological principles and fetal antiarrhythmic therapy. Ultrasound Obstet Gynecol 1:286–297

80. Krapp M, Baschat AA, Gembruch U, Geipel A, Germer U (2002) Flecainide in the intrauterine treatment of fetal supraventricular tachycardia. Ultrasound Obstet Gynecol 19:158–164

81. Allan L (1990) Fetal arrhythmias. In: Long W (ed) Fetal and neonatal cardiology. Saunders, Philadelphia, pp 180–184

82. Chan F, Woo S, Ghosh A et al. (1990) Prenatal diagnosis of congenital fetal arrhythmias by simultaneous pulsed Doppler velocimetry of the fetal abdominal aorta and inferior vena cava. Obstet Gynecol 76:200–205

83. Schade RP, Stoutenbeek P, deVries LS, Meijboom EJ (1999) Neurological morbidity after fetal supraventricular tachyarrhythmia. Ultrasound Obstet Gynecol 13:43–47

84. Rabinerson D, Gruber A, Kaplan B, Lurie S, Peled Y, Neri A (1997) Isolated persistent fetal bradycardia in complete A-V block: a conservative approach is appropriate. A case report and review of the literature. Am J Perinatol 14:317–319

85. Copel JA, Liang R, Demasio K, Ozeren S, Kleinman CS (2000) The clinical significance of the irregular fetal heart rhythm. Am J Obstet Gynecol 182:813–819

86. Singh GK, Shumway JB, Amon E, Marino CJ, Nouri S, Winn HN (1998) Role of fetal echocardiography in the management of isolated fetal heart block with ventricular rate of <55 bpm. Am J Perinatol 15:661–668

87. Cuneo BF, Strasburger JF (2000) Management strategy for fetal tachycardia. Obstet Gynecol 96:575–587

88. Tongsong T, Wanapirak C, Sirichotiyakul S et al. (1999) Fetal sonographic cardiothoracic ratio at midpregnancy as a predictor of Hb Bart disease. J Ultrasound Med 18:807–811

89. Simpson LL, Marx GR, D'Alton ME (1997) Supraventricular tachycardia in the fetus: conservative management in the absence of hemodynamic compromise. J Ultrasound Med 16:459–464

90. Leung WC, Oepkes D, Seaward G, Ryan G (2002) Serial sonographic findings of four fetuses with homozygous alpha-thalassemia-1 from 21 weeks onwards. Ultrasound Obstet Gynecol 19:56–59

91. Lam YH, Tang HY, Lee CP, Tse HY (1999) Cardiac blood flow studies in fetuses with homozygous alpha-thalassemia-1 at 12–13 weeks of gestation. Ultrasound Obstet Gynecol 13:48–51

92. Naulaers G, Barten S, Banhole C et al. (1999) Management of severe neonatal anemia due to fetomaternal transfusion. Am J Perinatol 16:193–196

93. Ranzini AC, Shen-Schwarz S, Guzman ER et al. (1998) Prenatal sonographic appearance of hemorrhagic cerebellar infarction. J Ultrasound Med 17:725–727

94. de Spirlet M, Goffinet R, Philippe HJ et al. (2000) Prenatal diagnosis of a subdural hematoma associated with reverse flow in the middle cerebral artery: case report and literature review. Ultrasound Obstet Gynecol 16:72–76

95. Stringini FA, Cioni G, Canapicchi R et al. (2001) Fetal intracranial hemorrhage: Is minor maternal trauma a possible pathogenetic factor? Ultrasound Obstet Gynecol 18:335–342

96. Brown DL, Benson CB, Driscoll SG et al. (1989) Twin-twin transfusion syndrome: sonographic findings. Radiology 170:61–63

97. Danskin FH, Neilson JP (1989) Twin-to-twin transfusion syndrome: What are the appropriate diagnostic criteria? Am J Obstet Gynecol 161:365–369

98. Shah DM, Chaffin D (1989) Perinatal outcome in very preterm births with twin–twin transfusion syndrome. Am J Obstet Gynecol 161:1111–1113

99. Urig MA, Clewell WH, Elliott JP (1990) Twin–twin transfusion syndrome. Am J Obstet Gynecol 163:1522–1526

100. Gonsoulin W, Moise KJ, Krishon B et al. (1990) Outcome of twin–twin transfusion diagnosed before 28 weeks of gestation. Obstet Gynecol 75:214–216

101. Mahony BS, Petty CN, Nyberg DA et al. (1990) The "stuck twin" phenomenon: ultrasonographic findings, pregnancy outcome, and management with serial amniocenteses. Am J Obstet Gynecol 163:1513–1522

102. Skupski DW, Chervenak FA (2001) Twin–twin transfusion syndrome: an evolving challenge. Ultrasound Rev Obstet Gynecol 1:28–37

103. Shah Y, Gragg L, Moodley S et al. (1992) Doppler velocimetry in concordant and discordant twin gestations. Obstet Gynecol 80:272–276

104. Degani S, Gonen R, Shapiro I et al. (1992) Doppler flow velocity waveforms in fetal surveillance of twins: a prospective longitudinal study. J Ultrasound Med 11:537–541

105. Achiron R, Rabinovitz R, Aboulafia Y et al. (1992) Intrauterine assessment of high-output cardiac failure with spontaneous remission of hydrops fetalis in twin–twin transfusion syndrome: use of two-dimensional echocardiography, Doppler ultrasound and color flow mapping. J Clin Ultrasound 20:271–277

106. Mari G, Wasserstrum N, Kirshon B (1992) Reduction in the middle cerebral artery pulsatility index after decompression of polyhydramnios in twin gestation. Am J Perinatol 9:381–384

107. MacLean M, Mathers A, Walker J et al. (1992) The ultrasonic assessment of discordant growth in twin pregnancies. Ultrasound Obstet Gynecol 2:30–34

108. Ropacka M, Markwitz W, Breborowicz GH (2001) The role of Doppler blood flow velocimetry in multiple pregnancy. Ultrasound Rev Obstet Gynecol 1:307–314

109. Matias A, Montenegro N, Areias JC (2001) Ductus venosus blood flow evaluation at 11–14 weeks in the anticipation of twin–twin transfusion syndrome in monochorionic twin pregnancies. Ultrasound Rev Obstet Gynecol 1:315–321

110. Gonsoulin W, Moise KJ, Krishon B et al. (1990) Outcome of twin–twin transfusion diagnosed before 28 weeks of gestation. Obstet Gynecol 75:214–216

111. Chandran R, Serra-Serra V, Sellers S et al. (1993) Fetal cerebral Doppler in the recognition of fetal compromise. Br J Obstet Gynecol 100:139–144

112. Ott WJ (1990) Comparison of dynamic image and pulsed doppler ultrasonography for the diagnosis of intrauterine growth restriction. J Clin Ultrasound 18:3–11

113. Rizzo G, Arduini D, Romanini C (1992) Inferior vena cava flow velocity waveforms in appropriate and small-for-gestational-age fetuses. Am J Obstet Gynecol 166:1271–1280

114. Rizzo G, Arduini D (1991) Fetal cardiac function in intrauterine growth restriction. Am J Obstet Gynecol 165:876–882

115. Al-Ghazali W, Chita S, Chapman M et al. (1989) Evidence of redistribution of cardiac output in asymmetrical growth restriction. Br J Obstet Gynaecol 96:697–704

116. Makikallio K, Jouppila P, Rasanen J (2002) Retrograde net blood flow in the aortic isthmus in relation to human fetal arterial and venous circulations. Ultrasound Obstet Gynecol 19:147–152

117. Rizzo G, Arduini D, Romanini C (1992) Accelerated cardiac growth and abnormal cardiac flow in fetuses in type I diabetic mothers. Obstet Gynecol 80:369–376

118. Rizzo G, Arduini D, Romanini C (1991) Cardiac function in fetuses of type I diabetic mothers. Am J Obstet Gynecol 164:837–843

119. Salvesen D, Higueras M, Brudenell M et al. (1992) Doppler velocimetry and fetal heart rate studies in nephropathic diabetics. Am J Obstet Gynecol 167:1297–1303

120. Salvesen D, Higueras M, Mansur C et al. (1993) Placental and fetal Doppler velocimetry in pregnancies complicated by maternal diabetes mellitus. Am J Obstet Gynecol 168:645–652

121. Weiner Z, Zloczower M, Lerner A, Zimmer E, Itskovitz-Eldor J (1999) Cardiac compliance in fetuses of diabetic women. Obstet Gynecol 93:948–951

122. Axt-Fliedner R, Hendrik HJ, Ertan K, Remberger K, Schmidt W (2001) Course and outcome of a pregnancy with a giant fetal cervical teratoma diagnosed prenatally. Ultrasound Obstet Gynecol 18:543–546

123. Wang RM, Shih JC, Ko TM (2000) Prenatal sonographic depiction of fetal mediastinal immature teratoma. J Ultrasound Med 19:289–292

124. Chisholm CA, Heider AL, Kuller JA et al. (1999) Prenatal diagnosis and perinatal management of fetal sacrococcygeal teratoma. Am J Perinatol 16:89–92

125. Eirich C, Longo S, Palmgren M, Finnan JH, Ross-Ascuitto N (2002) Unusual sonographic appearance of a large fetal cardiac rhabdomyoma. J Ultrasound Med 21:681–685

126. Tseng JJ, Chou MM, Lee YH, Ho ESC (1999) In utero diagnosis of cardiac hemangioma. Ultrasound Obstet Gynecol 13:363–365

127. Morine M, Takeda T, Minekawa R et al. (2002) Antenatal diagnosis and treatment of a case of fetal goitrous hypothyroidism associated with high-output cardiac failure. Ultrasound Obstet Gynecol 19:506–509

128. Lee TH, Shih JC, Peng SSF et al. (2000) Prenatal depiction of angioarchitecture of an aneurysm of the vein of Galen with three-dimensional color power angiography. Ultrasound Obstet Gynecol 15:337–340

129. Zalel Y, Weisz B, Gamzu R et al. (2002) Chorioangiomas of the placenta: sonographic and Doppler flow characteristics. J Ultrasound Med 21:909–913

130. Nakai Y, Nishio J, Tsujimura A et al. (1998) Management of large placental chorioangioma with Doppler flow velocimetry. Ultrasound Obstet Gynecol 11:80–81

131. Levy R, Matitiau A, Arie AB, Milman D, Or Y, Hagay Z (1999) Indomethacin and corticosteroids: an additive constrictive effect on the fetal ductus arteriosus. Am J Perinatol 16:379–383

132. Fisher D (1990) Cardiomyopathies. In: Long W (ed) Fetal and neonatal cardiology. Saunders, Philadelphia, pp 499–510

Chapter 36

Doppler Echocardiographic Studies of Deteriorating Growth-Restricted Fetuses

Domenico Arduini, Giuseppe Rizzo

Intrauterine growth restriction (IUGR) is associated with significant perinatal mortality and morbidity [1, 2]. Adequate management of this condition requires early recognition of small-for-gestational-age (SGA) fetuses, a differential diagnosis of the factors that induce a delay in growth, monitoring the fetal condition, and determining the time of delivery.

The differential diagnosis between these etiologies is complex, but the introduction of noninvasive (i.e., high-resolution ultrasound imaging and Doppler ultrasonography) and invasive (i.e., cordocentesis) techniques allows a differential diagnosis in most of the cases [3]. Doppler ultrasonography, by providing a unique tool with which to examine fetal and maternal circulations noninvasively, has greatly enhanced our knowledge of the circulatory adaptive mechanisms that occur with various complications of pregnancy including IUGR [4, 5]. In particular, the study of fetal intracardiac hemodynamics has clarified the pathophysiologic steps in progressive fetal deterioration, allowing better definition of the severity of fetal compromise. Accurate assessment of the fetal condition may have favorable effects on perinatal mortality and morbidity, as fetuses can be delivered before irreversible damage occurs. In this chapter we outline the importance of Doppler echocardiography for antenatal monitoring of IUGR fetuses, with special emphasis on the hemodynamic changes at the level of the fetal heart in the presence of progressive deterioration.

Pathophysiology

Although the pathophysiology underlying uteroplacental insufficiency is poorly understood, it is assumed that various maternal, uterine, placental, and perhaps fetal abnormalities cause a reduction in the supply of nutrients provided to the fetus through the placenta [5–7]. This situation induces Doppler-detectable modifications in various vascular districts. These changes may include increased impedance to flow at the level of the uterine arteries (believed secondary to failure or impairment of trophoblast invasion), which results

in poor uteroplacental blood perfusion [8, 9]. Similarly, impedance to flows is usually increased in the umbilical artery, which is considered an expression of high placental vascular resistance due to a reduction in the number of small muscular arteries in the tertiary stem villi or their obliteration [10–12]. Other explanations, such as increased fetal blood viscosity or reduced arterial blood pressure, have not been excluded [13, 14]. Irrespective of the underlying cause, the increased impedance in the uterine or umbilical arteries results in reducted delivery of oxygen and placental substrates to the fetus [5]. This condition causes differential changes of arterial vascular resistances in the fetal circulation with vasodilatation at the level of the brain and myocardium and constriction at the muscular and visceral level, resulting in the brain-sparing effect [15–17], a phenomenon long recognized in animal models [18]. Thus during the first stage of the disease, the supply of substrates and oxygen to vital organs is maintained at near-normal levels despite an absolute reduction of placental transfer.

The temporal sequence of Doppler-detectable modifications during a pregnancy with developing IUGR is still unknown. Sometimes abnormal uterine artery velocity waveforms are the first Doppler-detectable sign [19]. IUGR may occur even in the presence of normal uterine artery velocity waveforms, suggesting an etiology primarily related to abnormal placental function. Similarly, there is no evidence as to whether the abnormalities in the umbilical artery occur earlier, simultaneously, or later than those in fetal vessels [20]. As already stated, despite the common denominator of a reduced supply of nutrients, IUGR has multiple etiologies that may involve the uterine circulation, placenta, or fetal circulation.

Persistence of nutritional deprivation leads to progressive deterioration of the fetal condition with further hemodynamic changes mainly affecting cardiac function [21, 22] and causing abnormalities in the venous system [23]. Additional modifications include abnormalities in fetal motor behavior and heart rate patterns [6, 24]. Finally, if the fetus is not delivered in due course, fetal death ensues.

tween the first Doppler abnormalities in the umbilical or fetal circulation (i.e., brain-sparing effect) and delivery is usually wide. According to published data it may range from 1 to 9 weeks [49–52].

Knowledge of the temporal hemodynamic sequence in IUGR fetuses after establishment of the brain-sparing phenomenon has important clinical implications. In fact, there are reports that IUGR fetuses that are acidotic during intrauterine life or that have antepartum abnormal heart rate tracings exhibit poor neurologic development at 2 years [53, 54]. This finding has led some authors to suggest that IUGR fetuses should be delivered before the onset of abnormal fetal heart rate patterns (suggestive of fetal acidemia) in order to avoid the consequence of prolonged malnutrition and hypoxia on the brain [24]. Moreover, gestational age should be taken into account, as the anticipation of the time of delivery may increase the risk of prematurity-related neonatal complications [50, 51].

At present, irrespective of the criteria for timing the delivery of these fetuses, knowledge of the progressive hemodynamic changes in deteriorating IUGR fetuses may help to clarify their natural history and to predict the time left before the onset of abnormal heart rate patterns. Serial studies on IUGR fetuses followed from the diagnosis to the onset of heart rate late decelerations have allowed us to partly clarify the hemodynamic changes at various placental and fetal levels. A theoretic scheme of the temporal sequence of Doppler changes secondary to uteroplacental insufficiency is outlined in Table 36.1.

Table 36.1. Suggested hemodynamic steps during deterioration of IUGR fetuses and concomitant Doppler changes

Hemodynamic steps	Doppler findings
Brain-sparing phenomenon	Increased UA/MCA
Change of cardiac afterload	Increased pulmonary artery TPV Decreased aortic TPV
Redistribution of cardiac output	Decreased RCO/LCO
Decreased cardiac output	Decreased aortic PV Decreased pulmonary PV
Increased venous pressure	Increased percent reverse flow in IVC Increased S/A in DV UV pulsations
Decompensation	Abnormal FHR patterns

UA, umbilical artery; MCA, middle cerebral artery; TPV, time to peak velocity; RCO/LCO, right/left cardiac output; PV, peak velocity; IVC, inferior vena cava; S/A, systolic peak velocity/atrial madir ratio; DV, ductus venosus; UV, umbilical vein; FHR, fetal heart rate.

Umbilical Artery

Experimental animal models in which obliteration of the placenta is achieved through embolization of the umbilical artery with microspheres have been used to show that only after 50% occlusion is there an increase in Doppler-measured vascular impedance [55]. This concept, validated in vitro [56, 57], suggests that wide damage of the placental vascular bed is already present at the time of diagnosis. However, further changes may occur, usually increasing progressively and dramatically around the onset of abnormal fetal heart rate patterns [16].

Fetal Peripheral Vessels

Doppler studies on the fetal descending thoracic aorta and fetal renal artery have shown that after establishment of the brain-sparing phenomenon further modifications of the PI occur with a behavior similar to that described for the umbilical artery [16] (i.e., a slight increase during the first stage of the disease followed by a rapid increase at the last stage of the disease). Of particular interest are the relations between the fetal renal artery PI and fetal PO_2, urine production, and amniotic fluid volume [58, 59].

Cerebral Vessels

After establishment of the brain-sparing effect, additional changes occur in the cerebral circulation as assessed by the PI in the middle cerebral artery or internal carotid artery, but the trend of these changes differs from that described for the umbilical artery and fetal peripheral vessels [16, 17, 51]. Indeed, the PI decrease is progressive during the first stage of the disease, reaching a nadir at least 2 weeks before the onset of abnormal fetal heart rate patterns [16, 60]. Furthermore, it has been shown that a few hours before fetal death there is a loss of cerebral vasodilatation despite the persistence of high resistance in peripheral vessels [61, 62]. These terminal changes are consistent with those reported in animal models [63]. However, Hecher et al. [51] found that in fetuses delivered before 32 weeks' gestation, middle cerebral artery PI became progressively abnormal until delivery, which is in contrast to the findings of Arduini et al. [16], who found that PI of cerebral vessels did not change in the last week preceding fetal heart rate abnormalities, and Weiner et al. [63], who even found a normalization of middle cerebral artery PI before the occurrence of abnormal fetal heart rate. Johnson et al. [65] demonstrated that increased middle cerebral artery PI may also occur in absence of premorbid fetal state, particularly in very preterm IUGR fetuses.

The significance of the different trends between cerebral vessels and peripheral or umbilical vessels is obscure, but two hypotheses can be suggested. The first is related to different vascular sensitivities to fetal hypoxemia. The cerebral vessels may experience massive vasodilatation in reaction to a mild to moderate level of hypoxemia, whereas profound changes in fetal peripheral vessels may occur only after severe hypoxemia or acidosis [18]. This concept is validated by cordocentesis data showing that the relation between vasodilation in the middle cerebral artery and hypoxemia exists only if the hypoxemia is mild to moderate; with more severe hypoxemia and acidemia the reduction in PI reaches a nadir that has been suggested to represent maximal cerebral vessel dilatation [66]. Similarly, in fetal lamb models with progressively deteriorating fetal oxygenation, it has been shown that the modifications in cerebral blood flow occur at an early stage of hypoxemia, whereas only minimal changes are present in peripheral vascular areas [18]. With more severe hypoxemia vascular resistance and organ flow changes in peripheral vessels occur abruptly, associated with further small increases or even reductions in cerebral blood flow [63].

An alternative explanation is based on the impairment of fetal cardiac function at the last stage of the disease, leading to decreased cardiac output [51, 66, 67]. Because the PI is highly and inversely dependent on input pressure and therefore on cardiac output [68], a decrease in cardiac contractility may explain the increase in peripheral and umbilical vessels. Moreover, the autoregulatory mechanisms of the cerebral circulation may maintain the nadir of cerebral vasodilatation until impending fetal death when the PI values may increase [66, 69].

The implications of changes in middle cerebral artery blood flow on subsequent long-term neurodevelopment are unclear. Some follow-up studies have suggested that the brain-sparing effect is a benign adaptation in IUGR fetuses [70, 71]; however, further long-term studies are required to establish the natural history of such cases.

Fetal Cardiac Flows

Uteroplacental insufficiency greatly affects fetal cardiac function. The brain-sparing effect induces selective changes in cardiac afterload that occur in IUGR fetuses (i.e., decreased left ventricle afterload due to cerebral vasodilation and increased right ventricle afterload due to systemic vasoconstriction). Furthermore, hypoxemia may impair myocardial contractility and polycythemia, which is usually present [72], may alter blood viscosity and therefore the preload. As a consequence, IUGR fetuses exhibit impaired ventricular filling properties [67, 73], lower peak velocities in the aorta and pulmonary arteries [21, 74] (Figs. 36.1, 36.2), increased aortic and decreased pulmonary TPV [44], and a relative increase in left cardiac output associated with decreased right cardiac output [67]. These hemodynamic intracardiac modifications are compatible with a preferential shift of cardiac output in favor of the left ventricle, leading to improved perfusion to the brain; and they occur simultaneously with the changes in fetal peripheral vessels.

Serial recordings have allowed us to clarify the evolution of intracardiac modifications in IUGR fetuses [66]. TPV values and the ratio of right/left ventricular outputs remain stable during serial recordings in such fetuses, suggesting that there are no other significant changes in outflow resistance or cardiac output redistribution after establishment of the

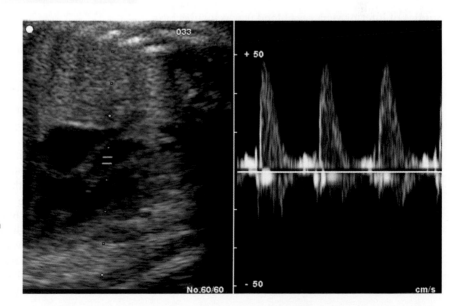

Fig. 36.1. Doppler tracing from the aortic outflow tract in an IUGR fetus at 29 weeks' gestation. The peak velocity is 48 cm/s (normal value for gestation is 64 cm/s)

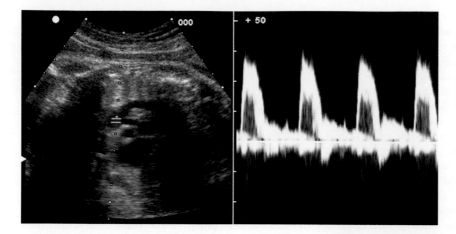

Fig. 36.2. Doppler tracing from the pulmonary artery in an IUGR fetus at 29 weeks' gestation. The peak velocity is 37 cm/s (normal value for gestation is 57 cm/s)

brain-sparing mechanism. However, peak velocities and cardiac output progressively decline, rather than rise with gestation as expected. The ventricular ejection force decreases in both ventricles and the different hemodynamic conditions in the vascular district (reduced cerebral resistance for the left ventricle and increased splanchnic and placental resistances for the right ventricle) can explain this decline in cardiac output. These changes may reflect decompensation of a normally protective mechanism responsible for the brain-sparing effect. According to this model, the fetal heart adapts to placental insufficiency in a manner that helps to maximize brain substrate and oxygen supply. With progressive deterioration of the fetal condition, this protective mechanism is overwhelmed by the decreased cardiac output, which may explain the reported changes in fetal peripheral vessels and the venous circulation.

Fetal Venous Flows

Studies of inferior vena cava blood flow velocities have demonstrated a characteristic pattern during fetal heart failure [75, 76]. Changes in venous blood velocity have been described during congestive heart failure with decreased diastolic blood velocity and increased reversal of flow during atrial contraction [76].

In IUGR fetuses an increase of reverse flow during atrial contraction may be present in the most severely compromised fetuses [23, 77] (Fig. 36.3). As a consequence of these abnormal venous flow patterns, the return of blood from the placenta to the heart is impaired, further reducing the supply of oxygen and nutrients. These findings are compatible with the decrease in both cardiac output and aortic and pulmonary peak velocities in deteriorating IUGR fetuses [50, 66, 78]. These changes are an expression of the sample phenomenon (i.e., cardiac decompensation) that impairs both the filling and the output of the heart. Concomitant changes are present in the ductus

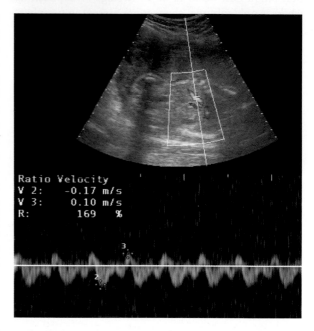

Fig. 36.3. Doppler tracing from the inferior cava in an IUGR fetus at 29 weeks' gestation. The percent reverse flow in the inferior vena cava is 16.9% (normal value for gestation is 7.4%)

venosus of IUGR fetuses, where the velocity during atrial contraction is significantly reduced or reversed [50, 62, 79] (Fig. 36.4).

It seems that the blood velocity waveform in the hepatic vein is an earlier predictor of intrauterine death than that of the ductus venosus [78]. This might be due to the fact that the hepatic vein is nearer the heart and blood flow from the right liver lobe flows mainly to the right side of the heart, while that from the ductus venosus flows mainly to the left ventricle in the foramen ovale. The fetal left ventricle in IUGR fetuses usually has to work against a lower afterload than the right ventricle, due to brain spar-

Fig. 36.4. Doppler tracing from the ductus venosus in an IUGR fetus at 27 weeks' gestation. (The PI normal value for gestation is 0.55)

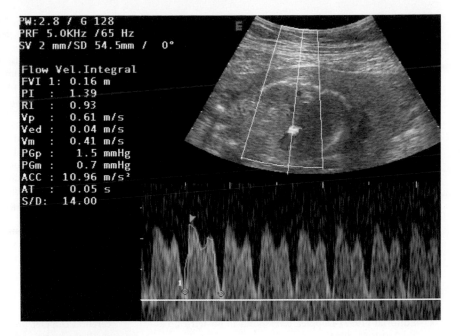

Fig. 36.5. Doppler tracing from the umbilical artery and vein in an IUGR fetus at 27 weeks' gestation. Note the absence of end-diastolic velocity in the umbilical artery and the end-diastolic pulsation in the umbilical vein

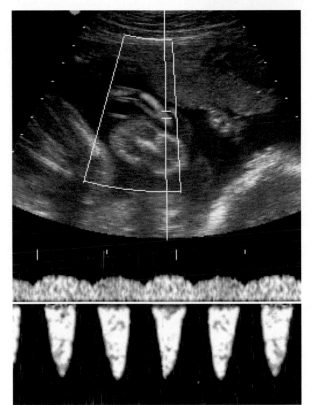

ing in chronic hypoxia. The differences in afterload might cause some differences in timing of signs of imminent heart failure in the two vessels. As flow from the right hepatic vein mainly enters the right ventricle, a compromised fetal state may therefore be expressed better in the hepatic vein than in the ductus venosus [79].

The presence of pulsations in the umbilical vein (Fig. 36.5) indicates severe cardiac compromise and imminent asphyxia. Double pulsation is known to be a more severe sign of fetal compromise and a direct reflection of pulsation in the central vein due to opening of the ductus venosus, either due to the hypoxia or increased central venous pressure [79, 80].

In IUGR fetuses the presence of pulsations in the umbilical vein is associated with a fivefold increase in perinatal mortality compared to IUGR fetuses with continuous umbilical flow [80, 81]. Actuarial analysis has demonstrated that of all the Doppler indices for IUGR fetuses, the pathological venous velocimetry in the vena cava, hepatic vein, and ductus venosus and the onset of umbilical vein pulsations are the events that best predict the onset of abnormal heart rate patterns [60, 79]. Hence, venous Doppler should be considered when timing delivery.

Conclusions

Examination of the fetal circulation by Doppler techniques provides evidence of some of the mechanisms of adaptation and decompensation of the IUGR fetus in response to uteroplacental insufficiency. At present, the condition of IUGR fetuses can be accurately assessed by sequential studies of Doppler waveforms from various vascular areas. Therefore the optimal timing of delivery to prevent intrauterine injury may be guided by combining multivessel Doppler ultrasounds. Combining Doppler, composite biophysical profile, and/or computerized fetal heart rate analysis will provide significant early indication for action in the management of severe IUGR fetuses.

References

1. Dobson PC, Abell DA, Beisher NA (1981) Mortality and morbidity of fetal growth retardation. Aust NZ J Obstet Gynaecol 21:69–72

2. McIntire DD, Bloom SL, Casey BM, Leveno KJ (1999) Birth weight in relation to morbidity and mortality among newborn infants. N Engl J Med 340:1234–1238

3. Wladimiroff JW (1991) Review of the etiology, diagnostic technique and management of IUGR, and the clinical application of Doppler in the assessment of placental blood flow. J Perinat Med 19:11–13

4. Editorial (1992) Doppler ultrasound in obstetrics. Lancet 339:1083–1084

5. Nicolaides KH, Rizzo G, Hecher K (2000) Doppler studies in fetal hypoxemic hypoxia. In: Nicolaides KH (ed) Placental and fetal Doppler. Parthenon Publishing London NewYork, pp 67–88

6. Visser GHA, Bekedam DJ, Ribbert LSM (1990) Changes in antepartum heart rate patterns with progressive fetal deterioration. Int J Biomed Comput 25:239–246

7. Pardi G, Marconi AM, Cetin I (2002) Placental-fetal interrelationship in IUGR fetuses – a review. Placenta 23[Suppl A]:S136–141

8. Schulman H, Fleisher A, Farmakides G et al (1986) Development of uterine artery compliance in pregnancy as detected by ultrasound. Am J Obstet Gynecol 155:1031–1036

9. Harrington K, Cooper D, Carpenter RG, Lees C, Hecher K, Campbell S (1996) Doppler ultrasound of uterine arteries: the importance of bilateral notching in the prediction of pre-eclampsia, placental abruption, or delivery of small for gestational age baby. Ultrasound Obstet Gynecol 7:182–188

10. Giles WB, Trudinger BJ, Baird PJ, Cook CM (1985) Fetal umbilical artery flow velocity waveforms and placental resistance: pathological correlation. Br J Obstet Gynaecol 92:31–36

11. Bracero LA, Beneck D, Kirshenbaum N et al (1989) Doppler velocimetry and placental disease. Am J Obstet Gynecol 161:388–393

12. Todros T, Sciarrone A, Piccoli E, Guiot C, Kaufmann P, Kingdom J (1999) Umbilical Doppler waveforms and placental villous angiogenesis in pregnancies complicated by fetal growth restriction. Obstet Gynecol 93: 499–503

13. Steel SA, Pearce JM, Nash G et al (1991) Correlation between the results of Doppler velocimetry with spectral analysis and the viscosity of cord blood. Rev Fr Gynecol Obstet 86:168–171

14. Fairle FM, Lang GD, Lowe GG, Walker JJ (1991) Umbilical artery flow velocity waveforms and cord blood viscosity. Am J Perinatol 9:250–253

15. Campbell S, Vyas S, Nicolaides KH (1991) Doppler investigation of the fetal circulation. J Perinat Med 19:21–26

16. Arduini D, Rizzo G, Romanini C (1992) Changes of pulsatility index from fetal vessels preceding the onset of late decelerations in growth retarded fetuses. Obstet Gynecol 79:605–610

17. Harrington K, Thompson MO, Carpenter RG, Nguyen M, Campbell S (1999) Doppler fetal circulation in pregnancies complicated by pre-eclampsia or delivery of a small for gestational age baby: 2. Longitudinal analysis. Br J Obstet Gynaecol 106:453–466

18. Peeters LLH, Sheldon RF, Jones MD, Makowsky EI, Meschia G (1979) Blood flow to fetal organ as a function of arterial oxygen content. Am J Obstet Gynecol 135:637–646

19. Harrington KF, Campbell S, Bewley S, Bower S (1991) Doppler velocimetry studies of the uterine artery in the early prediction of preeclampsia and intra-uterine growth retardation. Eur J Obstet Gynecol Reprod Biol 42[Suppl]:S14–S20

20. Severi FM, Bocchi C, Visentin A, Falco P, Cobellis L, Florio P, Zagonari S, Pilu G (2002) Uterine and fetal cerebral Doppler predict the outcome of third-trimester small-for-gestational age fetuses with normal umbilical artery Doppler. Ultrasound Obstet Gynecol 19:225–228

21. Groenenberg IA, Baerts W, Hop WC, Wladimiroff JW (1991) Relationship between fetal cardiac and extra-cardiac Doppler flow velocity waveforms and neonatal outcome in intrauterine growth retardation. Early Hum Dev 26:185–192

22. Rizzo G, Arduini D, Romanini C (1992) Doppler echocardiographic assessment of fetal cardiac function. Ultrasound Obstet Gynecol 2:434–445

23. Reed KL, Appleton CP, Anderson CF, Shenker L, Sahn DJ (1990) Doppler studies of vena cava flows in human fetuses: insights into normal and abnormal cardiac physiology. Circulation 81:498–505

24. Visser GHA, Stitger RH, Bruinse HW (1991) Management of the growth-retarded fetus. Eur J Obstet Gynecol Reprod Biol 42:S73–S78

25. Reuss ML, Rudolph AM (1980) Distribution and recirculation of umbilical and systemic venous blood flow in fetal lambs during hypoxia. J Dev Physiol 2:71–84

26. Burns PN (1987) Doppler flow estimations in the fetal and maternal circulations: principles, techniques and some limitations. In: Maulik D, McNellis D (eds) Doppler ultrasound measurement of maternal-fetal hemodynamics. Perinatology Press, Ithaca, NY, pp 43–78

27. Comstock CH, Riggs T, Lee W, Kirk J (1991) Pulmonary to aorta diameter ratio in the normal and abnormal fetal heart. Am J Obstet Gynecol 165:1038–1043

28. Stottard MF, Pearson AC, Kern MJ et al (1989) Influence of alteration in preload of left ventricular diastolic filling as assessed by Doppler echocardiography in humans. Circulation 79:1226–1236

29. Gardin JM (1989) Doppler measurements of aortic blood velocity and acceleration: load independent indexes of left ventricular performance? Am J Cardiol 64:935–936

30. Bedotto JB, Eichorn EJ, Grayburn PA (1989) Effects of left ventricular preload and afterload on ascending aortic blood velocity and acceleration in coronary artery disease. Am J Cardiol 64:856–859

Chapter

Eval
Feta
for |

James C

Studies
tion on
effects c
possible
long-ter
how the
siology
sess feti
clinical
the effe
tion. Th
circulat

In th
how tw
line, ai
niques
lation (
effects.
arterio:
this ty
the "se
and pr

Dop
sive to
gradier
fetal du
indom(
was de
ductal
ventric
pulmoi
nary h
echoca
manag
used t
medic

Feta

Fetal

Compl
volves
diogra

31. Brownwall E, Ross J, Sonnenblick EH (1976) Mechanism of contraction in the normal and failing heart, 2nd edn. Little, Brown, Boston, pp 92–129
32. Takaneka K, Dabestani A, Gardin JM et al (1986) Left ventricular filling in hypertrophic cardiomyopathy: a pulsed Doppler echocardiographic study. J Am Coll Cardiol 7:1263–1271
33. Kenny J, Plappert T, Doubilet P, Saltzam D, St John Sutton MG (1987) Effects of heart rate on ventricular size, stroke volume and output in the normal human fetus: a prospective Doppler echocardiographic study. Circulation 76:52–58
34. Rizzo G, Arduini D, Romanini C (1992) Inferior vena cava flow velocity waveforms in appropriate and small for gestational age fetuses. Am J Obstet Gynecol 166:1271–1280
35. Kiserud T, Eik-Nes LR, Blaas HG, Hellevik LR (1991) Ultrasonographic velocimetry of the ductus venosus. Lancet 338:1139–1145
36. Soregaroli M, Rizzo G, Danti L, Arduini D, Romanini C (1993) Effects of maternal hyperoxygenation on ductus venosus flow velocity waveforms in normal third trimester fetuses. Ultrasound Obstet Gynecol 3:115–119
37. Hecher K, Campbell S, Snijders R, Nicolaides K (1994) References for fetal venous and atrioventricular blood flow parameters. Ultrasound Obstet Gynecol 4:381–390
38. Rizzo G, Capponi A, Arduini D, Romanini C (1994) Ductus venosus velocity waveforms in appropriate and small for gestational age fetuses. Early Hum Dev 39:15–22
39. De Vore GR, Horenstein J (1993) Ductus venosus index: a method for evaluating right ventricular preload in the second trimester fetus. Ultrasound Obstet Gynecol 3:338–342
40. Rizzo G, Arduini D, Romanini C (1992) Pulsations in umbilical vein: a physiological finding in early pregnancy. Am J Obstet Gynecol 167:675–677
41. Baschat AA, Gembruch U, Weiner CP, Harman CR (2003) Qualitative venous Doppler waveform analysis improves prediction of critical perinatal outcomes in premature growth-restricted fetuses. Ultrasound Obstet Gynecol 22:240–245
42. Reed KL, Sahn DJ, Scagnelli S, Anderson CF, Shenker L (1986) Doppler echocardiographic studies of diastolic function in the human fetal heart: changes during gestation. J Am Coll Cardiol 8:391–395
43. Kitabatake A, Inoue M, Asao M et al (1983) Noninvasive evaluation of pulmonary hypertension by a pulsed Doppler technique. Circulation 68:302–309
44. Rizzo G, Arduini D, Romanini C, Mancuso S (1990) Doppler echocardiographic evaluation of time to peak velocity in the aorta and pulmonary artery of small for gestational age fetuses. Br J Obstet Gynaecol 97:603–607
45. Machado MVL, Chita SC, Allan LD (1987) Acceleration time in the aorta and pulmonary artery measured by Doppler echocardiography in the midtrimester normal human fetus. Br Heart J 58:15–18
46. Allan LD, Chita SK, Al-Ghazali W, Crawford DC, Tynan M (1987) Doppler echocardiographic evaluation of the normal human fetal heart. Br Heart J 57:528–533
47. De Smedt MCH, Visser GHA, Meijboom EJ (1987) Fetal cardiac output estimated by Doppler echocardiography during mid- and late gestation. Am J Cardiol 60:338–342
48. Rizzo G, Arduini D (1991) Cardiac output in anencephalic fetuses. Gynecol Obstet Invest 32:33–35
49. Bekedam DJ, Visser GHA, van der Zee AGJ, Snijders R, Poelmann-Weesjes G (1990) Abnormal umbilical artery waveforms patterns in growth retarded fetuses: relationship to antepartum late heart rate decelerations and outcome. Early Hum Dev 24:79–90
50. Hecher K, Campbell S, Doyle P, Harrington K, Nicolaides K (1995) Assessment of fetal compromise by Doppler ultrasound investigation of the fetal circulation. Arterial, intracardiac, and venous blood flow velocity studies. Circulation 92:129–138
51. Hecher K, Bilardo CM, Stigter RH, Ville Y, Hackeloer BJ, Kok HJ, Senat MV, Visser GH (2001) Monitoring of fetuses with intrauterine growth restriction: a longitudinal study. Ultrasound Obstet Gynecol 18:564–570
52. Baschat AA, Gembruch U, Harman CR (2001) The sequence of changes in Doppler and biophysical parameters as severe fetal growth restriction worsens. Ultrasound Obstet Gynecol 18:571–577
53. Soothill PW, Ajayi RA, Campbell S et al (1992) Relationship between acidemia at cordocentesis and subsequent neurodevelopment. Ultrasound Obstet Gynecol 2:80–84
54. Todds AL, Trudinger BJ, Cole MJ, Cooney GH (1992) Antenatal tests of fetal welfare and development at age 2 years. Am J Obstet Gynecol 167:66–71
55. Copel JA, Schlafer D, Wentworth R et al (1990) Does the umbilical artery systolic/diastolic ratio reflect flow or acidosis? Am J Obstet Gynecol 163:751–756
56. Guiot C, Pianta PG, Todros T (1992) Modelling the feto-placental circulation. 1. A distributed network predicting umbilical hemodynamics throughout pregnancy. Ultrasound Med Biol 18:535–544
57. Todros T, Guiot C, Pianta PG (1992) Modelling the feto-placental circulation. 2. A continuous approach to explain normal and abnormal flow velocity waveforms in the umbilical artery. Ultrasound Med Biol 18:545–551
58. Vyas S, Nicolaides KH, Campbell S (1989) Renal flow-velocity waveforms in normal and hypoxemic fetuses. Am J Obstet Gynecol 161:168–172
59. Arduini D, Rizzo G (1991) Fetal renal artery velocity waveforms and amniotic fluid volume in growth-retarded and post-term fetuses. Obstet Gynecol 77:370–374
60. Arduini D, Rizzo G, Romanini C (1993) The development of abnormal heart rate patterns after absent end diastolic velocity in umbilical artery: analysis of risk factors. Am J Obstet Gynecol 168:43–49
61. Mari G, Wasserstrum N (1991) Flow velocity waveforms of the fetal circulation preceding fetal death in a case of lupus anticoagulant. Am J Obstet Gynecol 164:776–778
62. Rizzo G, Capponi A, Pietropolli A et al (1994) Cardiac and extra-cardiac flow changes preceding intrauterine fetal death. Ultrasound Obstet Gynecol 4:139–143
63. Richardson BS, Rurak D, Patrick JE, Homan J, Carmichael L (1989) Cerebral oxidative metabolism during sustained hypoxemia in fetal sheep. J Dev Physiol 11:37–43
64. Weiner Z, Farmakides G, Schulman H, Penny B (1994) Central and peripheral hemodynamic changes in fetuses with absent end-diastolic velocity in umbilical artery: Correlation with computerized fetal heart rate pattern. Am J Obstet Gynecol 170:509–515

65.

66.

67.

68.

69.

70.

71.

72.

73.

The equipment for fetal Doppler examination is in a state of rapid evolution. At the present time, image-directed or color Doppler-directed pulsed-wave and continuous-wave Doppler ultrasonography is available to clinicians. Advances in several technologies have allowed progressive advances in this field. Better materials and an understanding of transducers and their design has led to improved acquisition of signals and an improved signal-to-noise ratio. The improvement in resolution for imaging also improves the spatial data collection for the Doppler setup and gives more confidence that the blood velocity came from the site where the sample volume was placed. Advances in broad-band amplifier design and phased-array and annular technologies affect modern obstetric Doppler equipment and allow the same transducer to be used efficiently for both Doppler sonography and imaging. Integration of imaging and Doppler sonography is now possible.

Color Doppler sonography is being applied to supplement other modes of ultrasonic scanning (see below). The color Doppler technique provides information about the flow of blood and specifically blood velocity in the structures being visualized.

The intensities of the various Doppler modalities are different. With a method of intensity assessment using the spatial peak temporal average (milliwatts per square centimeter, or mW/cm^2) as a measure of the heating potential of the ultrasound, the exposure for pulsed-wave, continuous-wave, and color Doppler technology can be compared [7].

Peripheral Doppler/Cardiac Doppler Sonography

The umbilical cord arterial Doppler pattern is characterized by a peak velocity during late systole, an end-diastolic velocity measured before the next upstroke, and the mean velocity, which is the average of the entire waveform over the cardiac cycle. The energy source for the umbilical waveform is the fetal heart. The left ventricle and (predominantly) the right ventricle pump blood to the placental circulation. The early part of the upstroke of the umbilical waveform gives information about the waveform passing from the heart to the peripheral circulation. It is determined by myocardial performance, large-vessel compliance and elastic properties, and arterial reflections along the fetal descending aorta. The rapidity of the upstroke should therefore relate to several factors that transmit a pressure waveform to the cord. Factors that would increase the rate of systolic velocity increase are increased myocardial inotropy, decreased compliance of the aortic wall, and high total impedance. The diastolic portion of the curve is not sharply demarcated but reflects the time when the semilunar valves are closed and the circulation propels blood based on its inertia and pressure

wave propagation during vascular relaxation. The principal determinant of the end-diastolic velocity is the distal resistance. The latter parameter is a consequence of both the systemic and parallel placental circulations. There is mor pulsation (pulsatility) in an umbilical waveform when the distal impedance is increased. Therefore cord pulsatility can be used as an indirect indicator of placental impedance. Waveforms with a high diastolic velocity are associated with high flow during diastole, and those with low or absent diastolic velocity have low diastolic flow.

The best index to use for analysis and communication of umbilical cord Doppler information is controversial. Several authors have presented arguments for the options [8], which include the pulsatility index (PI), the resistance (Pourcelot) index (RI), and the systolic/diastolic (S/D) ratio.

$$PI = (S - D)/\text{mean velocity}$$

$$RI = (S - D)/S$$

$$S/D \text{ ratio} = S/D$$

where S = peak systolic velocity and D = minimum diastolic velocity. Mean velocity equals the integrated mean over the cardiac cycle.

The PI is less susceptible to a variation in heart rate because the heart rate is an intrinsic factor in the mean velocity. This parameter requires digitalization of the entire waveform over one cycle and is the best parameter for longitudinal comparison. The RI and S/D ratio are popular because they require little computation. The PI of the peripheral circulation reflects the distal impedance and therefore is low with low impedance. In situations where there is kinetic energy release with discrete obstruction in the circulation, such as with carotid arterial obstruction or coarctation of the aorta, the PI may be used to describe the waveform changes. In this situation, a low PI is indicative of increased obstruction and pressure gradient and usually lower flow.

Cardiac Doppler examination is performed by placing the pulsed Doppler sample volume in the valve (arch) of interest during the examination as described below. The three major Doppler techniques (pulsed-wave, continuous-wave, and color) are complimentary in the fetal examination. All three are used during a complete examination of the heart and the peripheral vessels. Continuous-wave and pulsed-wave Doppler techniques have been applied to the assessment of fetal hemodynamics by detecting flow in the umbilical cord and studying the pulsatility of that waveform. The typical examination includes sampling many sites in the circulation.

Umbilical Cord

Optimal recordings in the umbilical cord have both arterial and venous tracings. The umbilical venous tracing is a low-velocity (20–30 cm/s) signal with high intensity. If there are cardiac pulsations in the umbilical venous trace, one should suspect increased venous pressures and cardiac failure.

Uterine Artery

Sampling the maternal circulation at the uterine artery provides a waveform that appears to correlate with uterine impedance. Early studies in these vessels suggested that detection of growth restriction is possible during pregnancy.

Descending Aorta

The pulsed sample volume should completely insonate the lumen of the descending aorta. The descending aorta has a high systolic velocity (50–100 cm/s) and a low diastolic velocity in the same direction as the systolic velocity. This waveform has been shown to change in the presence of growth restriction, probably indicative of increased total systemic resistance. In the extreme example of a fetus with advanced growth disturbance, there is an absence of end-diastolic flow.

Middle Cerebral Artery

The middle cerebral artery (MCA) is used as an indicator of brain vascular impedance. The normal pattern is similar to that in the umbilical cord at a lower velocity. The diastolic velocity can be elevated with severe intrauterine growth restriction (IUGR), presumably indicative of compensatory cerebral vasodilation, the brain-sparing effect.

Renal Artery

The renal artery waveform is obtained in transverse sections of the abdomen during visualization of the kidneys. Color Doppler sonography greatly improves the percentage of patients from whom high-quality data can be obtained. The waveform has a high systolic velocity and a low diastolic velocity, similar to that in the descending aorta. The normally pulsatile renal vein is often noted while interrogating the proximal renal artery.

Ductal and Aortic Arches

The aortic arch and ductal arch may appear similar, but systolic velocity is always higher in the ductal arch. Ductal constriction is characterized by an increase in both systolic and diastolic velocities (see below).

Pulmonary and Aortic Valves

Pulsed-wave Doppler sonography in the semilunar valves shows a pattern of systolic ejection with a rapid upstroke in the pulmonary value and a slower upstroke in the aortic valve. The peak velocities of ejection may be useful for assessing cardiac output indirectly. Integration of the waveform gives the time-velocity integral (TVI) and is proportional to the stroke volume. Correcting for heart rate, any change in valve flow can be studied by comparing the TVI-heart rate product before and after the intervention [9]. If valve stenosis is present, there will be evidence of turbulence and the peak velocity will be slightly increased. If valve regurgitation is present, there will be an abnormal turbulent jet back into the ventricle during diastole.

Atrioventricular Valves

The mitral and tricuspid valves are assessed using pulsed-wave Doppler sonography from an apical view. The 2-mm sample volume is placed at the valve annulus to obtain a biphasic pattern during diastole consisting of an E wave (corresponding to the rapid filling of the ventricle) and an A wave (corresponding to atrial contraction). Systolic velocity back into the atria suggests valvar regurgitation and is detected on the pulsed-wave evaluation; however, the use of continuous-wave Doppler sonography is helpful for interrogating the atrioventricular (A-V) valve area. Grading valvar regurgitation is qualitative, with a nonholosystolic jet being classed as trivial and a holosystolic jet as significant. Most fetal valve regurgitation is trivial or mild in the absence of other signs of fetal congestive heart failure, such as an abnormal venous Doppler result. Because the peak velocity of A-V valve regurgitation is so typical and is higher than any other velocity in the fetal circulation, the range ambiguity introduced by the use of continuous-wave Doppler sonography does not cause any confusion. On the contrary, continuous-wave Doppler sonography with high filter settings can detect a tiny jet of A-V valve regurgitation and characterize the timing of it and the nature of the early upstroke velocity. Such a jet is turbulent and creates an abnormal finding on color Doppler interrogation owing to the high peak velocity. The most common cause of tricuspid valve regurgitation in our practice is the effect of indomethacin on the fetal ductus arteriosus.

Inferior Vena Cava

The waveform in the inferior vena cava (IVC) is normally biphasic during flow to the heart with an additional brief period of reversal during atrial systole. This waveform is useful for detecting abnormal forward flow states in the fetal circulation. The abnormal presence of an increase in reversal of blood velocity during atrial contraction suggests a state of fetal congestive heart failure [10, 11].

Pulmonary Veins

Pulmonary venous waveforms are similar to systemic venous (IVC) waveforms. Reversal in this site could indicate A-V valvar regurgitation, myocardial failure, or an obstruction to emptying the atrium.

Pulmonary Artery

Fetal pulmonary resistance is high, and a typical waveform in the left pulmonary artery reflects this state with biphasic forward flow: midsystolic reversal and brief reversal during early diastole. The end-diastolic velocity at this site is useful for evaluating the state of the fetal pulmonary vasculature. The normal finding is low velocity of forward flow into the pulmonary vascular bed. This flow is of markedly low velocity and may not be detectable using standard high-pass filter settings on the current equipment. Absence of this flow or the finding of reversal of flow during diastole suggests abnormal peripheral vascular impedance.

Fetal Ductal Evaluation

An Acuson 128 scanner, in combination with 5.0- and 3.5-MHz probes, is used for the fetal cardiovascular examination. After evaluation of the cardiac anatomy, continuous-wave Doppler interrogation of the flow through the ductus arteriosus is performed using 5.0- or 3.5-MHz image-directed continuous-wave Doppler sonography in a sagittal plane showing the pulmonary artery, ductus arteriosus, and descending aorta simultaneously as previously described [1]. Power output is kept below 100 mW/cm^2 spatial peak temporal average at all times. Each study is recorded on standard VHS 0.5-inch video tape for later analysis, although on-line analysis of the waveform of the blood velocity of the ductus is performed for immediate clinical reporting (pulsatility index). All Doppler recordings are obtained in the absence of fetal breathing movements at an angle of less than 30° to flow, and color flow mapping is used for alignment of the Doppler beam. Waveforms are analyzed for maximal, end-diastolic, and mean velocities, respectively. The PI is calculated using the formula: (maximal velocity – end-diastolic velocity)/mean velocity,

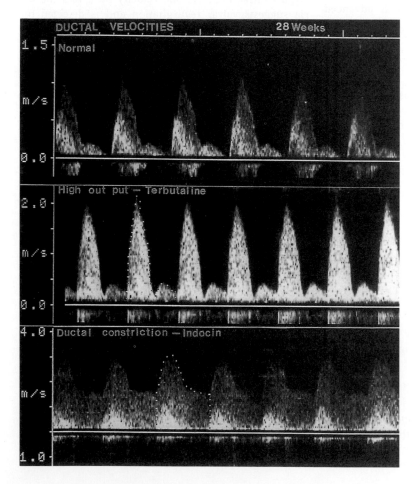

Fig. 37.1. Doppler waveforms in the fetal ductus arteriosus. *Top:* Normal waveform at 28 weeks shows a systolic velocity of approximately 1 m/s. *Middle:* During terbutaline administration to the mother, fetal Doppler sonography of the ductus shows increased peak velocity with little change in the end-diastolic velocity resulting in an increase in the pulsatility index (PI). *Bottom:* Fetal ductal constriction shows increased systolic and diastolic velocities and a decreased PI. (Reprinted from [13] with permission)

as described above. Therefore a decrease in the PI of the ductus arteriosus (below the normal values of 1.9–3.0) is suggestive of ductal constriction.

Normal Doppler Waveforms

The normal Doppler waveform in the fetal ductus arteriosus is characterized by high systolic velocity and low diastolic velocity from the main pulmonary artery to the descending aorta (Fig. 37.1). This velocity is the highest systolic one in the normal fetus that can be obtained by Doppler interogation of the fetal circulation and has a distinctive waveform. Color Doppler sonography is useful for obtaining continuous-wave Doppler images of the ductus in the ductal arch region where the velocity is highest. Aliasing in the ductal arch marks the site of peak velocity in a fetal sagittal imaging plane. It has been shown that maximal ductal blood velocity increases from 25 to 32 weeks' gestation [1], and data from our center based on a prospective longitudinal study from 121 examinations on 41 normal pregnant women showed a linear increase in systolic velocity from 14 to 40 weeks' gestation (Fig. 37.2). The ductal velocity was toward the descending aorta during systole (65–140 cm/s) and diastole (15–35 cm/s). The PI of the ductal velocity did not change with gestation (mean ± 2 standard deviations: 2.46 ± 0.52).

Ductal Constriction After Therapy for Preterm Labor

Second and third trimester fetuses have an increase in ductal blood velocities with increasing gestational age. The reasons for the increasing ductal blood velocity are complex: The ductal velocities are a function of multiple variables, including ductal wall caliber and compliance, systolic and diastolic ductal flow, and right ventricular function. Blood velocities of the fetal ductus arteriosus must be considered in relation to gestational age for correct interpretation.

Exposure to nonsteroidal antiinflammatory agents, with the prototype being indomethacin, can lead to constriction of the ductus and alterations in human cardiovascular physiology. This change is presumed due to inhibition of fetal prostaglandins. However, as-

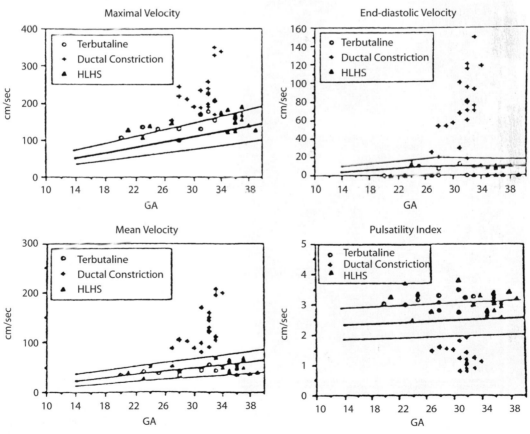

Fig. 37.2. Ductus ateriosus flow and pulsatility index in fetuses exposed to terbutaline ($n=10$), fetuses with ductal constriction ($n=22$), and fetuses with hypoplastic left heart syndrome ($n=14$) compared with normal range (mean ± 2 SD) versus gestational age. (Reprinted from [13] with permission)

say of the indomethacin levels in the maternal circulation (and presumably the fetal circulation) did not correlate with the presence or severity of ductal constriction [2]. Fetal ductal constriction is characterized by elevation of maximal end-diastolic ductal velocity resulting in a Doppler waveform similar to taht seen postnatally across coarctation of the aorta [1]. One may consider that fetal ductal constriction is really a hemodynamic coarctation of the ductus in utero. Typically, fetuses with structurally normal hearts presenting with preterm labor refractory to other agents with a gestational age of 23–32 weeks are treated with indomethacin in doses ranging from 25 to 50 mg every 4–6 h. After 24 h on indomethacin, increased ductal velocities consistent with constriction are found in 25%–40% of fetuses. Indications of constriction included increased systolic *and* diastolic velocities and a PI below 2.0 (Fig. 37.2). Evidence of constriction usually resolves within 1–5 days after discontinuation of indomethacin. Constriction also has been documented using ibuprofen or aspirin in this gestational age range.

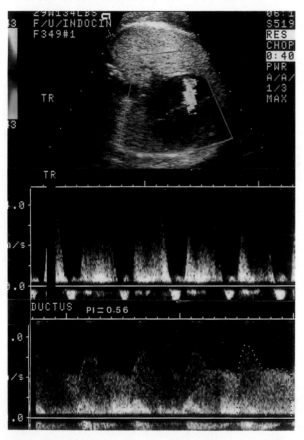

Fig. 37.3. *Top, middle:* Doppler patterns of ductal constriction with tricuspid valve regurgitation. Note the peak systolic velocity of 4 m/s. *Bottom:* The pattern of ductal constriction and the method of obtaining the mean velocity is shown with a pulsatility index of 0.56 (normal range 1.9–3.0)

Ductal constriction with the highest elevations of ductal systolic and diastolic velocity are often associated with the new finding of tricuspid regurgitation on Doppler examination (Fig. 37.3). It appears to be due to the fact that ductal constriction increases the right ventricular afterload (pulmonary artery pressure), thereby altering normal fetal tricuspid valve function. Fetal tricuspid valve regurgitation without cause is rare [12]. Marked decreases in the shortening of the right ventricle are also observed during severe constriction. Typical decreases in right ventricular shortening are from approximately 30% to 15%–20%.

Prolonged or severe constriction of the ductus may also be associated with tricuspid regurgitation and eventually right ventricular dysfunction and abnormal fetal perfusion. We recommended baseline fetal echocardiography on all women at the start of indeomethacin therapy (24–48 h after beginning therapy). Weekly echocardiograms should then be obtained for the duration of the therapy, specifically assessing the size and flow through the ductus, as well as the presence of tricuspid regurgitation. Venous Doppler examination is useful for detecting abnormal cardiac compensation [11]. Although tricuspid regurgitation in some settings is an ominous sign, in this setting it is of uncertain significance and in our experience has been transient [12]. Similar, ductal constriction has been observed but also resolves with discontinuation of indomethacin. Thus we do not alter indomethacin therapy solely on the basis of either ductal constriction (mild or moderate) or the finding of tricuspid regurgitation. Abnormal venous Doppler may indicate heart failure in this setting.

Hemodynamic Effects of Ductal Constriction

Fetal ductal constriction causes a significant change in the distribution of the cardiac output between the ventricles. Measurements using pulsed-wave Doppler sonography attempting to quantitate the semilunar valve outputs before and after ductal constriction have shown that the left ventricular output increases significantly with constriction of the fetal ductus (average 21%) relative to the baseline value. The ratio of aortic/pulmonary valve flow (time-velocity integral/heart rate product) increases. This redistribution of fetal flow to the left heart is the result of increased flow through the foramen ovale due to a decrease in right ventricular stroke volume and an increase in fetal pulmonary flow, which increases fetal pulmonary venous return.

Two to three days of fetal ductal constriction during tocolysis with indomethacin is well tolerated because cardiac flow redistributes to the left heart during constriction and combined cardiac output is maintained, therapy maintaining normal peripheral organ perfusion.

Clinical Implications of Ductal Constriction

Whether prolonged constriction of the ductus can lead to clinically significant hypertrophy of the smooth muscle in the pulmonary vascular bed is currently under investigation. The right ventricle develops hypertrophy rapidly during constriction, and little is known about its impact on gestation or the postnatal course. It seems prudent to evaluate a fetus exposed to chronic indomethacin at least weekly if there it no evidence of constriction and to increase the surveillance to daily examinations if ductal constriction is present with tricuspid regurgitation.

Ductal Occlusion

Ductal occlusion of 1–5 days duration was diagnosed by fetal echocardiography in our practice over 2 years in 6 of 115 fetuses exposed to indomethacin (mean gestational age 27.4 weeks) at 31–35 weeks' gestation. None was hydropic, and all six had (1) right ventricular enlargement with decreased shortening and tricuspid valve regurgitation; (2) increased main and branch pulmonary artery sizes; and (3) increased left ventricular shortening and aortic arch velocity. Ductal occlusion was differentiated from ductal constriction by an absence of flow in the ductus, seen by color Doppler ex-

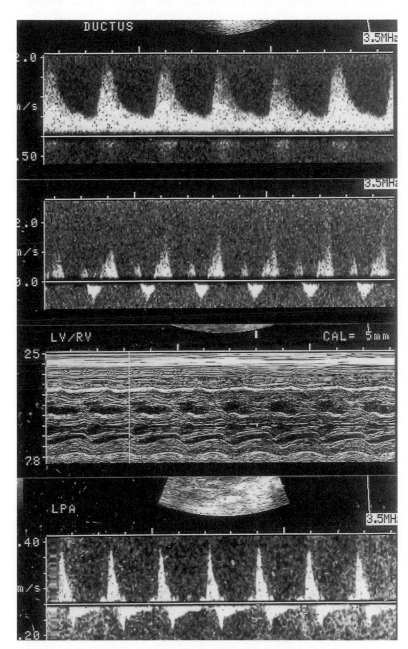

Fig. 37.4. Fetal echocardiography following fetal ductal occlusion of 1 week duration showing residual ductal constriction. *Top panel:* Ductal constriction is indicated by the persistently elevated velocities. *Second panel:* There is decreased forward flow in the pulmonary valve and slight pulmonary valve regurgitation, which is never seen in the normal fetus. *Third panel:* M-mode echocardiography shows residual thickening of the right ventricle. *Bottom panel:* Left branch of the pulmonary artery (*LPA*) Doppler velocity is abnormal, with diastolic reversal indicating elevated fetal pulmonary vascular resistance. The fetus resolved this pattern prior to birth and was delivered without complication

amination. Indomethacin was withdrawn when closure was diagnosed, and fetal echocardiography was repeated daily while terbutaline was used for tocolysis. The fetal ductus reopened 1–5 days after indomethacin withdrawal and was characterized by a period of ductal constriction varying from 1 to 10 days (median 2 days) (Fig. 37.4). All patients continued normal pregnancies, and none had postnatal pulmonary hypertension. The only residual finding after reopening was right ventricular hypertrophy in one pair of twins (both with closure that persisted 3 and 5 days, respectively, after two 50 mg doses at 32 weeks' gestation). One fetus with constriction was delivered without difficulty.

From this experience we concluded that the reopening of ductal occlusion occurred withint 2 weeks of indomethacin withdrawal without residual abnormality. Withdrawal is the optimal treatment if the gestation is premature. Additional studies are focus-

ing on myocardial adaptation of the fetal right ventricle to this increase in workload and the fetal pulmonary vascular response to this complication of indomethacin use.

Terbutaline

Fetuses whose mothers are treated with terbutaline for tocolysis have increased cardiac output [9], and we have noted markedly increased maximal ductal velocities in this setting. This drug, a sympathomimetic, increases the fetal heart rate and has a positive inotropic effect on the myocardium. Therefore all the peak systolic velocities in the fetal circulation are increased by maternal terbutaline administration (Fig. 37.5).

Clinically, mothers are often treated for preterm labor with terbutaline 5 mg PO every 4–6 h or by

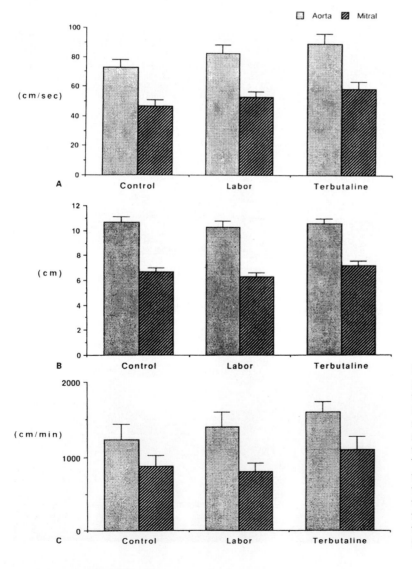

Fig. 37.5. Fetal left heart pulsed Doppler findings in fetuses with active preterm labor and others exposed to terbutaline transplacentally. There were significant group differences. *Top:* Peak systolic velocity in the aortic and mitral valves (centimeters per second). *Middle:* Time-velocity integrals of aortic and mitral valve Doppler sonography for the three groups. *Bottom:* Product of the time-velocity integral and heart rate for the aortic and mitral valves (equivalent to mean velocity) for the three groups. (Reprinted from [9] with permission)

continuous infusion. Terbutaline, and premature labor itself, has a positive inotropic effect on the fetal heart [9]. Increased right ventricular output causes a higher blood volume to be pumped from the main pulmonary artery to the descending aorta, resulting in an elevated maximal ductal blood velocity.

Terbutaline Effect Versus Ductal Constriction

An increase in ventricular stroke volume at times increases the ductal velocities such that the waveform may simulate ductal constriction. However, the PI increases in this situation, in contrast to a decreased PI with ductal constriction [13]. Terbutaline is not known to constrict the ductus, and we have not found such constriction. However, because it can increase fetal cardiac output and increase systolic velocities in the heart and arches, we have used the PI to distinguish these causes of increased systolic velocity (Fig. 37.1, 37.2). Ductal constriction lowers the PI to less than 2.0 owing to obstruction to flow and high velocities; increased fetal cardiac output elevates the PI to more than 3.0. This method of waveform analysis can therefore distinguish these two causes of increased ductal velocity.

When terbutaline fails to stop premature labor, indomethacin is frequently added as a second drug. Increased maximal velocity in these cases could be due to indomethacin-induced ductal constriction or the effect of terbutaline-induced increased right ventricular output. When using maximal ductal velocity alone, the latter case may be misinterpreted as fetal ductal constriction and could lead to discontinuation of an effective tocolysis regimen.

The flow pattern of a mildly constricted ductus and that of a wide open ductus with increased flow may have the same maximal systolic and end-diastolic velocities, but there is a significant difference in mean velocity and PI that clearly distinguishes the two etiologies.

The PI in peripheral vessels is thought to reflect peripheral impedance. In the ductus arteriosus, however, it is used only to help in the differential diagnosis of increased maximal velocity. Ductal constriction causes decreased pulsatility, with higher than normal velocities indicating obstruction; whereas decreased pulsability in the umbilical circulation, for example, is at low velocity and indicates increased flow and lower impedance [13]. Mean ductal blood velocity alone may be able to distinguish ductal construction from other causes of increased maximal velocity, but it has to be interpreted in relation to gestational age. The PI, on the other hand, does not change with gestational age and may therefore be a more useful parameter in clinical practice.

Fetal Pulmonary Assessment

Using Doppler, fetal pulmonary vascular status can be assessed. Pulsed Doppler has been shown to be obtainable in most pregnancies after 20 weeks' gestation. The typical blood velocity waveform with a systolic reversal pattern is obtained and can be quantitated with a PI. This approach was detailed by Rasanen [14] and showed that the pulmonary vascular resistance drops near 30 weeks' gestation and then rises near term. The fetal resistance is known to change with certain drugs such as indomethacin [15]. Reactivity of the human fetal pulmonary circulation to maternal hyperoxygenation was studied with advancing gestation and it was found that the fetal pulmonary circulation appeared to vasoconstrict after 31–36 weeks of gestation [16]. This technique has been applied in a cooperative study recently [17]. In this study, fetal pulmonary artery Doppler was used as a test during administration of 60% oxygen to the pregnant mother after 30 weeks' gestation to identify fetuses with pulmonary hypoplasia that would lead to perinatal death. A reactive test was defined as a decrease of at least 20% in the branch pulmonary PI with oxygen. Of the 14 fetuses who had a nonreactive hyperoxygenation test, 11 fetuses (79%) died of pulmonary hypoplasia. Of the 15 fetuses who had a reactive hyperoxygenation test, only one fetus (7%) died in the neonatal period (sensitivity, specificity, and positive and negative predictive values were 92%, 82%, 79%, and 93%, respectively).

We may speculate that application of this test could be of use in establishing the prognosis of fetuses at risk of pulmonary hypoplasia. Such a test has been performed in fetal lambs and the maternal hyperoxygenation test did predict those lungs with hypoplasia [18].

The test should be done by those with experience in normal and abnormal responses and may be technically difficult in some cases. Interventions designed to increase the pulmonary vascular bed cross-sectional area include occlusion of the trachea.

Summary

Treatment of preterm labor with nonsteroidal antiinflammatory agents can lead to acute, transient changes in the caliber of the fetal ductus arteriosus. These changes can be detected and quantitated using fetal echocardiography. This complication can be successfully managed with serial study of the fetus using Doppler techniques and may be indicated serially. The β-agonist sympathomimetic medications used to treat preterm labor, such as terbutaline, have an immediate effect on the fetal circulation and increase the heart rate and the inotropic state of the fetal myocardium. The future will see improved methods of fetal testing to assess the effects of both preterm labor and its treatment on the fetal circulation.

References

1. Huhta JC, Moise KJ, Fisher DJ et al (1987) Detection and quantitation of constriction of the fetal ductus arteriosus by Doppler echocardiography. Circulation 75:406–412
2. Moise KJ, Huhta JC, Sharif DS et al (1988) Indomethacin in the treatment of premature labor: effects on the fetal ductus arteriosus. N Engl J Med 319:727–731
3. Levin DL, Mills LJ, Parkey M, Garriott J, Campbell W (1979) Constriction of the fetal ductus arteriosus after administration of indomethacin to the pregnant ewe. Pediatrics 94:647–650
4. Huhta JC, Cohen A, Wood DC (1990) Premature constriction of the ductus arteriosus. J Am Soc Echocardiogr 3:30–34
5. Levin DL, Mills LJ, Weinberg AG (1979) Hemodynamic, pulmonary vascular, and myocardial abnormalities secondary to pharmacologic constriction of the fetal ductus arteriosus. Circulation 60:360–364
6. Momma K, Takao A (1989) Right ventricular concentric hypertrophy and left ventricular dilatation by ductal constriction in fetal rats. Circ Res 64:1137–1146
7. Wild LM, Nickerson PA, Morin III FC (1989) Ligating the ductus arteriosus before birth remodels the pulmonary vasculature of the lamb. Pediatr Res 25:251–257
8. Morin III FC (1989) Ligating the ductus arteriosus birth causes persistent pulmonary hypertension in the newborn lamb. Pediatr Res 25:245–250
9. Sharif DS, Huhta JC, Moise KJ, Morrow RW, Yoon GY (1990) Changes in fetal hemodynamics with terbutaline treatment and premature labor. J Clin Ultrasound 18:85–89
10. Gudmundsson S, Huhta JC, Wood DC et al (1991) Venous Doppler ultrasonography in the fetus with non-immune hydrops. Am J Obstet Gynecol 164:33–37
11. Tulzer G et al (1994) Doppler in hydrops non-immune fetalis. Ultrasound in Obstet Gynecol 4:279–283
12. Respondek ML, Kammermeier M, Ludomirsky A, Weil SR, Huhta JC (1994) The prevalence and clinical significance of fetal tricuspid valve regurgitation. Am J Obstet Gynecol 171:1265–1270
13. Tulzer G, Gudmundsson S, Sharkey A et al (1991) Doppler echocardiography of fetal ductus arteriosus constriction versus increased right ventricular output. J am Cell Cardiol 18:532–536
14. Rasanen J, Wood DC, Weiner S, Ludomirski A, Huhta JC (1996) Role of the pulmonary circulation in the distribution of human fetal cardiac output during the second half of pregnancy. Circulation 94:1068–1073
15. Rasanen J, Debbs RH, Wood DC, Weiner S, Huhta JC (1999) The effects of maternal indomethacin therapy on human fetal branch pulmonary arterial vascular impedance. Ultrasound Obstet Gynecol 13:112–116
16. Rasanen J, Wood DC, Debbs RH, Cohen J, Weiner S, Huhta JC (1998) Reactivity of the human fetal pulmonary circulation to maternal hyperoxygenation increases during the second half of pregnancy: a randomized study. Circulation 97:257–262
17. Broth RE, Wood DC, Rasanen J, Sabogal JC, Komwilaisak R, Weiner S, Berghella V (2002) Prenatal prediction of lethal pulmonary hypoplasia: the hyperoxygenation test for pulmonary artery reactivity. Am J Obstet Gynecol 187:940–945
18. Sylvester KG, Rasanen J, Kitano Y, Flake AW, Crombleholme TM, Adzick NS (1998) Tracheal occlusion reverses the high impedance to flow in the fetal pulmonary circulation and normalizes its physiological response to oxygen at full term. J Pediatr Surg 33:1071–1074; discussion 1074–1075

Chapter 38

Three-Dimensional Doppler Ultrasound in Gynecology

Ivica Zalud, Lawrence D. Platt

Three-dimensional (3D) reconstruction of ultrasound images was first demonstrated nearly 15 years ago but only now is becoming a clinical reality. In the meantime, methods for 3D reconstruction of computed tomography (CT) and magnetic resonance imaging (MRI) have achieved an advanced state of development, and 3D imaging with these modalities has been applied widely in clinical practice. Three-dimensional applications in ultrasound have lagged behind CT and MRI, because ultrasound data is much more difficult to render in 3D, for a variety of technical reasons, than either CT or MRI data. Only in the past few years has the computing power of ultrasound equipment reached a level adequate enough for the complex signal processing tasks needed to render ultrasound data in three dimensions. Within the past years several new ultrasound techniques have appeared. Three-dimensional ultrasound scanning, in which there has been great interest, is one of them [1]. Especially within obstetrics and gynecology several papers on that topic describe promising results. Gynecologic diagnostics relying on morphologic signs and accurate distance and volume measurements is one of the areas believed to benefit from 3D ultrasound; however, until now only few prospective works have been published, most of them counted as preliminary. One of the main reasons might be the huge technologic challenge. It is proposed that technologic progress over the next few years will allow feasible real-time 3D scanning. Gynecologic ultrasound scanning will thereby undoubtedly take another giant leap forward.

Why do we need 3D ultrasound in gynecology? Great strides have been made in gynecology secondary to the development of high-performance transvaginal ultrasound (TVS) instruments; however, even this advanced technology can provide only two-dimensional (2D) views of three-dimensional (3D) structures. Although an experienced examiner can easily piece together sequential 2D planes for creating a mental 3D image, individual sectional planes cannot be achieved in a 2D image because of various difficulties. Presently, 3D TVS can portray not only individual image planes, it can also store complex tissue volumes which can be digitally manipulated to display a multiplanar view, allowing a systematic tomographic survey of any particular field of interest. The same technology can also display surface rendering and transparency views to provide a more realistic 3D portrayal of various structures and anomalies.

Technique

Since the end of the 1980s, 3D ultrasound has become a major field of research in gynecology. The technique of acquiring 3D data involves making a set of consecutive 2D ultrasound slices by moving the transducer and continuously storing the images. These ultrasound data must be converted into a regular cubic representation before presentation in different 3D visualization modes. The creation of new ultrasound sections from the 3D block, and also the surface shading of a structure of interest, promise improvement in the diagnosis of congenital uterine anomalies and pelvic masses. In addition, the possibility of volume calculation by 3D ultrasound has to be considered as a clear innovation. At present, almost all of the diagnoses illustrated by 3D ultrasound can be made by 2D ultrasound, and this will continue to be so in the foreseeable future. Recently, computer-assisted treatment of sonographic images has permitted 3D reconstruction in gynecology. This is achieved by scanning a given volume containing the organ of interest. Two practical options exist. Some ultrasound probes are equipped with an automatic scanning device while others use manual scanning, electronically normalized or not. Both approaches make use of an electronic matrix, i.e., a pile of 2D sonographic images. Secondary cuts are possible through the electronic matrix, including plans not normally accessible to ultrasound scanning because of anatomical limitations. One of the secondary cuts most clinically useful is the frontal plane of the uterus. This enables one to visualize the organ lying flat as it is commonly drawn on medical sketches. Studying the frontal plane of the uterus acquired electronically from a 3D matrix improves the visualization of possible interactions between structures such as uterine fibroids and the endometrium. The

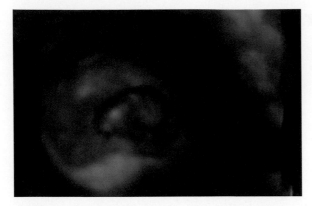

Fig. 38.1. Three-dimensional ultrasound surface rendering of ectopic pregnancy

frontal plane of the uterus also offers marked improvements for studying uterine malformations.

Three-dimensional ultrasound offers several options extending conventional 2D scanning. Various imaging modes are available. Three perpendicular planes displayed simultaneously can be rotated and translated in order to obtain accurate sections and suitable views needed for diagnosis and geometric measurements. Three-dimensional ultrasound tomography combines the advantages of ultrasound, e.g., safety, simplicity of application and inexpensiveness, with the advantages of sequentially depictable sections in numerous rotatable and translatable sections. Surface rendering gives detailed plastic images if there are surrounding layers of different echogenicity allowing for the definition of a certain threshold. Transparent modes provide an imaging of structures with a higher echogenicity in the interior of the object. A combination of the two modes sequentially definable by the sonographer allows for the optimal viewing of structures. These imaging modes are innovative features that have to be evaluated for clinical applicability and usefulness (Fig. 38.1). Digital documentation of whole volumes enables full evaluation without loss of information at a later point. The 3D technology provides an enormous number of technical options that have to be evaluated for their diagnostic significance and limitations in obstetrics and gynecology.

3D Doppler Measurements

Doppler methods are routinely used to study the vascular system. Flow and tissue motion information can be obtained by frequency and time-domain processing. Instruments range in complexity from simple continuous-wave devices without imaging capability through advanced real-time 2D color-flow scanners and intra-vascular devices. A 3D display is now avail-

able. Contrast agents can be used to increase the detectability of blood flow signals. The properties of the tissue impose an envelope on achievable ultrasonic imaging. Doppler studies can provide information about flow velocity profile, vessel compliance, wall shear rate, pressure gradient, perfusion, tumor blood flow, and the presence of emboli. These capabilities can be integrated into a holistic picture of ultrasonic vascular studies [2, 3].

Three-dimensional Doppler ultrasound has the potential to study pelvic blood flow and process of neovascularization. The 3D Doppler superimposed to 3D gray scale can detect early vasculogenesis within the uterine or adnexal mass. Traditionally, we defined blood flow information as (a) quantitative, i.e., volume flow measurements (cc/min), and (b) semiquantitative, i.e., pulsed Doppler waveform analysis (RI, PI, S/D index).

Three-dimensional power Doppler introduces a new way to look at blood flow detection and analysis. Using the computer-generated VOCAL imaging program (*v*irtual *o*rgan *c*omputer-aided *a*nalysis), different patterns of blood flow can be described:
1. Vascularization index (VI)
2. Flow index (FI)
3. Vascularization flow index (VFI)

Vascularization index gives information (in percentage) about the amount of color values (vessels) in the observed organ or area (e.g., uterus, ovary, or mass). Flow index is a dimensionless index (0–100) with information about intensity of blood flow. It is calculated as a ratio of weighted color values (amplitudes) to the number of color values. Vascularization flow index (VFI) is combined information of vascularization and mean blood flow intensity. It is also a dimensionless index (1–100) that is calculated by dividing weighted color values (amplitudes) by the total voxels minus background voxels. Three-dimensional Doppler was used to acquire volumes (Fig. 38.2). VOCAL was then used to delineate the 3D areas of interest (Fig. 38.3) and the "histogram facility" employed to generate three indices of vascularity: the VI; the FI; and the VFI (Fig. 38.4). The ultrasonographer should be aware that 3D Doppler is prone to the same artifacts and pitfalls as 2D Doppler. This information should be taken into account when any assessment of pelvic or tumor blood flow is made.

3D Doppler in Human Reproduction

Three-dimensional Doppler ultrasound is a new modality finding its way into clinical practice. We discuss recent publications related to 3D Doppler applications in human reproduction, gynecologic oncol-

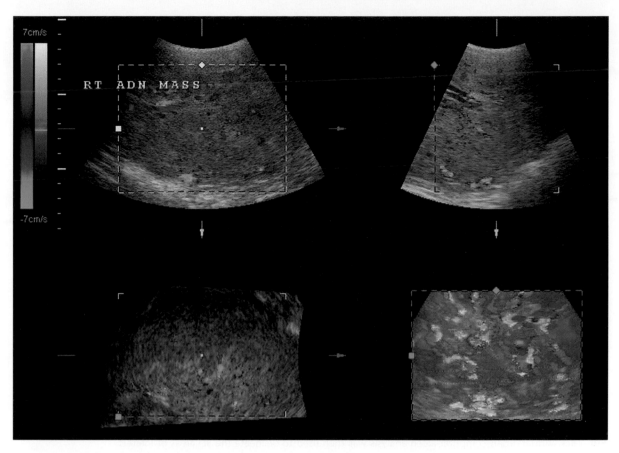

Fig. 38.2. Three-dimensional Doppler was used to acquire volumes

ogy, and in the field of benign gynecology. Pan et al. aimed to test the hypothesis that the decreased ovarian sensitivity to gonadotropins observed in women embarking on an in vitro fertilization (IVF) treatment may be due to changes in ovarian stromal blood flow [4]. They used 3D power Doppler ultrasonographic indexes to quantify ovarian stromal blood flow and vascularization in poor responders. Forty patients undergoing an IVF cycle were collected and divided into two groups, a poor responder group ($n=17$; estradiol <600 pg/ml or ≤3 oocytes retrieved) and normal responder group ($n=23$), based on their response to a standard down-regulation protocol for controlled ovarian stimulation. During ovarian stimulation, on the day of administration of human chorionic gonadotropin (HCG), patients underwent hormonal (serum E2), ultrasonographic (follicular number and diameter), and 3D power Doppler (ovarian stromal blood flow) evaluation. Compared with poor responders, the serum estradiol levels on the day of administration of HCG, the number of follicles >14 mm, the number of oocytes retrieved, the number of embryos transferred, and the pregnancy rate were significantly higher in normal responders. The vascularization in-

dex, flow index, and vascularization flow index were significantly lower in the poor responders compared with the women with a normal response. They concluded that the 3D power Doppler indexes of ovarian stromal blood flow in poor responders was significantly lower than those of normal responders. This may help to explain the poor response during HCG administration in controlled ovarian stimulation.

The British group used 3D power Doppler to examine the periodic changes in endometrial and sub-endometrial vascularity during the normal menstrual cycle in 27 women without obvious menstrual dysfunction or subfertility [5]. Doppler exam was performed on alternate days from day 3 of the cycle until ovulation and then every 4 days until menses. Virtual organ computer-aided analysis and shell imaging were used to define and to quantify the power Doppler signal within the endometrial and sub-endometrial regions producing indices of their relative vascularity. Both the endometrial and sub-endometrial VI and VFI increased during the proliferative phase, peaking approximately 3 days prior to ovulation before decreasing to a nadir 5 days post-ovulation; thereafter, both vascular indices gradually increased

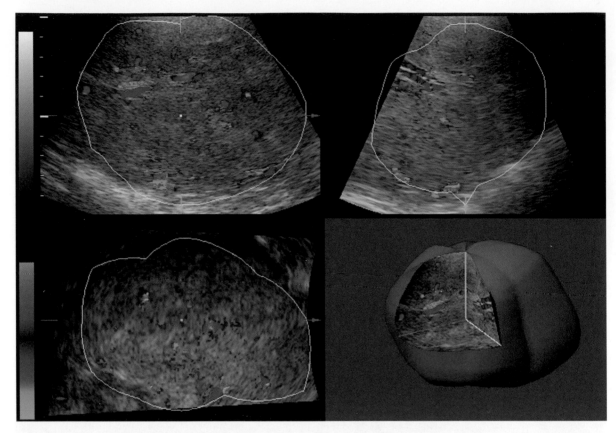

Fig. 38.3. Virtual organ computer-aided analysis was then used to delineate the 3D areas of interest

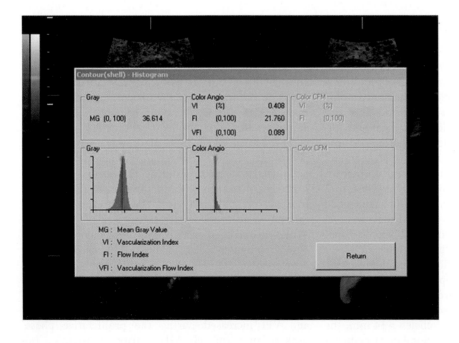

Fig. 38.4. The "histogram facility" was employed to generate three indices of vascularity: the vascular index; the flow index; and the vascularization flow index

during the transition from early to mid-secretory phase. The FI showed a similar pattern but with a longer nadir post-ovulation. Smoking was associated with a significantly lower VI and VFI. The FI was significantly lower in women aged ≥31 years and significantly higher in parous patients. The authors concluded that endometrial vascularity, as assessed by 3D Doppler, varies significantly during the menstrual cycle and is characterized by a pre-ovulatory peak and post-ovulatory nadir during the peri-implantation window.

Three-dimensional power Doppler has been largely used for the subjective assessment of vascular patterns, but semiquantification of the power Doppler signal is now possible. Raine-Fenning et al. addressed the intraobserver and interobserver error of the semiquantification of pelvic blood flow using 3D Doppler, VOCAL, and shell imaging [6]. The 3D Doppler was used to acquire 20 ovarian and 20 endometrial volumes from 40 different patients at various stages of in vitro fertilization treatment. The VOCAL was then used to delineate the 3D areas of interest and the "histogram facility" employed to generate three indices of vascularity: the VI; the FI; and the VFI. Intraobserver and interobserver reliability was assessed by two-way, mixed, intraclass correlation coefficients (ICCs) and general linear modeling was used to examine for differences in the mean values between each observer. The intraobserver reliability for both observers was extremely high and there were no differences in reliability between the observers for measurements of both volume and vascularity within the ovary or endometrium and its shells. With the exception of the outside sub-endometrial shell volumes, there were no significant differences between the two observers in the mean values obtained for either endometrial or ovarian volume and vascularity measurements. The interobserver reliability of measurements was equally high throughout with all measurements obtaining a mean ICC of above 0.985. They concluded that 3D Doppler and shell imaging offer a reliable, practical, and non-invasive method for the assessment of ovarian, endometrial, and sub-endometrial blood flow. Future work should concentrate upon confirming the reliability of data acquisition and the validity of the technique before its predictive value can be truly tested in prospective clinical studies.

Vlaisavljevic et al. wanted to study whether they might predict the outcome of unstimulated in vitro fertilization/intracytoplasmic sperm injection (IVF/ICSI) cycles with quantitative indices of perifollicular blood flow assessed with 3D reconstruction of power Doppler images [7]. This prospective study included an analysis of 52 unstimulated cycles. Color and power Doppler ultrasound examinations of a single dominant preovulatory follicle were performed on the day of oocyte pick-up. With 3D reconstruction and processing, quantitative indices were obtained, i.e., the percentage of volume showing a flow signal (VFS) inside a 5-mm capsule of perifollicular tissue and the percentage of VFS of each of the three largest vessels in this capsule. These indices as well as pulsed Doppler indices were compared between the groups of cycles with different outcomes using a one-way analysis of variance test. In nine cycles no oocyte was retrieved (group A), in seven cycles no fertilization occurred (group B), and in 30 cycles no implantation occurred (group C). Six cycles resulted in pregnancy (group D). There were no statistically significant differences in pulsed and power Doppler indices between these groups; however, the percentage of VFS in the capsule was higher than average in cycles with implantation and the percentage of VFS in the main vessel exhibited lower than average values in cycles with implantation, but only reached borderline statistical significance. It can be hypothesized that the follicles containing oocytes able to produce a pregnancy have a distinctive and more uniform perifollicular vascular network.

Other authors also looked at 3D Doppler of the ovary and relationship with hormonal status in IVF patients. Wu et al. investigated, in a retrospective study, whether the quantification of ovarian stromal blood flow and/or leptin concentration are predictive of IVF outcomes in women after laparoscopic ovarian cystectomy for large endometriomas [8]. Twenty-two women undergoing IVF after laparoscopic surgery for ovarian endometriomas (>6 cm) comprised the study group. Twenty-six women with tubal factor infertility constituted the control group. Ovarian stromal blood flow was evaluated by 3D power Doppler ultrasound imaging using VOCAL. Serum and follicular fluid (FF) leptin concentrations were quantified using an enzyme-linked immunosorbent assay kit. There were significantly decreased ovarian stromal blood flow parameters (including VI, FI, and VFI) in the endometriosis group without an evident difference in total ovarian volume on the day of human chorionic gonadotropin. The value of FF leptin demonstrated a negative correlation with ovarian stromal FI in the control group, but there was a loss of this effect in the endometriosis group. It appeared that the quantification of ovarian stromal blood flow by 3D power Doppler ultrasound in women with endometriosis may provide an important prognostic indicator in those undergoing IVF.

Kupesic and Kurjak designed the study to evaluate whether ovarian antral follicle number, ovarian volume, stromal area, and ovarian stromal blood flow are predictive of ovarian response and IVF outcome [9]. A total of 56 women with normal basal serum FSH concentrations who had no history of ovarian surgery and no ovarian and/or uterine pathology

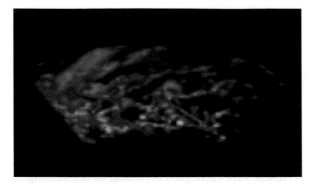

Fig. 38.6. Tumoral vessels network in ovarian mass reconstructed by 3D Doppler

of this new technique include the analysis of vascular anatomy and the potential assessment of organ perfusion. The latest application is intra-vascular study. Some catheters with an ultrasound transducer in the tip have been tested for intra-vascular studies. Just like conventional transducers, they provide 2D images which are then postprocessed into longitudinal 3D or volume reconstructions. The former resemble angio-

graphic images and can be viewed 3D rotating the image along its longitudinal axis. Volume images, which are more complex and slower to obtain, can be rotated on any spatial plane and provide rich detailing of the internal vascular lumen. The clinical importance of intravascular ultrasound with 3D volume reconstructions lies in the diagnosis of vascular conditions and the assessment and monitoring of intravascular interventional procedures, e.g., to detect inaccurate deployment of intravascular stents and endoluminal grafts during the maneuver. Three-dimensional reconstructions involve geometric data assembly and volumetric interpolation of a spatially related sequence of tomographic cross sections generated by an ultrasound catheter withdrawn at a constant rate through a vascular segment of interest, resulting in the display of a straight segment; therefore, particular care is needed and there are some useful hints to avoid mistakes.

Three-dimensional reconstructions of B-mode and Doppler images are no longer a work in progress and their clinical importance and possible applications are both established and ever-increasing. On the

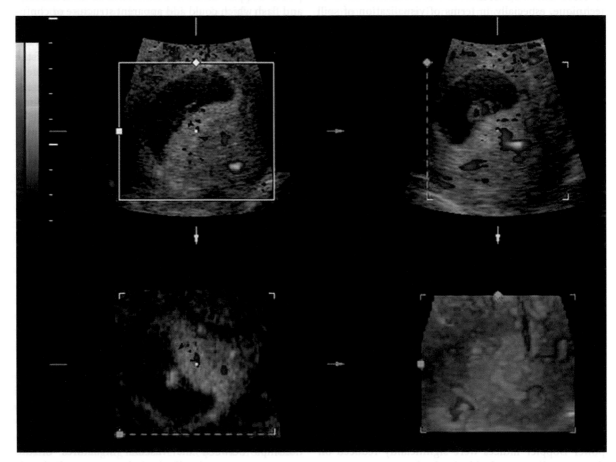

Fig. 38.7. The spatial relationships between the vascular structures of ectopic pregnancy and Fallopian tubes as studied by 3D Doppler ultrasound

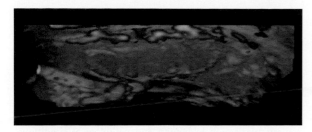

Fig. 38.8. Ovarian artery and vein and intraovarian vascular network as seen by 3D Doppler

other hand, independent of the different types of energy used, also computed tomography and magnetic resonance 3D reconstructions are very useful from a clinical viewpoint and they have become an established routine technique for both these methods. It is very likely that 3D volume reconstructions in ultrasound will find numerous applications in the near future (Fig. 38.8). They may help to increase the diagnostic confidence and to facilitate diagnosis, intraprocedure monitoring in interventional radiology, and follow-up and also to reduce the number of invasive examinations with iodinated contrast agents.

Conclusion

At this point in time, the clinical application of 3D Doppler ultrasound is likely to advance rapidly, as improved 3D rendering technology becomes more widely available. In the past 10 years, gynecological ultrasonography has proliferated rapidly, and is by some gynecologists considered an integral part of the gynecological exam. Abnormalities are detected in asymptomatic women at a high rate, resulting in a number of surgical interventions due to suspected malignancy. Present evidence is insufficient to determine the medical and economical value, if any, of surgical removal. Such intervention may in fact be as detrimental as leaving an abnormality in place. Gynecologic ultrasonography should therefore be performed on strict medical indications. Proper training of operators is also vital. In the past decade, research investigators and commercial companies have further advanced ultrasound imaging with the development of 3D ultrasound. This new imaging approach is rapidly achieving widespread use with numerous applications in human reproduction, gynecologic oncology, and benign gynecology. The major reason for the increase in the use of 3D ultrasound is related to the limitations of 2D viewing of 3D anatomy, using conventional ultrasound. This occurs because:

1. Conventional ultrasound images are 2D, yet the anatomy is 3D; hence, the diagnostician must integrate multiple images in his mind. This practice is

inefficient, and may lead to variability and incorrect diagnoses.
2. The 2D ultrasound image represents a thin plane at some arbitrary angle in the body. It is difficult to localize the image plane and reproduce it at a later time for follow-up studies.

Three-dimensional Doppler ultrasound is a new modality finding its way into clinical practice. Most of the major ultrasound vendors are now developing 3D ultrasound capabilities. We expect that, although 3D ultrasound will not replace 2D ultrasound, many additional benefits will be identified and its use will continue to grow, especially when 3D Doppler is used. The ability to evaluate pelvic anatomy, pathology, and blood flow with multiplanar and surface-rendered images provides physicians additional valuable clinical information. Volume data allows for a specific point in space to be evaluated from many different orientations by rotating, slicing, and referencing the slice to other orthogonal slices. It also allows for new volume-rendering displays that show depth, curvature, and surface images not available with conventional methods. The current limitations of image resolution, intuitive interfaces for obtaining and displaying optimal images, and technologic limitations for data storage and manipulation (including real-time 3D ultrasound) will surely be overcome in the near future. As 3D Doppler ultrasound continues to develop, the presence of real time 3D (or 4D) imaging equipment in the clinical setting will expand and stimulate new areas of investigation and identify new frontiers where 3D ultrasound can further enhance clinical care.

References

1. Campani R, Bottinelli O, Calliada F, Coscia D (1998) The latest in ultrasound: three-dimensional imaging. Part II. Eur J Radiol 27 (Suppl 2):S183–S187
2. Fleischer AC (2001) New developments in the sonographic assessment of ovarian, uterine, and breast vascularity. Semin Ultrasound CT MR 22:42–49
3. Wells PN (1998) Doppler studies of the vascular system. Eur J Ultrasound 7:3–8
4. Pan HA, Wu MH, Cheng YC, Wu LH, Chang FM (2004) Quantification of ovarian stromal Doppler signals in poor responders undergoing in vitro fertilization with three-dimensional power Doppler ultrasonography. Am J Obstet Gynecol 190:338–344
5. Raine-Fenning NJ, Campbell BK, Kendall NR, Clewes JS, Johnson IR (2004) Quantifying the changes in endometrial vascularity throughout the normal menstrual cycle with three-dimensional power Doppler angiography. Hum Reprod 19:330–338
6. Raine-Fenning NJ, Campbell BK, Clewes JS, Kendall NR, Johnson IR (2003) The reliability of virtual organ computer-aided analysis (VOCAL) for the semiquantification of ovarian, endometrial and subendometrial perfusion. Ultrasound Obstet Gynecol 22:633–639

7. Vlaisavljevic V, Reljic M, Gavric Lovrec V, Zazula D, Sergent N (2003) Measurement of perifollicular blood flow of the dominant preovulatory follicle using three-dimensional power Doppler. Ultrasound Obstet Gynecol 22:520–526

8. Wu MH, Tsai SJ, Pan HA, Hsiao KY, Chang FM (2003) Three-dimensional power Doppler imaging of ovarian stromal blood flow in women with endometriosis undergoing in vitro fertilization. Ultrasound Obstet Gynecol 21:480–485

9. Kupesic S, Kurjak A (2002) Predictors of IVF outcome by three-dimensional ultrasound. Hum Reprod 17:950–955

10. Schild RL, Holthaus S, d'Alquen J, Fimmers R, Dorn C, van der Ven H, Hansmann M (2000) Quantitative assessment of subendometrial blood flow by three-dimensional-ultrasound is an important predictive factor of implantation in an in-vitro fertilization program. Hum Reprod 15:89–94

11. Kurjak A, Kupesic S, Sparac V, Prka M, Bekavac I (2003) The detection of stage I ovarian cancer by three-dimensional sonography and power Doppler. Gynecol Oncol 90:258–264

12. Czekierdowski A, Smolen A, Bednarek W, Kotarski J (2002) Three dimensional sonography and 3D power angiography in differentiation of adnexal tumors. Ginekol Pol 73:1061–1070

13. Cohen LS, Escobar PF, Scharm C, Glimco B, Fishman DA (2001) Three-dimensional power Doppler ultrasound improves the diagnostic accuracy for ovarian cancer prediction. Gynecol Oncol 82:40–48

14. Kurjak A, Kupesic S, Sparac V, Kosuta D (2000) Three-dimensional ultrasonographic and power Doppler characterization of ovarian lesions. Ultrasound Obstet Gynecol 16:365–371

15. Sparac V, Kupesic S, Kurjak A (2000) What do contrast media add to three-dimensional power Doppler evaluation of adnexal masses? Croat Med J 41:257–261

16. Suren A, Osmers R, Kuhn W (1998) 3D Color power angio imaging: a new method to assess intracervical vascularization in benign and pathological conditions. Ultrasound Obstet Gynecol 11:133–137

17. Platt LD, Santulli T Jr, Carlson DE, Greene N, Walla CA (1998) Three-dimensional ultrasonography in obstetrics and gynecology: preliminary experience. Am J Obstet Gynecol 178:1199–1206

18. Yaman C, Ebner T, Jesacher K (2002) Three-dimensional power Doppler in the diagnosis of ovarian torsion. Ultrasound Obstet Gynecol 20:513–515

19. Sladkevicius P, Ojha K, Campbell S, Nargund G (2000) Three-dimensional power Doppler imaging in the assessment of Fallopian tube patency. Ultrasound Obstet Gynecol 16:644–647

20. Chan CC, Ng EH, Li CF, Ho PC (2003) Impaired ovarian blood flow and reduced antral follicle count following laparoscopic salpingectomy for ectopic pregnancy. Hum Reprod 18:2175–2180

21. Nelson TR, Pretorius DH, Hull A, Riccabona M, Sklansky MS, James G (2000) Sources and impact of artifacts on clinical three-dimensional ultrasound imaging. Ultrasound Obstet Gynecol 16:374–383

Doppler Ultrasonography for Benign Gynecologic Disorders, Ectopic Pregnancy, and Infertility

Ivica Zalud

Doppler ultrasound has the potential to study patterns of pelvic flow and hence identify functional changes. The availability of pulsed Doppler instruments has made it possible to sample the signals at a chosen depth and thus to direct flow in any selected deep pelvic vessel. Transvaginal color Doppler is a system that uses pulsed Doppler that performs flow analysis at multiple points along each scan line of echo data. Flow information is then color-coded and displayed on the entire corresponding anatomical image. The main advantage of this color Doppler system is rapid and definitive determination of the position of the small vessel, accuracy of the measurements, and precise indication of flow direction and velocity. After simultaneous visualization of morphological and blood flow information, a pulsed Doppler gate is placed over the area of interests to provide flow velocity waveforms which may be analyzed in a conventional fashion.

This chapter presents the application of the various modalities of Doppler ultrasound for investigating benign gynecological conditions, ectopic pregnancy and infertility.

Examination Technique

A brief explanation is required to ensure acceptance of this scanning technique and full cooperation by the patients. By comparing insertion of the probe with insertion of a tampon, speculum examination, or pelvic bimanual examination, a patient's fears are usually dispelled. The entire procedure can be done in a relaxed atmosphere without the inconvenience of the patient having a full bladder. All patients in fact should have a completely empty urinary bladder. Thus the patient and examiner do not have to wait for the slowly filling bladder in order to obtain satisfactory pelvic images. This point is important in case of an emergency, such as an ectopic pregnancy, acute pelvic inflammatory disease, or other pathology where the patient is a potential surgical candidate and consequently may not be permitted to drink in order to fill the bladder.

A regular gynecologic examination table with heel support is adequate for vaginal scanning, but a flat examination table can also be used. The patient is scanned in the lithotomy position with a slight reverse Trendelenburg tilt to localize free fluid in the pouch of Douglas. If present, this fluid creates tissue-fluid interfaces, which improves the outline of pelvic structures. In some instances, a Trendelenburg position helps to displace the bowel from the pelvic structures.

Normal menstruating women are best scanned during days 3–10 of the cycle to exclude changes in intraovarian blood flow that are known to occur during formation of the mature follicle and corpus luteum. The 5- to 10-MHz transvaginal transducer procedures a sector angle of 90°–320° to allow a satisfactory view of the pelvic organs. Before it is used, the probe should be covered with a coupling ultrasound gel, inserted into a condom, and gently inserted into the vagina. Pelvic structures may be brought closer to the acoustic focal range by placing the second hand on the patient's abdomen as for a bimanual examination. The scanning is done systematically, starting with the uterus as a landmark. The ovaries are next, then the fallopian tubes (not always seen), and finally the cul-de-sac. Various planes and depths are reached by the operator by tilting and angling the tip of the probe, thereby introducing various structures into the acoustic focal range. The morphology and size of the pelvic structures should be assessed.

After visualization of pelvic anatomy by B-mode sonography, color Doppler sonography is used to locate blood flow in normal or newly formed pelvic vessels. Subsequently, structures of particular interest are examined for prominent areas of vascularization, probably reflecting neovascularization. These vessels usually appear as continuously fluctuating color rather than the pulsating color seen with normal arteries. The color flow pattern of interest can be explored with the Doppler sample volume until the typical spectral waveform is seen. The angle of the transducer should be moved to obtain the maximum waveform amplitude and clarity. Pulsed repetition frequency for color and pulsed-wave Doppler examination should be properly set separately. The color and pulsed-wave Doppler gain, color gate, sample volume, and wall filter must also be adjusted. Automatic default settings can be used to speed up the examination. However, manual adjustments of all mentioned parameters are needed to detect and differentiale low-velocity and high-velocity vessels. If inadequate Doppler settings are used, low-velocity vessels might not be visualized at all and high-velocity vessels might exhibit an artifact known as aliasing. Unfortunately, there are no universal guidelines for Doppler studies in gynecology, one reason being the large variety of Doppler ultrasound instruments that use different technical setups for blood flow visualization and measurement. Another more unfortunate reason is the lack of standardization of Doppler measurements. The setups are often not mentioned in the literature, making comparisons of studies impossible. Reports of these studies with precise information about the Doppler settings are rare. Moreover, the results reported vary widely and are sometimes controversial, which may ultimately compromise and devalue this relatively new ultrasound technique. Standardization of Doppler measurements is urgently needed.

Color flow can be quantified by pulsed-wave Doppler waveform analysis. The peak systolic (A) and end-diastolic (B) Doppler shift frequency can be recorded; and the A/B ratio, Pourcelot resistance index (RI), the pulsatility index (PI), and other indices may be calculated. The RI is a useful way of expressing blood flow impedance distal to the point of sampling. Each parameter is angle-dependent, but once they are in proper relation the RI becomes independent of the angle between the investigated vessels and the emitted ultrasound beam. Although the volume flow measurement would be of more benefit than Doppler waveform analysis, this approach requires precise measurement of the angle of insonation and the diameter of the vessel. If achieved, the volume (milliliters) of blood passing through a certain vessel during a particular time unit can be calculated. To avoid these measurement difficulties, waveform analysis offers semiquantizative assessment of the quality of blood flow. Because the systolic and diastolic blood flows are expressed as a ratio, measuring one or the other of these blood flows is not sufficient to report it as high-velocity or low-velocity flow: The flows cannot be observed and interpreted separately. This point is particularly important for randomly dispersed small vessels, for which the angle of insonation and the diameter of the vessel are almost impossible to determine. The basic question is whether the color signal represents a single small vessel or it is a summary of flow from an unknown number of small vessels. It is believed that the increased RI value results from increased peripheral vascular resistance. For each measurement, at least three cardiac cycles must be recorded and the mean value of the RI calculated. The mean duration of examination is usually no longer than 15 min in experienced hands. The spatial peak temporal average intensity should not exceed 100 mW/cm^2, which is the highest limit of insonation energy permitted by the US Food and Drug Administration (FDA) for use in fetal medicine.

Normal Pelvic Blood Flow

Transvaginal color Doppler (TVCD) sonography and pulsed-wave Doppler sonography provide a unique noninvasive method for the evaluation of normal and abnormal conditions in the female pelvis [1]. Transvaginal ultrasonography displays uterine, iliac, and ovarian blood flow in pregnant and nongravid women and identifies physiologic flow patterns. Blood flow in the main pelvic vessels can be easily visualized and recognized. The artery and vein are distinguished according to the pulsation and brightness of color flow (Fig. 39.1). The internal iliac vessels can be visualized in the entire population. The iliac vein is most commonly seen immediately below the ovary. The ability to view iliac veins is an excellent way to document patency or thrombosis. The iliac arteries at the bifurcation have characteristic waveforms. The common and external iliac arteries, which are part of the aortofemoral segment, show plug flow, a window under the waveform, and a reversed component during diastole. The internal iliac artery, in contrast, has parabolic flow with an even distribution of velocities within the waveform. Internal iliac vessels can usually be observed in the side wall of the pelvis, often lying deep and close to the ovary. The internal iliac artery produces prominent, pulsating color flow at high velocity, typically with reverse flow and high impedance of flow.

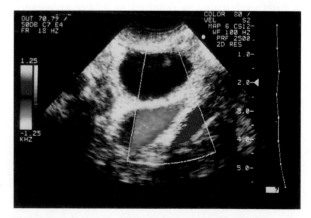

Fig. 39.1. The internal iliac artery (*red*) and vein (*blue*) are distinguished by color Doppler according to the brightness of the color and pulsation, not by the color itself

Fig. 39.2. Uterine artery spectral Doppler waveform has high systolic flow, high resistance, low diastolic flow, and a characteristic notch during diastole. The uterine vein Doppler pattern is shown *below the zero line*

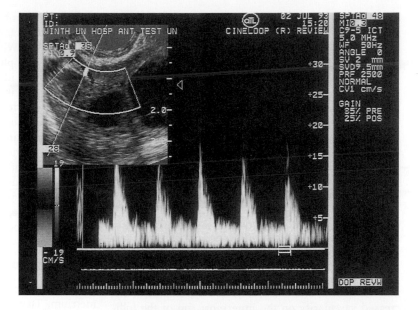

The color Doppler signal from the main uterine vessels may be seen in all patients lateral to the cervix. The transvaginal transducer clearly displays all the vessels coursing from the sides of the cervix, up to the lateral wall of the uterus, along the fallopian tube, and terminating above the ovaries. Branches of the uterine artery can be followed as they enter the myometrium, and even endometrial perfusion can be studied. The uterine artery spectral Doppler waveform in both nongravid and first-trimester pregnant women has high impedance (low diastolic flow) with a characteristic notch during diastole. Uterine flow states can be determined by the Doppler spectrum (Fig. 39.2). The impedance to blood flow depends on age, phase of the menstrual cycle, and special conditions (e.g., pregnancy, tumor). It is usually a high resistance system.

The ovarian artery is a tributary of the upper aorta and reaches the lateral aspect of the ovary through the infundibulopelvic ligament. In some patients, these vessels are not clearly visualized and the sample volume should be moved across the ligament and then through the substance of the ovary until the arterial signal is identified. Signals from the ovarian artery are characterized by the low Doppler shifts of a small vessel with low velocity [2]. The waveform shape varies with the state of activity of the ovary. Studies of ovarian artery blood flow show the difference in the vascular resistance between the two ovarian arteries depending on the presence of the dominant follicle or corpus luteum. A longitudinal study of the ovarian artery throughout the menstrual cycle will usually show decreased PIs and RIs, reflecting vascular impedance and implying increased flow to the ovary containing the dominant follicle or corpus

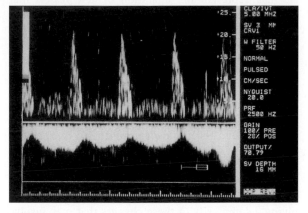

Fig. 39.3. Ovarian artery visualized in the lateral upper pole of the right ovary. Color flow is usually not prominent, velocity is low, and resistance varies greatly according to menstrual cycle

luteum. The ovarian artery of the "inactive" ovary in this cycle would show low end-diastolic flow or absence of diastolic flow. A rise in end-diastolic flow in the "active ovary" is most obvious around day 21 and suggests that the corpus luteum acts as a low-impedance shunt. The increased blood supply to the functioning corpus luteum is essential for delivery of precursors involved in steroidogenesis and for distribution of progesterone.

The ovarian artery is a high-pressure system with blood flow characteristics very different from intraovarian circulation (Fig. 39.3). Near the ovarian hilus the penetrating vessels are coiled and tortuous. This type of vascularity demonstrates high-resistance blood flow [3]. Every month during the woman's reproductive life, one oocyte is released from the single

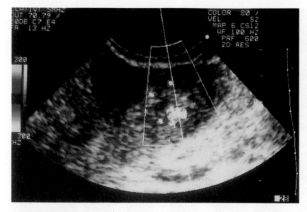

Fig. 39.4. Corpus luteum vascularization detected by color Doppler sonography. Such small randomly dispersed vessels are difficult to study without color as a guide

mature follicle that has completed development. Increased vascularity on the innermost rim of the follicle may represent the dilatation of new vessels that have developed between the relatively vascular theca cell layer and the normally hypoxic granulose cell layer of the follicle. It is hoped that information on ovarian perfusion may be used both to predict ovulation and to investigate ovulatory dysfunction.

Color flow is more easily obtainable from ovarian tissue in the luteal phase. The qualitative postovulatory changes in intraovarian blood flow are characterized by increased turbulent flow accompanying morphological changes in the intraovarian vascular network and appearance of numerous arteriovenous shunts during the luteal phase (Fig. 39.4). In summary, changes in the intraovarian blood flow occur before ovulation, implying a complexity of these changes that may involve both angiogenesis and hormonal factors, while postovulatory vascular accommodation is potentially important in the luteal phase. Using transvaginal color Doppler, corpus luteum blood flow, characterized by low impedance and high flow requirements, can easily be detected in normal early pregnancy, ectopic pregnancy, and nonpregnant women.

Benign Uterine Pathology

Transabdominal ultrasonography permits gross visualization of the uterine corpus through the distended urinary bladder. Estimates of size in terms of the sagittal, anteroposterior, and transverse diameters are easily obtained. In the clinical setting of an enlarged uterus (e.g., leiomyomata uteri) transabdominal scanning may be helpful.

Transvaginal scanning permits close examination of a structure of interest within the corpus or cervix of the normal or slightly enlarged uterus. Proximity and high-

er-frequency probes provide improved imaging and infrastructural detail not possible with the transabdominal approach. With the advent of color Doppler analysis, additional physiologic/functional and pathologic states may be identifiable. The blood supply to the uterus, the uterine arteries, are direct branches of the hypogastric artery and have a typically high-resistance/low-diastolic-flow velocity waveform. Pulsed-wave Doppler analysis of the uterine artery has been described previously. Color Doppler analysis allows identification of the small vessels within the myometrium (e.g., arcuate arteries and their branches). Again, the age of the patient, phase of the menstrual cycle, pregnancy state, and pathologic conditions influence the type of velocity waveform obtained.

Fibroids/Leiomyomas

Leiomyomas are benign tumors of the uterine myometrium. They are derived from the mitotic division of a smooth muscle cell within the uterine wall. Among a screened population of women over 40 years of age, 25%–30% exhibit findings of intramural leiomyomas. They are often incidental findings, as they may occur in a uterus of overall normal size. Utilizing two-dimensional transvaginal scanning in the sagittal and transverse planes, leiomyomas can be described as intramural, submucous, subserosal, fundal, cervical, or intracavitary; anterior or posterior; lateral left or right. A variety of sonographic images are seen in leiomyomas. The internal echogenicity depends on the amount of smooth muscle and fibrous tissue, degeneration, and vascularity. Leiomyomas can undergo cystic degeneration (echo-lucent) or, conversely, calcific degeneration (echogenic) with shadowing, as well as the spectrum in between.

The addition of color Doppler analysis facilitates determination of the predominance of myometrial vessels feeding a leiomyoma and the type of flow present. The Zagreb group studied uterine flow and myometrial vessel flows in women with fibroids [4]. Diastolic flow is present in the myometrial vessels and is usually increased relative to that seen in the uterine arteries. Uterine artery flow velocity in the normal uterus has a mean RI of 0.84. In women with leiomyomas a slight decrease in the mean RI to 0.74 was observed. The mean RI of myometrial blood flow in these patients was 0.54.

In the clinical setting localization and flow determinations of leiomyomas may be helpful. Such information might influence one's surgical approach. In addition, the utility and effectiveness of new treatment modalities may become subjects of color Doppler analysis.

Investigations on the use of gonadotropin-releasing hormone (GnRH) analogs for treatment of leiomyoma uteri and endometriosis are reported in increasing numbers. The effect of GnRH analogs, essentially a medically induced menopause, might be assessed in a semiquantitative manner using transvaginal sonography and color Doppler flow analysis. It has been our observation that women distant from menopause exhibit an increased resistance flow pattern and higher RI [5]. The utility of this modality for exploring benign conditions of the uterus continues to expand.

Endometrium

Transvaginal sonography greatly enhances imaging of the uterine cavity and endocervix. It is now possible to identify small submucous myomas, endometrial polyps, distortions of the endometrial cavity, and the exact location of an intrauterine device (IUD). Measurement of the total thickness of the endometrium is facilitated by transvaginal scanning (Fig. 39.5). The measurement should be obtained in the sagittal plane and reported in millimeters. Literature accumulated to dat suggests that endometrial thickness in the postmenopausal, non-hormone-replaced individual should be less than 6 mm (Table 39.1). A thickness of 6 mm or more is suspect [6, 7]. Pathologic conditions seen in the setting of increased endometrial thickness include endometrial hyperplasia, endometrial polyps, and adenocarcinomas of the endometrium (Fig. 39.6). Among a screened population at our institution, more than 2,000 women underwent transvaginal sonography and color Doppler analysis, with assessment of the endometrial cavity as well. There were 20 asymptomatic women who underwent endometrial sampling or biopsy based on a report of the endometrium being greater than 6 mm. None of the women had symptoms (i.e., postmenopausal bleeding or staining) (Table 39.2). There were three cases of adenocarcinoma

Table 39.1. Previous studies on endometrial thickness

Study	Reason for consult	No.	Cutoff thickness (mm)	Result (disease)
Klug and Leitner[a]	Referred	215	10	Benign (<10)
Nasir and Coast[b]	Referred	90	6	Sensitivity 91%
Osmers et al.[c]	Study	155	4	Sensitivity 81%
Goldstein et al.[d]	Bleeding	30	6	6/17 Abnormal
Smith et al.[e]	Bleeding	96	8	Sensitivity 100%, specificity 61%
Osmers et al.[f]	Bleeding + control	872	4	20% Asymptomatic
Current study	Asymptomatic	841	6	13/20 Abnormal

[a] Klug PW, Leitner G (1989) Comparison of vaginal ultrasound and histologic findings of the endometrium. Geburts Frauenheilk 49:797–802.
[b] Nasri MN, Coast GJ (1989) Correlation of ultrasound findings and endometrial histopathology in postmenopausal women. Br J Obstet Gynaecol 96:1333–1338.
[c] Osmers R, Volksen M, Rath W, Kuhn W (1990) Vaginosonographic detection of endometrial cancer in postmenopausal women. Inter J Obstet Gynecol 32:35–37.
[d] Goldstein SR, Nachtigall M, Snyder JR, Nachtigall L (1990) Endometrial assessment by vaginal ultrasonography before endometrial sampling in patients with postmenopausal bleeding. Am J Obstet Gynecol 163:119–123.
[e] Smith P, Bakos O, Heimer G, Ulmsten U (1991) Transvaginal ultrasound for identifying endometrial abnormality. Acta Obstet Gynecol Scand 70:591–594.
[f] Osmers R, Volksen M, Kuhn W (1992) Evaluation of the endometrium in postmenopausal women by means of vaginal ultrasound. Rev Fran Gynecol Obstet 87:309–315.

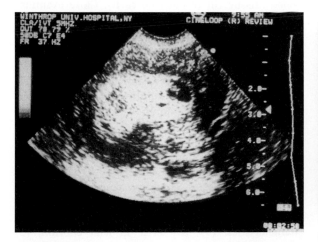

Fig. 39.5. Thick endometrium visualized by transvaginal ultrasonography. A small submucous myoma can also be seen

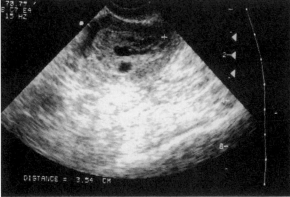

Fig. 39.6. Irregularly shaped thick endometrium in a postmenopausal woman without hormonal replacement therapy. Endometrial carcinoma was confirmed on histopathology

Table 39.2. Data on women having endometrial biopsies

Histology	Age (years)	No.	Thickness (cm)
Adenocarcinoma	65–73	3	0.83–1.10
Adenomatous hyperplasia	51–60	5	0.68–1.10
Polyps	56–69	7	0.89–3.73
Disordered endometrium	54–56	2	0.60–1.08
Atrophic	59–62	3	0.67–1.14
No biopsy	53–79	4	0.60–1.34
Lost to follow-up	49–68	6	0.69–1.12

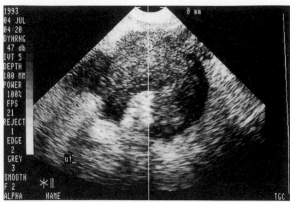

Fig. 39.8. Transvaginal sonography from a case of septic abortion. The patient had undergone elective termination of pregnancy at 16 weeks' gestation. Ten days later she presented with pelvic pain, fever, and bleeding. Transvaginal sonography of the uterus showed "tissue" in the uterine cavity. Close examination of the ultrasound image shows intraabdominal contents entering the left fundus

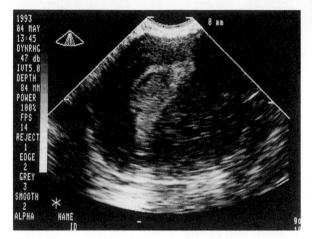

Fig. 39.7. Myometrial invasion in the case of an advanced stage of endometrial cancer seen by transvaginal ultrasonography

of the endometrium, five hyperplasias (one with atypia), and seven polyps (one with hyperplasia). There was no cutoff value, however, whereby benign versus malignant conditions could be discriminated. In one of the adenocarcinoma cases abnormal blood flow was observed in the uterine artery and the myometrial vessels by waveform analysis. Attention should be given to the endometrial-myometrial interface, as myometrial invasion can be visualized (Fig. 39.7). Others have also evaluated the use of color Doppler analysis for assessing endometrial cancer [8–11].

When hormone replacement therapy is used, a cutoff value of 6 mm cannot be used as an accurate criterion for suspicion. In the case of breakthrough bleeding on hormone therapy, these authors utilize transvaginal sonography and color Doppler analysis to assess the endometrium [12, 13]. If a thin echo is seen at 2–3 mm and color Doppler velocimetry is normal, the patient may be able to avoid repeated endometrial biopsies. In the case of an endometrial thickness of more than 6 mm, sampling for breakthrough bleeding (i.e., endometrial sampling) is suggested and supported.

Retained Products of Conception

Transvaginal sonography can be valuable when evaluating a postabortal patient. After a spontaneous abortion the uterine cavity may be inspected for retained products of conception, determining if surgical completion is required. In the case of elective termination of pregnancy (TOP) or postsurgically completed abortion, postoperative bleeding can be assessed for retained tissue. The application of color Doppler analysis is new and uncertain in this setting.

Transvaginal sonography proved vital in a case of septic abortion presenting to the emergency room at our hospital. The patient had undergone an elective TOP at 16 weeks' gestation at another institution. Ten days later she presented with pelvic pain, fever, and bleeding. Transvaginal sonography of the uterus revealed "tissue" in the uterine cavity. Close examination of the ultrasound image showed intraabdominal contents entering at the left fundus (Fig. 39.8). A color flow analysis may have been interesting in this case, looking for bowel motility within the cavity. More than likely, however, any bowel would have "ileus", or diminished motility. Laparotomy confirmed a left fundal perforation, with omentum and transverse colon within the defect. Reinstrumentation of this patient would have been harmful and potentially fatal. Ultrasound findings in this case were paramount to the management.

The other uterine condition connected to pregnancy is gestational trophoblastic disease (GTD). This term describes a group of tumors that share several characteristics: (1) they arise in fetal chorion; (2) they produce human chorionic gonadotropin (hCG); and (3) they respond well to chemotherapy. The incidence of hydatidiform mole appears to be about 1 per 1,000 pregnancies in most parts of the world, with that figure perhaps twice as high in Japan [14]. Choriocarcinoma is much less common, and estimates of the incidence are highly variable.

Ultrasonography is one of the most valuable non-invasive diagnostic methods for diagnosing GTD. Molar pregnancy can be easily diagnosed by ultrasonography by its typical snowstorm pattern. However, ultrasonography is thought to be unreliable for distinguishing a noninvasive mole from an invasive one or from choriocarcinoma, as the sonographic appearance is almost the same for all three lesions. The clinical management and prognosis depend on a correct diagnosis [15]. Other diagnostic modalities, such as the β-hCG level and its dynamics, computed tomography (CT), and magnetic resonance imaging (MRI), or even an invasive procedure such as pelvic arteriography or hysterectomy, are performed to confirm clinical suspicion.

Many patients with persistent GTD have been treated without ever demonstrating the site of the persistent trophoblastic focus. TVCD ultrasonography has been reported to be able to accurately map uterine blood flow during pregnancy. The arcuate, radial, and spiral arteries can be precisely localized by color flow analysis and studied by pulsed-wave Dopplr waveform analysis [16–18].

GTD is a clinically complex, diagnostically challenging condition. It might be fatal if it turns malignant. Fortunately, the disease is considered a treatable malignant tumor, with a survival rate approaching 100% [15]. The prognosis is highly dependent on early, reliable diagnosis. Ultrasonography has played a major role in differential considerations when GTD is suspected [19–21].

The ultrasonographic appearance of molar pregnancy varies with the gestational age at which the examination is performed. During the first trimester a hydatidiform mole may mimic a missed abortion, an incomplete abortion, or a blighted ovum. In most cases an accurate diagnosis can be made. Myometrial invasion can also be estimated by ultrasonography, but the degree of invasion is usually arbitrary. The ultrasound features of choriocarcinoma are difficult to distinguish from those of an invasive mole. Othr diagnostic techniques, usually more invasive and risky, are employed to solve the dilemma.

Color Doppler sonography was reported as an accurate way to distinguish the various segments of uterine vascularization during pregnancy [16]. Color flow analysis is used to locate the arcuate, radial, and spiral arteries. Pulsed-wave Doppler sonography is then used to study the various flow patterns of the visualized vessels. We described abnormal early pregnancies and the vascular changes in the uterus, and

we noted that some of the blighted ova were richly vascularized [22]. It was speculated that the intensity of color flow corresponds to trophoblast activity. Abundant color possibly indicates which blighted ovum would undergo molar changes. Different patterns of blood flow (intensity of color, number of vessels, degree of myometrial invasion, velocity, and waveform analysis) might reflect different aspects of gestational trophoblastic disease. We concluded that because there has been no typical ultrasound marker that can be used for differentiating between choriocarcinoma and invasive mole, color Doppler characterization might be of diagnostic value.

The level of myometrial invasion by trophoblastic tissue can be assessed by color flow sonography. It is obvious in patients with choriocarcinoma and invasive mole: The normal vascular network is changed, and as the process progresses the spiral and radial arteries are either incorporated in the tumor tissue or destroyed by invasive disease. The latter condition is probably more common. The basis for abundnat color flow relies almost entirely on neovascularization. All six patients with choriocarcinoma in our study showed this disturbed, markedly changed intrauterine blood flow. One of two patients with proved invasive mole also presented with the same chaotic blood flow pattern.

Such a change suggests two prognostic possibilities when the invasive mole is considered: destructive invasion of the myometrium and metastasis or spontaneous regression. These possibilities are supported by clinical experience. Carter et al. used TVCD sonography to study GTD [23]. They evaluated blood flow characteristics of the uterine artery and intratumoral vessels. The uterine artery PI correlated significantly with age, uterine size, and β-hCG titer. The intratumoral PI correlated significantly only with uterine size. Regression analysis of β-hCG titers in the uterine artery and intratumoral PI revealed a linear association. They concluded that the PI is strongly associated with prognosis and correlates with the β-hCG titers.

It seems now that ultrasonography may be able to distinguish reliably between the forms of gestational trophoblastic disease. Because of its noninvasiveness and relatively simple, easily performed technique, TVCD sonography can be of considerable clinical value. The other important point is that the study results are available immediately for clinical judgment.

Benign Adnexal Pathology

Functional cysts are the most common source of adnexal masses in women of reproductive age. The two main types of functional cyst, follicle and corpus luteum cysts, are benign and derived from either an unruptured follicle or the cystic degeneration of a corpus luteum, respectively. Typically, these cysts are unilateral and are less than 6 cm in diameter, and during pelvic examination they feel smooth and cystic. On sonograms, the cysts appear unilocular and fluid-filled, without evidence of solid components or excrescences. It seems that transvaginal color Doppler is helpful in the differential diagnosis of different causes of acute abdomen and in the detection of torsion of the functional cyst [24]. Torsion affects blood supply to the ovary both from the ovarian artery and the ovarian branch of the uterine artery. Below a morphologically recognized point, no blood supply was detected. Hemorrhage from a ruptured corpus luteum cyst can be severe enough to be mistaken for a ruptured ectopic pregnancy. This new technique enhances our ability to distinguish between these two conditions and to select the patients for surgical intervention when necessary.

Mature teratomas (dermoid cysts) occur commonly in women of reproductive age. They contain elements of mature adult structures derived from all three embryonic layers: endoderm, mesoderm and, peripherally, ectoderm. These structures include hair, teeth, bone, skin, and calcified components that give focal, high-amplitude reflectors with acoustic shadowing. Unfortunately, these high-amplitude reflectors may simulate bowel gas; therefore, these lesions may be camouflaged and sometimes even large lesions can go undetected on sonograms.

Serous and mucinous cystadenomas are also common lesions. Serous cystadenomas may be unilocular but they are mostly multilocular, with or without papillary growth into the cavity. Mucinous cystadenomas may attain a huge size, and several have been reported to weigh 45–90 kg. Grossly, they present as rounded or ovoid masses with a smooth capsule that is usually translucent or bluish-whitish gray. Mucinous cystadenomas are thin-walled and mostly multilocular. Papillary formations may be present, but they are less common than in serous cystadenomas. Sonographic evaluation whether alone or in combination with tumor markers cannot determine the nature of the lesion before Doppler assessment. This is not surprising, because it can be difficult to distinguish a benign ovarian tumor from a malignant or borderline one by macroscopic inspection of the specimen or even by microscopic evelation.

Fibromas, thecomas, and Brenner's tumors are solid, benign tumors found in premenopausal and postmenopausal patients. Small, solid tumors are difficult to detect on sonograms because they are similar in echo texture to the normal ovary. If a solid lesion is observed in the adnexa of a premenopausal woman, it is more likely to be a pedunculated or broad ligament leiomyoma than a solid ovarian neoplasm. Transvaginal color Doppler is useful in differentiating fibroids from solid ovarian masses on the basis of their vascularity. Within or on the periphery of the uterine mass, even when it is out of the contour of the uterus, it is possible to detect waveform signals that are typical for the uterine vascular network. In such cases, blood flow is usually similar to normal myometrial perfusion, originating from terminal branches of the uterine artery. On the other hand, small vessels that feed a growing ovarian tumor are of ovarian vasculature origin.

Endometriosis

Endometriosis is a condition in which abnormal growth of tissue, histologically resembling endometrial tissue, occurs outside the uterus, including the surfaces of the bowel, bladder, or abdominal wall. The ovary represents a relatively unique site of implantation, as the levels of steroids surpass those in the circulation, and hence this affords an ideal environment for implantation of endometrial growth. It seems that the surface epithelium and the proximity of the tubal ostia influence transplantation production. When endometrial cells enter the ovarian stroma, large endometrial cysts filled with viscous chocolate-colored liquid may be formed. There is usually a well-demarcated separation between the endometrial cyst wall and the normal adjacent ovarian stroma. The most prominent vascular area in these common benign cysts is at the level of the ovarian hilus. This type of neovascularization was often seen with endometriomas. It seems that low-impedance/high-diastolic flow is present when there is a hemorrhage during the menstrual phase of the cycle. Therefore, it is recommended to study the ovarian endometrioma vascularity during the late follicular phase. It is postulated that the effect of medical treatment is highly dependent on the metabolically active implants arriving via a blood-supplying network. Conservative treatment has encouraging potential and can be successfully used in patients with an optimal vascular pattern. Surrounding inflammation and fibrotic changes that may disturb this process can be detected by transvaginal color Doppler. Based on some experience, avascular ovarian lesions could be best removed surgically.

Pelvic Inflammatory Disease

Ultrasonography is often used to exclude intrauterine and ectopic pregnancy or to document the presence of an adnexal mass. Sonography shows a predominantly cystic collection with internal echoes that may have multiple loculations. Occasionally, distinction from fluid-filled loops of bowel may be difficult. In this instance, a water enema may be helpful because the movement of water through the bowel will be observed on real-time ultrasound. Because the inflammatory process in the ovary involves both structural and vascular changes, color Doppler ultrasound can be a useful tool in its diagnosis and management. Edema of the fallopian tubes and dilatation of the blood vessels in their walls characterize the early phase of the disease. The inflamed ovaries are enlarged and filled with multiple cysts, which represent infected follicles, or corpus luteum cysts. Intraovarian vessels can easily be identified and show usually moderate resistance to blood flow.

It is well known that the sonographic appearance of a complex adnexal mass should be interpreted in the context of the clinical setting. For example, in the febrile patient, a thick-walled mass containing echogenic fluid is likely to be an abscess. In this advanced and most severe form of pelvic inflammatory disease, it is difficult to identify the pelvic anatomy. Ovaries are usually adherent to the pelvic sidewall or to the uterus, and the scarring process can alter their endocrine function and circulation. Based on our experience, dynamic use of color Doppler ultrasound in patients affected with pelvic inflammatory disease is important for accurate diagnosis, follow-up, and evaluation of the ovulatory function and ovarian perfusion.

Color Doppler ultrasound is a useful tool in the diagnosis of pelvic inflammatory disease. It helps distinguish between dilated vessels and a fluid-filled hydrosalpinx, and it can be useful in the differential diagnosis of tubo-ovarian abscess. Measurements of the intraovarian resistance in the acute phase of the disease reveal the ovarian involvement and function, as these relate to the rapidly changing pattern of the disease. An increased resistance to blood flow in the chronic phase is probably related to the extensive scarring. This condition of reduced perfusion may have long-term effects on the endocrine function of the ovary.

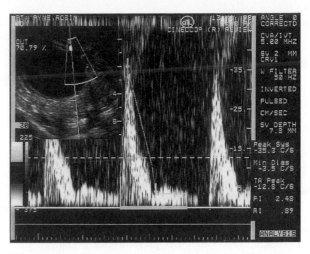

Fig. 39.10. Pulsed-wave Doppler waveform of the same ovarian vessels as shown in Fig. 39.9, with typically high resistance blood blow. A benign ovarian cystadenoma was found on histopathology

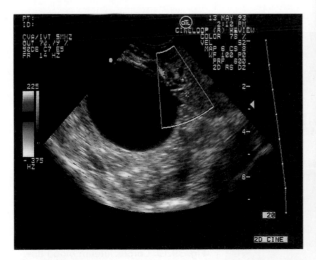

Fig. 39.9. Transvaginal color Doppler of an ovarian cyst with feeding vessels

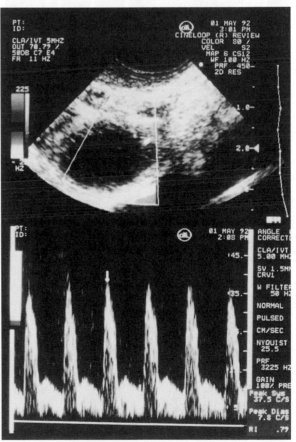

Fig. 39.11. Color and pulsed-wave Doppler findings in the case of a benign ovarian mass

Previous studies have suggested that ovarian ultrasound morphology is not precise for diagnosing ovarian neoplasms; sensitivities vary from 70% upward [25, 26]. Standard ultrasound criteria that suggest a benign condition are well known: unilocular, cystic, unilateral, absence of internal echoes. Conversely, malignant tumors have been characterized as complex: multilocular, cystic-solid, bilateral, with positive free fluid in the peritoneal cavity. Using these criteria both false negatives and false positives are encountered. In a premenopausal population these morphologic criteria may be misleading. Certain pathologic conditions, though benign, appear sonographically with malignant morphology. Examples are dermoid cysts, endometriosis, corpus luteum, and hemorrhagic cysts. Color Doppler waveform analysis provides additional information (Figs. 39.9–39.11). If a high-resistance velocity wave pattern is observed, one may be more confident that the lesion is benign (Fig. 39.12). In the case where a high-velocity/low-resistance pattern is seen the examination must be repeated during the next cycle. Recall that the corpus luteum or luteal flow may exhibit a low-resistance waveform pattern (Fig. 39.13).

Several investigators are now applying a scoring system to both morphologic criteria and color Doppler waveform analysis [27, 28]. Table 39.3 shows the scoring system used by the Zagreb group. This study is the largest series of adnexal tumors analyzed by color Doppler velocimetry [28]. The data yielded a Pourcelot RI cutoff of 0.40 as a discriminatory value for benign versus malignant lesions.

Application of color flow analysis may have important implications with respect to clinical management. Traditionally, the standard of care for an adnexal mass has been laparotomy with surgical excision. For a lesion where the morphology and Doppler analysis suggest a benign condition, conservative therapeutic options may be entertained. Advances in video-endoscopic laparoscopy offer a conservative surgical approach to removing an ovarian cyst.

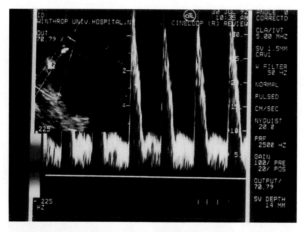

Fig. 39.12. Tumor feeding vessel with typical high-resistance blood flow in the case of benign multilocular ovarian enlargement

Doppler Ultrasound and Ectopic Pregnancy

Ectopic pregnancy is defined as implantation of the fertilized ovum anywhere outside the normal uterine cavity. It accounts for 2% of all pregnancies in the United States, with its incidence is reported to be increasing over the past two decades [29, 30]. Ectopic pregnancy is associated with a high maternal mortality and morbidity, accounting for 9%–13% of all pregnancy-related deaths [31]. The most common site

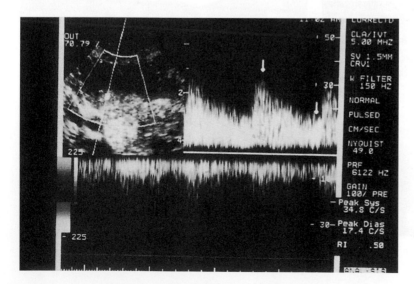

Fig. 39.13. Corpus luteum blood flow may imitate a Doppler pattern that suggests malignancy

Table 39.3. Ovarian tumor B-mode ultrasonography and color Doppler velocimetry scoring system

Classification		
Mass	**Fluid**	**Internal borders**
Unilocular	Clear (0) Internal echoes (1)	Smooth (0) Irregular (2)
Multilocular	Clear (1) Internal echoes (1)	Smooth (1) Irregular (2)
Cystic-solid	Clear (1) Internal echoes (2)	Smooth (1) Irregular (2)
Papillary projections	Suspicious (1)	Definite (2)
Solid	Homogeneous (1)	Echogenic (2)
Peritoneal fluid	Absent (0)	Present (1)
Laterality	Unilateral (0)	bilateral (1)

Ultrasound score

≤2 or less	Bening
3–4	Questionable
>4	Suspicious for malignancy

Color Doppler
No vessels seen (0)
Regular separate vessels (1)
Randomly dispersed vessels (2)

Pulsed Doppler (RI index)
No Doppler signal (0)
>0.40 or more (1)
<0.40 (2)
Note: If suspected corpus luteum blood flow, repeat scan during next menstrual cycle in proliferative phase.

Color Doppler score
≤2 Benign
3–4 Quesionale for malignancy

for an ectopic pregnancy is the fallopian tube; rare types include interstitial, cervical, ovarian and abdominal pregnancy. The management of ectopic pregnancy has metamorphosed impressively from a period in the 1970s and early 1980s when laparotomy was the only choice, to the present period of advances in operative laparoscopy and ultimately high-resolution ultrasonography. This was in step with sensitive quantitative β-hCG determinations, when earlier diagnosis of ectopic pregnancy not only allowed greater use of conservative therapy, but also drastically reduced maternal mortality rates from 35.5 per 10,000 women with ectopic pregnancy in 1970 to 3.8 in 1989 [31]. Ruptured ectopic pregnancy cannot be managed conservatively, and acute cases require emergency laparotomy. Women who have one ectopic pregnancy are at increased risk for another such pregnancy and for future infertility. Early detection and subsequent surgical and medical intervention may account for this reduction in mortality. The exact cause of blastocyst implantation and development outside the endo-

metrial cavity is unknown. Abnormal tubal morphology, alterations in the hormonal environment affecting tubal motility, uterine abnormalities, foreign bodies, and defects of the fertilized ovum are associated with its occurrence. Early recognition of the symptoms and risk factors attributed to ectopic pregnancy and prompt application of advanced technology gives a quicker diagnosis and allows initiation of conservative therapy to reduce the morbidity.

The diagnosis of ectopic pregnancy remains a challenge to the clinician despite advances in ultrasound and biochemical technology. Contemporary practice requires an understanding of the normal sonographic features and hormonal profiles as well as the pathogenesis of an ectopic nidation. Frequently, the diagnosis remains uncertain until laparoscopy or dilatation and curettage has been performed.

The practicing gynecologist should consider all relevant factors, including the patient's clinical history and predictive risk factors, symptoms, and physical findings, serum β-hCG level, and the ultrasound scans, before deciding whether operative intervention is indicated and necessary. Nevertheless, further improvement in imaging techniques may aid in enhancing preoperative certainty and possibly eliminate or reduce the performance of unnecessary surgery. For this purpose, transvaginal Doppler ultrasonography was introduced to add more information by looking at the blood flow characteristics in the adnexa (Figs. 39.14–39.23).

Color and pulsed Doppler flow imaging capabilities have been added to transvaginal sonography (TVS) in an effort to improve sonographic diagnosis. The technique consists of identifying the site of vascular color in a characteristic placental shape called "ring of fire" pattern and a high-velocity, low-impedance flow pattern of placental perfusion. When this pattern is seen outside the uterus while the uterine

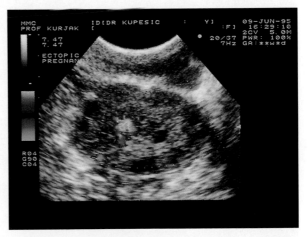

Fig. 39.14. Small gestational sac measuring 1 cm with prominent blood flow signals obtained from its periphery

cavity is "cold" with respect to blood flow, diagnosis of ectopic pregnancy is confirmed. It has been reported to increase the diagnostic sensitivity of sonography for ectopic pregnancy from 71% to 87% [32–34]. It also helps eliminate the problem of false positives, except in rare situations of ovarian pregnancy.

Kurjak et al. have reported on the difference between the RI of the corpus luteum blood flow and peritrophoblastic flow of the ectopic pregnancy. The cutoff value for the RI of corpus luteum blood flow has been described to be 0.4 and the RI of peritrophoblastic blood flow below 0.4 [34]. Kirchler has described the use of Doppler blood flow in measuring the RI in tubal branches of the bilateral uterine ar-

teries. The vessel with low-resistance flow indicates the side of the ectopic pregnancy [35].

Endometrial color flow/image-directed Doppler imaging has also been reported to reduce the false-positive TVS examinations which occur in 5%–10% of patients with high-risk findings. Ectopic pregnancy has no intrauterine trophoblastic activity, hence the presence of trophoblastic flow (arterial blood flow within the endometrium) lowers the risk of ectopic pregnancy whether an intrauterine gestational sac is present or not. However, care must be taken to ensure that arterial and not venous flow signals are obtained. The Doppler cursor should be completely within the endometrium to ensure that the signal is endometrial

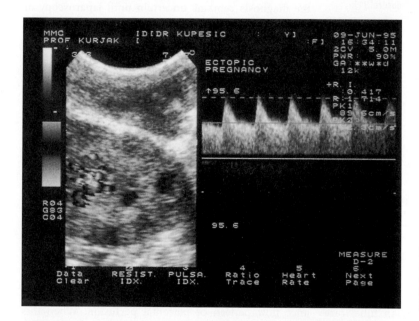

Fig. 39.15. High-velocity/low-impedance (RI = 0.42) blood flow signals are obtained from the color-coded area and represent active, invasive trophoblast

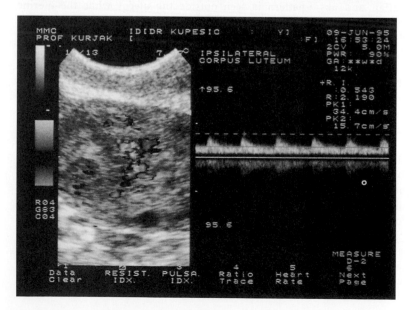

Fig. 39.16. Blood flow signals isolated from ipsilateral corpus luteum demonstrate a moderate to high resistance index (RI = 0.54)

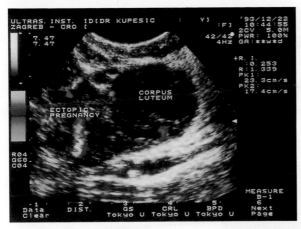

Fig. 39.17. Complex adnexal mass representing an ectopic pregnancy (prominent color signals on the *left*) and a corpus luteum cyst on the *right*

and not from the endometrium-myometrial junction. Further, correlation with serum β-hCG levels is essential [36].

Kemp et al. have reported on the use of Doppler sonographic criterion, i.e., the presence of a signal-intensive ring of vessels (correlated to neovascularization of the tube) for differentiating between a viable ectopic pregnancy with trophoblastic activity and a dissolving tubal abortion [37]. This may help decide about the optimal management, since surgical methods or injection of drugs must arrest chorionic activity, while tubal abortion may be managed expectantly in a clinically stable patient. However, further studies are needed to determine the efficacy of this approach in management of tubal ectopic pregnancy.

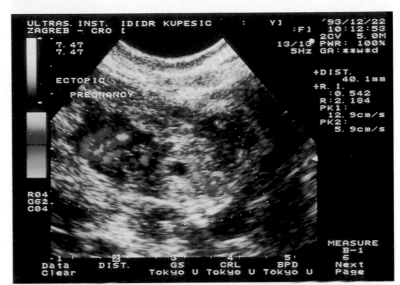

Fig. 39.18. Gestational sac 1 cm in diameter with peripheral vascularization indicating invasive trophoblast

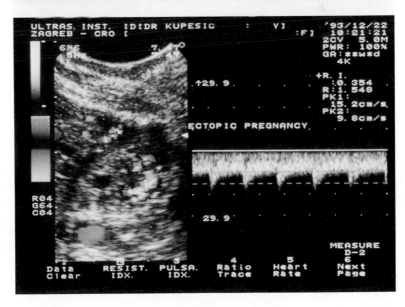

Fig. 39.19. Same patient as shown in Fig. 39.5. The pulsed-wave Doppler waveform analysis demonstrates low impedance to blood flow (RI = 0.35)

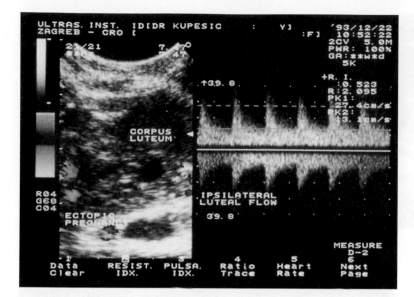

Fig. 39.20. Ipsilateral corpus luteum shows significantly higher impedance to blood flow (RI=0.52) and can be distinguished from signals obtained from the periphery of the gestational sac

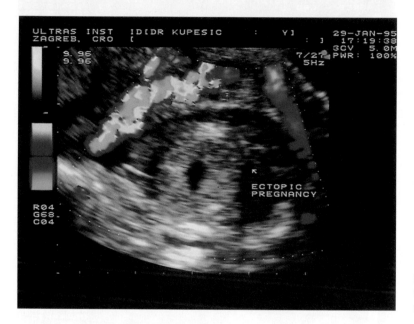

Fig. 39.21. Ectopic gestational sac in the left adnexal region surrounded by a "ring of fire" (nearby vessels)

Other Types of Ectopic Pregnancy

Interstitial/Cornual Pregnancy

These two terms are used interchangeably, though strictly speaking the term cornual pregnancy should be reserved for pregnancy in a rudimentary uterine horn. Only 2%–4% of ectopic pregnancies develop in the interstitial portion of the fallopian tube [38]. The surrounding myometrium permits the pregnancy to progress to an advanced age (12–16 weeks) before it ruptures. Severe hemorrhage ensues leading to a significantly higher mortality and morbidity.

High-resolution ultrasound along with the color flow Doppler equipment enables an early and accurate diagnosis to be made. Sonographic findings include eccentric location of the gestational sac and myometrial thinning. Ackerman et al. have described the "interstitial line" sign in cases where the visible myometrium completely surrounds the gestational sac, making the diagnosis difficult. They proposed that since interstitial pregnancy grows within the lumen of the tube, the endometrial cavity or interstitial portion of the tube can be traced directly to the eccentric gestational sac. This sign was reported to be 80% sensitive and 99% specific for the interstitial pregnancy [39].

Fig. 39.22. Blood flow signals isolated from the periphery of an ectopic gestational sac demonstrate low impedance to blood flow (RI = 0.43)

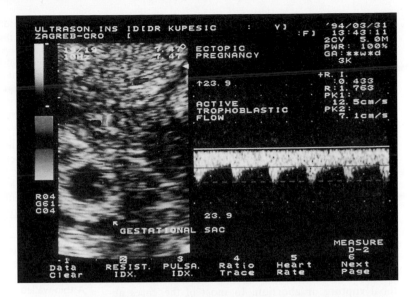

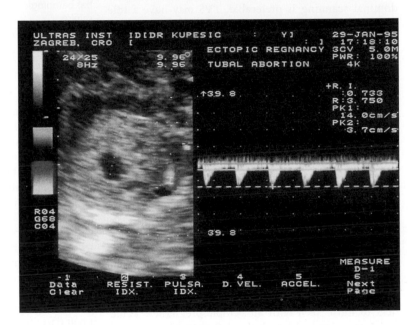

Fig. 39.23. Pulsed-wave Doppler waveform analysis obtained from an ectopic pregnancy in a regression phase demonstrates significantly higher impedance to blood flow (RI = 0.73)

Cervical Pregnancy

Cervical pregnancy is a rare condition accounting for approximately 0.15% of all ectopic pregnancy [40]. When undiagnosed, it leads to massive hemorrhage requiring an emergency hysterectomy. In 1978, Raskin presented the first report of a sonographic diagnosis of a cervical pregnancy [41]. Subsequently other workers have reported on use of TVS in early diagnosis of cervical pregnancy [42, 43]. Location of the gestational sac within the endocervical canal is the cardinal sonographic sign. This leads to cervical enlargement and the classically described "hourglass appearance" of the uterus [44]. With the advent of

TVS, cervical pregnancies can be diagnosed early in gestation at less than 7 weeks of menstrual age, enabling prompt treatment.

Ovarian Pregnancy

Ovarian pregnancy is an uncommon type of ectopic pregnancy. Its incidence has been reported to be 1 per 7,000 pregnancies and it accounts for 1%–6% of all ectopic pregnancies [45]. Presenting symptoms are similar to those of tubal pregnancy. A causative relationship with an intrauterine device has been recognized [46]. It is difficult to preoperatively diagnose ovarian pregnancy clinically [47].

However, recent advances in hCG determination and ultrasound, especially TVS, have helped in its early diagnosis and correct localization [48, 49]. TVS has been reported to be of diagnostic value in differentiating ovarian pregnancy from tubal pregnancy [50]. The image of ovarian mass is characterized by a double hyperechoic ring surrounding a small hypoechogenic field. A case of twin ovarian pregnancy diagnosis on TVS has also been reported [51]. Bontis et al. have evaluated the criteria for diagnosis of ovarian pregnancy based on currently available diagnostic methods [52].

Abdominal Pregnancy

It accounts for 0.03% of ectopic pregnancies [40]. Its diagnosis is often missed on TVS or delayed, as most of these are secondary implantations occurring after tubal rupture or abortion. In most of the cases abdominal scanning is preferable. TVS may have a role in suspected abdominal pregnancy by virtue of clear depiction of the gestation sac outside the uterus. The endocervical canal does not extend up to the placenta but is present either posterior or anterior to it. Walls of the lower uterine segment are seen opposed to each other and not separated by the gestational sac.

Diagnostic Difficulties

The ultrasonologist should be aware of conditions causing false-positive or false-negative Doppler ultrasound diagnosis of ectopic pregnancy [32], which are listed in Table 39.4. A false-positive diagnosis predominantly comes from corpus luteum, but other adnexal tumors may also be a source of error. Malignant ovarian or tubal masses, endometriosis, or inflammation can be a diagnostic challenge. Corpus luteum can produce color and pulsed-wave Doppler patterns that are similar and sometimes almost identical to those seen with an ectopic pregnancy. Zalud and Kurjak studied luteal blood flow in pregnant and nonpregnant women [53]. Typical luteal low-impedance blood flow was detected in 82.8% cases of normal early pregnancy, 80.8% cases of ectopic pregnancy, and 69.3% cases of nonpregnant women during the luteal phase of the menstrual cycle. The lowest RI (0.42 ± 0.12) of luteal flow was found in nonpregnant women, and the highest RI (0.53 ± 0.09) was seen with an early intrauterine pregnancy. The RI in cases of ectopic pregnancy was 0.48 ± 0.07. In 86.4% of patients with proved ectopic pregnancy, luteal flow was detected on the same side as the ectopic pregnancy. This observation can be used as a guide when searching for an ectopic pregnancy.

A false-negative result may arise from technical inadequacy of the performed ultrasound scan, lack of

Table 39.4. Conditions affecting Doppler ultrasound findings for ectopic pregnancy

False-positive findings
- Corpus luteum [a]
- Endometriosis
- Pelvic inflammatory disease
- Other adnexal masses or structures [b]
- Ovarian cancer

False-negative findings
- Very early ectopic pregnancy
- Avascular ectopic gestation
- Lack of experience of the technician
- Technical difficulties
- Nonvascularized ectopic pregnancy
- Patient noncompliance [c]

[a] The corpus luteum may create the impression of a sac-like structure because it is eccentrically located within the ovary and surrounded by ovarian tissue.
[b] A thin-walled ovarian follicle; the small intestine; and tubal pathologic conditions such as a fluid-containing hydrosalpinx.
[c] Patient is not lying very still.

experience, or the patient's noncompliance. Another possibility is a nonvascularized ectopic gestation. Noting that one-third of ectopic pregnancies showed no evidence of detectable vascularity, Meyers and associates investigated the hypothesis that this group represented nonviable ectopic pregnancies [54]. They studied them by comparing the serum β-hCG levels in women with vascular and nonvascular ectopic pregnancies. A statistically significant difference was seen between the serum hCG level of those women with ectopic pregnancies with vascularity compared with those women without vascularity. The avascular ectopic pregnancies showed low levels of serum β-hCG, suggesting a nonthriving or dying embryo. We diagnosed ectopic gestations routinely by color Doppler sonography when the β-hCG level was below 1,000 IU/L. The impact of these observations on possible conservative therapy has yet to be considered.

Management

Conservative Management

Initiation of conservative therapy for ectopic pregnancy requires fulfillment of strict selection norms [4]. The established criteria for patient selection are listed in Table 39.5.

Conservative management of ectopic pregnancy includes: (a) tubal-conserving surgery which is usually performed laparoscopically; (b) expectant management; and (c) medical management. The conservative laparoscopic procedures for treatment of ectopic preg-

Table 39.5. Criteria for conservative management of ectopic pregnancy

- β–hCG level is indicative of ectopic pregnancy[a]
- Ectopic gestation has been identified on a sonogram
- Ectopic gestation has not ruptured
- Gestational sac size is less than 4 cm (preferably without embryonal cardiac activity)
- Hemoglobin level and hematocrit are in the normal range
- Patient is compliant[b]
- Patient is hemodynamically stable

[a] An increase of less than 66% of an initial value over a 48-h period is indicative of either an ectopic pregnancy or a missed abortion.

[b] Patient is able to reliably and precisely follow postoperative instructions (usually at home) for very early signs of unsuccessful conservative management (e.g., ruptured ectopic pregnancy with pelvic pain and intraabdominal or vaginal bleeding).

nancy include salpingostomy, injection of antimetabolites (e.g., methotrexate) or lytic agents (e.g., potassium chloride). The operative manipulations can be achieved with use of endoscissors, endocoagulation, electrocautery, laser, endoloops, and endosutures.

Ultrasound imaging, used in conjunction with serum β-hCG estimation, is indispensable for conservative management of ectopic pregnancy. It helps in (a) early diagnosis of ectopic pregnancy and selection of cases, (b) execution of local treatment, and (c) monitoring the response to treatment and follow-up of the patients managed conservatively.

Expectant Management

Here, asymptomatic women with declining or stable β-hCG levels and small adnexal masses at transvaginal sonography (TVS) are monitored without intervention. Monitoring involves clinical evaluation and repeated ultrasound and β-hCG estimations. The basis of expectant management is that a substantial number of ectopic pregnancies are diagnosed at a very early stage when some may be expected to resolve spontaneously – "involuting ectopic pregnancy." In 1955, Lund first reported on a conservative nonsurgical approach to the treatment of tubal pregnancies [55]. Subsequently several other workers have reported on expectant management of ectopic pregnancy [56].

Strict ultrasound parameters have been used as inclusion criteria. Trio et al. expectantly managed 67 stable patients with (a) no adnexal embryonic cardiac activity, (b) no adnexal mass greater than 4 cm in diameter, and (c) cul de sac fluid estimated to be less than 100 ml. In total, 73% of their patients showed complete resolution of ectopic pregnancy; however,

success depended on a low initial HCG level [57]. Stovall and Ling restricted expectant management to tubal ectopic pregnancies with a diameter not greater than 3.5 cm and reported a 48% spontaneous resolution rate [58]. However, the safety and efficacy of this management are questionable and it remains a controversial mode of treatment. A longer time to resolution and need for intensive monitoring are inconvenient, but the subsequent repeat ectopic rate is not increased.

The role of ultrasound in medical management of ectopic pregnancy was first proposed in 1982 by Tanaka et al. using methotrexate (MTX) [59]. Since then a large number of studies have reported on intramuscular and local injection of MTX and other agents like potassium chloride (KCl), prostaglandin E2 and F2a, and hyperosmolar glucose [60–62]. Medical treatment with MTX is cost-effective and it is estimated that a cost saving of 265 million dollars/year can be achieved in the United States if 30% of all patients with ectopic pregnancy are eligible for this therapy [63].

Studies reporting on systemic MTX employ ultrasound imaging for selection of cases, the important criteria being an adnexal mass less than 3.5 cm in diameter in a hemodynamically stable patient [64]. The other important application of ultrasound is local MTX injection into the tubal gestational sac (salpingocentesis) by the transvaginal route under transvaginal sonographic guidance, first reported by Feichtinger et al. in 1987 [65]. Transabdominal puncture under transabdominal sonography has also been reported for both tubal and interstitial pregnancies [66]. However, the transvaginal route offers the advantage of accurate needle placement and is the route of choice for intrasac injection in most cases of ectopic pregnancy. Accurate placement of the needle into the gestational sac enables use of MTX locally and avoids side effects of systemic treatment. Success rates with this procedure vary from 60%–100%, and patients should be carefully instructed to report if signs and symptoms of worsening pain or rupture of the ectopic pregnancy occur [67].

Ultrasound-guided salpingocentesis can be performed using manual needle insertion or an automated puncture device. For manual needle insertion analgesia and sometimes local anesthesia is used and the procedure is performed with guidance of a 5–7.5-MHz vaginal transducer probe through a fixed needle guide attached to the probe shaft. This permits easier visualization of the entire length of the needle and better control for accurate needle placement. Amniotic fluid is aspirated from the ectopic gestational sac followed by injection of MTX or another chosen agent. Usually a single 50-mg injection of MTX is used but as little as 5 mg has been used successfully

[60]. If a 50-mg dose is used, it is usually followed by a single dose of folinic acid to prevent systemic side effects. When using KCl, approximately 0.25–0.5 ml of the solution (2 mEq/l) is injected in the area of the beating fetal heart and observed for 10 min.

At completion of the procedure and after an observation period of 2–3 h, the pelvic structures and cul de sac are observed sonographically to detect possible internal bleed or any other complication.

An automated puncture device is more accurate and potentially less painful than manual needle introduction. This spring-loaded device, when mated to the shaft of the vaginal probe, provides extreme accuracy and precision and its high-velocity release makes the procedure virtually painless thus obviating the need for anesthesia.

Interstitial Pregnancy

Systemic chemotherapy with MTX can be used for nonsurgical management of interstitial pregnancy. MTX or KCl solution can also be used for local injection into the gestational sac under sonographic guidance. Some additional sonographic parameters have been defined to refine patient selection and posttreatment monitoring [68]. These are: (a) Peritrophoblastic blood flow – a solid "ring of fire" sign suggests a highly vascularized implantation which may respond better to direct intrasac therapy than systemic MTX. Color flow Doppler may also indicate resolution if blood flow can be shown to decrease with treatment [69]. Persistent trophoblastic blood flow may be associated with increased risk of spontaneous rupture and deferral of subsequent pregnancy might be considered until the blood flow pattern returns to normal. (b) Myometrial thickness assessed akin to that described for lower uterine segment thickness in patients with previous cesarean section [70]. When it is less than 3.5 mm the patient may be at an increased risk for rupture and this may be a pertinent parameter for guiding the management. The precise predictive value of these parameters is, however, uncertain and requires further evaluation.

Cervical Pregnancy

Local intrasac injection of MTX or KCl has been described. Paltzi et al. used a combination of MTX given intracervically followed by intramuscular injection [71]. Kaplan et al. used transabdominal sonography to guide injection of MTX into the amniotic sac of a cervical pregnancy [72]. Timor-Tritsch et al. used transvaginal sonography-guided MTX injection with an automated puncture device and 21G needle in five cases of viable cervical pregnancy [73]. Frates et al. used TVS-guided injection of KCl into the embryo or gestational sac in six cases of cervical pregnancy of less than 7.9 weeks' gestation [74]. Success was reported in all the cases. Thus, when cervical pregnancy is diagnosed early, ultrasound-guided local therapy is safe and effective. It involves minimal patient discomfort and recovery time and preserves the patient's reproductive potential.

Ovarian Pregnancy

Traditional treatment for ovarian pregnancy involves ipsilateral oophorectomy. Koike et al. reported the first successful case of an unruptured ovarian pregnancy treated medically by local injection of 0.5 mg prostaglandin F2 with an additional dose of prostaglandin E2 (dinoprostone) administered orally for 14 postoperative days [75]. Subsequently systemic MTX has been used for medical management of ovarian pregnancies [76]. The response to treatment can be assessed by ultrasound imaging, as described for tubal pregnancy.

Heterotopic Pregnancy

Ultrasonography helps in conservative management of heterotrophic pregnancies. Unlike MTX, KCl is only embryotoxic and not antitrophoblastic therefore ultrasound-guided local injection of KCl into the ectopic sac is used to avoid harm to the coexistent intrauterine pregnancy.

Ultrasound Monitoring of Conservative Management

Ultrasonography is crucial to follow up along with β-hCG estimations every 3–5 days. Real-time sonography is carried out to observe the decrease in size of the adnexal mass. Color Doppler is used to assess vascularity and normalization of the RI. Disappearance of adnexal/ectopic pregnancy mass usually occurs by day 30–40, with the RI normalizing by day 5–20. β-hCG levels gradually fall rapidly to normal levels by 2 weeks to a maximum of 8 weeks. Following systemic or intratubal MTX, a visible adnexal mass may persist on TVS for more than 3 months, even after a β-hCG test yields negative results. It is not uncommon for these to transiently enlarge and have increased Doppler flow signal [67].

Ultrasound imaging thus helps in monitoring the response to treatment and evaluation of potential complications both during and after the therapy. In the literature, a few patients treated by salpingocentesis underwent hysterosalpingography and were found to have patent fallopian tubes [60]. A rise in β-hCG levels and an increase in ectopic pregnancy mass associated with persistent or acute upon subacute clinical symptoms apprise of possible failure of conservative treatment.

Doppler Ultrasound and Infertility

Uterine Blood Flow during Menstrual Cycle

Transvaginal color Doppler (TVCD) sonography provides an opportunity to visualize and quantify pelvic blood flow in relation to hormonal changes during the menstrual cycle. The follicle and corpus luteum of the ovary and endometrium are the only areas in the normal adult where angiogenesis occurs [77, 78]. Uterine artery waveform analysis shows high to moderate flow velocity (Figs. 39.24 and 39.25). The resistance index (RI) depends on the patient's age, the

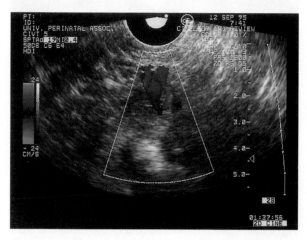

Fig. 39.24. Uterine artery and vein visualized by transvaginal color Doppler sonography

phase of the menstrual cycle, and specific conditions such as pregnancy and uterine tumors.

Transvaginal color Doppler sonography can be used to obtain flow velocity waveforms at any time during the menstrual period. Apparently there are complex relations between the concentration of ovarian hormones in peripheral blood and uterine artery blood flow parameters [79, 80]. In most women there is a small amount of end-diastolic flow in the uterine artery during the proliferative phase. Collins and co-workers reported that diastolic flow in the uterine artery disappeared during the day of ovulation [81]. Goswamy et al. found an increasing RI and systolic/diastolic (S/D) ratio during the postovulatory drop in the serum estradiol concentration [79]. Steer et al. reported increased uterine artery impedance 3 days after the luteinizing hormone (LH) peak [82]. Scholtes and colleagues recorded the highest pulsatility index (PI) value in the uterine artery on cycle day 16 [83]. These findings may be explained by increased uterine contractility and compression of the vessels transversing the uterine wall, which decreases their diameter and causes a consequent higher resistance to flow.

During the normal menstrual cycle there is a sharp increase in end-diastolic velocity between the proliferative and secretory phases of the menstrual cycle. It is particularly interesting that the lowest blood flow impedance occurs at the time of peak luteal function, during which time implantation is most likely to occur. It is logical that the blood supply to the uterus should be high during the late luteal phase as reported by Kurjak, Goswamy, Steer, Battaglia, and their colleagues [78, 79, 82, 84]. During anovulatory cycles these changes are nor present, and a continu-

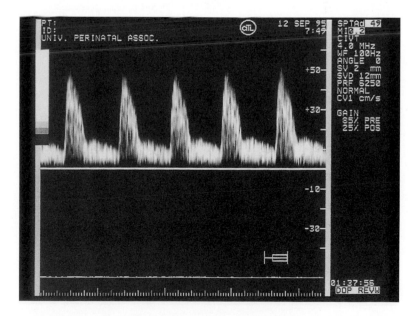

Fig. 39.25. Typical pulsed-wave Doppler waveform of the uterine artery during the luteal phase of a normal menstrual cycle

ous increase in the RI is not seen. In some infertile patients the end-diastolic flow is not present [80]. There are no data yet on which to base speculation whether absent diastolic flow is associated with infertility or poor reproductive performance. It seems that transvaginal Doppler sonography may be used as a noninvasive assay of uterine receptivity; it would enable clinicians to cryopreserve the embryos if uterine conditions are adverse and reduce the number of transferred embryos when conditions are optimal. Uterine artery blood flow could be used to predict a hostile uterine environment before embryo transfer [82]. Those women with poor uterine perfusion could then be advised that pregnancy is unlikely during their treatment cycle and so have their embryos cryopreserved for transfer at a later date.

One of the major problems associated with current in vitro fertilization (IVF) is the need to use multiple-embryo transfer to increase the pregnancy rate, which results in an increase in multiple pregnancies. This increase may contribute to increased obstetric risk and diminished perinatal outcome compared to singleton pregnancies. It is well known that the probability of pregnancy is strongly related to embryo quality and uterine receptivity. Instead of performing an endometrial biopsy, which may cause trauma and bleeding at the implantation site, uterine receptivity could be assessed by color Doppler ultrasonography. This noninvasive technique is rapid, is easy to perform, and may predict the likelihood of implantation, thereby minimizing the risk of multiple pregnancy. Circulatory changes similar to those observed in the main uterine artery are seen in the minute arteries (radial and spiral) (Figs. 39.26–39.28). The endometrium has an exceptional capacity to undergo changes in structure and

function during the menstrual cycle. Histologic changes include the striking development of blood vessels, the spiral arteries becoming more developed during the menstrual cycle. The increased endometrial vascularity during the menstrual cycle depends on changes in the uterine, arcuate, and radial artery blood flow. Changes in blood flow velocity waveform of the spiral arterises during a normal ovulatory cycle have been demonstrated for the first time by TVCD sonography [85]. Endometrial perfusion may be used to predict implantation success and to reveal unexplained infertility problems.

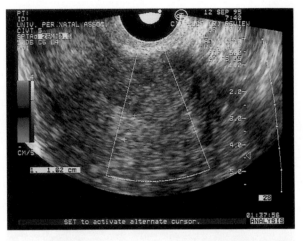

Fig. 39.26. Color Doppler mapping of the radial and spiral arteries. The spiral arteries are closer to endometrium (endometrial thickness 1.02 cm is shown)

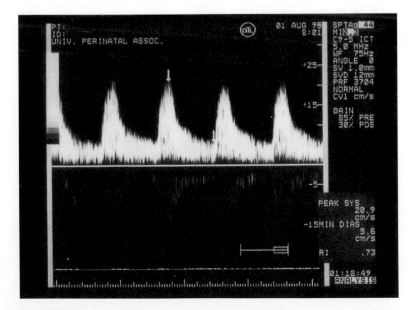

Fig. 39.27. Pulsed-wave Doppler waveform of the radial artery

Fig. 39.28. Doppler analysis of blood flow in the spiral artery in the same patient as shown in Fig. 39.27. Note the lower velocity but almost the same impedance to blood flow

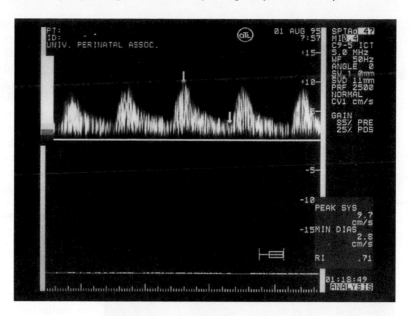

Ovarian Blood Flow during Menstrual Cycle

Using the same method it is possible to assess intraovarian blood flow during the menstrual cycle (Figs. 39.29–39.37). Color Doppler imaging facilitates detection of small vascular areas in the ovarian stroma and follicular rim [86]. Pulsed-wave Doppler sonography has become available on high-resolution vaginal ultrasound probes for studying ovarian blood flow. Doppler studies of ovarian blood flow are based on semiquantitative analysis of Doppler flow waves recorded over the ovarian artery at their entry into the ovary and color Doppler mapping of intraovarian vessels. Semiquantitative analysis of the ovarian artery Doppler flow waves is frequently insufficient for identifying the ovarian artery, particularly in multiparous women. Mapping intraovarian vessels, however, appears to be a promising feature of vaginal Doppler imaging for studying ovarian blood flow, provided the proper ultrasound equipment is used. Specifically, TVCD sonographic mapping of intraovarian vessels allows positive visual detection of the onset of the ovulatory process prior to follicular rupture. Thus color Doppler sonographic mapping of ovarian vessels provides an improved, simplified approach to timing intercourse and inseminations in infertile patients. With controlled ovarian hyperstimulation used for IVF, mapping of intraovarian vessels by color Doppler sonography offers a fascinating insight into normal and pathologic responses of ovarian follicles to human chorionic gonadotropin (hCG). Finally, color Doppler imaging seems to be a promising adjunct to transvaginal ultrasonography for distinguishing suspicious ovarian cysts from their benign counterparts.

Blood flow from the follicle can be seen when the follicle reaches 10–12 mm in diameter and may be a hemodynamic parameter of its growth, maturation, and ovulation. The RI is approximately 0.54 ± 0.04 until ovulation approaches. A decline begins 2 days before ovulation and reaches a nadir (0.44 ± 0.04) at ovulation. At the time of presumed ovulation there is increased vascularity on the inner wall of the follicle and a coincident surge in blood velocity just before eruption. These changes may represent dilatation of new vessels that have developed between the relatively vascular theca cell layer and the normally hypoxic granulosa cell layer of the follicle [87]. These vascular changes compound the effect of the oxygen concentration across the follicular epithelium. Immediately after follicular rupture, there is another dramatic increase in the velocity of blood flow to the early corpus luteum. The RI remains at that level for 4–5 days and then gradualy climbs to 0.50 ± 0.004, which is still lower than that seen during the proliferative phase. Collins et al. found that the changes of PI observed from the wall of the dominant follicle and corpus luteum were less marked than the changes in blood velocity [81]. Merce and coworkers obtained Doppler shift waveforms from the parenchyma adjacent to the dominant follicle or corpus luteum in the dominant ovary [87]. They noted that the blood flow velocity index in the dominant ovary was lower during the luteal phase than during the follicular phase. Increased resistance was observed during the late luteal phase.

These blood flow changes reflect changes in vascularization and function of the corpus luteum. Increased blood flow supply to the ovary that contains the dominant follicle and corpus luteum is necessary for delivery of steroid precursors to the ovary and production of progesterone. Therefore changes in flow velocity occur in the uterine and ovarian vessels before ovulation, implying that these changes are complex and not purely secondary to progesterone action. Undoubtedly, many other vasoactive compounds, such as prostaglandins, are involved in regulation of the vasculature.

Clinical Application

Transvaginal ultrasonography depicts anatomic and physiologic parameters that are important to the management of female infertility. Specifically, follicular development into functional corpus luteum, uter-

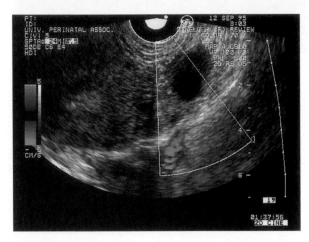

Fig. 39.29. Follicular blood flow visualized by color Doppler sonography in the left ovary. The internal iliac vessel is also shown (*blue*)

ine perfusion prior to implantation, studies of uterine integrity, and tubal potency are areas for clinical application of this relatively new diagnostic modality. Other applications involve detection of abnormally located or distended parauterine vessels. These vessels should be avoided during guided needle aspiration. Similarly, dilated uterine and ovarian veins are seen in some patients with pelvic congestion. Pelvic Doppler sonography has been useful for assessing blood flow to leiomyomas prior to initiation of hormonal suppression therapy. Perhaps those that have an intact blood supply are more likely to respond than those that are relatively avascular. Other possible applications for Doppler sonography in regard to infertility include diagnosis of endometriosis, ovarian hyperstimulation, ovarian torsion, pelvic inflammatory disease, and ectopic pregnancy.

A logical extension of this technology is its usefulness in the evaluation of infertile women [88–95]. In an earlier study, TVCD sonography was used to analyze uterine and ovarian blood flow during the menstrual cycle [78]. This study was carried out on 100 infertile women and the results compared to those from 150 women attending the clinic for annual checkups. Uterine flow velocity has an RI of 0.88 during the proliferative phase and starts to decrease the day before ovulation. A nadir of 0.84 ± 0.04 is reached on day 18 and remains at that level for the rest of the cycle. These changes do not occur in anovulatory cycles. Some women with primary infertility showed a marked reduction in uterine flow velocity. Ovarian artery flow velocity is usually detected when the dominant follicle reaches 12–15 mm. The RI is 0.54 and declines on the day before ovulation. A nadir of

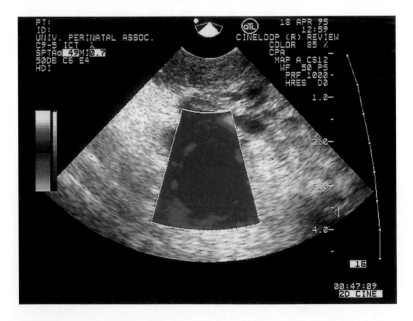

Fig. 39.30. Small vessels around the mature follicle can also be visualized by color Doppler sonography

Fig. 39.31. Intraovarian blood flow during the proliferative phase of the normal menstrual cycle

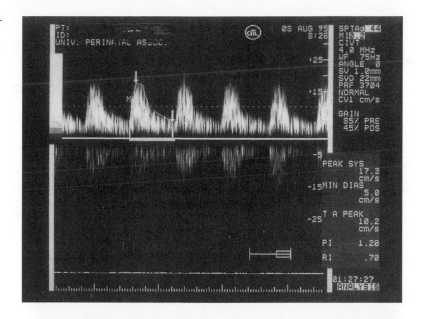

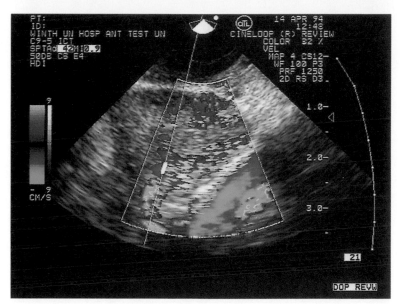

Fig. 39.32. Corpus luteum blood flow during the early secretory phase. The rich vascular supply shown here by color Doppler sonography is typical

0.44±0.04 is reached 4–5 days later and then slowly rises to 0.05–0.04 before menstruation. Because the changes in the uterine and ovarian flow velocities begin prior to ovulation, it can be conjectured that these changes involve angiogenesis as well as hormonal factors. Our own study with color flow sonography confronted an important question. In most women there is a small amount of end-diastolic flow in the uterine arteries during the proliferative phase. In our study end-diastolic flow was not present in some infertile women. Currently, we are unable to determine whether absent end-diastolic flow is associated with infertility or poor reproductive perfor-

mance. A prospective study design is necessary to establish this point. These studies raised the interesting question of whether blood flow changes play a role in infertility. Could failure of adequate flow result in early pregnancy loss? Is it possible that endometrial defects could be hormonal or deficient on the basis of inadequate vascular support? Similarly, could inadequate vascularization play a role in the luteal phase defect? It is not clear at present whether the small but significant changes noted in this study can provide a sensitive enough differential to answer these questions.

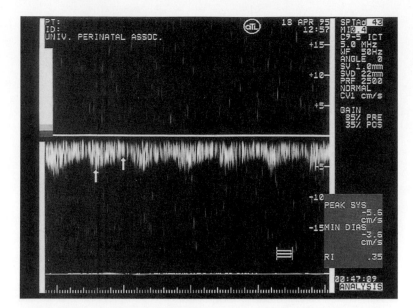

Fig. 39.33. Pulsed-wave Doppler waveform analysis typical for corpus luteum neovascularization

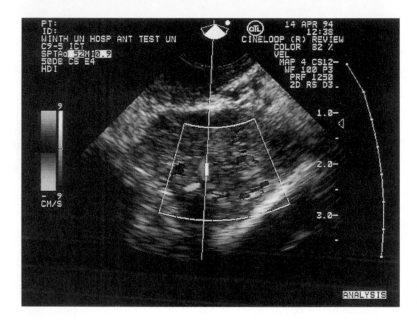

Fig. 39.34. Reduced intraovarian blood flow during the late secretory phase

Conclusion

Transvaginal ultrasonography and the Doppler technique have become available diagnostic modalities for evaluating patients with various gynecological conditions. The addition of color Doppler sonography has added to the diagnostic potential of the ultrasound armamentarium. In addition to improved morphologic detail inherent in the use of the transvaginal probe, new information is gained on perfusion and the pathophysiologic changes associated with abnormal pelvic blood flow. Color Doppler sonography has exposed small and randomly dispersed vessels that could not be seen with the real-time technique, and pulsed-wave Doppler is becoming a diagnostic tool for quantifying and comparing different blood flow detected by color flow analyses. The conditions amenable to such investigations include benign gynecological disorders such as leiomyomas, endometrial hypoplasia, and benign adnexal masses.

Ultrasound imaging, especially transvaginal sonography, and color and pulse Doppler flow imaging contribute to accurate diagnosis of ectopic pregnancy and selection of patients for conservative management. This helps in decreasing the mortality rate of

Fig. 39.35. Hyperstimulated right ovary. Color Doppler velocimetry shows the intraovarian blood flow

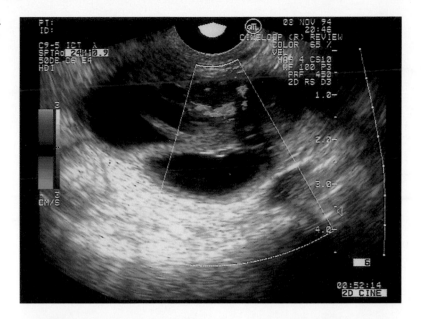

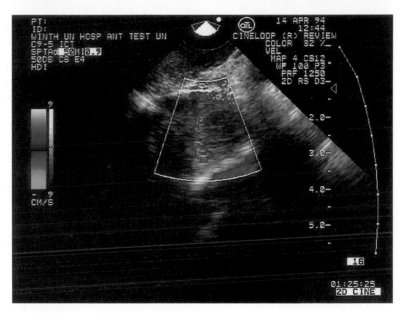

Fig. 39.36. Corpus luteum blood flow visualized by color Doppler velocimetry is usually semilunar in appearance

ectopic pregnancy. It also reduces the morbidity associated with surgery and anesthesia and is more cost-effective than surgical management. Unlike laparoscopy, it is a procedure that is non-invasive, can be repeated, and is easily available. Further studies may help identify more accurate sonographic parameters for better patient selection and post-treatment follow-up.

Transvaginal ultrasonography has brought the pelvic organs into closer view than ever before. Color Doppler sonography has exposed small vessels that could not be seen with the B-mode technique alone, and pulsed-wave Doppler imaging is becoming an important adjunct in the assessment of many physiologic and pathologic states. Vascular changes of the ovary and uterus during the menstrual cycle are now being followed during infertility protocols. They are also bein investigated to determine the viability of an early pregnancy and may increase our confidence in the diagnosis of an ectopic pregnancy in selected cases. Color Doppler ultrasonography has been used to gain insight into the physiologic processes and pathologic conditions involving the female reproductive tract. The ability to assess uteroovarian blood flow with transvaginal color Doppler ultrasonography has several applications for the assessment of women

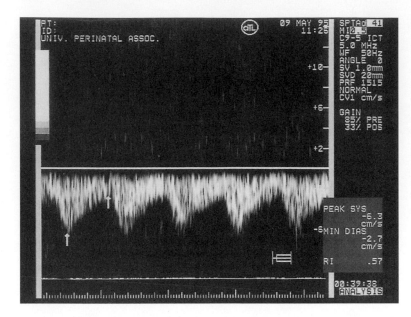

Fig. 39.37. Luteal blood flow waveform analysis

with fertility problems. It extends the scope of sonographic imaging from an anatomic to a physiologic modality. The changes in ovarian and uterine perfusion during spontaneous or induced menstrual cycles can be assessed and thereby optimized, allowing embryo transfer to take place when conditions are most favorable for implantation. Color Doppler processing also enhances detection of flow in nonvascular structures, such as contrast medium injected into the tubes to assess their potency. Although much of this work is preliminary, transvaginal Doppler ultrasonography has tremendous potential for assessment of infertility. In conclusion, we think that vaginal Doppler imaging should be considered a marvelous refinement of ultrasonography rather than a truly new diagnostic tool. Vaginal color Doppler imaging has the potential for markedly improving the sensitivity and specificity of vaginal ultrasonography in the assessment of infertility.

References

1. Kurjak A, Kupesic S (2000) An Atlas of transvaginal color Doppler, 3rd edn. Parthenon Publishing, New York London
2. Zalud I (2002) Doppler evaluation of the ovary: clinical applications and challenges. Contemp Obstet Gynecol 47:37–59
3. Oyelese Y, Kucek AS, Barter J, Zalud I (2002) Asymptomatic postmenopausal simple ovarian cyst. Obstet Gynecol Survey 57:803–809
4. Kurjak A, Kupesic-Urek S, Miric D (1992) The assessment of benign uterine tumor vascularization by transvaginal color Doppler. Ultrasound Med Biol 18:645–649
5. Zalud I, Conway C, Schulman H, Trinca D (1993) Endometrial and myometrial thickness and uterine blood flow in postmenopausal women: the influence of hormonal replacement therapy and age. J Ultrasound Med 12:737–741
6. Gull B, Karlsson B, Milsom I, Granberg S (2003) Can ultrasound replace dilation and curettage? A longitudinal evaluation of postmenopausal bleeding and transvaginal sonographic measurement of the endometrium as predictors of endometrial cancer. Am J Obstet Gynecol 188:401–408
7. Warming L, Ravn P, Skouby S, Christiansen C (2002) Measurement precision and normal range of endometrial thickness in a postmenopausal population by transvaginal ultrasound. Ultrasound Obstet Gynecol 20:492–495
8. Bourne TH (1991) Transvaginal color Doppler in gynecology. Ultrasound Obstet Gynecol 1:359–373
9. Merce LT, Garica L, De La Fuente F (1991) Doppler ultrasound assessment of endometrial pathology. Acta Obstet Gynecol Scand 70:525–530
10. Bourne TH, Campbell S, Steer CV et al (1991) Detection of endometrial cancer by transvaginal ultrasonography with color flow imaging and blood flow analysis: a preliminary report. Obstet Gynecol 40:253–259
11. Kurjak A, Shalan H, Sosic A et al (1993) Endometrial carcinoma in postmenopausal women: evaluation by transvaginal color Doppler sonography. Am J Obstet Gynecol 169:1597–1603
12. Kurjak A, Zalud I (1991) Uterine masses. In: Kurjak A (ed) Transvaginal Color Doppler. Parthenon, Lancaster, UK, pp 123–135
13. Bourne T, Hillard TC, Whitehead MI et al (1990) Oestrogens, arterial status, and postmenopausal women. Lancet 335:1470
14. Palmer JR (1994) Advances in the epidemiology of gestational trophoblastic disease. J Reprod Med 39:155–162
15. Anonymous (1993) Management of gestational trophoblastic disease: ACOG technical bulletin number 178 – March 1993. Int J Gynaecol Obstet 42:308–315

16. Jurkovic D, Jauniaux E, Kurjak A et al (1991) Transvaginal color Doppler assessment of the uteroplacental circulation in early pregnancy. Obstet Gynecol 77:365–369

17. Jaffe R, Warsof SL (1991) Transvaginal color Doppler imaging in the assessment of uteroplacental blood flow in the normal firsttrimester pregnancy. Am J Obstet Gynecol 164:781–785

18. Kurjak A, Zalud I, Predanic M, Kupesic S (1994) Transvaginal color and pulsed Doppler study of uterine blood flow in the first and early second trimester of pregnancy: normal vs. abnormal. J Ultrasound Med 13:43–47

19. Smith DB, O'Reilly SM, Newlands ES (1993) Current approaches to diagnosis and treatment of gestational trophoblastic disease. Curr Opin Obstet Gynecol 5:84–91

20. Schneider DF, Bukovsky I, Weintraub Z, Golan A, Caspi E (1990) Transvaginal ultrasound diagnosis and treatment follow-up of invasive gestational trophoblastic disease. J Clin Ultrasound 18:110–113

21. Crade M, Weber PR (1991) Appearance of molar pregnancy 9.5 weeks after conception: use of transvaginal ultrasound for early diagnosis. J Ultrasound Med 10:473–474

22. Kurjak A, Zalud I, Salihagic A, Crvenkovic G, Matijevic R (1991) Transvaginal color Doppler in the assessment of abnormal early pregnancy. J Perinat Med 19:155–165

23. Carter J, Fowler J, Carlson J et al (1993) Transvaginal color flow Doppler sonography in the assesment of gestational trophoblastic disease. J Ultrasound Med 12:595–599

24. Pena JE, Ufberg D, Cooney N, Denis AL (2000) Usefulness of Doppler sonography in the diagnosis of ovarian torsion. Fertil Steril 73:1047–1051

25. Fleischer AC, Rodgers WH, Kepple DM, Williams LL, Jones III HW (1993) Color Doppler sonography of ovarian masses: a multiparameter analysis. J Ultrasound Med 12:41–46

26. Campbell S, Bhan V, Royston P et al (1989) Transabdominal ultrasound screening for early ovarian cancer. BMJ 199:1363–1367

27. Kurjak A, Zalud I, Jurkovic D et al (1989) Transvaginal color Doppler for the assessment of pelvic circulation. Acta Obstet Gynecol Scand 68:131–135

28. Kurjak A, Zalud I, Alfirevic Z (1991) Evaluation of adnexal masses with transvaginal color ultrasound. J Ultrasound Med 19:295–299

29. Fylstra DL (1998) Tubal pregnancy: a review of current diagnosis and treatment. Obstet Gynecol Surv 53:320–328

30. James WH (1996) Increasing rate of ectopic pregnancy. Hum Reprod 11:233–244

31. Goldner TE, Lawson HW, Xia Z, Atrash HK (1993) Surveillance for ectopic pregnancy – United States, 1970–1989. Mortal Wkly Rep CDC Surveil Summ 42:73–85

32. Zalud I, Collea J (1999) Diagnosis and management of ectopic pregnancy. Hosp Physician 5:1–14

33. Emerson DS, Cartier MS, Altieri LA et al (1992) Diagnostic efficacy of endovaginal color Doppler imaging in an ectopic pregnancy screening program. Radiology 183:413–420

34. Kurjak A, Zalud I, Schulman H (1991) Ectopic pregnancy: transvaginal color Doppler of trophoblastic flow in questionable adnexa. J Ultrasound Med 10:685–689

35. Kirchler HCh, Seebacher S, Alge AA et al (1993) Early diagnosis of tubal pregnancy: changes in tubal blood flow evaluated by endovaginal color Doppler sonography. Obstet Gynecol 82:561–565

36. Dubinsky TJ, Parvey HR, Maklad N (1997) Endometrial blood flow/image-directed Doppler imaging: predictive value for excluding ectopic pregnancy. J Clin Ultrasound 25:103–109

37. Kemp B, Funk A, Hauptmann S, Rath W (1997) Doppler sonographic criteria for viability in symptomless ectopic pregnancy. Lancet 349:1220–1221

38. Kelchman GG, Meltzer RM (1966) Interstitial pregnancy following homolateral salpingectomy: report of two cases and review of literature. Am J Obstet Gynecol 96:1139–1144

39. Ackerman TE, Levi CS, Dashefsky SM et al (1993) Interstitial line: sonographic finding in interstitial (cornual) ectopic pregnancy. Radiology 189:83–87

40. Hill GA, Herbert III CM (1993) Ectopic pregnancy. In: Copeland LJ, Jarrell JF, McGregor JA (eds) Textbook of gynecology. WB Saunders, Philadelphia, pp 242–260

41. Raskin MM (1978) Diagnosis of cervical pregnancy by ultrasound: a case report. Am J Obstet Gynecol 130:234–235

42. Bennett S, Waterstone J, Parsons J et al (1993) Two cases of cervical pregnancy following in-vitro fertilization and embryo transfer to lower uterine cavity. J Assist Reprod Genet 10:100–103

43. Weissman A, Hakim M (1993) Diagnosis and treatment of cervical pregnancy. A case report. J Reprod Med 38:656–658

44. Werber J, Prasadarao PR, Harris VJ (1983) Cervical pregnancy diagnosed by ultrasound. Radiology 149:279–280

45. Riethmuller D, Sautiere JL, Benoit S et al (1996) Ultrasonic diagnosis and laparoscopic treatment of an ovarian pregnancy. A case report and review of the literature. J Gynecol Obstet Biol Reprod Paris 25:378–383

46. Ferro PL, Badway SZA, Berry CJ, Rooney M (1996) Laparoscopic resection of an ovarian pregnancy in a patient using the Copper T intrauterine device. J Am Assoc Gynecol Laparosc 3:329–332

47. Salas Valien JS, Reyero Alvarez MP, Gonzalez Moran MA et al (1995) Ectopic ovarian pregnancy. An Med Intern 122:192–437

48. Sidek S, Lai SF, Lim Tan SK (1994) Primary ovarian pregnancy current diagnosis and management. Singapore Med J 35:71–73

49. Sidek S, Lai SF, Lim Tan SK (1993) Primary unruptured ovarian pregnancy: a case report. An Acad Med Singapore 22:964–965

50. Honigl W, Reich O (1997) Vaginal ultrasound in ovarian pregnancy. Ultraschall Med 1815 J:233–236

51. Marret H, Hamamah S, Alonso S, Pierre F (1997) Case report and review of the literature: primary twin ovarian pregnancy. Hum Reprod 12:1813–1815

52. Bontis J, Grimbizis G, Tarlatzis BC, Miliaros D, Bili H (1997) Intrafollicular ovarian pregnancy after ovulation induction/intrauterine inservination; pathophysiologi-

cal aspects and diagnostic problems. Hum Reprod 12: 376–378

53. Zalud I, Kurjak A (1990) The assessment of luteal blood flow in pregnant and non-pregnant women by transvaginal color Doppler. J Perinat Med 18:215–221

54. Meyers M, Feyock A, Holland S, Taylor KJW (1989) Correlation of duplex Doppler and hCG levels in ectopic pregnancy. Radiology 173:247–250

55. Lund JJ (1955) Early ectopic pregnancy. J Obstet Gynecol Br Emp 62:70

56. Sjarlot Kooi, Kock CLV (1992) Review of literature on nonsurgical treatment in tubal pregnancies. Obstet Gynecol Surv 47:739–749

57. Trio D, Strobelt N, Picciolo C et al (1995) Prognostic factors for successful expectant management of ectopic pregnancy. Fertil Steril 63:469–472

58. Stovall TG, Ling FW (1992) Some new approaches to ectopic pregnancy. Contemp Obstet Gynecol 37:35

59. Tanaka T, Hayashi H, Kutsuzawa T et al (1982) Treatment of interstitial ectopic pregnancy with methotrexate: report of a successful case. Fertil Steril 37:851–852

60. Feichtinger W, Kemeter P (1989) Conservative treatment of ectopic pregnancy by needling of sac and injection of methotrexate or PG E2 under transvaginal sonographic control: report of 10 cases. Arch Gynecol Obstet 246:85–89

61. Lindbolm B, Hahlin M, Kallfelt B et al (1987) Local prostaglandin F2a injection for temrination of ectopic pregnancy. Lancet 1:776

62. Lang PF, Weiss PAM, Major HO et al (1990) Conservative treatment of ectopic pregnancy with local injection of hyperosmolar glucose solution or PGF2a: a prospective randomised study. Lancet 336:78

63. Crenin MD, Washington AE (1993) Cost of ectopic pregnancy management: surgery versus methotrexate. Fertil Steril 60:963–969

64. Stovall TG, Ling FW (1993) Single dose methotrexate: an extended clinical trial. Am J Obstet Gynecol 168: 1759–1765

65. Feichtinger W, Kemeter P (1987) Conservative management of ectopic pregnancy by transvaginal aspiration under sonographic control and methotrexate injection. Lancet 1:381

66. Rovertson DE, Mage MA, Hansen JN (1987) Reduction of ectopic pregnancy by injection under ultrasound control. Lancet 1:974

67. Atri M, Bret BM, Tulandi T, Senterman MK (1992) Ectopic pregnancy: evaluation after treatment with transvaginal methotrexate. Radiology 185:749–753

68. Fisch JD, Ortiz BH, Tazuke SI et al (1998) Medical management of interstitial ectopic pregnancy: a case report and literature review. Hum Reprod 13:1981–1986

69. Bernardini L, Valenzano M, Foglia G (1998) Spontaneous interstitial pregnancy on a tubal stump after unilateral adnectomy followed by transvaginal color Doppler ultrasound. Hum Reprod 13:1723–1726

70. Tanik A, Ustun C, Cil E, Arslan A (1996) Sonographic evaluation of the wall thickness of the lower uterus segment in patients with previous cesarian section. J Clin Ultrasound 24:355–357

71. Paltzi Z, Rosenn B, Goshen R et al (1989) Successful management of a viable cervical pregnancy with methotrexate. Am J Obstet Gynecol 161:1147–1148

72. Kaplan BR, Bradt T, Javaheri G et al (1990) Nonsurgical treatment of a viable cervical pregnancy with intraamniotic methotrexate. Fertil Steril 53:941–943

73. Timor-Tritsch IE, Monteagudo A, Mandeville EO et al (1994) Successful management of viable cervical pregnancy by local injection of methotrexate guided by transvaginal sonography. Am J Obstet Gynecol 170: 737–739

74. Frates MC, Benson CB, Doubilet PM et al (1994) Conservative management of cervical ectopic pregnancy. Radiology 191:773

75. Koike H, Chuganji Y, Watanabe H et al (1990) Conservative treatment of ovarian pregnancy by local prostaglandin F2d injection. Am J Obstet Gynecol 163:696

76. Raziel A, Golan A (1993) Primary ovarian pregnancy successfully treated with methotrexate. Am J Obstet Gynecol 169:1362–1363

77. Findlay JK (1986) Angiogenesis in reproductive tissue. J Endocrinol 111:357–361

78. Kurjak A, Kupesic-Urek S, Schulman H, Zalud I (1991) Transvaginal color flow Doppler in the assessment of ovarian and uterine blood flow in infertile women. Fertil Steril 56:870–873

79. Goswamy RK, Williams G, Steptoe PC (1988) Decreased uterine perfusion – a cause of infertility. Hum Reprod 3:955–959

80. Goswamy RK, Steptoe PC (1988) Doppler ultrasound study of uterine artery in spontaneous ovarian cycle. Hum Reprod 3:721–726

81. Collins W, Jurkovic D, Bourne T, Kurjak A, Campbell S (1991) Ovarian morphology, endocrine function and intrafollicular blood flow during the peri-ovulatory period. Hum Reprod 3:319–322

82. Steer CV, Mils CV, Campbell S (1991) Vaginal color Doppler assessment on the day of embryo transfer accurately predicts patient in an in vitro fertilization programme with suboptimal uterine perfusion who fail to be pregnant. Ultrasound Obstet Gynecol 1:79–83

83. Scholtes MCW, Wladimiroff JW, van Rijen HJM, Hop WCJ (1989) Uterine and ovarian velocity waveforms in the normal menstrual cycle: a transvaginal study. Fertil Steril 52:981–984

84. Battaglia C, Larocca E, Lanzani A, Valentini M, Genazzani AR (1990) Doppler ultrasound studies of the uterine arteries in spontaneous and IVF cycles. Gynecol Endocrinol 4:245–248

85. Kupesic S, Kurjak A (1993) Uterine and ovarian perfusion during the periovulatory period assessed by transvaginal color Doppler. Fertil Steril 60:439–443

86. Kurjak A, Zalud I, Jurkovic D, Alfirevic Z, Miljan M (1989) Transvaginal color Doppler for the assessment of pelvic circulation. Acta Obstet Gynecol Scand 68:131–135

87. Merce LT, Garces D, Barco MJ, de la Fuente F (1992) Intraovarian Doppler velocimetry in ovulatory, dysovulatory and anovulatory cycles. Ultrasound Obstet Gynecol 2:197–200

88. Kurjak A, Zalud I, Kupesic S, Predanic M (1995) Transvaginal color Doppler. In: Dodson M (ed) Transvaginal ultrasound. Raven Press, New York, pp 325–340

89. Nargund G (2002) Time for an ultrasound revolution in reproductive medicine. Ultrasound Obstet Gynecol 20:107

90. Kupesic S, Hafner T, Bjelos D (2002) Events from ovulation to implantation studied by three-dimensional ultrasound. J Perinat Med 30:84–98

91. Sladkevicius P, Ojha K, Campbell S, Nargund G (2000) Three-dimensional power Doppler imaging in the assessment of Fallopian tube patency. Ultrasound Obstet Gynecol 16:644–647

92. Sterzik K, Abt M, Grab D, Schneider V, Strehler E (2000) Predicting the histologic dating of an endometrial biopsy specimen with the use of Doppler ultrasonography and hormone measurements in patients undergoing spontaneous ovulatory cycles. Fertil Steril 73: 94–98

93. Battaglia C, Sgarbi L, Salvatori M, Maxia N, Gallinelli A, Volpe A (1998) Increased anticardiolipin antibodies are positively related to the uterine artery pulsatility index in unexplained infertility. Hum Reprod 13:3487–3491

94. Brown JM, Schwartz LB, Olive D, Lange R, Laufer N, Taylor KJ (1997) Evaluation of Doppler ultrasonography as a means of monitoring in vitro fertilization and embryo transfer cycles: preliminary results and findings. J Ultrasound Med 16:411–416

95. Cacciatore B, Simberg N, Tiitinen A, Ylikorkala O (1997) Evidence of interplay between plasma endothelin-1 and 17 beta-estradiol in regulation of uterine blood flow and endometrial growth in infertile women. Fertil Steril 67:883–888

Chapter 40

Doppler Ultrasonography for Gynecologic Malignancies

Ivica Zalud

Ultrasonography has an important role in the evaluation of patients with a suspected or palpable pelvic mass. The origin, size, location, internal consistency, and definition of the walls of the mass, as well as the presence or absence of ascites or other metastatic lesions, are the main features determined by ultrasonography.

In clinical practice pelvic tumors are most commonly divided into three categories: cystic, solid, and complex. Each category has a relative specificity and should be viewed within the framework of other clinical findings as well. Prediction of whether a mass is benign or malignant according only to its sonographic appearance is moderately reliable, depending on the ultrasonographic findings of the septa, papillary projections, and inhomogeneous solid parts of the tumor.

The number of false-positive and false-negative sonograms of adnexal masses has been too high. Most errors of the sonographic evaluation of pelvic masses can be attributed to the misinterpretation of displayed tumor features on the ultrasound monitor.

Ovarian cancer is of particular interest to ultrasonographers and oncologists since it is the leading cause of gynecological malignancy mortality in the United States, affecting 1 in 56 women and causing about 14,500 deaths annually [1]. The natural history of this disease remains poorly understood; thus, there has been no reduction in mortality from this cause in the past 60 years [1]. Ovarian cancer usually presents late, greatly reducing the chances of curative therapy. The 5-year survival rate for stage I disease is approximately 75%, whereas the survival rate for stage IV is <5% [1]. Older women are more likely to present with advanced disease, and their relative 5-year survival rates are less than half that for women under 65 [1]. Thus the postmenopausal woman must be the target of any effective screening for ovarian cancer. In the quest to diagnose ovarian cancer early, various methods have been advocated for screening in the asymptomatic postmenopausal woman. In 1971 Barber and Graber [2] described the postmenopausal palpable ovary syndrome. At the time, before the widespread use of ultrasound, they stated that "a pelvic mass found during a pelvic examination is the only practical and consistent method available to us to detect an ovarian tumor."

The first report of an attempt to screen women for ovarian cancer by transabdominal ultrasonography was by Campbell et al. [3]. The overall specificity of such a screening procedure was high, but abdominal ultrasonography as a predictor of malignancy in postmenopausal women had low specificity [4]. High-frequency probes and the vicinity of the explored organs provided the possibility of exploring small details. Hence abdominal ultrasonography was abandoned and transvaginal ultrasonography has been used extensively. Color Doppler ultrasonography as a method for transvaginal imaging to assess pelvic pathology has now been described by many investigators [5–9]. The absence of intratumoral neovascularization and a high pulsatility index (PI) can be used to exclude the presence of invasive carcinoma [5]. On the other hand, a low resistance index (RI) value was reported in the case of adnexal malignancies [8, 9]. The authors agree that low impedance to blood flow with high blood speed within arteriovenous shunts is suggestive of malignancy, whereas moderate to high impedance to blood flow is correlated to benign tumors.

On the basis of our experience, morphology alone is of limited value for characterizing adnexal masses. All ovarian neoplasms should be precisely classified according to the ultrasound appearance determined by the shape, size, and inner cystic echoes (e.g., from the septa, papillary projections, irregularities of the wall) as well as the echogenicity and loculations. Transvaginal application of color Doppler (TVCD) sonography allows visualization of the small vessels that feed the growing tumor. Color Doppler parameters (vascular location as peripheral or central; vascular quality as regular, separated vessels or randomly dispersed vessels; and Doppler waveform type by means of low values for the RI or PI) should be combined with the morphologic tissue characterization to differentiate benign from malignant pelvic tumors.

The amount and vascularity of the stroma vary greatly among tumors. Slowly growing tumors are less vascularized than tumors with a high growth potential. In general, rapidly growing tumors, particularly sarcomas, have a highly vascularized stroma with little connective tissue.

Angiogenesis in Tumors of Low Malignant Potential

Ultrasonography has been widely used to detect, characterize, and evaluate ovarian tumors. The principle of the diagnostic imaging study is based on macropathology. Thick septae, irregular solid parts within a mass, indefinite margins, and presence of ascites are regarded as malignant patterns. Some authors have reported that ovarian tumors of low malignant potential presented the same patterns as malignant tumors. On the other hand, other authors mentioned that borderline tumors had an appearance similar to that of benign tumors and it was difficult to differentiate them from their benign counterparts. Therefore, assessment of vascular changes and the resistance to blood flow would be required in the ovarian tumor presenting either benign or malignant features by conventional ultrasound [10]. Blood flow velocity waveforms obtained from borderline tumors are of relatively high diastolic flow and low resistance. Doppler features are extracted from large arterioles or sinusoids with no muscles in their walls. This is a possible hemodynamic response to the tumor angiogenesis factor produced from low-malignant-potential cells. Therefore the preoperative assessment of the adnexal mass by ultrasonography would include the size, consistency, and blood flow to determine the likelihood of malignancy [8, 11–13].

Angiogenesis in Malignant Ovarian Masses

The advent of vaginal ultrasound screening methods for ovarian cancer has made the ovaries more accessible [14]. Dramatic changes in ovarian tissue vascularity during oncogenesis are mediated by numerous angiogenic factors and can be detected by using flow data from color Doppler (Figs. 40.1–40.4). Malignant tumor vessels are usually dilated, saccular, and tortuous, and may contain tumor cells within the endothelial lining of the vessel wall. Other features include the presence of arteriovenous shunting (large and direct communications, or microscopic communications in the tumor microcirculation) and bizarre thin-walled tortuous vessels lined by tumor cells that end in amorphous spaces constituting "tumor lakes" with or without associated necrosis. Arteriovenous shunts are remarkable because of extreme velocities that occur at sites of high-pressure gradients. This type of vessel is usually situated on the periphery of the tu-

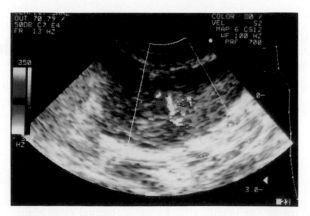

Fig. 40.1. Randomly dispersed small vessels detected by color Doppler in the central portion of a solid adnexal mass

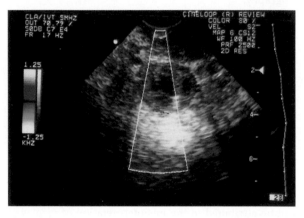

Fig. 40.2. Small vessel visualized on the periphery of the solid-cystic adnexal tumor

mor. New vessels are continually produced on the periphery of the tumor, creating the potential for its proliferation and growth. The second type of signal, exhibiting little systolic-diastolic variation, is usually present in the central vessels within the malignant tumor. This is, most probably, their response to the angiogenic activity of tumor cells. These vessels have a relative paucity of smooth muscle in their walls in comparison with their caliber and "behave" more like capillaries than true arteries or arterioles. Vessels deficient in their muscular elements present diminished resistance to flow and thereby receive a larger volume of flow than vessels with high impedance. It seems that distribution of the vessels and impedance to blood flow are dependent on tumor type and size. Tumors gradually begin to compress their own blood vessels when they continue growing beyond a certain size. The absence of functional lymphatic vessels in the tumor stroma, and the increase in cell mass and tumor vessel permeability, result in an increase in the interstitial pressure in the tumor core and lead to the

Fig. 40.3. Pulsed-wave Doppler findings in a case of malignant ovarian tumor. *Arrows* indicate the peak systolic and diastolic velocity on the Doppler waveforms

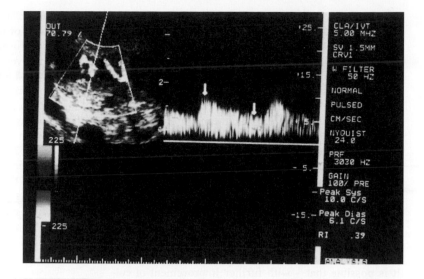

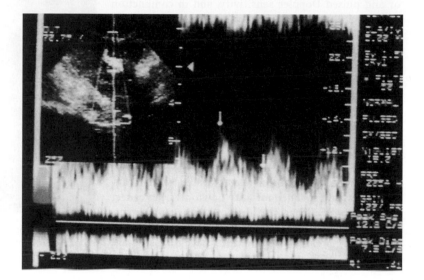

Fig. 40.4. Example of Doppler findings for a dominantly solid ovarian mass. Doppler sonography was essential to visualize newly formed vessels. Pulsed-wave Doppler was used to quantify blood flow in these vessels. Low resistance blood flow is a typical finding

occlusion of centrally located tumor vessels. This causes prolonged cessation of flow in the center of the tumor, followed by central necrosis. It seems that low resistance in centrally located vessels is a consequence of a response to the angiogenic activity of the tumor cells and to the differences in necrotic processes. Another important parameter for the assessment of tumor vascularity is the vascular arrangement. Randomly dispersed vessels within the solid part of malignant tumors were seen four times more than regularly separated vessels.

Color and pulsed Doppler sonography demonstrates the vascularity of an adnexal mass. Blood flow data should be considered to indicate the angiogenic intensity of a tumor, rather than indicating malignancy itself [15–17]. It seems clear that initial attempts to classify ovarian tumors solely on the basis of their impedance to blood flow have been too simplistic. This problem

has been partly solved by the introduction of other "vascular parameters" such as blood vessel arrangement and location, shape of the pulsed Doppler waveform, and appearance of an early diastolic notch, as well as assessment of blood flow velocities. However, the difference in flow parameters in benign versus malignant lesions may not always be sufficient to form the basis of a firm diagnostic impression [18–21]. A common criticism of color Doppler is that the operator is never blind to the B-mode image: there is a tendency to search harder for low-impedance blood flow patterns in lesions with a malignant appearance rather than in simple adnexal cysts. However, when applied by expert operators and in a disciplined fashion, it may significantly add to diagnostic information about an adnexal mass and its morphological appearance. If blood flow data are treated as providing an insight into the pathology of a tumor, they give reassurance when masses have a benign appearance, while giving confirmation of malignancy in adnexal masses with suspicious morphological features.

It is important to emphasize that the areas of overlap in benign versus malignant pelvic lesions tend to involve nonneoplastic masses that contain vasodilated vessels, owing to local or general hormonal imbalances. Whereas some malignant tumors elicit sparse angiogenesis and may appear avascular, and therefore benign, in terms of color Doppler sonography. Obese women and women with irregular cycles and hormonal disturbances may produce ovarian blood flow patterns with typical low vascular resistance to blood flow. Therefore, measurements of estradiol and progesterone serum levels on the day of the transvaginal color Doppler examination should be performed when low vascular impedance to blood flow is found. It is possible that – with further improvement of color and pulsed Doppler sensitivity, and in conjunction with clinical findings, gray-scale ultrasound imaging, and serum hormonal levels when necessary – a better distinction between malignant and benign pelvic tumors will be made. Contrast agents are another possibility for enhancing both color and power Doppler examinations by increasing the detection rate of small vessels [22].

Ovarian Cancer

Among gynecologic cancer-related deaths, ovarian cancer heads the list. The mortality due to ovarian cancer exceeds that of all uterine cancers, endometrial and cervical, combined. More than 65% of women with cancer of the ovary present with advanced-stage disease (stage III or greater). The 5-year survival rates for stage III and IV carcinoma of the ovary are 13% and less than 5%, respectively. Morbidity and mortality rates remain high despite improvements in surgical technologies, chemotherapy, and imaging techniques. There is presently no adequate screening tool for this disease.

The Zagreb group has studied the largest series of patients to date. Among approximately 14,000 women, more than 700 cases of adnexal pathology were detected [8], 624 were benign masses. Color flow was typically present in about one-third of the lesions. In all but one of the cases the RI was greater than 0.40. Color flow was present in more than 95% of ovarian malignancies, and the RI ranged from 0.28 to 0.40. Figures 40.5 and 40.6 show a malignant tumor with a high-velocity/low-resistance Doppler velocimetry pat-

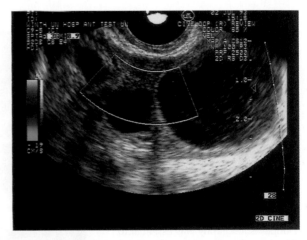

Fig. 40.5. Complex, dominantly cystic adnexal mass with blood flow detected by color Doppler in the septal portion

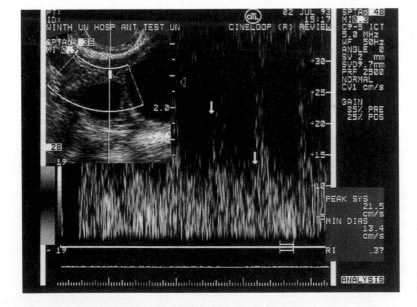

Fig. 40.6. Same patient as in Fig. 40.5. Pulsed-wave Doppler sonography showed high-velocity/low-resistance blood flow. *Arrows* indicate the peak systolic and diastolic velocity on the Doppler waveforms

tern. This original study was followed by a prospective series in which 1,000 postmenopausal women were examined by TVCD ultrasonography [9]. In these women, 74% of the lesions were detected by screening studies; the other patients were referred with a history. A total of 83 of the women underwent surgery, and 29 malignant neoplasms were found. Color flow was found in 27 of the 29 malignant tumors and in 36% of the benign tumors. The same cutoff value for the RI (0.41) yielded the best discriminatory value: sensitivity 96% and specificity 95%. The same scoring system as described previously was applied to these data. Morphology alone has poor sensitivity, as might be expected. When morphology and color Doppler indices were combined, the sensitivity improved to 90% (only 48% for morphology).

Bourne et al. studied 50 women referred because of a significant history [5]. Thirty of these women had normal ovaries, ten of whom were premenopausal and examined during the follicular phase. All of these had normal color Doppler analyses. Of the 20 women with surgical pathology in whom a positive color Doppler screen was noted, 2 had hydrosalpinges, 10 had benign tumors, and 8 had primary ovarian cancer. The PI of the nonmalignant masses ranged from 3.2 to 7.0, with no areas of suspicious neovascularization. Seven of the eight patients with ovarian cancer had clear areas of neovascularization, and the PI values ranged from 0.3 to 1.0. There was one false negative with an intraepithelial serous cystadenocarcinoma in a small ovary (< 5 ml volume); it had no sign of neovascularization and the PI for the feeding vessel was 5.5. It was the conclusion of this study that color Doppler flow analysis proved useful for identifying malignant conditions. Fleischer et al. reported color Doppler flow studies in women with malignant neoplasms and color flow Doppler indices suggestive of high-velocity/low-impedance indices [23]. Timor-Tritsch et al. reported on a series of adnexal masses with a similar scoring system whereby the diagnostic sensitivity was increased with the application of color Doppler analysis [24].

Transvaginal sonography has also been combined with measurements of serum CA-125, a tumor-associated antigen found in some women with ovarian cancer. Jacobs and colleagues obtained high sensitivity (99%) when the CA-125 assay and ultrasonography were used in combination [25]. The number of cases was small, and there was only one ovarian cancer detected. The CA-125 assay alone has routinely demonstrated inadequate sensitivity but may prove more helpful when added to color Doppler analysis.

Malignant Uterine Conditions

Malignant conditions of the uterine corpus are often difficult to distinguish from benign conditions (i.e., leimyoma uteri). Both may present as enlarged uterine masses with typical or atypical echogenicity when assessed by ultrasound imaging techniques. The Zagreb group did observe leiomyosarcomas with significant increased blood flow patterns [26]. It is a rare tumor, and so large numbers of patients are not available. At our institutions, uterine sarcoma was diagnosed preoperatively by ultrasonography and color Doppler velocimetry. The pattern seen was consistent with the presence of many aberrant vessels with high-velocity/low-resistance flow.

Endometrial cancer, the most common gynecologic cancer, often presents with abnormal bleeding, which leads to its diagnosis, versus primary detection by ultrasonography. In the postmenopausal, non-hormone-replacement individual the endometrium should measure less than 6 mm. Studies in the literature have proposed a discriminatory cutoff value for endometrial neoplasms. Many of these patients have symptoms. Color Doppler analysis was also performed in the screening population alluded to previously, wherein three asymptomatic endometrial cancers were diagnosed. In only one of the patients was an aberrant blood flow pattern seen. Low resistance vessels were observed in the myometrium and within the uterine arteries. The Zagreb group observed abnormal Doppler velocimetry in several cases as well [27]. Bourne and colleagues have studied the blood flow in women with endometrial cancer [28]. They used a PI cutoff value of 1.5 as a positive suspicious result. They studied the uterine vessels and concluded that in postmenopausal women who present with symptoms (i.e., bleeding) the predictive value of a positive test is 94%. It would be interesting to determine if sensitivity is better with color Doppler analysis of myometrial "feeding" vessels or intratumoral vessels. Again this modality may not significantly affect the diagnostic capability, as endometrial cancer is accompanied by symptoms in its early stage. The impact of such testing may not be as dramatic as with ovarian screening because of the many women who bleed early in the course of their disease. Early-stage endometrial cancer has a high cure rate, and most of the morbidity is related to the perioperative treatment. Data on carcinoma of the endometrium and color Doppler analysis are accumulating.

Potential of Screening

The next obvious question is whether this modality might prove useful in a screening capacity (Table 40.1). Ovarian cancer is significant in terms of dis-

Table 40.1. Comparative analysis: organ sites and screening programs

Site	Prevalence (1991)	Deaths per year	Screening method	Significant disease per 1,000	Cancer (no. per 1,000)
Cervix	13,000	4,500	Cytology	19	5.0
Breast	175,000	44,500	Radiography	16	5.0
Ovary	20,700	12,500	TVS, color flow	10	0.4
Endometrium	33,000	5,500	TVS	20	3–6

TVS, transvaginal sonography.

Table 40.2. Ovarian tumor B-mode ultrasonography and color Doppler scoring system

Classification		
Mass	**Fluid**	**Internal borders**
Unilocular	Clear (0) Internal echoes (1)	Smooth (0) Irregular (2)
Multilocular	Clear (1) Internal echoes (1)	Smooth (1) Irregular (2)
Cystic, solid	Clear (1) Internal echoes (2)	Smooth (1) Irregular (2)
Papillary projections	Suspicious (1)	Definite (2)
Solid	Homogeneous (1)	Echogenic (2)
Peritoneal fluid	Absent (0)	Present (1)
Laterality	Unilateral (0)	Bilateral (1)

Ultrasound score
≤2 Benign
3–4 Questionable
>4 Suspicious for malignancy

Color Doppler
No vessels seen (0)
Regular separate vessels (1)
Randomly dispersed vessels (2)

Pulsed Doppler (RI index)
No Doppler signal (0)
≥0.40 (1)
<0.40 (2)

Note: If corpus luteum blood flow is suspected, repeat the scan at the next menstrual cycle during the proliferative phase

Color Doppler score
2 or less Benign
3–4   Questionable for malignancy

ease morbidity and mortality, but it remains a low-prevalence disease in terms of screening. The annual pelvic examinations contributes little to the detection of ovarian neoplasms.

Pinotti et al. examined 499 women prior to ultrasound evaluation [29]. Bimanual detection of 4- to 6-cm cysts was approximately 33%. Only 75% of cysts measuring 6–8 cm were palpated. One of the first attempts to assess the utility of ultrasonography as a screening procedure for early detection of ovarian neoplasms was by Campbell et al. [3], who used transabdominal ultrasonography and ovarian volumes. Although the pathology correlated with the ultrasound findings in terms of the presence of a tumor and its size, it did not distinguish benign from malignant lesions. The addition of color Doppler analysis may provide this much needed utility – a discriminator of benign versus malignant disease (Table 40.2). There are several factors to consider when attempting to apply a new modality as a screening tool. As already stated, ovarian cancer is a low-prevalence condition. Large numbers of women have to be screened to report significant results. The eligibility of those who should undergo this type of screening must be considered. Ideally, in any screening program the screening test should not lead to an excess of interventions. The cost-effective issue must be raised as well.

Three-Dimensional Ultrasound

The three-dimensional capability has been extended to various diagnostic ultrasound modalities. In the case of ovarian tumor vascularity, the three-dimensional display allows the physician to visualize multiple overlapping vessels and to establish their relationship to other vessels and tumors or other surrounding tissues. The implementation of the three-dimensional display permits the physician to view structures in three dimensions interactively, rather than assembling the sectional images mentally. The three-dimensional power Doppler system may enable physicians to study the region of interest in more detail (Figs. 40.7, 40.8). Although power Doppler has several advantages over conventional color Doppler ultrasound, it is still a kind of color Doppler imaging and therefore subject to some of the limitations of the conventional technique. For example, various parameters of color Doppler ultrasound, such as pulse repetition frequency, wall filter, priority, power gain, color persistence, and frame rate, must be optimized for

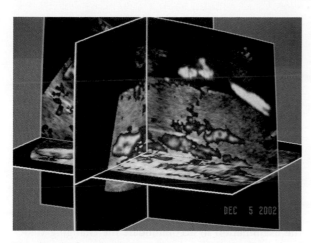

Fig. 40.7. Three-dimensional power Doppler in the case of malignant ovarian tumor

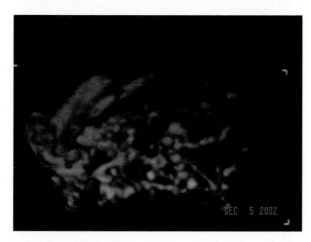

Fig. 40.8. The same patient as in Fig. 40.7 with detailed three-dimensional display of tumor vessels by power Doppler

less, there is a distinct impression from some reports that the distribution and branching pattern of blood vessels that supply fast-growing tumors differ from those of the normal blood supply to normal organs. This means that the blood vessel distribution seems to carry additional information that is missed by the present diagnostic approaches. However, describing branching structures such as the blood vessel tree is a mathematically complicated task. Microvessel density in ovarian cancers has been correlated with the likelihood of recurrence. The density (determined histologically) of microvessels, irrespective of their distribution, was found also to have significant implications for recurrence. In color Doppler studies the density can be determined by counting the number of color spots in a tumor area.

Different types of angiogenesis in different physiological and pathological conditions have been described. Physiological angiogenesis is seen in folliculogenesis, embryogenesis and implantation, chronic inflammation, and some benign neoplasms. According to some authors the luteal vessels are usually fewer and seldom have complicated branching or encircle the cyst, in contrast to the findings in a malignant neoplasm. In simple cysts the vessels are usually straight and regularly branching, whereas in "chocolate" cysts vessels usually branch from a hilar vessel then run along the surface of the tumor. Similar vascular anatomy is detected in dermoid cysts. In cases of malignant ovarian neoplasm the tumor vessels are usually randomly dispersed within the stroma and periphery, and some of them form several tangles or coils around the surface. The course of the main tumor vessel is usually irregular with more complicated branching. The diameter of these vessels is felt to be more uneven and "thorn-like." These findings can be compared to previous studies with conventional color Doppler ultrasound. However, the appeal of the three-dimensional display is that it is more comprehensive and allows physicians to understand the three-dimensional architecture of the microcirculation interactively. In addition, the resolution of current power Doppler is sufficient to detect vessels of around 1 mm in diameter. In an attempt to systematize the extent of perfusion, four regions of different perfusion states can be recognized: a necrotic region (central portion); a seminecrotic (ischemic) region; a stabilized microcirculation; and the hyperemic region within the outermost area. Different pathological types, tumors with different growth rates, primary tumors, or metastases can all exhibit different perfusion patterns.

three-dimensional display, as well as for qualitative and quantitative analysis of these power Doppler data. A change in color setting may lead to a totally different three-dimensional vascular image and dissimilar quantitative results. In addition, since now both color and power Doppler can be combined with more complex computing, the frame rate will be significantly reduced when the power/color Doppler mode is active. Therefore, if a mechanical three-dimensional probe is used, some very small vessels may escape from image capture. The effects of ultrasound attenuation can sometimes cause different "power intensity" and hence vessel detection between nearer and deeper parts of the tissue being explored.

Morphological analysis of the blood vessel system represents another approach to tumor diagnosis that, so far, has not been extensively evaluated. Neverthe-

The results reported in the recent literature on three-dimensional color and/or power Doppler raise many new questions about the regulation of tumor angiogenesis, the density of tumor vessels, and the differences between vessel architecture in benign and malignant ovarian growths [22, 30]. Improved detection and classification of tumor architecture after instillation of contrast agents might contribute to better diagnostic accuracy.

Pitfalls and Artifacts

It is well known that artifacts can be observed during ultrasound examinations. The same is true for color and pulsed-wave Doppler images of blood flow [31, 32]. Recognizing these artifacts is important so as to avoid image misinterpretation and, when possible, to overcome them by modifying the technique, the unit settings, or both. Most manufacturers have introduced, and many diagnostic units have obtained, color Doppler scanners. However, as with any new technology, color scanning is being used by many without a complete understanding of how the instrument can be optimally adjusted to provide the best possible diagnostic information. The examiner must have good working knowledge of the instrument controls that affect the color display and how these controls interact with each other. In addition, knowledge of Doppler physics, the basics of image display formats, and the hemodynamics of blood flow is essential to optimize color and pulsed-wave Doppler examinations.

Two basic colors – red and blue by convention – are assigned to represent the direction of blood flow relative to the ultrasound transducer. This rule assumes an ideal situation, where the artery and vein lie parallel to the skin surface and are straight, long tubes with blood flow parallel to the vessel walls. In reality, vessels do not follow these rules. They do not lie parallel to the skin surface. They are branched and tortuous, and their diameters often change. The flow pattern can be complicated. The combination of these features makes interpretation of the direction of blood flow difficult under ideal circumstances. The most important tip for determining the direction of flow is always to know where the ultrasound beams are coming from and how they are intersecting the vessels.

The length of the color or pulsed-wave Doppler bar represents the range of frequencies obtainable at a designated pulsed repetition frequency (PRF). The PRF is adjustable but is limited by the depth of the image. The Doppler bar is divided into maximum positive frequency and minimum frequency, with each assigned relative color or pulsed-wave Doppler assignments. The color shading can be selected by the operator in most systems. Once a "color map" is chosen, it should remain constant for each type of examination. The range of the Doppler scale is displayed as either the frequency or the velocity. The velocity values are calculated using a standard angle, usually $0°$. The numbers displayed are not quantitative values because most vessels examined to not lie parallel to the probe. These values are used, rather, in a qualitative manner; that is, as the numbers increase, the PRF increases and the ability do detect higher frequencies without aliasing is increased. The color frequency does not represent a peak frequency but a mean or mode frequency. The frequency displayed by the color is a single representative frequency between the maximum and minimum frequencies, as would be seen on a spectral waveform. These values should not be used for peak frequency or velocity measurements as is traditionally done with spectral waveforms.

The PRF should be changed constantly throughout the examination to accommodate the changing velocity patterns that may be present in the observed pelvic vessels. As a general rule, one should be aware that if the PRF is set too high the lower frequencies may not be detected; and if the PRF is set too low the higher frequencies are aliased. Color flow is essentially a guide for pulsed-wave Doppler exploration of solid tissue perfusion (i.e., uterus and ovary and tumor vascularization). Basically, if there is no color flow, waveform analysis is not done. The presettings of the instrument may be the reason for false-negative Doppler findings.

Aliasing refers to generation of one of the most common Doppler artifacts. It is a low-frequency component in the signal spectrum when the PRF of the instrument is less than two times the Doppler signal frequency. Doppler spectral waveforms display the aliased frequencies beginning at the opposite end of the scale and moving toward the zero baseline. Color Doppler sonography shows aliasing in the same manner: The aliased frequencies are displayed as the opposite color within the flow. In the display, dark color next to dark color usually indicates a directional change, but this color pattern also may occur with severe aliasing. Here the aliased frequencies are so high they go through the opposite color and cross the zero baseline into the dark shade of the original color. It is displayed as an apparent directional change and may be falsely interpreted. Aliasing occurs in areas where the frequency is increased owing to vessel obstruction or the angle of the vessels approaching $0°$ relative to the transducer. Therefore aliasing is often mistaken for true flow phenomena (e.g., turbulence or eddying) rather than a display artifact. Increased PRF, adjusted zero baseline, and decreased image depth can help to avoid aliasing.

The colors displayed can be chosen by the operator in most instruments. Usually manufacturer-preset maps are available, as is a method for creating personally selected maps. Experimentation with different maps for different studies is recommended to allow the operator to choose the most demonstrative colors and shadings for each area of study. These maps can be stored and used again. Some instruments offer a "green tag" function, which allows the operator to tag, in green, a specific velocity/frequency or to set a threshold level above which all the velocities are colored green. The green tag is often used to help identify areas of increased velocity more rapidly or to aid identification of aliasing by making more obvious the highest frequency before the alias point.

The wall filter is a high-pass filter that allows the higher frequencies to be detected and allows the operator to selectively remove low frequencies due to motion of the tissue. The filter is usually displayed in hertz units. Some wall filters are directly connected to the PRF and increase automatically as the PRF is increased; they may need to be manually decreased with decreasing PRF. It is generally suggested to keep the wall filter as low as possible during most pelvic studies, although the wall filter may need to be increased to reduce color "flash" from bowel noise or transmitted pulsation from large pelvic vessels.

The gain is a front panel control that adjusts the amplification of the displayed Doppler signal. Color and pulsed-wave Doppler gains should be constantly adjusted throughout the examination to accommodate the changing signal strengths. If the gain is set too low, some Doppler information may not be detected, or if it is set too high too much "noise" is observed. Increased color gain is suggested in situations of suspected low-velocity blood flow. An "overgain" adjustment may be useful in areas of questionably low flow or no flow, as this change can enhance any flow that may be present. Power settings also affect the gain; that is, increasing the power allows lower gain settings.

As mentioned earlier, aliasing, the mirrorimage artifact, consists of a similar time-velocity spectrum appearing above and below the zero line (Fig. 40.9). It occurs at large angles of interrogation, particularly at low signal-to-noise, when a large receiver gain is used to detect weak Doppler signals. It results in saturation of one quadrate phase detector due to strong clutter signals from stationary scatters.

Flow direction artifacts occur in tortuous vessels, such as the uterine or umbilical artery. Hence the same vessel can produce diverse color signals, depending on the temporary position of the vaginal probe. As the angle of insonation decreases at each end of the scan the velocity appears to increase. Experience allows us to recognize such artifacts. In a color Doppler study, any movement is modulated into color, which may produce an artifactual impression of blood flow. Bowel loop movements, such as peristalsis, can produce such an artifact, called color modulation of biologic movement. Several studies have presented the most common Doppler pitfalls and artifacts [33–37]. Potential solutions to avoid artifacts are also suggested. There is an urgent need for more standardization of the Doppler technique.

Artifacts in color and spectral Doppler imaging can be confusing and lead to misinterpretation of blood flow information. Inappropriate equipment settings, anatomic factors, and physical and technical limitations of the modality are the major causes. Incorrect gain, wall filter, or velocity scale settings can cause loss of clinically important information or distortion of the tracing. Reflection of the Doppler signal from highly reflective surfaces can create a color Doppler mirror image. Vascular motion can introduce

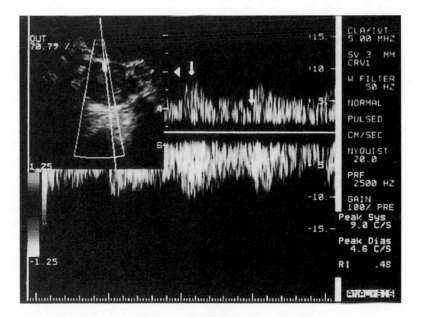

Fig. 40.9. Aliasing is a common artifact in Doppler studies. The mirror-image artifact shown here is at least as common. *Arrows* indicate the peak systolic and diastolic velocity on the Doppler waveforms

artifactual variation in velocity as the sample volume passes through different velocities in a laminar flow state. Unintentional motion can cause a generalized Doppler shift. Increasing the angle of Doppler interrogation degrades the quality of the tracing and gives the impression of spectral broadening. As angulation approaches 90°, directional ambiguity can occur, suggesting bidirectional flow. Recognition of these artifacts is essential for proper interpretation of Doppler information and for rendering a correct diagnosis. It is obvious that the display of color and pulsed-wave Doppler information is a complicated, sometimes confusing technology because of the many controls and their interactions. Understanding what each of these controls does independently and how the image is affected by adjustment and change is essential. More importantly, a permanent awareness of which control to sacrifice and which to enhance for the particular pelvic vessel is critical for obtaining the most diagnostically useful Doppler information.

Conclusions

The color Doppler modality provides a valuable approach to the pathology of female reproductive organs. The results reported in the recent literature on three-dimensional color and/or power Doppler are indeed provocative and, not surprisingly, raise many new questions about the regulation of tumor angiogenesis, the density of tumor vessels, and the differences between vessel architecture in benign and malignant growths. Three-dimensional power Doppler depiction of tumor angiogenesis has many clinical implications, including early detection of ovarian and endometrial cancers. Improved detection and classification of tumor architecture after instillation of contrast agents might contribute to better diagnostic accuracy. Early detection of ovarian carcinoma is still the most attractive argument for conducting additional studies.

References

1. DiSaia PJ, Creasman WT (1997) Clinical gynecologic oncology, 5th edn. Mosby, St. Louis
2. Barber HRK, Graber EA (1971) The PMPO syndrome. Obstet Gynecol 38:921–922
3. Campbell S, Bhan V, Royston P et al (1989) Transabdominal ultrasound screening for early ovarian cancer. BMJ 199:1363–1367
4. Luxman D, Bergman A, Sagi J, Manachem D (1991) The postmenopausal adnexal mass: correlation between ultrasonic and pathologic findings. Obstet Gynecol 77:726–729
5. Bourne T, Campbell S, Steer C et al (1989) Transvaginal color imaging: a possible new screening technique for ovarian cancer. BMJ 199:1376–1379
6. Weiner Z, Thaler I, Beck D et al (1992) Differentiating malignant from benign ovarian tumors with transvaginal color flow imaging. Obstet Gynecol 79:159–163
7. Kawai M, Kano T, Kikkawa F et al (1992) Transvaginal Doppler ultrasound with color flow imaging in the diagnosis of ovarian cancer. Obstet Gynecol 79:163–167
8. Kurjak A, Zalud I, Alfirevic Z (1991) Evaluation of adnexal masses with transvaginal color ultrasound. J Ultrasound Med 10:295–299
9. Kurjak A, Schulman H, Sosic A, Zalud I, Shalan H (1992) Transvaginal ultrasound, color flow and Doppler waveform of the postmenopausal adnexal mass. Obstet Gynecol 80:917–921
10. Fleischer AC (2001) New developments in the sonographic assessment of ovarian, uterine, and breast vascularity. Semin Ultrasound CT MR 22:42–49
11. Kinkel K, Hricak H, Lu Y, Tsuda K, Filly RA (2000) US characterization of ovarian masses: a meta-analysis. Radiology 217:803–811
12. Brown DL, Doubilet PM, Miller FH et al (1998) Benign and malignant ovarian masses: selection of the most discriminating gray-scale and Doppler sonographic features. Radiology 208:103–110
13. van Nagell JR Jr, DePriest PD, Reedy MB, Gallion HH, Ueland FR, Pavlik EJ, Kryscio RJ (2000) The efficacy of transvaginal sonographic screening in asymptomatic women at risk for ovarian cancer. Gynecol Oncol 77:350–356
14. Takac I (1998) Analysis of blood flow in adnexal tumors by using color Doppler imaging and pulsed spectral analysis. Ultrasound Med Biol 24:1137–1141
15. Aslam N, Tailor A, Lawton F, Carr J, Savvas M, Jurkovic D (2000) Prospective evaluation of three different models for the pre-operative diagnosis of ovarian cancer. BJOG 107:1347–1353
16. Schelling M, Braun M, Kuhn W, Bogner G, Gruber R, Gnirs J, Schneider KT, Ulm K, Rutke S, Staudach A (2000) Combined transvaginal B-mode and color Doppler sonography for differential diagnosis of ovarian tumors: results of a multivariate logistic regression analysis. Gynecol Oncol 77:78–86
17. Zalud I (2002) Doppler evaluation of the ovary: clinical applications and challenges. Contemp Obstet Gynecol 47:37–59
18. Fleischer AC, Cullinan JA, Peery CV, Jones HW (1996) Early detection of ovarian carcinoma with transvaginal color Doppler ultrasonography. Am J Obstet Gynecol 174:101–116
19. Lerner JP, Timor-Tritsch IE, Federman A, Abramovich G (1994) Transvaginal ultrasonographic characterization of ovarian masses with an improved, weighted scoring system. Am J Obstet Gynecol 170:81–85
20. Timmerman D, Valentin L, Bourne TH, Collins WP, Verrelst H, Vergote I; International Ovarian Tumor Analysis (IOTA) Group (2000) Terms, definitions and measurements to describe the sonographic features of adnexal tumors: a consensus opinion from the International Ovarian Tumor Analysis (IOTA) Group. Ultrasound Obstet Gynecol 16:500–505
21. Orden MR, Gudmundsson S, Kirkinen P (2000) Contrast-enhanced sonography in the examination of benign and malignant adnexal masses. J Ultrasound Med 19:783–788

22. Cohen LS, Escobar PF, Scharm C, Glimco B, Fishman DA (2001) Three-dimensional power Doppler ultrasound improves the diagnostic accuracy for ovarian cancer prediction. Gynecol Oncol 82:40–48

23. Fleischer AC, Rodgers WH, Kepple DM, Williams LL, Jones III HW (1993) Color Doppler sonography of ovarian masses: multiparameter analysis. J Ultrasound Med 12:41–46

24. Timor-Tritsch IE, Lerner J, Monteagudo A, Santos R (1992) Transvaginal sonographic characterization of ovarian masses using color-flow directed Doppler measurement. Ultrasound Obstet Gynecol 2:171–175

25. Jacobs I, Prys Davies A, Bridges J et al (1993) Prevalence screening for ovarian cancer in postmenopausal women by CA 125 measurement and ultrasonography. Br Med J 306:1030–1034

26. Kurjak A, Shalan H, Kupesic S et al (1993) Transvaginal color Doppler sonography in the assessment of pelvic tumor vascularity. Ultrasound Obstet Gynecol 3:137–154

27. Kurjak A, Zalud I (1991) Characterization of uterine tumors by transvaginal color Doppler. Ultrasound Obstet Gynecol 1:50–55

28. Bourne TH, Campbell S, Whitehead MI et al (1990) Detection of endometrial cancer in postmenopausal women by transvaginal ultrasonography and color flow imaging. BMJ 299:369–373

29. Pinotti JA, De Franzin CM, Marussi EF, Zeferino LC (1988) Evaluation of cystic and adnexal tumors identified by echography. Int J Gynaecol Obstet 26:109–114

30. Pairleitner H, Steiner H, Hasenoehrl G, Staudach A (1999) Three-dimensional power Doppler sonography: imaging and quantifying blood flow and vascularization. Ultrasound Obstet Gynecol 14:139–143

31. Kremkau FW (1992) Doppler color imaging: principles and instrumentation. Clin Diagn Ultrasound 27:7–60

32. Taylor KJW, Holland S (1990) Doppler ultrasound. Part I. Basic principles, instrumentation, and pitfalls. Radiology 174:297–307

33. Winkler P, Helmke K, Mahl M (1990) Major pitfalls in Doppler investigations. Part II. Low flow velocity and colour Doppler application. Pediatr Radiol 20:304–310

34. Pozniak MA, Zagzebski JA, Scanlan KA (1992) Spectral and color Doppler artifacts. Radiographic 12:35–44

35. Derchi LE, Giannoni M, Crespi G, Pretolesi F, Oliva L (1992) Artifacts in echo-Doppler and color-Doppler. Radiol Med 83:340–352

36. Mitchell DG (1990) Color Doppler imaging: principles, limitations, and artifacts. Radiology 177:1–10

37. Jaffe R (1992) Color Doppler imaging: a new interpretation of the Doppler effect. In: Color Doppler Imaging in Obstetrics and Gynecology, R Jaffe, SL Warsof (eds). McGraw-Hill, New York, pp 17–34

Subject Index

3

Printing and Binding: Stürtz GmbH, Würzburg